To prof.

the great

many thanks.

Ahmad Ali
20.11.2008

Bone in Clinical Orthopedics

AO Publishing

Geoff Sumner-Smith

Bone in Clinical Orthopedics

with a foreword by Robert Bruce Salter

Executive Editor

Gustave E. Fackelman

Thieme
Stuttgart · New York 2002

Design & typesetting: AO Publishing, CH-8600 Dübendorf
Scans: ComArt, CH-6330 Cham
Cover illustration: AO Research Institute, CH-7270 Davos
Index: Jill Halliday, GB-Diss, Norfolk IP21 4QT

Library of Congress Cataloging-in-Publication Data is
available from the publisher.

Copyright © 2002, by AO Publishing
Stettbachstrasse 10, CH-8600 Dübendorf
Exclusive distribution right by
Georg Thieme Verlag, Rüdigerstrasse 14, D-70469 Stuttgart, Germany, and
Thieme New York, 333 Seventh Avenue, New York, NY 10001, USA

"Bone in Clinical Orthopaedics: A Study in Comparative Osteology"
First published in 1982 © by W.B. Saunders Co.

Printed in Germany by Staudigl, Donauwörth

ISBN 3-13-125721-0 (GTV)
ISBN 0-86577-829-9 (TNY)

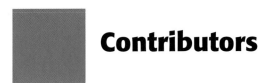

Contributors

Editor

Geoff Sumner-Smith, DVSc (Liv.),
BVSc, MSc, FRCVS,
University Professor Emeritus
Department of Clinical Studies
University of Guelph
CDN-Guelph, Ont. N1G 2W1

Executive editor

Gustave E. Fackelman, Prof., DVM,
Dr. med. vet.
PO Box 10
USA-Rockwood, ME 04478

Authors

Dennis R. Carter, PhD
Professor and Biomedical Engineer
Rehabilitation Research and
Development Center
Veteran's Affairs Palo Alto HCS
3801 Miranda Ave.
USA-Palo Alto, CA 94304-1200

Joanne R. Cockshutt, MSc, DVM,
Dip ACVS
Associate Professor (Retired)
Department of Clinical Studies
University of Guelph
CDN-Guelph, Ont. N1G 2W1

Howard Dobson, BVM&S, DVSc,
Cert. EO. Dip ACVRS
Associate Professor, Department of
Clinical Studies
Chief Radiologist Veterinary
Teaching Hospital
University of Guelph
CDN-Guelph, Ont. N1G 2W1

Stina Ekman, DVM, PhD, Dip ECVP
Associate Professor
Swedish University of Agricultural
Sciences
Department of Pathology
PO Box 7028
S-750 07 Uppsala

John R. Field, MSc, BVSc, DVSc,
   PhD
   Associate Professor of Surgery
   (Orthopedics)
   Department of Surgery
   Flinders University
   AUS-Adelaide, SA 5041

Lawrence Friedman, MVBCh,
   FFRAD (D) SA, FRCPC, FACR
   Clinical Associate Professor
   Department of Radiology
   Guelph General Hospital
   115 Delhi Street
   CDN-Guelph, Ont. N1E 4J4

Harold M. Frost, BA, MD, DrSc
   Department of Orthopedic Surgery
   Southern Colorado Clinic
   2002 Lake Ave.
   USA-Pueblo, CA 81004

John E.F. Houlton, MA, VetMB,
   DVR, DSAO, MRCVS, DipECVS
   Consultant Cambridge University
   Empshill Robins Lane
   Lolworth
   GB-Cambridge, CB3 8HN

Lance E. Lanyon, BVSc, PhD DSc,
   MRCVS
   Principal, The Royal Veterinary
   College
   Royal College Street
   GB-London, NW1 0TU

Johannes Müller, MD (deceased)

Sydney Nade, DSc, MD, MB, BS,
   BSc (Med), FRCS, FRACS, MRCP
   (UK) FAOrthA
   Department of Surgery
   The University of Sydney
   PO Box R168
   Royal Exchange
   AUS-Sydney, NSW 1225

Sten-Erik Olsson, Prof. (deceased)

Matthew J. Pead, BvetMed, PhD,
   CertSAO, MRCVS
   Department of Small Animal
   Medicine and Surgery
   The Royal Veterinary College
   Hawkshead Lane
   North Mymms
   GB-Hatfield Herts, AL9 7TA

Berton A. Rahn, Prof. Dr. med.,
   Dr. med. dent.
   AO Research Institute
   Clavadelerstrasse
   CH-7270 Davos Platz

Joseph Schatzker, MD, BSc,
   FRCS(C)
   Professor of Orthopedic Surgery
   University of Toronto
   Sunnybrook Health Science Centre
   2075 Bayview Avenue, Suite A315
   CDN-Toronto, Ont. M4N 3M5

Robert K. Schenk, Prof. Dr. med.
   Department of Oral Surgery
   Freiburgstrasse 7
   CH-3010 Bern

Dan M. Spengler, MD
   Professor and Chairman
   Department of Orthopaedics and
   Rehabilitation
   Vanderbilt University Medical
   Center
   USA-Nashville, TN 37232

Alastair J.S. Summerlee, BSc,
   BVSc, PhD, MRCVS, Prof.
   Department of Biomedical Sciences
   Ontario Veterinary College
   University of Guelph
   CDN-Guelph, Ont. N1G 2W1

Geoff Sumner-Smith, DVSc (Liv.),
   BVSc, MSc, FRCVS,
   University Professor Emeritus
   Department of Clinical Studies
   University of Guelph
   CDN-Guelph, Ont. N1G 2W1

Brigitte von Rechenberg, PD Dr.
   med. vet., Dipl. ECVS
   Musculoskeletal Research Unit
   Dept. of Veterinary Surgery
   University of Zürich
   Winterthurerstrasse 260
   CH-8057 Zürich

Hans Willenegger, Prof. (deceased)

James W. Wilson, DVM, MS,
   DipACVS
   PO Box 51523
   USA-Livonia, MI 48151

James Wilson-MacDonald, FRCS
   The John Radcliffe Hospital
   Headlay Way
   GB-Oxford, OX3 9DU

Dedication

Stephan M. Perren
Prof. Dr. med. Dr. sci. (h.c.)

Stephan Perren has significantly affected the lives of many who
have worked in fields associated with the study of orthopedics.
His influence on research, in many parts of the world, has been
significant and to the benefit of all concerned. His advice has,
and still is, given with the convictions of an honest scientist and
always with the utmost courtesy and charm.

This edition of Bone is affectionately dedicated to Stephan
Perren, a gentleman in orthopedics.

Geoff Sumner-Smith
2001

Foreword

Having been an Honorary Member of the Veterinary Orthopaedic Society (North America) for over a decade, I continue to be greatly impressed by the importance of the relevance of basic knowledge and clinical practice in animals on the one hand and in humans on the other hand. This relevance is especially true with respect to disorders and injuries of the musculoskeletal system including orthopedics, fractures, joint injuries, rheumatology, metabolic bone disease, and dentistry.

Those of us who are privileged to work as orthopedic surgeon-scientists in musculoskeletal research laboratories are extremely grateful to our veterinary colleagues who give us such sagacious advice as we develop animal models of human disorders and injuries and who also provide essential supervision of our animal laboratory facilities.

Now, thanks to the second edition of this splendid book entitled "Bone in Clinical Orthopedics", we can also be grateful to Professor Geoffrey Sumner-Smith—one of the world's most distinguished academic orthopedic veterinarians—and his 24 additional contributing authors for providing a bridge between those who treat humans and those who treat animals.

The horizontal double column format of this 496 page comprehensive and comprehendible book makes for easy reading and the 335 illustrations, many in color, are both clear and informative. Unlike a reference book, this textbook in its logical sequence, is intended to be read and savoured by the reader from beginning to end. The targeted readership of this outstanding book includes postgraduate students, in both veterinary and human orthopedics, as a solid scientific basis for understanding the tissues with which they will be working throughout their professional careers.

In the millennium within academic orthopedics, both for animals and for humans, we live in a milieu of increasing specialization and the creation of subspecialists as well. Historically, 50 years ago one individual person, for example a histologist such as the renowned late Professor Arthur Haru, could have written a credible book on the broad subject of "bone". By contrast, today the preparation of such a book requires a multitude of specialist and subspecialist authors including embryologists, anatomists, histologists, physiologists, biochemists, pathologists, geneticists, molecular biologists, epidemiologists, diagnostic imagers (radiologists) and clinical orthopedic surgeon-scientists.

The antiquated "one-man-band" of the past has been replaced by a symphonic orchestra of widely varied musical specialists. Of course, every such orchestra must be led by a talented conductor who understands the entire group of the musicians. In his role of conductor, Professor Geoffrey Sumner-Smith, has assembled all of the necessary musculoskeletal specialists who are pivotal in his creating and editing this outstanding book. His intrinsic fine thread of exquisite and elegant English is woven throughout the fabric of the text. He has indeed been fortunate in having Professor Gustave E. Fackelman in the role of "concert master".

Solomon, one of the greatest teachers of all times, has written: "Give me facts but, above all, give me understanding". My assessment of this opus magnus is that Professor Sumner-Smith, and his other contributing authors, have given us not only the facts but also the understanding and have thereby done all of us an enormous service.

Indeed, I am confident that this book will be become a classic in its field.

Robert Bruce Salter
2001

CC, O ONT, FRSC, MD, MS (Tor), FRCSC, FACS, Hon Dr med (Uppsala), Hon D Sc (Memorial), Hon LL D (Dalhousie), Hon D Litt S (Wycliffe, Toronto), Hon FRCPS (Glasg), Hon FRCS (Edin), Hon FCSSA (S Africa), Hon FRCS (Eng), Hon FRACS (Aust), Hon FRCS (Ire), Hon MCFPC

University Professor of the University of Toronto
Professor of Orthopaedic Surgery, University of Toronto

Preface to the first edition

The intention behind the production of this work is to form a bridge, or more properly a "firm callus", between the literature available for undergraduate students of orthopedics and those intending to study bone in more depth. Many texts already exist for the undergraduate and also for the student of advanced orthopedic surgery. It is hoped that this book will set the stage for graduate training in orthopedics for surgeons in the medical, dental, and veterinary fields. It is my belief that no one should undertake a detailed study of orthopedics as a subject before familiarizing themselves with much of the material presented herein. Some of it is in outline form, but in other areas the contributor has taken the theme to considerable depth. In some chapters, the material is not of a nature that is often altered by new contributions to the particular subject being described. I hope this type of text permits recent findings to be put before the reader in a succinct form.

It is a matter of particular pleasure and pride to me, as the editor of this text, to be able to present such a galaxy of experts. The fact that each contributor responded, readily and with enthusiasm, to the invitation to contribute convinced both the publishers and me that there is a need for such a text. The reception of the results of the contributions of so many people by you, the reader, will prove us right or wrong.

The production of a multi-authored text is not without its difficulties; naturally there is some overlap of subjects of one chapter with another. I believe this to be a healthy situation and, even though opinions may differ in minor details, it serves to show the serious student of orthopedics that all is not quite so cut and dried as one might have been led to believe from undergraduate teaching.

Geoff Sumner-Smith
1982

Preface to the second edition

It is now nineteen years since the publication of the first edition of this book by Saunders, Philadelphia. Many individuals have requested copies of that text, which, unfortunately, went out of print in 1984. Much of that which I wrote in 1982 is still pertinent to this second edition, and the intent for the material to form a "bridge" between the literature available for undergraduate students of orthopedics and those intending to study bone in depth still stands.

Some of the authors are contributing for the first time, and my initial statement that "I am proud to present such a galaxy of experts" is still valid. The whole text has been enlarged from eleven to fifteen chapters and has been rewritten to reflect current knowledge. Some chapters have been deleted and replaced with fresh material. The original chapter concerned with the hormonal control of bone has been deleted. This has been done after much soul searching. The decision was taken in the light of the explosion of knowledge in that area. Many texts on the subject are currently available to those interested in that material. However, the new edition of "Bone" gives the reader a "taste" of the local factors that affect the life of bone and cartilage cells.

Although many orthopedists are likely to use the text as a reference, one would wish to reiterate that it is initially intended for the new graduate, entering the professions of human, dental, or veterinary orthopedics.

Geoff Sumner-Smith
2001

1 Bone formation and development

—In memory of Richard N. Smith

Alastair J.S. Summerlee

1 Introduction

There are two critical phases in the development of bone. The first occurs in utero when bone tissue starts to form. Centers of ossification develop in the approximate positions that will determine the basic skeletal pattern of the adult. The fetus is born with many ossified precursors of adult bone already in place. The second phase of development occurs in postnatal life as the animal starts to grow. During this time bones elongate and change shape to assume the adult form. This phase will determine the external appearance of the animal and underlie the differences observed in physical form, for example, whether or not this animal will be mouse, man, or mastodon. But bone is not static, even when fully mature. There is a constant, if much slower, rate of modeling and remodeling that continues throughout life and is affected by a variety of external and internal factors. Before discussing the prenatal and postnatal development of bone it is important to establish some of the gross anatomical and histological features that characterize adult bone.

2 Basic anatomy of bone

Descriptive anatomy divides bones into two major groups: long bones and flat bones. Initially, this classification was based solely on the gross appearance of the types of bone. The long-bone category was extended to include two further types of bone that were neither flat nor long: short bones and irregular bones. Later, it was observed that bones of the skull (which comprise the majority of the flat bones of the body) and bones of the appendicular skeleton were derived from different embryonic tissues, which strengthened the emerging view that long and flat bones developed by different processes. During the 1980s, this classic view of bone development was challenged. Despite their apparently different embryological origins, bones throughout the body develop by an identical process, and this has important implications for the organization and management of reparative processes.

A long bone consists of a compact shaft (diaphysis), an intermediate area (metaphysis), and a terminal portion (epiphysis). Each of these areas has a specific gross appearance (Fig. 1-1) and histological appearance (Fig. 1-2). The diaphysis is a hollow cylinder of compact bone which contains a medullary cavity. In contrast, the epiphysis consists of spongy or cancellous bone surrounded by a thin eggshell of compact bone. Cancellous bone is characterized by a delicate interweaving of spicules of bone known as trabeculae. In young animals a growth plate lies between these two regions of bone. This plate consists of layers of cartilage cells and matrix, blood vessels, and newly formed bone. Uniting the growth plate to the diaphysis is an intermediate region, the metaphysis, comprising columns of spongy bone. The growth plate and the metaphyseal region represent the growth component of the bone and can be seen clearly in bones of young animals. In the adult, the plate is absent, and the cancellous bone of the epiphysis becomes continuous with the cancellous bone of the diaphysis with a small white line of compact bone between them. Limb bones are classic examples of long bones.

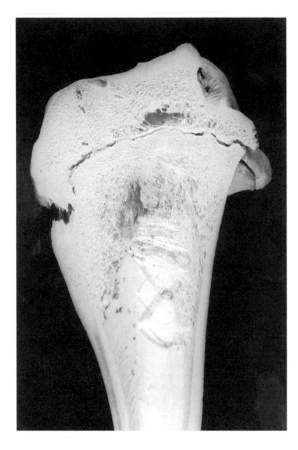

Fig. 1-1: A median section through the proximal end of an ox tibia showing the variation in the thickness of the shell of compact cortical bone and the lattice-work, honey-combed appearance of the cancellous bone. During the drying process to prepare this specimen the growth plate has separated, emphasizing the position of the epiphysis *(above)* and the metaphysis *(below)*. Within the diaphysis the medullary cavity is clearly visible.

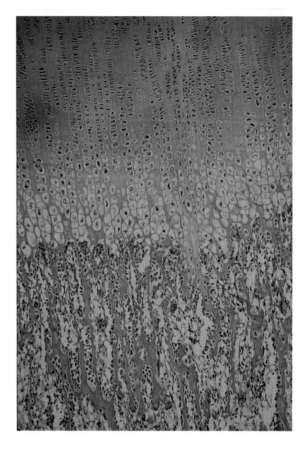

Fig. 1-2: Low-power magnification of a section through the cartilaginous growth plate between the epiphysis and the metaphysis *(below)* at the proximal end of a dog femur. A series of changes from the zones of multiplication of the cartilage *(above)*, to hypertrophic layers, formation of columns, and matrix formation with partial chondrolysis to the ossifying front are shown. (H and E stain: magnification ×250; courtesy of Dr Yamashiro, Biomedical Sciences, Ontario Veterinary College.)

Flat bones are predominantly found in the skull and comprise two layers of compact bone separated by a layer of cancellous bone. Short and irregular bones consist primarily of a core of cancellous bone bounded by a cortex of compact bone of variable thickness. Many of the carpal and tarsal bones are considered to be examples of short or irregular bones.

In general, strength of bone depends on the hardness of the compact cortical bone and on the underlying scaffolding effect of the trabeculae of cancellous bone. The orientation of the trabeculae reflects the directions of maximum stresses exerted on the bone, and changes in the disposition of the mechanical forces applied to the bone will result in major remodeling of these spicules of cancellous bone.

The entire surface of bone, except where articular cartilage is present, is covered by specialized dense connective tissue known as periosteum. This layer is attached to the cortical bone below by a series of collagenous bundles known as Sharpey fibers and the strength of these attachments varies between different bones. The internal surface of bone, which includes the medullary cavity, cavities of the haversian system of compact bones and the trabeculae of cancellous bone, is lined with another connective layer, endosteum. Sandwiched between the periosteum and the outer layer of cortical bone and between the endosteum and the inner layers of bone are osteoblasts which are vital in growing bone for osteogenesis and for reparative processes throughout life. Rasmussen and Bordier [1] produced evidence to indicate that remodeling of bone in adult life is a very slow process, but osteoblasts below the endosteum are more active than those below the periosteum.

The histological structure of compact bone is similar for all types of bones, whether they are long, short, flat, or irregular, and reflects its mode of development. The basic construction unit is known as an osteon (haversian system). Each osteon (**Fig. 1-3**) comprises a central canal, containing blood vessels and a small amount of connective tissue, with interconnecting channels surrounded by concentric layers of bone, the lamellae. Intercalated into the bone substance are cavities with trapped osteocytes, lacunae. The lacunae communicate with each other and with the canal of the osteons through a ramifying network of canaliculae. The lacunae and canaliculae are extracellular and contain tissue fluid and interstitial substances for maintenance of the osteocytes. Presumably, therefore, nutrients and other essential molecules reach their targets by diffusion. There is a similar structural arrangement in the trabeculae of cancellous bone, but the osteons are not present.

There are three major cell types associated with mature bone: the osteoblast, which participates in the ossification process and is present when new bone is being formed; the osteoclast, which is commonly found in sites where bone is being resorbed; and the osteocyte, which is found trapped within the bone lacunae as described above and is active in constant remodeling of bone. These cell types are all derived from mesenchymal stem cells. An understanding of the lineage

of osteoblasts, particularly in the postfetal skeleton, is fundamental to our appreciation of growth and reparative processes but is a subject of debate. Progenitor cells are presumably present within the marrow or in the periosteal or endosteal connective tissue, and there is some evidence to suggest that there is a continuum of cells throughout bone spaces [2]. Certain of these cells lie on or near the bone surface and exist as preosteoblasts, and there are indications that these are derived from specific stem cells [3]. The latter, however, are uncharacterized except for their potential to regenerate and differentiate into all types of progeny characteristic of the particular cell line [4]. There is still debate as to whether these precursors are present as part of a generalized body system of generating stromal cells or are already differentiated sufficiently to be designated specifically for the osteoblastic lineage [5]. Our understanding of the lineage is further complicated by the presence of fibroblastic precursor cells in the blood circulation [6–8]. However, fibroblastic stromal cells from certain organs, including marrow, do appear to express different antigenic markers from other organ-specific systems, which may be

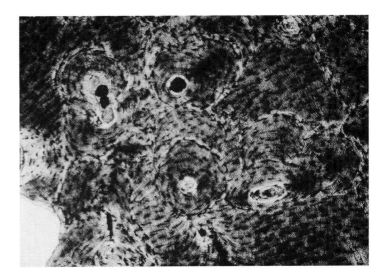

Fig. 1-3: Transverse ground section of compact bone from femoral shaft of dog. Note the variation in size and shape of osteons and their surrounding canals and the distribution of lacunae. (Courtesy of Dr Yamashiro, Biomedical Sciences, Ontario Veterinary College.)

related to functional requirements for each organ [8]. As will be discussed later, development of bone is dependent upon the interaction between hemopoietic and osteogenic tissues, and the possible cell lines for differentiation of the two cell populations are critical for the successful development and subsequent growth of bone. A putative lineage of stem-cell lines is shown in **Fig. 1-4**. Recent evidence compels us to reconsider the traditional view of bone formation and development and the difference between these two cell lines.

Normal bone formation occurs when "committed" stem cells and their progeny are stimulated to proliferate and differentiate. These "committed" cells are referred to as the osteogenic progenitor cells [3]. When they are removed mechanically with bone marrow and transplanted heterotopically they differentiate spontaneously into bone [9–11]. Similar cells probably reconstitute the medullary cavity following injury and ablation [12–14].

Fig. 1-4: Diagram to illustrate the origin and fate of cells in mature bone.
(Diagram taken from Williams P, Warwick R, Dyson M, et al., 1989, Gray's Anatomy, Churchill Livingstone.)

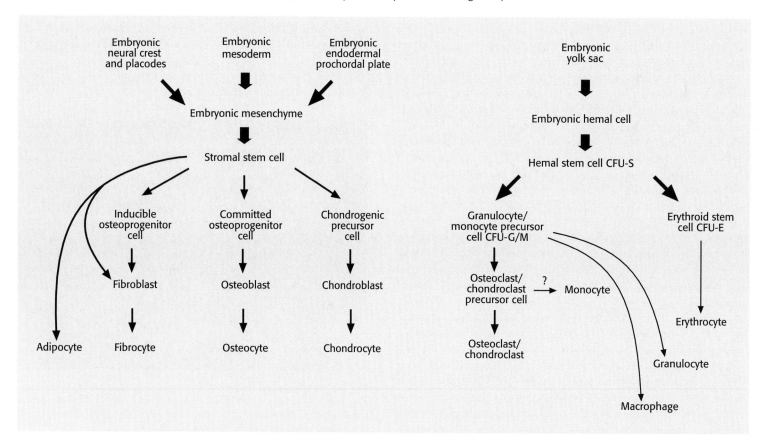

3 Early bone formation

Caplan et al. [15] described the process of development, maturation, and aging as a continuum of sequential cellular and molecular events of replacement. This is a useful concept to discuss because the changes observed in bone represent cells and matrix that are slowly and progressively replaced by structures with an ever-decreasing capacity for differentiation but with an increased degree of specialization. Some of the new structures are simply variants of their predecessor, a type of evolutionary change, while others represent the development of a novel structure that may be unique to a particular site. Whatever the process, there are three fundamental principles that govern these changes [16]:

1) The genomic repertoire of the organism sets the limits of the developmental and maturational possibilities. The shape, size, and presence of particular tissues are genetically programmed. For example, differences in the shape and size of the femur of a mouse, man, or an elephant are appropriately proportioned for the animal. Another example might be the lack of teeth in birds whose prehistoric ancestors possessed teeth.

2) Developmental outcomes are progressive and irreversible. There is a correct sequence of developmental changes that follow each other and these changes are not reversible. Even in crisis, for example during repair, there is no dedifferentiation of tissue [17]. Once differentiated, a cell type will produce particular progeny or specialized molecules, but the descendants are committed to the parental lineage. Therefore, to affect repair, undifferentiated stem cells must be activated (and/or even brought to the site: see **Fig. 1-4**), to provide the cells necessary for reparative processes.

3) Local environmental factors are of paramount importance in the rate and extent of development, maturation, and reparative processes. Such factors, which include cellular components and molecular products of those cells, may influence and hence determine the process of further cellular differentiation and expression. For example, a mesenchymal stem cell may differentiate into either an osteoblast or a chondrocyte by virtue of factors present in the immediate environment.

These three principles determine that, despite apparent similarities, the process of embryonic development is unique. Despite superficial similarities between the processes of bone formation, maturation, and repair, the mechanism of embryonic development cannot be recapitulated. The maturation and repair will take place in an environment profoundly modified by the existing structure. Therefore, an understanding of the embryological development of bone may explain how the tissue arises, but it cannot predict how the maturation process will continue, nor how regenerative mechanisms will operate.

The rest of this chapter will be devoted to a description of the process of embryonic development of bone: growth and maturation, the modeling and remodeling process, ectopic bone formation, and a brief discussion of the reparative processes.

3.1 Theories of bone formation

Until recently there has been a firmly established view that bone development occurred by one of two processes: either by direct transformation of connective tissue, known as intramembranous ossification, or by replacement of a previously formed cartilaginous model, endochondral or intracartilaginous ossification. In some bones it was accepted that both processes occurred simultaneously. In both intramembranous and endochondral ossification, the biochemical and the physiological processes were identical and involved activation of osteoblasts. The arguments for two separate methods of bone formation relied on the following observations:

- Endochondral ossification occurred where a rod of cartilage was seen to develop in the expected final position of the bone. This rod appeared to mimic the general shape of the adult bone and was considered as a precursor or template for the adult structure.

- There was an anatomical difference between bones that formed by endochondral ossification (predominantly long bones and occasionally short and irregular bones) and those that developed by intra-membranous ossification (flat bones of the skull and the subperiosteal layer of the diaphysis of long bones).

- Cranial/facial bones and bones in the rest of the body have distinct embryological origins: bones of the skull are derived from ectomesenchyme (neural crest cells) while other bones are derived from lateral plate mesenchyme [18].

Recently, however, considerable data has accumulated, primarily from work on the chicken tibia, to suggest that our concepts of these alternative approaches to ossification should be challenged [16].

3.2 Classical view of ossification

3.2.1 Intramembranous ossification

Bone develops within stromal connective tissue that is characterized by mesenchymal stem cells, connected by thin cell processes, lying in a matrix of haphazardly arranged collagenous fibrils. Immediately before ossification commences two changes are observed; the mesenchymal stem cells proliferate and start to differentiate, finally forming osteoblasts, and the intercellular matrix becomes more dense and homogeneous. These changes alone are sufficient to induce a suitable environment for early calcification to commence, and the mineral content of the matrix increases rapidly. The osteoblasts augment the process by producing more matrix that is calcified, and some of these cells will become trapped in the tissue and will transform into osteocytes. Until the bone has reached the final size, a layer of osteoblasts remain on the periosteal surface. The same process occurs for flat bones and on the periosteal surface of the diaphyses of long bones.

3.2.2 Endochondral ossification

Endochondral ossification occurs where bones elongate at a growth plate. This plate is arbitrarily divided into specific regions for descriptive purposes. At the epiphyseal front there is a layer of hyaline cartilage formed by cartilage cells, some of which may be embedded in matrix. The older cartilage cells begin to multiply and form into columns separated by wide parallel bands of interstitial substance. The cells are separated from each other by a thin capsule of matrix. These cells hypertrophy and incorporate stores of glycogen. Providing there are adequate concentrations of minerals available, the intercellular matrix then starts to calcify, particularly between adjacent columns of cells. This zone forms a provisional structural framework between the growth plate and the cancellous bone of the metaphysis. Loops of blood vessels then invade the connective tissue and penetrate into the vertical columns. The interstitial tissue is removed, leaving calcified vertical columns of matrix known as the primary spongiosa. This primary spongiosa is considered to be the necessary scaffolding upon which the bone matrix can be deposited. In this way the newly formed endochondral bone mirrors the cartilage model which it has replaced. The key feature of this hypothesis is that the cartilage model forms first and the bone is laid down onto that model. As bone matrix is laid down upon the primary spongiosa they are transformed into secondary spongiosa, a more permanent set of trabeculae. These will be modified by the joint action of osteoblasts and osteoclasts to form the thickened adult trabeculae, which are clearly visible upon gross examination of the cut surface of bone.

The pattern of mineralization at the growth plate can be clearly demonstrated by autoradiography and is of some interest. Comar et al. [19] showed that soon after calcium 45 (^{45}Ca) administration heavy deposits of radioactive ion are seen in the growth plate and adjacent trabecular bone of the metaphysis. Thirty days after ^{45}Ca administration, the radioactive content of the plate is relatively low and concentration in the trabecular bone is less than on day one. By 60 days, osteoclastic activity has removed and remodeled almost all the newly formed bone and the level of radioactivity observed is low in all areas.

Once an animal achieves skeletal maturity, bone stops growing in length and there is no further new formation of bone. The skeleton continues to be modeled and remodeled but the rate of change is considerably less than during the growth phase. Radioactive calcium introduced into bone at this stage may take years to be resorbed and removed. This underlines concerns about the hazards from certain radionuclides, for example strontium 90 (^{90}Sr) or strontium 89 (^{89}Sr), which have been shown to accumulate selectively in the skeleton [20, 21].

3.2.3 Ossification revisited

Over the last decade, data have been emerging to support a reconsideration of the process of bone formation. Based on work on the chicken tibia, it is now proposed that the initial steps in the formation of long bones are different from those of previous theories. The critical differences between the two explanations of development are related to the role of the cartilage model that was thought to be a predeterminant of bone formation: the new hypothesis argues that a collar of bone-producing cells in the mid-diaphyseal region arises first. This collar gradually spreads to lie around the whole of the newly forming bone and defines the size of the cartilage rod (once thought to be the scaffold upon which the bone was laid down). Finally, the cartilage rod is then eroded and modified to form the medullary cavity of the adult bone.

The timing of events is summarized in **Tab. 1-1**. The critical mass of cells that will initiate the process of development is not the cartilage model but a group of four to six cells that are arranged as a stack in the mid-diaphyseal region. The stacked cells are arranged as a collar that will come to lie around a cartilaginous center, which will develop later. The cells of this collar are referred to as the stacked cell layer. These early stages include another important feature, the exclusion of vascular elements from the developing layers of cells. Vasculature is sandwiched between the collar of stacked cells and the chondrocytes that will form the cartilage rod that lies in a position similar to the final position of the adult bone [22, 23]. The cells of the stacked layer will differentiate at the interface with the developing vasculature into osteogenic progenitor cells that

will further differentiate into osteoblasts. These osteoblasts secrete the unique matrix, type-1 collagen-rich osteoid, that produces a rigid collar around the developing cartilaginous center. Caplan [16] speculates that this rigid collar forms a physical barrier for nutrients and other vascular-derived molecules that are diffusing into the avascular cartilage core. He speculates further that these physical limitations may initiate the observed hypertrophy of core chondrocytes. As the collar of osteoid begins to spread toward the ends of the long bone, the mid-diaphyseal region undergoes further mineralization and becomes bone.

The next stage of development may be the most significant. The stacked cell layer is invaded and penetrated by vascular elements that are positioned just outside the central region of the newly formed bone [23]. The capillaries invade through the osteogenic precursor layer and come to make a network of vessels over the first layer of mineralized bone. Lying between these invading capillaries and perpendicular to the first layer of newly formed bone, further osteoid struts are formed and are subsequently mineralized. Deposition of a second layer of bone, parallel to the first, completely surrounds the developing capillaries which are locked between the two layers of bone that are in turn connected by strengthening struts, the bony trabeculae. Fundamental to this process is the relationship between the capillary endothelium and the osteoblasts. Histological evidence suggests that these early osteoblasts have specific orientation with the base of the cells in contact with the capillary endothelium and secretion of osteoid occurring at the apex. The highly active secretory process, carried out by the osteoblasts, is clearly related to the direction of transport across the cell from the blood. Caplan [16] suggests that this unique relationship may explain the production of unique, large-diameter collagen fibrils which are observed in osteoid. The relationship between endothelium, its basement membrane and osteoblast may be of fundamental importance in our understanding of the process of development and might be significant for our appreciation of the role of vascular supply in regenerative/restorative processes in the adult. It has already been shown that the presence of vasculature at the site of breakage determines the method of repair. If there is a stable fracture site, and vasculature continuity can be established between the broken fragments, then the mesenchymal repair blastema will differentiate directly into trabecular bone. If the fracture is not stable, an avascular repair blastema arises, characterized by the formation of a wedge of cartilage that plugs the gap between the fragments. Until recently, the key role of the vasculature at repair sites was thought to be related to nutrient supply, especially oxygen, to the area. The dependence of bone development on the endothelial/osteoblast relationship may indicate that the vascular elements in the reparative processes have an additional, and perhaps more significant, role to that of simply bringing extra nutrients and oxygen to the site of repair. Moreover, devising methods that stimulate this unique partnership between the lining cells of

the capillaries and the bone-producing cells may be important developmental approaches for bone healing in the future.

The role of the cartilage model, which lies at the core of the developing bone and scaffolding theory of bone building, is now open for negotiation. While the collars of bone develop around the central group of cartilage precursor cells, these chondrocytes start to undergo differentiation and expansion. These changes in birds and mammals follow, not lead, the formation of the stacked cell layer of osteogenic precursor cells. Whether or not the chondrocytes begin to hypertrophy in response to starvation when the first layer of osteoid is laid down remains to be proven. Initially, these hypertrophied cells begin to secrete unique products such as large chondroitin

Table 1-1: The sequence of bone formation. A comparison between events in chicken, mouse, and where possible human fetus. (Data taken from Caplan AI, Pechak DG, Cell and Molecular Biology of Vertebrate Hard Tissues; 1988.)

	Sequential stage of development	Days of development		
		Chick	**Mouse**	**Human**
Stage 1	Formation of limb buds	3		
Stage 2	Commitment of mesenchymal cells to osteogenic lineage	4	12	40
Stage 3	Commitment of mesenchymal cells to chondrogenic lineage	4	13	40
Stage 4	Expression of phenotypic characteristics	4.5	14	40
Stage 5	Formation of cartilage core	4.5–7	14	40
Stage 6	Osteoprogenitor cells of the Stacked Cell layer	4.5	15	40
Stage 7	Production of mid-diaphyseal osteoid	6	15	50
Stage 8	Phase boundary between osteoid and cartilage core	6.5	15	50
Stage 9	Initiation of hypertrophy in cartilage core	6.5	15	50
Stage 10	Progressive proximal and distal spreading of osteoid layer	7.0–16	15–16	50
Stage 11	Mineralization of osteoid	7.5	15	50
Stage 12	Vascular invasion onto the mineralized collar	8	15	50
Stage 13	Cartilage hypertrophy culmination (cessation of synthesis of anti-angiogenesis factors)	9	14–15	50–55
Stage 14	Formation of vertical struts between capillaries	8.5	16	56–57
Stage 15	Initiation of second layer of trabecular osteoid	9	16	57–58
Stage 16	Marrow elements associated with vascular collar	8.5	16	60
Stage 17	Mid-diaphyseal invasion of first bone by osteoclasts	9	–	56
Stage 18	Vascular penetration and erosion of cartilage	9	15	56
Stage 19	Cartilage replaced by vasculature and marrow	9–14	16–17	60
Stage 20	Continued sequential formation of 12 more layers of trabecular bone	9–19	–	–
Stage 21	Dissolution of the first layer of bone by marrow elements	11	–	–

sulfate proteoglycan [24] and type-X collagen [25], but eventually they die; if they are rescued and maintained in an organ bath, they will continue to secrete these unique products for many months [26]. Furthermore, Caplan [16] argues that the histological appearance of developing cartilage is suggestive of pressure restrictions on growth within the cartilage core: chondrocytes in the center of the cartilage core are normally round cells, while those near the periphery are flattened at the bone–cartilage interface as if they have been compressed against the rigid walls of the collar of developing bone.

In mammals the core of hypertrophic cartilage is calcified for most bones, although in some sites the calcified cartilage is encapsulated with newly formed bone. The process is different in the chicken; the hypertrophic cartilage is not calcified or covered with bone. The next process is, however, common to mammals and birds. The cartilage core is replaced by marrow and vascular elements, not by bone [22]. This cartilage core, once considered to be the scaffold for new bone, is, however, a scaffold for the marrow cavity. It is therefore not surprising that the cartilage model at the core of the developing bone defines precisely the initial size of the marrow cavity of the bone.

The consequences of the shift in our understanding of the process of bone formation can be summarized:

- Formation of long bones and flat bones (endochondral and intramembranous ossification) occurs by the same process.
- The relationship between endothelial cells of invading vasculature and the first osteoblasts is fundamental to the process of development and may be vital for reparative processes.

4 Ectopic bone formation

Cells located in sites removed from bone surfaces, in extra-skeletal sites, have the capacity for true bone formation [27–29]. The differentiation of an unspecialized mesenchymal cell population into bone tissue is initiated by a process known as bone induction. Huggins [30] demonstrated bone induction in a series of classic experiments almost 60 years ago by transplanting urinary epithelium into various connective-tissue sites in dogs and rabbits. Subsequently, other living epithelial cells were found to have similar properties [31, 32]. Transplanting bone fragments into non-skeletal sites also results in the induction of bone formation, indicating that bone tissue contains endogenous factors that regulate and control the formation of ectopic bone. Goldhaber [33] demonstrated that normal mouse bone synthesizes and secretes a bone-inducing factor capable of inducing bone formation. A similar substance was later discovered in certain mouse and human osteosarcomas [34–37]. Urist [38] was the first to show that devitalized bone contains an osteoinductive agent, which he named bone morphogenic protein (BMP).

It is important to identify and characterize osteoinductive agents as these would allow basic studies on osteogenic induction and osteogenesis at the cellular level and, more importantly, allow an assessment of their mechanisms of action in abnormal bone growth and healing processes. Based on the original techniques for producing soluble fractions containing osteoinductive factors [39], there have been several attempts at biochemical isolation of the materials [39–42]. These factors from a variety of sources have been shown to be non-collagenous proteins of low molecular weight; for example, human BMP and bovine BMP are said to have molecular weights of approximately 18,000 and to have characteristics of acidic proteins [43–45]. These substances have not been sequenced or, as Triffitt [2] suggests, if they have been sequenced, the results are closely guarded commercial secrets. Despite similarities in size between various osteogenic factors, there may be differences in composition; for example, osteosarcoma-derived BMP is a basic protein [2]. Levels of monoclonal antibodies to the major protein in purified bovine fractions with BMP activity in normal patients have been compared with those in patients affected by a variety of bone diseases [44, 46]. Despite clear differences in serum between individuals, data on the full characterization of the antibodies are not available.

Histologically, formation of bone from a transplanted bone chip resembles the classic picture of endochondral ossification. The initial phase is characterized by attraction of mesenchymal stem cells to the site of implantation. These stem cells surround the chip and within 1–3 days there is a powerful wave of mitogenic activity followed by differentiation into cartilage around the bone fragment. The cartilage becomes calcified, and new bone forms. It has been accepted that this process demonstrates the cartilage model system for bone formation, but closer inspection of the temporal events has revealed otherwise. Caplan [16] reports that there is a layer of osteogenic cells that form a sheet covering the bone chip and that this layer of cells, in intimate contact with invading capillaries, forms the first osteoid which is mineralized onto the surface of the bone fragment. The hypertrophic cartilage is, however, replaced by marrow, and there are accounts of marrow formation associated with these bone chips [47].

5   Development and maturation of bone

There are differences in the timing of appearance of secondary centers of ossification, their positions and rates of growth between species, but comparative analysis can be useful in establishing trends. In man, with a gestation period of 275 days, the ossification centers can be detected initially at 63 days, toward the middle of the first trimester of pregnancy. The centers develop rapidly and their position and extent for the eleventh week of gestation is shown diagrammatically in **Fig. 1-5a**. Although centers of ossification develop in a similar pattern in the dog, they are found much later. Gestation in the bitch lasts 63 days but the centers of ossification do not appear until at least day 28 of pregnancy. These centers are shown for day 33 of pregnancy in **Fig. 1-5b**. In consequence, during the second half of pregnancy, fetal puppies undergo massive skeletal development that continues into the neonatal period. The rate of development is clearly related to the immediate functional needs of the neonate. Calves, foals, fawns, and many other animals are born with all of their secondary ossification centers actively engaged in growth and almost all of the appendicular and axial skeleton at least partly ossified. These newborn animals are expected to stand within minutes or hours of birth,

follow their mothers, and even run to escape predators. Marsupials show perhaps the most spectacular form of differential development of the skeleton. The minuscule fetal marsupial is born with fully functional weight-bearing forelimbs and axial skeleton as far distal as the first few thoracic vertebrae. The remaining caudal vertebrae and the primitive limb buds that represent the final position of the hindlimbs are hardly developed at all. In this partly developed condition, they crawl, with the aid of their head, neck, and forelimbs, from the vulva into their mother's pouch and attach to a waiting nipple where they can continue growth.

5.1   Axial skeleton

5.1.1   Skull

There are many modifications and adaptations of the skull throughout the animal kingdom, with some spectacular evolutionary switches in the function of various components of the skull. For example, Hamilton and Mossman [48] showed that the ear ossicles, which are used to transmit sound waves in higher mammals, are derived from structures that support the gills in primates and chordates, and form part of the jaw in fish, reptiles, and amphibia.

Within a species there can be considerable variation in the shape and size of the skull. For example, there are racial differences in facial bone structure in man [49–53], and there have even been contentious claims of racial traits and even abilities associated with cranial vault size, which have been discredited. In cattle, there are vast differences in breed, size, and shape of the head, perhaps best exhibited by comparing beef and dairy breeds, or polled and horned breeds. It is, though, in dogs, where man's intervention has exaggerated the differences by selective breeding, that such differences can be seen so clearly. Consider the difference between the wide, squat-nosed, massive, heavy face of the Bulldog, a brachycephalic breed, and the elongated, fine, pointed head of a dolicocephalic breed such as the Afghan. It is interesting to note that these clear-cut differences, between the skulls of brachy-

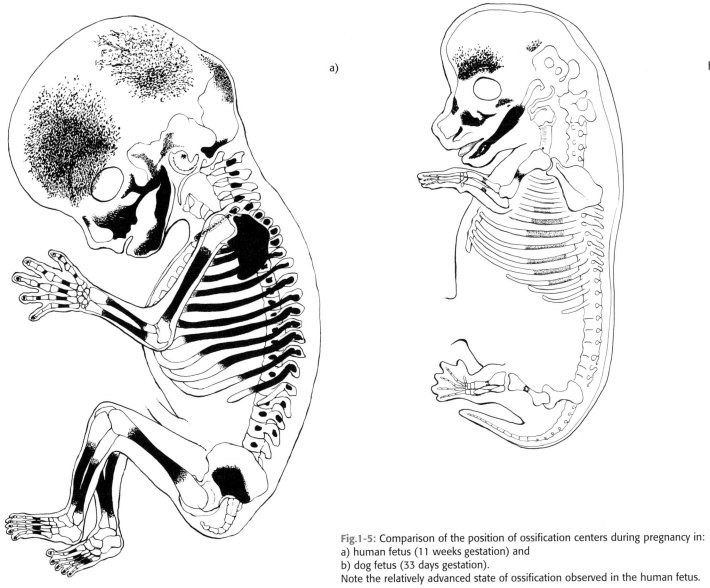

a)

b)

Fig.1-5: Comparison of the position of ossification centers during pregnancy in:
a) human fetus (11 weeks gestation) and
b) dog fetus (33 days gestation).
Note the relatively advanced state of ossification observed in the human fetus.

cephalic and dolicocephalic breeds, are not present at birth. Puppies are generally born with a common, basic head shape that will undergo genetically determined modifications as the puppy matures.

In general, the larger the head at birth, the less the bones of the skull are completely ossified. This is observed to the greatest degree by comparing the skull of a newborn child with that of a newborn puppy. The head of a human baby is approximately a quarter of the total length of the newborn. Delivery of the head represents the greatest hurdle during birth in humans and it is vital that the head can be molded to the shape of the birth canal. In consequence, the cranial vault is not completely ossified in newborn infants and patent fontanelles are present. Fontanelles are also seen during development in other species but the gaps between cranial bones have been closed and many, if not all, of the bones of the skull have undergone ossification by the time of birth. After delivery, a child's head progressively decreases proportionally in size compared with the rest of the body until it represents only a sixth or perhaps a seventh of the total body length of the human adult. There is less difference in the comparative size of the neonatal dog and the adult. However, some species, particularly the dolicocephalic breeds, will show substantial elongation of the facial bones during early postfetal life.

5.1.2 Vertebral column

Development of the vertebral column in higher vertebrates is initiated by the axial notochord. This primitive structure is surrounded by mesoderm during early embryonic life and condenses into sections to form somites. From these somites concentrations of mesenchyme develop, known as sclerotomes, that will form the vertebrae and, where appropriate, the ribs. The basic shape of individual vertebrae is similar, irrespective of whether they will develop into cervical or lumbar vertebrae. Typically, each vertebra has three centers of ossification, one for the centrum and one for each of the two neural arches. From the midline fusion of these two arches the dorsal spinous process will develop. Later, the transverse and costal (if appropriate) processes will develop from the position

where the ossification centers of the neural arches fuse to the developing centrum. For each region of the vertebral column, with the exception of the cervical region (where there are always seven vertebrae with only one or two exceptions, even for the long-necked giraffe), higher mammals have different numbers of vertebrae, but the characteristic shape of a vertebra from each region is consistent across species. For example, lumbar vertebrae have well-developed transverse processes to support the lateral and ventrolateral abdominal wall; the thoracic vertebrae have more pronounced dorsal spines and costal foveae for articulation with the ribs. The first two cervical vertebrae are, however, different from the others in their regional grouping: the body of the atlas (cervical vertebra one, C1) fuses to the body of the axis (cervical vertebra two, C2) forming the dens.

The appearance of the three ossification centers for each vertebra does not occur simultaneously, nor is a craniocaudal wave of development observed [54]. In general, the centers develop first and there is logical sequence from C1 through to thoracic vertebra seven (T7). Initiation of the centers for these vertebrae is rapidly followed by the appearance of the centers for the neural arches of the same segments. Then, for an unknown reason, the sequence is interrupted, and ossification centers for the caudal (coccygeal) vertebrae five to seven (Co 5–7) appear, followed by their respective arches. The craniocaudal sequence of development then resumes in the midthoracic region.

Lateral costal processes develop from the precursor thoracic vertebrae into the spaces between developing myotomes. These will separate from the developing vertebrae and form the ribs, each with a separate true articulation with the vertebrae at the proximal end and a cartilaginous articulation with the sternum at the distal end.

In addition to its functional support for the animal, flexibility of the spine is a prerequisite for locomotion. There are approximately 40 joints throughout the vertebral column whose movement is limited by conformation of the articular surfaces and ligaments involved. Most of these joints are limited to flexion, extensions and lateral movement. Only the occipito-atlantoaxial unit is different. Together, the articulations between these bones function more like a universal joint and afford greater ranges of movement. The unique movements, exhibited by these cranial articulations of the spine, are related to the specialized form of the bones and articulations involved. There are differences between species but, in general, the same basic shapes can be seen in all species. The occipital bone terminates at the occipitoatloid joint by two condyles with very large surface areas permitting considerable excursions of movement. The atlas, unique among vertebrae by its lack of a body, has two large lateral processes, wings, that serve for muscle attachment. In turn, the atlas articulates with condyles of the axis and rotates around the dens of the axis. The pivoting movement between C1 and C2 determines whether the face can be rotated 180° (man), greater than 240° (owls), or less than 100° (cattle).

5.1.3 Ribs

Embryological origins of the ribs have been discussed above. There is considerable variation between species in the number of ribs present and the presence or absence of false ribs (not connected to the sternum). In general, higher mammals possess nine ribs that are connected directly to the sternum and between three to eight ribs that are either linked to the sternum by cartilage or may be completely unconnected. Together, the double rows of ribs form the bony cage that protects the thoracic viscera. The shape of this thoracic cage differs according to the posture and size of the animal and reflects the stresses exerted on the thorax.

5.1.4 Sternum

The sternum develops from two midline ventral (anterior in man) condensations of mesenchyme in the thoracic region of the embryo. Each side of the sternum is known as a hemisternum and is curved in two directions: boat-shaped along the ventral surface of the embryo, and curved away from the midline as the condensation progresses caudally. As the ventral surface of the embryo closes, so the two hemisterna move closer together and fuse, at least at the cranial end. There is considerable species difference in the degree of fusion ob-

served. Laterally, the hemisterna attract the distal ends of the developing ribs, but they do not fuse in a craniocaudal sequence. Usually, ribs 2–7 fuse before the first rib unites with the sternum, followed by the last two true ribs. Anomalies of closure of the two hemisterna, and of fusion of the last two true ribs, are relatively commonly occurrences.

As the sternum grows there is considerable variation in shape and size between species. In man, the sternum expands to form a flat plate of bone that might be considered important in protection of the thorax. The same structure is elongated, thin, and clearly reflects its segmental origin in the dog, while in the horse and cow the sternum retains its original boat-shaped appearance and even grows to form a ventral projection akin to a keel that serves for muscle attachment.

5.2 Appendicular skeleton

For orthopedic purposes, postnatal development of the appendicular skeleton is of paramount importance. Centers of ossification in man are relatively consistent over the time of their appearance and fusion, which means that it is possible to make predictions about bone length and assessment of age with reasonable accuracy. The same is not true for dogs. Breed variation in size and shape makes it impossible to use bone length as an accurate guide to age. Sumner-Smith [55] compares the time of fusion of epiphyses throughout the skeletal system with age. This produces a reasonable correlation, but there is still considerable variation in the earliest and latest time fusion for one particular epiphysis (**Tab. 1-2**). There appears to be a relatively consistent chronological order to the sequence of fusion. It may be useful to list a number of factors that cannot be related consistently to the timing of fusion of epiphyses in dogs; for example, variation between siblings is commonplace, there is no predominance shown by male, female, or neutered animals, and breed size does not effect time of fusion.

Table 1-2a: A comparison of the time of appearance of ossification centres and growth plate fusion in man and dog—pectoral limb.

	Man				Dog	
	Ossification centre		Growth plate fusion		Ossification centre	Growth plate fusion
Scapula						
Coracoid	1		18–21		–	–
Acromion	15–18		18–19		–	–
Glenoid cavity	18		19		–	–
Supraglenoid tubercle	prenatal		15		12 wk	5 mo
Clavicle	17		18–24		absent	–
Humerus						
Proximal						
Head	fetal		centres fuse together 4–6		only one centre	
Greater tubercle	6 mo–2		fuse to shaft		present at birth	fuse to shaft
	3 mo–1		19–21			13–14 mo
Lesser tubercle	3–5		18–20			
Distal						
Medial epicondyle	7	5	18	15	3–4 mo	fuse to shaft
Trochlea	9	8	fuse together at puberty		one centre	5–8 mo
Lateral epicondyle	12	11	fuse to shaft		prenatal	
Capitulum	5 mo	4 mo	17	14	prenatal	
Ulna						
Olecranon	10	8	15–17	14–15	3–4 mo	5–9 mo
Distal epiphysis	6	5	19	17	3–4 mo	6–8 mo
Radius						
Head	5	4	13–17	14–15	prenatal	5–8 mo
Radial tuberosity	10–12		14–18		absent	partial fusion to ulna 11 mo
Distal epiphysis	1		19	17	prenatal	6–9 mo
Carpus						
Accessory	6 mo		4		3–4 mo	5–6 mo
Radial	6		–		3 mo	–
Intermediate	4		–		3 mo	–
Ulna	12		–		3–4 mo	–
I	5		5		3 mo	–
II	4		–		3 mo	–
III	6 mo		–		3 mo	–
IV	6 mo		–		3 mo	–
Metacarpals						
I	2	1²/₃	14–21		absent	–
II–V	1–1½		14–21		3–4 mo	5–8 mo
Phalanges						
Proximal	5 mo–2½		14–21		3–4 mo	5 mo
Middle	5 mo–2½		14–21		3–4 mo	5 mo
Distal	5–2 (except I 1½ 1)		14–21		3–5 mo	5 mo

Table 1-2b: A comparison of the time of appearance of ossification centres and growth plate fusion in man and dog—hip bones.

	Man		Dog	
	Ossification centre	Growth plate fusion	Ossification centre	Growth plate fusion
Hip				
Acetabular	10–13		6–8 wk	4–6 mo
Ischium	60 wk (fetal)		25 wk (fetal)	
Pubis	60 wk (fetal)	fuse at puberty (12–13)	20 wk (fetal)	fuse 1–2
Illium	60 wk (fetal)		10 wk (fetal)	
Iliac crest	puberty		4 mo	1–2,5
Ischial arch	13–15		5–8 mo	8–12 mo
Ischial tuberosity	13–15		2,5–4 mo	6–10,5 mo
Symphyseal cartilage	13–20		4–10 mo	fusion symphysis (1–5)

Table 1-2c: A comparison of the time of appearance of ossification centres and growth plate fusion in man and dog—pelvic limb (excluding hip bones).

	Man				Dog	
	Ossification centre		Growth plate fusion		Ossification centre	Growth plate fusion
Femur						
Greater trochanter	3		16–17		3–4 mo	9–11 mo
Lesser trochanter	12	11	16–17		3–4 mo	9–10 mo
Head	4 mo		17–18	16–17	3–4 mo	6–9 mo
Distal epiphysis	36 wk (fetal)		18–19	17	3–4 mo	6–8 mo
Tibia						
Proximal epiphysis	40 wk (fetal)		18–19	16–17	3–4 mo	6–11 mo
Tibial tuberosity	7–15		19		3–4 mo	8–11 mo
Distal epiphysis	6 mo		17–18		3–4 mo	5–11 mo
Fibula						
Proximal epiphysis	4	3	18–20	16–18	3–4 mo	6–10 mo
Distal epiphysis	1	9 mo	17–18		3–4 mo	5–8 mo
Tarsus						
Calcaneus	24–26 wk (fetal)	12–22			prenatal	4–7 mo
Talus	26–28 wk (fetal)					
Navicular	2					
Cuboid	40 wk (fetal)	variable			variable	
Cuneiforms I–II	1–2					
III	3–6 mo					

All times are given in years except where indicated.
Reference sources: Arey LB, A Textbook and Laboratory Manual of Embryology, WB Saunders Co.; 1974. Hare WCD, The ages of which the centres of ossification appear roentgenographically in limb bone of the dog, Am J Vet Res; 1961. Riser WH, Growth and development of the normal canine pelvis—Hip joints and femurs from birth to maturity, J AM Vet Radiol Soc; 1973. Smith RN, Radiological observations on the limbs of young greyhounds, J Small Anim Prac; 1960. Smith RN, The pelvis of the young dog, Vet Rec; 1964. Smith RN, Alcock J, Epiphyseal fusion in the greyhound, Vet Rec; 1960. Sumner-Smith G, Observations of epiphyseal fusion of the canine appendicular skeleton, J Small Anim Prac; 1966. Turek SL, Orthopaedic principles and their application, JB Lippincott Co.; 1977.

5.2.1 Pectoral limb

Scapula

The position of the scapula and its relation to the thorax differs substantially in man from other animals. It forms part of the true pelvic girdle while in quadrupeds the pectoral limb is attached to the axial skeleton by a synsarcosis. In both man and dog, the body of the scapula is present at birth, derived from one major center of ossification. This major center also gives rise to the spine and acromion of the scapula. Shortly after birth, a second center appears in man [56] and dog [57], which gives rise to the supraglenoid tubercle. In dogs fusion takes place slowly with the rest of the scapula, and the cartilage plate is usually eroded by 28 weeks postpartum. In cats and horses, there is another secondary center of ossification adjacent to the glenoid cavity which fuses shortly after birth.

Clavicle

This bone is an important part of the pectoral girdle. It is therefore present in many quadrupeds that climb or dig. Most of the common domestic species only possess a bony (cat) or cartilaginous (dog) remnant of this bone, which is intercalated into the brachiocephalic muscle. In man, an ossification center for the clavicle is among the first to develop in the fetus [58]. The secondary ossification center, however, develops much later (at about 11–14 years of age) on the sternal end of the bone.

Humerus

The shaft of the humerus is present at birth. Arey [56] reports that the shaft is present as early as the seventh week of pregnancy in man. In addition, an ossification center is present at the head of the humerus at birth. Appearance of this center during fetal life can be used to identify accurately fetal age since it develops in the human fetus during week 38 of gestation [59]. There is species variation in the number of centers of ossification present. In man, the proximal center divides during childhood to give rise to two centers that will form the greater and lesser tubercles of the proximal end of the bone. These centers fuse together before uniting with the shaft of the humerus. The major increase in bone length, seen during childhood, occurs at the proximal end of the bone [58]. Three centers of ossification develop during childhood for the distal end of the shaft. These correspond to the medial and lateral parts of the distal condyle and one for the medial epicondylar region. In dogs, there is only one proximal center of ossification for the humerus. From this single area the greater and lesser trochanters are formed. The cartilaginous growth plate, between the proximal center and the shaft, remains intact until the 43rd week of life. This might suggest that in dogs the major region for growth in length of the humerus occurs at the proximal end of the bone, similar to that reported in man. By 51 weeks only remnants of the plate are seen and gradually, over the next 8 weeks, the plate is removed completely. Distally, three centers develop which start to fuse from the 21st week of life onwards and fusion is completed by the 33rd week.

Radius

Initially, this bone appears as a long cylinder, which develops spherical-shaped centers of ossification at both ends in early childhood (man), or within the first 4 weeks (dog). Gradually, the centers broaden out and assume the characteristic shape of the adult bone. Fusion occurs in children aged 8–11 years and in puppies between 45–47 weeks.

Ulna

Formation of the ulna is more complex. In many of the domestic species the bone is partly or completely fused to the radius during development. The most extreme example is the horse where the olecranon and proximal third of the bone are present: the latter decreases substantially in size distal to the elbow joint and is completely fused to the radius from birth. In man and dog, the ulna is present at birth as a long cylinder on the caudolateral aspect of the rudimentary radius. Shortly after birth, the characteristic semilunar trochlear notch develops at the proximal end and starts to interact with the developing proximal radius and distal humerus to form the elbow joint.

In dogs, proximal and distal centers of ossification appear at 8 weeks. The distal epiphysis grows rapidly in an uneven manner; two spurs of developing bone grow on the medial and lateral sides of the ulnar metaphysis. This uneven rate of growth continues and by 12 weeks the cartilage separating the metaphysis and epiphysis has adopted a V-shaped appearance. The distal epiphysis swells and becomes larger in diameter than the shaft of the ulnar diaphysis. Complete fusion of the distal center is achieved by the 47th week while the proximal epiphysis fuses to the shaft earlier, during the 37th week. In both man and dog small foci of ossification associated with the anconeal process have been identified. Almost as soon as these foci appear fusion starts to occur, although there are many documented cases where failure of fusion leads to a pathological, non-united anconeal process which will be associated with elbow dysplasia.

Coordination between the growth rates of the radius and ulna are important in the normal development of the forearm. In animals where the bones are linked together there are fewer reported conditions of uncoordinated growth, but in man and dog premature closure of one of the growth plates will result in malformation of the forearm, and possibly the elbow and carpus. Problems associated with premature or failed closure of the proximal ulna plate are relatively common but will not affect conformation of the forearm. Premature closure of the distal growth plate of the ulna is the most common condition that will distort the bones; the manus will deviate laterally and the forearm will curve. Premature closure of the distal plate of the radius is less common and is not usually associated with bowing of the forearm: quite the contrary, the forearm is reported straighter than normal, but the patient experiences elbow joint pain. (The elbow pain is usually greater in quadrupeds as the condition is exacerbated by weight bearing.) Failure of closure of the proximal radius growth plate is rare: accompanied by no change in the conformation of the forearm, an increase in the humeroradial space that can be detected radiographically and joint pain, especially upon palpation.

Carpus

Carpal centers of ossification are not present in either man or dog at birth. There is a similar sequence for the appearance of these centers in both species but a considerable difference in time scale. Centers for the intermediate and accessory carpal are the first to develop, followed quickly by centers for the other five bones. There is partial fusion of the bones in the carpus of the dog, and the initially separate centers of ossification for the radial and intermediate carpal bones in the dog quickly fuse and are completely united by the 12th week of life. A second center of ossification appears for the accessory carpal bone in both man and dog. In general, complete fusion of the epiphyses has occurred by the age of 6 months in dogs and by 10 years in children.

Manus

Shafts representing the rudimentary metacarpals and phalanges are present at birth for the major digits present (four in dog, five in man). Each of the bones and the sesamoids that develop subsequently on the palmar aspects of the metacarpophalangeal joints develop one center of ossification. In general, the metacarpal centers remain active for longer than the phalangeal centers, but there is great variability in the timing and sequence of closure of the plates between digits.

5.2.2   Pelvic limb

Hip bones

Despite major differences in the shape and form of the hip bones between species, there are underlying trends that outline development. Considering the hip bones of dog and man, the most notable differences are the lateral divergence of the wings of the ilia in man compared with the almost cranio-caudal direction in the dog. Nevertheless the bones start to form in much the same manner. At birth, in both species, there are three major centers of ossification that will develop into the three major bony components of the pelvis: ilium, ischium, and pubis (paired structures). A center develops during weeks 6–7 in dogs, or during the third trimester in man, which will form the acetabular bone. The components of the acetabulum fuse together and other centers of ossification for parts of the ischial tuber, iliac crest, and eventually the symphysis develops. Complete ossification of the pelvic symphysis occurs up to age 6 in dogs and during late teens or early twenties in man.

Femur

Again, the shaft of this bone is present in almost all species at birth. For animals that are expected to stand and walk within minutes or hours of birth other components are also present, such as proximal and distal centers of ossification, which allow contact to be made and rudimentary joints to be established with respective bones. In dogs, an epiphysis develops within 2 weeks of birth at either end of the shaft. By 8 weeks a further pair of centers develops at the proximal end of the femur which will form the greater and lesser trochanters. The first proximal center forms the head of the femur and takes a considerable length of time to fuse to the shaft. This period and the integrity of the head are critical for normal conformation to be attained. The single distal center develops into the complex trochlea, condyles, and epicondylar regions of the distal end of the femur. Closure of the growth plates occurs between the 41st and 47th week in dog. At approximately 32 weeks of life the center for the patella, followed 20–30 weeks later by small foci for the fabellae, develops. There are subtle differences in the shape of the human femur, including a longer femoral neck, wider distal condylar region, and less pronounced lesser trochanteric region, but the pattern and sequence of development is similar. The timescale of development is extended into late childhood for complete fusion to occur.

Tibia

With the shaft ossified at birth, the tibia grows in length with the appearance of a single proximal and a distal epiphysis. There are peculiarities about the changes observed at both these centers. The proximal center develops first and a small notch appears in the cranial aspect of the center. Development of the distal epiphysis then occurs, rapidly followed by the appearance of a third center which is responsible for the tibial tuberosity. Ossification at the distal center does not occur by circumferential growth but seems to develop primarily on the medial aspect of the bone and spreads around the periphery of the cartilage plate. Fusion of the three plates usually occurs first in the distal center, followed by the tibial tuberosity and lastly by the proximal center, although they may be in various stages of closure simultaneously.

Fibula

Animals from species that retain a fibula during development are born with an ossified shaft. Following a now fairly familiar pattern, two centers of ossification appear at either end of the bone: the proximal epiphysis appears first and is the first to fuse, the distal appearing and fusing slightly later. The central portion of the diaphysis in the dog fuses for a short but individually variable distance to the developing tibia. In most breeds of dog the shaft of the fibula is straight but is twisted laterally around the tibia in man [58].

Tarsus

There are striking differences between the tarsal regions of bipedal and quadrupedal animals. The plantigrade locomotion of man produces concussive forces on the tarsal region that are not experienced by quadrupeds. However, the pattern of ossification and development of the two regions is similar between bipedal and quadrupedal animals; for example, animals are born with the centers developed for the calcaneus and talus, followed shortly after birth by centers for the central, third, and fourth tarsal bones. The appearance of a second growth area for the calcaneus usually occurs at the time that centers for the first and second tarsal bones develop. Many of the domestic species show varying degrees of fusion between tarsal bones. Like their counterparts in the carpus, the early development of separate centers for each of the tarsal bones is rapidly followed in these species by immediate fusion of these centers giving rise, for example, to a fused central and fourth tarsal in the ox, or a fused first and second tarsal in the horse.

Pes

With the exception of the longer length of the metatarsal bones in most species, in comparison with the metacarpals in the same animal, the sequence and rate of development of the pes is similar to that described for the manus.

6   Bone modeling and remodeling

Overall conformation of adult bone is determined genetically. Once maturity is achieved bone ceases to grow, but mechanical stresses of weight bearing, muscle attachment, and applied loads will all result in constant adaptation of the internal structure and external appearance of bone. There is a vast panoply of factors that are known to affect bone growth and modeling; some of these are more important in the initiation of bone growth, others in the growing process itself or in the modeling process, while some are vital for reparative processes (see **Chapters 7** and **9**).

Bone resorption, the primary function of osteoclasts, occurs predominantly on the endosteal surface. Tunnels are eroded into the bone at right angles to the shaft and are occupied by osteoblasts and vascular elements. Quickly, layers of lamellar bone are laid down and the osteoblasts are stranded and enclosed in matrix, becoming osteocytes within lacunae. In this way a progression of osteons are formed, each layer breaking through established bone.

The mechanics of resorption are not completely understood. Osteoclastic activity is fundamental to the process. These cells are present, at all times, on the surfaces of bone; yet bone is not continuously eroded and resorbed at all sites. This argues that: Either the osteoclasts are not always active and have to be goaded into action or the bony structures are protected by a lining of condensed connective tissue or perhaps a very thin layer of bone-lining cells. The last of these possibilities is considered most likely [60]. The following sequence is suggested:

- The barrier which protects the bone itself has to be removed.
- The exposed matrix attracts mononuclear phagocytes to the bone surface.
- Resorption is initiated.
- The mononuclear phagocytes fuse together and form histologically recognizable osteoclasts.

The exact process of resorption has yet to be elucidated. The osteoclasts have a ruffled or brush border in contact with the bone surface and it is suggested that the following process might occur:

- Components of the bone matrix are released first by a variety of hydrolytic enzymes, including collagenase.
- These mineral components and collagen fragments are phagocytized by the osteoclast.
- Complete enzymatic dissolution of the matrix is achieved within osteoclastic vacuoles.

7 Bibliography

Blue references indicate links to abstracts
of articles available online:
http://www.aopublishing.org/BONE/1.htm

1. **Rasmussen H, Bordier P** (1974)
*The Physiological and Cellular Basis of
Metabolic Bone Disease.* Baltimore:
Williams & Wilkins.

2. **Triffitt JT** (1987) Initiation and
enhancement of bone formation. A
review. *Acta Orthop Scand;*
58 (6): 673–684.

3. **Friedenstein A** (1973) Determined
and inducible osteogenic precursor
cells. *Hard Tissue Growth, Repair and
Remineralization:* Ciba Foundation
Symposium (New Series), 169–182.

4. **Hendry J** (1985) Mathematical
aspects of colony growth, trans-
plantation kinetics and cells survival.
In: Pottan CS, Hendry JH, editors.
Cell Clones. Edinburgh: Churchill
Livingstone.

5. **Owen N** (1985) Lineage of
osteogenic cells and their relationship
to the stromal system. In: Peck WA,
editor. *Bone and Mineral Research:*
Elsevier; 3:1–25.

6. **Maximow A** (1928) Cultures of
blood leucocytes: from lymphocyte
and monocyte to connective tissue.
Arch Exp Zellforsch; 5:169–268.

7. **Luria EA, Panasyuk AF,
Friedenstein AY** (1971) Fibroblast
colony formation from monolayer
cultures of blood cells. *Transfusion;*
11 (6):345–349.

8. **Piersma AH, Ploemacher RE,
Brockbank KG, et al.** (1985)
Migration of fibroblastoid stromal
cells in murine blood. *Cell Tissue Kinet;*
18 (6):589–595.

9. **Patt HM, Maloney MA** (1972)
Evolution of marrow regeneration as
revealed by transplantation studies.
Exp Cell Res; 71 (2):307–312.

10. **Tavassoli M, Crosby WH** (1968)
Transplantation of marrow to
extramedullary sites. *Science;*
161 (836):54–56.

11. **Friedenstein AJ, Piatetzky S, II,
Petrakova KV** (1966) Osteogenesis
in transplants of bone marrow cells.
J Embryol Exp Morphol; 16 (3):381–390.

12. **Branemark PI, Brine U,
Johansson B, et al.** (1964)
Regeneraton of bone marrow: A
clincal and experimental study
following removal of bone marrow
by currettage. *Acta Anat;* 50:1.

13. **Maloney M, Patt HM** (1969) Bone
marrow restoration after localized
depletion. *Cell Tissue Kinet;* 2:29–38.

14. **Patt HM, Maloney MA** (1975)
Bone marrow regeneration after local
injury: a review. *Exp Hematol;*
3 (2): 135–148.

15. **Caplan AI, Fiszman MY,
Eppenberger HM** (1983) Molecular
and cell isoforms during development. *Science;* 221 (4614): 921–927.

16. **Caplan AI** (1988) Bone Development.
In: Caplan AI, Pechak DG, editors.
*Cell and Molecular Biology of Vertebrate
Hard Tissues:* Ciba Foundation
Symposium (New Series), 3–21.

17. **Caplan AI, Ordahl CP** (1978)
Irreversible gene repression model for
control of development. *Science;*
201 (4351):120–130.

18. **Hall B** (1978) *Developmental and
cellular skeletal biology.* New York:
Academic Press.

19. **Comar C, Lotz WE, Boyd GA**
(1952) Autoradiographic studies of
calcium, phosphorus and strontium
distribution in the bones of the
growing pig. *Am J Anat;* 90:113–125.

20. **McLean F, Budy AM** (1964)
Radiation, Isotopes and Bone. New York:
Academic Press.

21. **Comar C, Wasserman RH** (1964)
Strontium. In: Comar CI, Bronner F,
editors. *Mineral Metabolism Part A.*
New York: Academic Press.

22. **Caplan AI, Pechak DG** (1987) The
cellular and molecular embryology of
bone formation. In: Peck WA, editor.
Bone and Mineral Research.
Elsevier; 5:117–184.

23. **Pechak DG, Kujawa MJ, Caplan
AI** (1986) Morphological and
histochemical events during first
bone formation in embryonic chick
limbs. *Bone;* 7 (6):441–458.

24. **Carrino DA, Weitzhandler A,
Caplan AI** (1985) Proteoglycans
synthesized during the cartilage to
bone transition. In: Butler WT, editor.
The Chemistry of Mineralized Tissues.
Birmingham, AL: EBSCO Media,
197–208.

25. **Schmid TM, Linsenmayer TF**
(1985) Immunohistochemical
localization of short chain cartilage
collagen (type X) in avian tissues.
J Cell Biol; 100 (2):598–605.

26. **Syftestad GT, Weitzhandler M,
Caplan AI** (1985) Isolation and
characterization of osteogenic cells
derived from first bone of the
embryonic tibia. *Dev Biol;*
110 (2):275–283.

27. **Connors J** (1983) *Soft tissue
ossification.* Berlin: Springer-Verlag.

28. **Smith R, Triffitt JT** (1986) Bones
in muscles: the problems of soft tissue
ossification. *Q J Med;* 61 (235):985–990.

29. **Urist MR, DeLange RJ, Finerman
GA** (1983) Bone cell differentiation
and growth factors. *Science;*
220 (4598):680–686.

30. **Huggins C** (1930) Experimental
osteogenesis. *Proc Soc Exp Biol Med;*
27:349–351.

31. **Anderson HC** (1976) Osteogenetic
epithelial-mesenchymal cell interactions. *Clin Orthop;* (119):211–223.

32. **Wlodarski K** (1969) The inductive
properties of epithelial established cell
lines. *Exp Cell Res;* 57 (2):446–448.

33. **Goldhaber P** (1961) Osteogenic
induction across millipore filters in
vivo. *Science;* 131:2065–2067.

34. **Hanamura H, Higuchi Y, Nakagawa M, et al.** (1980) Solubilization and purification of bone morphogenetic protein (BMP) from Dunn osteosarcoma. *Clin Orthop;* (153):232–240.

35. **Amitani K, Nakata Y, Stevens J** (1974) Bone induction by lyophilized osteosarcoma in mice. *Calcif Tissue Res;* 16 (4):305–313.

36. **Heiple KG, Herndon CH, Chase SW, et al.** (1968) Osteogenic induction by osteosarcoma and normal bone in mice. *J Bone Joint Surg [Am];* 50 (2):311–325.

37. **Bauer FC, Urist MR** (1981) Human osteosarcoma-derived soluble bone morphogenetic protein. *Clin Orthop;* (154):291–295.

38. **Urist MR** (1965) Bone: formation by autoinduction. *Science;* 150 (698): 893–899.

39. **Urist MR, Mikulski AJ** (1979) A soluble bone morphogenetic protein extracted from bone matrix with a mixed aqueous and nonaqueous solvent. *Proc Soc Exp Biol Med;* 162 (1): 48–53.

40. **Urist MR, Conover MA, Lietze A, et al.** (1981) Partial purification and characterization of bone morphogenetic protein. In: Cohn DV, Talmage RV, Matthews JL, editors. *Hormonal Control of Calcium Metabolism.* Amsterdam: Excepta Medica, 307–314.

41. **Urist MR, Lietze A, Mizutani H, et al.** (1982) A bovine low molecular weight bone morphogenetic protein (BMP) fraction. *Clin Orthop;* (162): 219–232.

42. **Sampath TK, Reddi AH** (1981) Dissociative extraction and reconstitution of extracellular matrix components involved in local bone differentiation. *Proc Natl Acad Sci USA;* 78 (12):7599–7603.

43. **Urist MR, Sato K, Brownell AG, et al.** (1983) Human bone morphogenetic protein (hBMP). *Proc Soc Exp Biol Med;* 173 (2):194–199.

44. **Urist MR, Huo YK, Brownell AG, et al.** (1984) Purification of bovine bone morphogenetic protein by hydroxyapatite chromatography. *Proc Natl Acad Sci USA;* 81 (2):217–375.

45. **Urist MR, Chang JJ, Lietze A, et al.** (1987) Preparation and bioassay of bone morphogenetic protein and polypeptide fragments. *Methods Enzymol;* 146:294–312.

46. **Urist M, Hudak RT, Huo YK, et al.** (1985) Osteoporosis: a bone morphogenetic protein autoimmune disorder. In: *Normal and Abnormal Bone Growth: Bone and Clinical Research.* New York: Alan R. Liss Inc., 77–96.

47. **Reddi AH, Kuettner KE** (1981) Vascular invasion of cartilage: correlation of morphology with lysozyme, glycosaminoglycans, protease, and protease-inhibitory activity during endochondral bone development. *Dev Biol;* 82 (2):217–223.

48. **Hamilton WJ, Mossman HW,** (1972) *Human Embryology 4th Edition.* Baltimore: Williams & Wilkins.

49. **Meredith HV, Spurgeon JH** (1976) Comparative findings on the skelic index of black and white children and youths residing in South Carolina. *Growth;* 40 (1):75–81.

50. **Meredith HV** (1978) Secular change in sitting height and lower limb height of children, youths, and young adults of Afro-black, European, and Japanese ancestry. *Growth;* 42 (1):37–41.

51. **Spurgeon JH, Meredith EM, Meredith HV** (1978) Body size and form of children of predominantly black ancestry living in West and Central Africa, North and South America, and the West Indies. *Ann Hum Biol;* 5 (3):229–246.

52. **Spurgeon JH, Meredith HV** (1979) Body size and form of black and white male youths: South Carolina youths compared with youths measured at earlier times and other places. *Hum Biol;* 51 (2):187–200.

53. **Walker A** (1976) *The Hominids of East Turkanan.* San Francisco: WH Freeman.

54. **Bagnall KM, Harris PF, Jones PR** (1977) A radiographic study of the human fetal spine. 2. The sequence of development of ossification centres in the vertebral column. *J Anat;* 124 (3):791–802.

55. **Sumner-Smith G** (1966) Observations on epiphyseal fusion of the canine appendicular skeleton. *J Small Anim Pract;* 7 (4):303–311.

56. **Arey LB** (1974) Developmental Anatomy. In: Arey LB, editor. *A Textbook and Laboratory Manual of Embryology.* 7th ed. Philadelphia: WB Saunders Co.

57. **Hare W** (1961) The ages at which the centres of ossification appear rotentgenographically in limb bone of the dog. *Am J Vet Res;* 22:825–835.

58. **Williams P, Warwick R, Dyson M, et al.** (1989) *Gray's Anatomy.* Edinburgh, Melbourne & New York: Churchill Livingstone.

59. **Kuhns LR, Sherman MP, Poznanski AK, et al.** (1973) Humeral-head and coracoid ossification in the newborn. *Radiology;* 107 (1):145–149.

60. **Wasserman RH** (1984) Bones. In: Swenson MJ, editor. *Duke's Physiology of Domestic Animals.* Ithaca & London: Cornell University Press, 467–485.

2 Blood supply to developing, mature, and healing bone

James W. Wilson

1 Introduction

1.1 Importance of knowledge of bone blood supply

Bones may be compared to the girders in a building; they have the consistency of brick, and broken pieces can fit together in a way similar to pieces of a broken china cup. The appearance of bone is very deceptive. To stay alive, bones must have an adequate blood supply. All physiologic processes within bone, including the ability to repair itself, are dependent upon its blood supply. Bones can degenerate or die, their appearance may change, their function may alter, healing may be delayed or cease due to damage to this blood supply through inappropriate therapy or poor surgical technique. Thus, for the orthopedists, knowledge of the normal blood supply to bone and its response with injury is imperative.

1.2 Historical survey

Information on the circulation of blood in bones can be traced to the beginnings of modern science. In 1678, the Dutch merchant Anton van Leeuwenhoek, the founder of microscopy, reported that bone was composed of subunits, that it had longitudinal channels, and that vessels could be found on the outer surface. In 1691, the English physician Clopton Havers described the penetration of the cortex by the nutrient artery and the metaphyseal arcade. He observed the lamellar pattern of cortical bone and described the canals that bear his name: haversian canals. His complete report suggested a centrifugal nutrition of cortical bone. Havers was not sure whether the canals in bone contained blood vessels or "medullary oil". In 1757, Albinus, using vascular injections, was able to demonstrate fine blood vessels in haversian canals. He identified vessels entering and leaving the bone from both periosteal and endosteal surfaces. The theory of dual blood supply to cortical bone, from periosteal and medullary vessels, was introduced.

1.3 Methodology utilized in study

Recent investigations employ many techniques. The techniques utilized, and the results obtained from investigations, may conveniently be divided into anatomical representations of the vasculature and physiologic measurements of blood flow, using miscellaneous techniques. The experimental animal most commonly used is the dog, which, among the common laboratory animals, appears to have an osseous blood supply closest to that of man [1, 2].

1.3.1 Anatomical methods

The methods of microangiography in use today [3–5] are a modification of techniques developed for bone by Trueta et al. [6] and Barclay [7].

The technique entails perfusion with finely divided barium sulfate, serial sawing of the perfused bone, and production of stereoscopic radiographs on high-resolution photographic plates or film. The arterial tree under investigation is usually infused at the animal's normal systolic blood pressure; thus, there is physiologic filling of the arteries and capillaries functional at the time of the infusion. Afferent vessels, as small as 10 μm in diameter, are demonstrable by soft radiography in decalcified tissue slices. It is the "micro" radiographic technique, used to produce the angiograms of the tissue slices, that gives rise to the terms microangiography and microangiogram. Production of microangiograms does not damage the tissue slice, and each slice can then be embedded and sectioned by microtome. This exacting technique is the only one known that allows demonstration of both the microcirculation and the histologic morphology within a single slice of tissue. By visually stacking serial tissue slices, the microvascular and correlated histologic patterns of areas can be observed. In addition, microangiograms give an excellent qualitative measure of blood flow, which has been found to correlate with microsphere-measured blood flows [8]. At the present time, a method to quantify microangiograms is under study [9].

A second popular technique, commonly referred to as the Spalteholz technique, involves arterial injection of India ink and clearing of the harvested tissues with solutions [10]. The vessels, when viewed under a bright-field microscope, appear black against a clear transparent background [8, 11–14]. An example is depicted in **Fig. 2-1**. If a dissecting microscope is utilized, 3-D relationships can be appreciated. The clearing process precludes histologic processing; thus cellular morphology is lost. Spalteholz clearing of tissues has also been utilized following arterial injections of barium sulfate [15] or silicone rubber [16, 17]. Eitel et al. used both India ink and barium sulfate as the infusate and evaluated thin decalcified sections rather than cleared specimens [17].

Vascular perfusion with plastics, followed by corrosion of the bone, produces a display of vessels that can be examined by bright-field or scanning electron microscopy. This technique has seen only limited use in the study of blood supply to bone [18–20]. As with the Spalteholz technique, direct examination of the histologic nature of the tissues is lost; however, an imprint of cells of the vessel wall can be seen on the casts. The electron microscope has seen limited use [20, 21].

Fig. 2-1: Photograph of a Spalteholz preparation (×7) showing the distribution of the afferent vascular system to the normal mid-diaphyseal canine tibia. Medullary arterioles penetrate the endosteal surface circumferentially. Periosteal arterioles enter the anterior surface, *above*, and at the posterior corners, *below* [119].

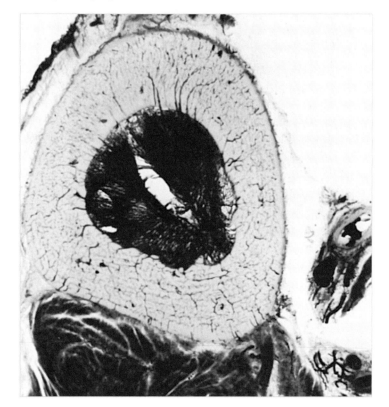

1.3.2   **Blood flow methods**

Pioneer organ-perfusion studies, in the early 1900s, estimated blood flow to an organ by collection and measurement of the entire venous outflow from the organ under study. Today a number of improved techniques are in use. Most have in common the injection and measurement of a radioactive tracer. The specific tracers involve inert gases, soluble elements, labeled compounds, or labeled particulate matter. Measurement of activity and calculation of blood flow are performed by scintigraphy, clearance, washout, or entrapment.

The rate of disappearance of an injected small volume of diffusible tracer from an organ is termed "washout". A concentration-versus-time graph can be constructed and a disappearance-rate constant obtained from the graph. Assuming that the rate of disappearance is proportional to blood flow, flow can be calculated if the volume of distribution of the tracer is known. Tracers used in bone-flow washout studies are iodoantipyrine I 125 [22], argon 41 (^{41}Ar) [23, 24], xenon 133 (^{133}Xe) [25, 26], and hydrogen [27–31]. Accuracy and precision of flow calculations are influenced by heterogeneity of flow created by surgical intervention, by recirculation of the tracer, and by binding of the tracer within the marrow. Recently Kiaer et al. reported that a comparison of freon and argon washout measurement of bone blood flow correlated significantly with microsphere measurement [32]. With both techniques, measured perfusion to bone was reduced by 80% following arterial occlusion whereas a lesser and inconsistent reduction was recorded with venous occlusion.

Clearance differs from washout in that the rate of disappearance of a radioisotope from the blood, not the organ of interest, is measured. If the element injected is selectively accumulated by the tissue of interest, then the rate of disappearance from the blood can be related to organ blood flow. In dogs, the clearance of strontium 85 (^{85}Sr), an analogue for calcium, has been shown not to be significantly different than the clearance of calcium 47 (^{47}Ca) [33]. Thus, ^{85}Sr clearance has been utilized to estimate blood flow to bone [34–37]. Flow calculation requires assumption that the tissue of interest is homogenous, that the equilibration between blood and tissue is immediate, and that clearance of isotope is affected only by

flow. Unfortunately, extraction of ^{85}Sr is only about 43% and is flow dependent. Extraction of the isotope is less at high flows than at low flows [38]. The clearance of flourine 18 (^{18}F) was also found to be flow dependent and removal of unbound tracer was not complete during a single passage [39].

Scintigraphy has its greatest use as a non-invasive, non-destructive method to determine gross changes in vascularity to an organ. A relative measure of flow, compared to normal or to different regions, can be obtained. Accurate quantitative measurements of blood flow are not possible. Technetium 99 (^{99}Tc), bound to diphosphonate [15], hydroxymethylene diphosphonate [34, 40, 41], or sodium pertechnetate [42] is commonly utilized. A static phase scan of the clearance of radioisotope is obtained by single image analysis at some time, minutes to hours after injection of the radioisotope. This static scan may be used as an indication of relative vascularity, but not as a direct measure of flow. At flow rates 50% greater than normal, there is a non-linear relationship between uptake and flow [38]. The normal rate of diffusion of tracer from blood to extracellular fluid and then to bone is such that an increase in blood flow is without marked effect on bone uptake. A dynamic scan to some extent overcomes this diffusion limitation. This scan is obtained by transposing a single static scan onto each of multiple sequential scans. The resultant individual sequential scan counts are then plotted versus time to obtain an uptake curve, which can provide a semi-quantitative measure of bone blood flow. Nutton et al. noted that uptake of ^{99}Tc may be increased in woven bone [41]. Using microautoradiographic techniques, Einhorn et al. reported technetium methylene diphosphonate T 99 to be clearly localized along mineralization fronts [43]. The isotope was occasionally found in the substance of osteoid but never within the osteoblasts, osteocytes, or osteoclasts. Osteocytic lacunae, but not Howship lacunae, occasionally had the isotope at their borders.

The radioactive tracer microsphere method, first described by Prinzmetal et al. in 1947 [44] has become one of the most widely accepted and utilized methods to evaluate blood flow to bones since Kane and Grim [45] and Lunde and Michelsen [46] first applied it. Simplified, the technique involves injection of uniform-diameter radio-labeled beads into the systemic circulation. The organ under study is harvested, and the beads that have become entrapped in vessels of small diameter within the organ are counted. Flow to the organ can then be calculated by comparison to counts and flow within a known reference organ. Maki et al. reported on a method of selective local injection of microspheres with good correlation of measured flows compared to standard systemic injection [47]. This technique may be worth consideration when systemic injection of microspheres results in insufficient numbers of microspheres being deposited in the study tissue. Microspheres in use today are made of styrenedivinylbenzene resin and are labeled as one of the following: scandium 46 (^{46}Sc), chromium 51 (^{51}Cr), cobalt 57 (^{57}Co), ^{85}Sr, niobium 95 (^{95}Nb), ruthenium 103 (^{103}Ru), stannum 113 (^{113}Sn), ^{125}I, or cerium 141 (^{141}Ce), although other labels could also be used. Microspheres are not metabolized by the body; thus sequential flow measurements, hours to days apart, within a bone are possible.

The size of microsphere utilized must be chosen with consideration of the vasculature of the organ under study. The microspheres should be large enough to be trapped in capillaries and not be phagocytized, yet small enough to not block larger vessels. For calculated flow rates to be accurate, there should be no bypass or non-entrapment of microspheres. Non-entrapment of microspheres in an organ can be measured by counting the number of spheres present in the venous return from that organ, or by counting the number of microspheres trapped from the venous circulation by the lungs. Microspheres 15 µm in diameter are considered to be the most suitable for study of blood flow to bones. Microspheres 9 µm in diameter are able to pass through the vasculature of bones and result in an underestimate of flow [48]. However, 11 µm microspheres were found to yield flows similar to 15 µm microspheres [49]. Niv et al. found similar flows in dogs, using simultaneous hydrogen washout and microspheres [27]. Non-entrapment, for the whole body, of heart-injected 15 µm microspheres in dogs, has been found to be less than 5% [50]. When injected into the tibial nutrient artery, 14% of the administered number were found in the femoral vein and 0.5% in the lungs [50]. However, if the percentage of cardiac output delivered to the skeleton is estimated at 7.7%, then marked non-entrapment could occur without noticeable lung microsphere count [51].

Non-entrapment may also be effected by, and increase with, periods of ischemia [52]. In a study directed at evaluating the potential release of tumor cells from a biopsy site, Robertson et al. found that 15 µm microspheres moved rapidly from a surgically deposited femoral site to the lungs, but not to regional lymph nodes [53].

Accuracy of flow estimation is dependent on the mixing, injection, distribution, and number of microspheres entrapped within the collected sample. Buckberg et al. determined that a minimum of 384 microspheres within a soft-tissue sample was necessary to obtain a 10% error at a 95% confidence level [54]. Li et al. found that, with their technique, flow estimates in bones with either high or low microsphere counts were not significantly different, with a percentage error of near 5% [55]. They suggested a minimum count of 250. To obtain sufficient numbers of microspheres in a bone sample, either a large number of microspheres needs to be injected or a large sample of bone needs to be collected. Sample size may be limited by study design, thus making injection numbers important. The number of microspheres injected varies in reported studies from 9×10^4 spheres/kg body weight of study animal to 2×10^7. A dose of 3×10^6 spheres/kg is common. Li et al. suggested that a dose of 5×10^5 spheres/kg body weight of study animal is sufficient [55]. Measurement error was found to be less than 10% using this lower dose and after normalizing the results [56]. Electrocardiographic and respiratory rate changes, with several deaths, were reported with injection of greater than 3×10^6 microspheres/kg [8]. It has been suggested that microvascular skimming may cause uneven distribution of microspheres in bone and that considerable arteriovenous shunting may occur [57]. Both these conditions could affect accuracy of measured flow values. Serial estimates of bone blood flow can also be affected by anesthesia, suggesting the need to normalize results [56].

It has been proposed that desmethylimipramine (DMI), a noradrenaline antagonist, could function as a "molecular microsphere" and in theory provide potential advantages over conventional microspheres in the measurement of blood flow in bone. McCarthy reported that, in studies conducted on rabbits, data indicates that either DMI is not completely extracted during a single passage in some tissues or that there is some release of extracted DMI over time [58]. He found that DMI estimated greater blood flow to cortical bone than the microsphere method.

Recently, colored microspheres have been successfully utilized to assess blood flow to injured knee ligaments in rabbits [59]. Colored microspheres are markedly less expensive than radio-labeled spheres; there is no hazard to laboratory personnel and no radioactive waste to dispose of. Flow rates can be determined by spectrophotometric analysis of hydrolyzed samples compared to a reference tissue. Flow distribution can also be determined by microscopic identification of microspheres in histologic samples using either bright-field or fluorescent light.

Another method to determine blood flow in bone is laser Doppler flowmetry (LDF). A hand-held laser probe records the Doppler shift in reflected light caused by movement of blood cells within an illuminated hemispheric $0.27-7.0$ mm^3-volume of tissue. Blood cell flux is measured and recorded as volts. Although the signal can be correlated to flow, it cannot be directly converted to units of flow within a tissue. Measurement and recording are effected by probe motion, probe positioning, and hemorrhage. Only a very small volume of tissue is measured. The maximum depth at which the laser Doppler probe can evaluate flow was found to be approximately 2.9 mm in cortical bone, 3.5 mm in bone covered by 1 mm cartilage, and 3.5 mm in trabecular bone [60, 61].

Like scintigraphy, LDF seems to have its greatest potential use as a qualitative comparative measure of relative blood flow. In the mandible, simultaneous ^{133}Xe washout and laser Doppler recordings showed virtually no correlation [25]. In a study in rabbits, correlation between LDF recordings and microsphere measurement for femoral-head blood flow approached, but did not achieve, statistical significance [62]. A later study in sheep found a low correlation for all data between laser Doppler recordings and microspheres [63]. Lausten et al. reported similar results [61]. They reported a coefficient of variation of 0.15 for multiple measurements of the same site and added that, since LDF measurements are relative, data from individual animals cannot readily be pooled for analysis. They did find a good correlation between microsphere-measured and LDF-measured variations in altered flow states. Zero flow states (devascularized bone and post-euthanasia animals) register about 60 mV due to no-flow red blood cell fluxes and other physiologic factors [64]. LDF was used to identify postischemia hyperemia in an in vivo porcine model [65]. Blood flow was recorded and changes charted only in millivolts as measured directly from the flowmeter. Schemitsch et al. reported on the development of an implantable fiber LDF system that could, potentially, provide long-term assessment of bone microcirculation [66].

In a preliminary study, the laser speckle method, a non-contact method for evaluation of 2-D flow, has been used to measure subchondral bone blood flow through articular cartilage and was found to correlate with paired hydrogen-washout measurements [67]. This may prove to be a superior alternative to LDF.

Bone blood flow changes have also been assessed using magnetic resonance imaging (MRI) [68, 69]. MRI was capable of detecting decreases in bone blood flow, but was not found to be able to quantify the magnitude of change [69]. An increase in both T_1 and T_2 MR signal intensity was seen in avascular non-united, canine femoral-head osteotomies, contrasting sharply with a decreased MR signal in healing revascularized femoral heads [68].

Lastly, bone-marrow blood flow has been assessed using positron emission tomography (PET) [70]. Although the study focused on assessing bone-marrow cellularity in patients with hematological disorders, this report may herald future studies on bone blood flow. No relationship between bone-marrow cellularity and bone-marrow blood flow was found. Kimori et al. found PET-measured vascular-bed volume of human-volunteer, whole femoral heads ranged from 1.5–4.5 mL/100g [71]. They found regional differences in vascular bed volume, which was usually lower in the upper regions. Kubo et al. found femoral-head vascular-bed volume ranged from 1.67–2.54 mL/100g in their human volunteers [72]. Femoral-head blood flow was estimated at 2.21–6.68 mL/min/100g.

1.3.3 Blood gases

Kiaer et al. measured "intraosseous" blood gases of bone through cannulas inserted into the femoral condyles of pigs and found significant correlation between intraosseous blood samples and on-line spectrometer measurement of oxygen and carbon dioxide [73]. Arterial occlusion resulted in severe hypoxia, whereas a more moderate change followed venous occlusion. Normal Po_2 using either technique measured ±35 mm Hg and Pco_2 measured ±50 mm Hg.

2   Blood supply of immature bone

Formation of primary and secondary centers of ossification in the developing skeleton is initiated by vascularization of the cartilage anlage. In the primary center, the invading vessels become the principal nutrient artery and vein to that bone. In the secondary centers, cartilage canals play an important role in bony development [74].

The major growth in length of long bones occurs at cartilaginous disks located near their ends. Increased length is achieved by transformation of this cartilage into metaphyseal bone (endochondral ossification). These growth plates, sandwiched between epiphyseal and metaphyseal bone, have a well-organized polar morphology, characterized by a columnar arrangement of chondrocytes. The histologic appearance represents a still image of the dynamic process that leads to elongation of the bone. There are two major differences between the vasculature of mature and immature bones. Vessels do not traverse the actively growing physeal plate; thus the epiphyses and the metaphyses of growing long bones have separate blood supplies. Also, the osteogenic layer of the periosteum is actively depositing sequential osseous lamellae, which requires an extensive vascular supply not necessary in the mature individual.

A vascular circle, the epiphyseal-metaphyseal arcade, covers the end of the growing long bone. Vasculature to the physis consists of two afferent supplies, with physiologically distinct functions (**Fig. 2-2**). Only a few large arterioles penetrate to supply the epiphysis. They usually originate as branches, which approach the epiphysis in localized areas at joint-capsule attachments (**Fig. 2-3**). At the rim of the physeal plate, an arborization of finely branching and anastomosing vessels perforates the epiphysis. These are in addition to the numerous vessels that arise to supply the joint capsule itself. Numerous capillaries then sprout toward the reserve zone of cartilage, and end in bulbous terminal sacculations (**Fig. 2-4**). This arcade alone is adequate blood supply for approximately 97% of longitudinal growth [75]. In the femoral head, it was once thought that vasculature to the epiphysis was also supplied by the ligamentum teres. This was shown not to be true in the dog (**Fig. 2-5**) [76]. In the femoral condyles, the posterior vessels have been found to be the major vascular supply [77]. These posterior vessels were sufficient to supply the entire epiphysis if all other soft-tissue structures were excised, whereas the medial and lateral vessels individually provided an inadequate supply. Destruction of the posterior vessels was not found to produce any significant area of ischemia as long as both medial and lateral supply was intact. Blood supply to the greater trochanter (a traction apophysis) remains from extraosseous vessels arising in the gluteals even after fusion with the proximal femur at maturity. Greater trochanter osteotomy, gluteal damage, careless dissection, or excessive tension can seriously jeopardize postfixation healing [78].

An exception to the normal picture of physeal vasculature worth noting is recognized in the fetus, and in some young postpartum animals: Firth and Poulos identified many large vessels crossing all parts of the growth plate in foals prior to 44 days of age [79, 80]. With increasing age, fewer vessels were seen. Over 70 days of age, crossing vessels were seen only at the periphery. Short blunted vessels entered, but did not cross, some physes up to 120 days of age. Similar vessels have been seen in calves [81] and in pigs [82]. Firth and Poulos thought these vessels might play an important role in metaphyseal blood supply. More likely, their presence is linked to remnants of cartilage canals or to overgrowth of vascularization to the forming secondary ossification center.

In the fetus, the metaphyseal side of the growth plate is supplied by vessels originating from the principal nutrient artery. During development, arteries perforate the growing bone in the region of the metaphysis and become increasingly prominent. These arteries are larger than those of the epiphysis. They perforate at numerous sites through foramina encircling the metaphysis near the growth plate. Branches of the metaphyseal and nutrient vessels anastomose to form innumerable small arterioles that course perpendicularly toward the physis. Here, it has traditionally been thought, they make a "hair-pin bend" and retreat back upon themselves, forming capillary loops. Plastic corrosion casts [20] and the author's recent stereoscopic microangiograms, suggest that the terminal metaphyseal vessels, at the level of the last hyper-

trophic chondrocyte, are saccular projections arising from an anastomosing series of singular capillary sprouts (**Fig. 2-6**), not capillary loops. A similar situation is found in the endplates of vertebral bodies for nutrition of the intervertebral disk [83]. Venous return is by way of venous sinuses. This microvascular organization would suggest that low flow and/or pooling are possible and could be instrumental in the genesis of growth deformities and hematogenous osteomyelitis.

During the period of bone growth, the osteogenic layer of the periosteum provides an increase in girth by appositional

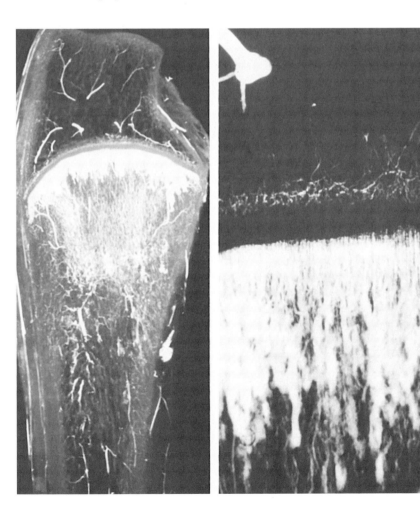

Fig. 2-2: Normal immature canine radius. Photomicroangiograph (×5) of distal epiphysis, metaphysis, and adjacent diaphysis, showing the overall afferent vascularization. The only vascular connections between metaphysis and epiphysis are along the periosteum [119].

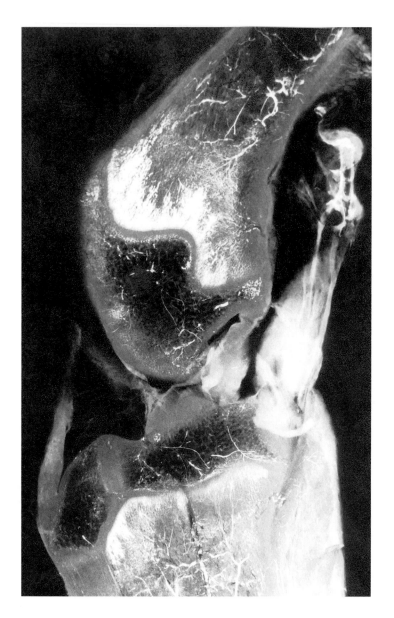

Fig. 2-3: Photomicroangiograph (×2.5) from the knee of a 6-month-old dog, with sagittal view of femur above and tibia below. Vasculature within the epiphyses of both distal femur and proximal tibia can be seen to originate from vessels entering at the posterior joint-capsule attachment.

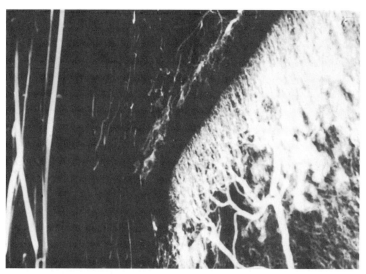

Fig. 2-4: Enlargement (×20) of Fig. 2-2 at the junction of growth plate and periosteum. The periosteal vessels are at the far-left side of the photomicroangiograph [119].

growth. An abundant blood supply can be demonstrated (Fig. 2-7). Many arteries run longitudinally over the periosteal surface with innumerable smaller radiating vessels perforating the newly formed bone. Upon cessation of growth, this vascularity atrophies to the minimal vestiges seen in the mature bone.

In 10-week-old and 20-week-old piglets, Nakano et al. found that microsphere-measured mean flows to femoral and tibial cancellous bone were respectively 17.6 and 21.3 mL/min/100gm, compared to 10.9 and 7.5 mL/min/100gm for cortical bone [84]. In epiphyseal cancellous bone, flow was significantly greater in the 2-mm surface layer than in the remaining bone. No significant age effect on the rate of flow to cancellous bone was found; however, the two sample periods were both within a phase of marked longitudinal growth in swine. Flow levels to articular cartilage decreased from the 10-week-old to the

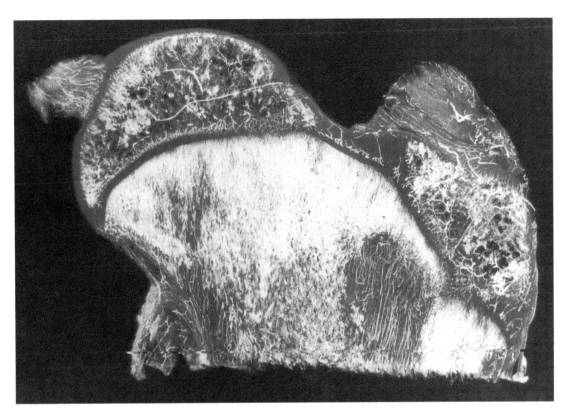

Fig. 2-5: Photomicroangiograph (×6) from the proximal femur of a 5-month-old dog. A large artery can be seen entering the epiphysis at the joint-capsule attachment at the right. Note that no vessels within the ligamentum teres enter the capitus.

20-week-old piglets and correlated with a decrease in histologic vascularity, chondrocyte density, and cartilage thickness. Morris and Kelly, using microspheres in mature and immature dogs, concluded that a greater proportion of cardiac output reaches the bone with an open physis [51]. They found, however, that proportionately more blood went to the cortical midshaft region and attributed this to rapid periosteal appositional growth. The age of the dogs used by Morris and Kelly was not stated. It is therefore possible that the data from piglets is representative of flows during a phase of rapid longitudinal growth, whereas the data from the dogs represents flows at a later age in which longitudinal growth has slowed markedly, yet bone diameter is still increasing. In immature rats, Kirkeby and Berg-Larsen found highest blood flow rates in the ilium and metaphyses, with lower flows in the diaphyses and epiphyses [85]. Epiphyseal blood flow was half the measured flow in the metaphyses. The sequential change in microsphere-measured bone flow from the neonate to the mature has been observed in several bones of the dog [86].

Thus, immature bones have a unique and extensive vasculature associated with active growth. Blood flow is greater than in mature bones and greatest to areas of endochondral ossification and appositional growth. Because of the number of active vessels, the multiple sites of entrance into the bone, and the high blood flow, healing is usually rapid. Clinically, the delicate supply to the epiphysis requires special surgical care and the juxtaepiphyseal circulation may be of anatomical significance in growth deformities and infection.

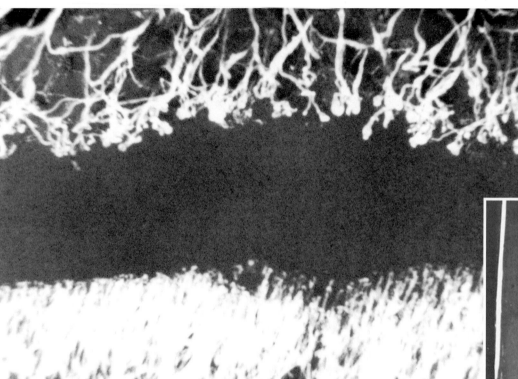

Fig. 2-6: Enlarged photomicro-angiograph (×50) from the capital physis of a 22-week-old puppy. *Above:* epiphyseal arterioles project toward the proliferating chondrocytes, terminating in globular capillary masses. *Below:* innumerable saccular projections, originating from terminal metaphyseal vessels, invade the zone of hypertrophic chondrocytes.

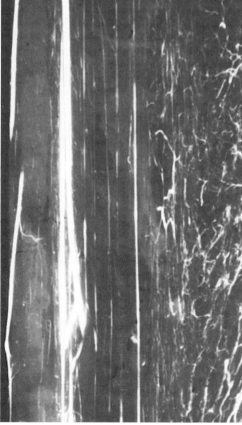

Fig. 2-7: Normal longitudinal periosteal arterioles of the immature canine radius (×20) [119].

3 Blood supply of irregular and flat bones

Blood supply to irregular and flat bones has generally been poorly studied. This is partially due to the ease with which fractures heal in these bones.

Bones of the tarsus and carpus are structurally similar to the epiphyseal ends of long bones. Each consists of a small mass of cancellous bone covered with articular cartilage, and limited areas of thin compact bone at regions of ligamentous attachments. Vessels usually enter these bones at multiple sites rather than at a major nutrient foramen, with nutrient veins being more numerous than arteries. Revascularization following trauma can proceed from several directions, thus allowing for rapid healing. One exception to this is the radial carpal bone. In some, but not all cases, the nutrient vessels supplying this bone enter at foramina concentrated near the tubercle. Fracture may therefore lead to devascularization of the proximal pole and resultant delayed union or non-union.

Although many aspects of the blood supply to the flat bones of the skull are still disputed, it is agreed that the vascularity is diverse. Arteries pierce the inner surface of cranial bones at one or more nutrient foramina and enter the outer surface at innumerable fine foramina near the suture borders. Venous drainage accompanies the arteries through nutrient and juxtasutural foramina, as well as through diploic veins and capillaries leaving both the inner and outer surfaces. Venous communication exists between meningeal, cranial, and pericranial vessels. The success of osteoplastic flaps, employed in brain surgery, further demonstrates the abundance of blood supply to cranial bones by showing that either dural or pericranial vasculature alone is sufficient to sustain the bone.

Fractures of the mandible are of particular importance to the veterinary orthopedic surgeon. Vascular compromise following repair is implicated in bone resorption, tooth loss, osteomyelitis, and non-union. A branch of the maxillary artery enters each mandible caudally at the mandibular foramen. This artery, the inferior alveolar artery, runs the length of the mandible and exits at the rostral mental foramina. Smaller arterioles radiate from this central artery to supply all of the cortical bone [87]. These arterioles traverse the mandibular marrow space in radial fashion, enter the cortex perpendicular to the endosteal surface, arborize within the cortical bone, and are drained at the periosteal surface. Dental, interdental, and interradicular branches of the inferior alveolar artery supply the teeth, periodontal ligament, and alveolar bone (**Fig. 2-8**). Multiple arteries were seen to enter the apical foramen of some teeth (**Fig. 2-9**). No periosteal contribution to normal cortical blood supply was seen. Near the symphysis, both medullary and periosteal arteries were seen to penetrate the mandible, thus giving a microangiographic picture similar to that of the metaphysis of a long bone. No vessels were seen to cross the fibrous syndesmosis. Blood flow within the mandible, under normal conditions, appeared to be centrifugal. Roush and Wilson [88] found that, following midbody osteotomy, extra-

osseous vasculature was seen to augment normal circulation very similar to that seen in long-bone healing (see **Section 6.2**). Intraosseous anastomosis of blood supply across the syndesmosis was not seen, even under conditions of vascular compromise to one mandible.

A large nutrient artery pierces the scapula and the ilium. Smaller foramina are found near the glenoid, the coracoid and spine of the scapula, and the acetabulum and iliac crest. In addition, these flat bones have extensive muscle attachments with additional extraosseous blood supply at these sites.

Although the ribs would seem anatomically similar to long bones, their blood supply is more extensive, resembling that of the ilium and scapula. Blood vessels enter at a principal nutrient foramen and at similar foramina on the head, neck, and tubercle. In addition, capillaries traverse the entire cortex, providing venous drainage from the hematopoietic marrow vasculature.

The blood supply to each vertebra is derived from the extensive vascular complex supplying the whole vertebral column. Many branches from large peripheral arteries ensure afferent blood supply, while a venous network provides drainage. Bidirectional flow of venous blood is possible due to the lack of venule valves. Although adequate blood supply to individual vertebrae appears ensured, damage to a single vertebra may adversely affect the blood supply to adjacent vertebrae.

A vertebra can be visualized as a long bone (the body) connected to a flat bone (the neural arch). Blood supply to the body consists of a principal nutrient artery and vein entering the midbody, and an epiphyseal-metaphyseal supply entering the cranial and caudal ends at numerous sites. The blood supply to the neural arch is extensive. There is a single nutrient artery originating from the spinal artery, and many smaller vessels enter through numerous small foramina scattered over the surface. The vasculature to the dorsal spinous process arises from a single major arteriole, which branches off arteries of the neural arch. This principal artery ascends the spinous process, arborizes into many smaller arterioles, and supplies the entirety of the spinous process (**Fig. 2-10**). There is little contribution to normal blood supply from muscles attaching to the spinous process. Rischen et al. have shown that blockage of flow at the surface of the spinous process by a bone plate did not result in disruption of blood supply or in devitalization of the underlying bone [89]. Using scanning electron microscopy, Oki et al. identified end-arteriole arborization and microvascular loops located at the vertebral endplates which, they suggested, play a major role in the nutrition of the intervertebral disks [83].

Fig. 2-8: Photomicroangiograph (×14) of a longitudinal section from the mandible of a mature dog. Three teeth are seen in transverse section with vascular roots and periodontal attachments. Interradicular and interdental vessels can be seen near the fourth premolar. The radial direction of blood supply to the mandibular cortex is evident.

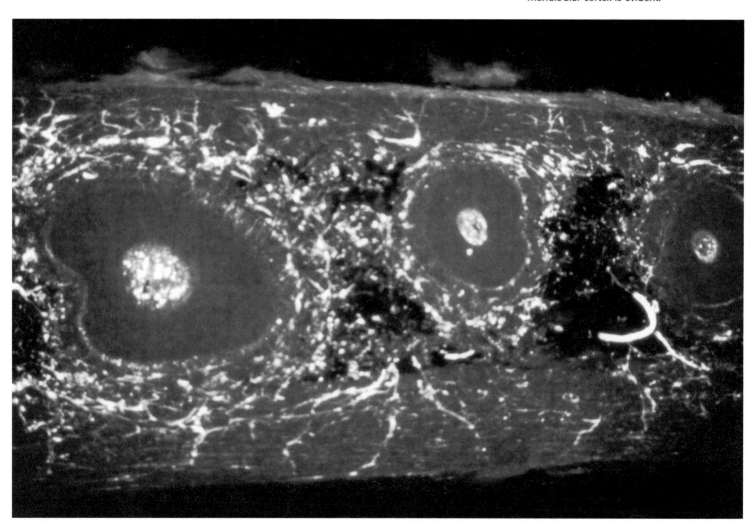

In an investigation looking at microsphere distribution to the skeleton, Tothill and MacPherson looked at total blood flow to several membranous bones [51]. A dimensionless "blood-flow index" was calculated to show variation of flows between specific bones. In dogs, the ribs, sternum, pelvis, spine, and scapulae had flow indices markedly greater than the long bones.

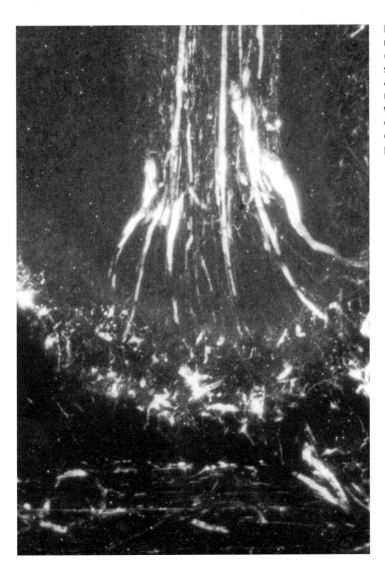

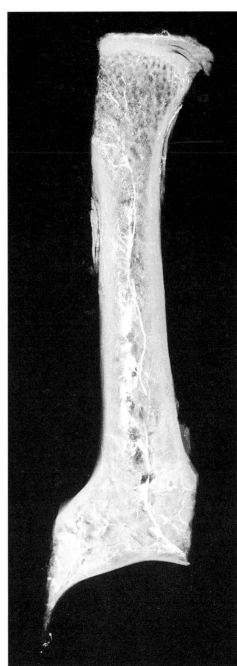

Fig. 2-9: Photo-microangiograph (×33) of a sagittal section showing the apical foramen of a mature canine molar with numerous dental arterioles entering the tooth pulp [87].

Fig. 2-10: Transverse photomicroangiograph (×5) of a normal canine dorsal spinous process. Vasculature arises from a principal artery originating within the underlying dorsal lamina [89].

4 Blood supply of normal long bones

4.1 Direction of blood flow through cortex

Studies by Brookes and Harrison [90], MacNab [91, 92], MacAuley [93], Jackson and MacNab [94], Nelson et al. [95], Brookes [75, 96, 97], and Rhinelander [1] have substantiated that the direction of normal blood flow through the diaphyseal cortex of a long bone is centrifugal—from medulla to periosteum. The intravascular pressure is higher in the medulla than in the periosteal area, and this pressure gradient is the chief factor in maintaining the flow centrifugally [75]. Brookes believed that the intramedullary pressure was probably in the order of 60 mm Hg. Recently, Bauer and Walker measured the intramedullary pressure in a large number of normal dogs [98]. Measured pressures were markedly lower than stated by Brookes. Mean diaphyseal pressure for the femur, humerus, and tibia was approximately 26 mm Hg. Metaphyseal pressures were significantly lower, with a mean pressure of approximately 16 mm Hg for the three bones. Intramedullary pressure variation in this study did not correlate with variations in blood pressure.

Evidence of the centrifugal flow of blood through cortex can be seen when periosteum is elevated. In **Fig. 2-11a** periosteum has been elevated by sharp dissection in preparation for experimental osteotomy. The nutrient artery, situated more proximally, was avoided. Slow, scattered, punctate bleeding from the exposed periosteal surface 3 minutes later can be seen in **Fig. 2-11b**. Under pathological conditions the pressure in the

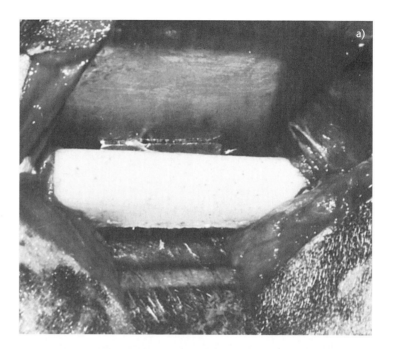

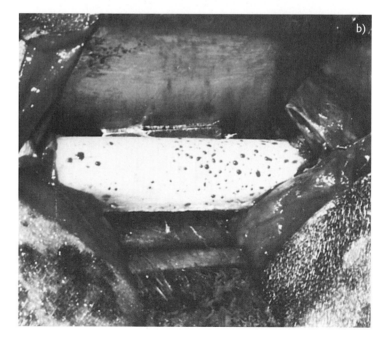

Fig. 2-11: Photographs of a normal mature canine femur after lateral exposure and complete circumferential stripping of the periosteum around the mid-diaphysis [119].
a) Immediately after wiping blood from the exposed cortical surface.
b) Venous blood effluent after 3 minutes.

medulla may be reduced, with the result that the flow of blood through the cortical vascular channels is reversed, becoming centripetal. This has been shown by Brookes in human occlusive vascular disease and osteoarthritis, and experimentally in the rabbit after ligation of the nutrient artery [75]. The reversal of flow is apparently through the normal vascular channels in the cortex. Results of experiments by Branemark on the rabbit fibula, using vital microscopy, suggest that venous blood from cortical bone returns normally to the medullary cavity [99]. However, in these experiments, there was nowhere else for the observed blood cells to go because all cortical bone, except for a paper-thin layer at the endosteal surface, had been ground away in the experimental preparation. This observation represents a pathological reversal of the normal direction of blood flow in cortex.

4.2   Vascular systems

The blood vessels constituting the normal circulation of a long bone may be referred to according to their anatomical location or physiologic function. The three functional vascular entities are:

1) The afferents (arteries and arterioles)
2) The efferents (veins and venules)
3) The intermediate vascular system (capillary-sized vessels in rigid bony canals connecting the afferent and efferent systems) [1, 100].

4.2.1   Afferent vascular system

The afferent vascular system is of most frequent concern in orthopedics. Consistent with the theory of centrifugal cortical blood flow, afferent supply to a long bone is almost exclusively into the medullary cavity. The basic components of this medullary supply are: 1) the principal nutrient artery, and 2) the proximal and distal metaphyseal arteries. These two components anastomose freely with each other at each end of the medullary cavity. Metaphyseal vessels can be seen following selective injection of contrast material into the nutrient artery [75]. Tothill et al. have also shown the duality of flow, following systemic injection of microspheres with occlusion of the nutrient artery compared with selective injection of microspheres into the nutrient artery [101]. This redundant,

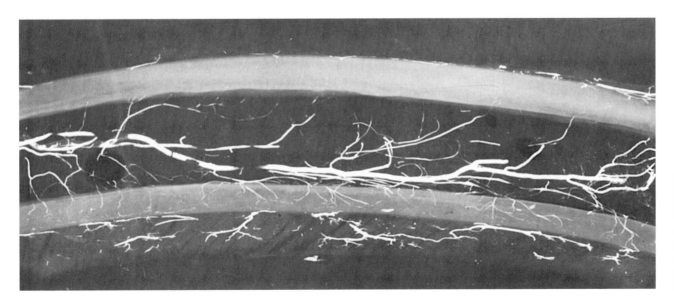

Fig. 2-12: Photomicro-angiograph (×3) of a normal mature canine radius with circulation in a resting state [196].

dual set of arteries forms an excellent medullary source of flow to the cortex.

The principal nutrient artery (which may be dual, as in the human femur) enters the cortex along a major fascial attachment. It traverses the cortex, without giving off branches, to enter the medullary cavity. Once in the medullary cavity it divides into ascending and descending medullary arteries. These divide further and enter all areas of the endosteal surface to provide the main blood supply to all of the diaphysis (**Fig. 2-12**). Shim et al. [102] and Tothill et al. [101] have estimated that 70% of flow to the diaphysis and 30% of flow to the entire tibia is normally provided by this vessel.

The metaphyseal arteries are multiple and enter all sides of the proximal and distal metaphyses (**Fig. 2-13**). They emanate from the periarticular plexuses, which form the epiphyseal-metaphyseal arcade of immature bones. Their terminal branches directly supply metaphyseal bone and anastomose with terminal branches of ascending or descending medullary arteries at each end of the medullary cavity. Under resting conditions, this anastomosis is exclusively at the capillary level [75]. Normal contribution of metaphyseal arteries to medullary circulation is minimal. However, when the nutrient artery is injured or compromised, the metaphyseal arteries have the capacity to take over the medullary supply completely by hypertrophy of existing anastomoses and creation of new vascular channels. Tothill et al. found that acute occlusion of nutrient artery flow resulted in a 30% decrease in total tibial microsphere-measured flow but with measurable flows still within the diaphysis [101]. Together, the nutrient and metaphyseal arteries compose the medullary arterial supply, which is the major afferent supply to the entire diaphyseal cortex and to the marrow elements.

Marrow and cortex have parallel, separate circulations. The two systems are not in series. Each is supplied by separate terminal branches of the nutrient artery. It has been suggested that approximately 70% of nutrient artery flow is directed to the cortex, and 30% to the marrow [22]. In human volunteers [70] mean marrow flow to the posterior iliac crest, measured by PET, was 10 mL/min/100 cm³. Arterioles supplying the marrow are short and branch off the nutrient artery close to the endosteal surface. They quickly and profusely arborize and

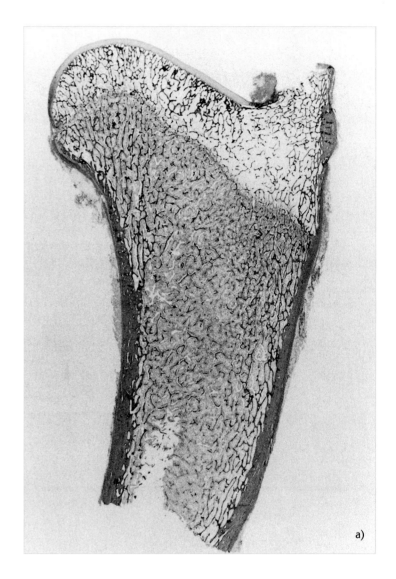

a)

Fig. 2-13: Longitudinal sections from a normal mature canine proximal humerus.
a) Photomicrograph (Picro-Sirius Red stain; ×5) showing the cancellous and cortical structure of the bone.
b) Corresponding photomicroangiograph (×5) illustrating resting metaphyseal and medullary arterial circulation. Anastomosis is by small vessels, which are faintly visible.

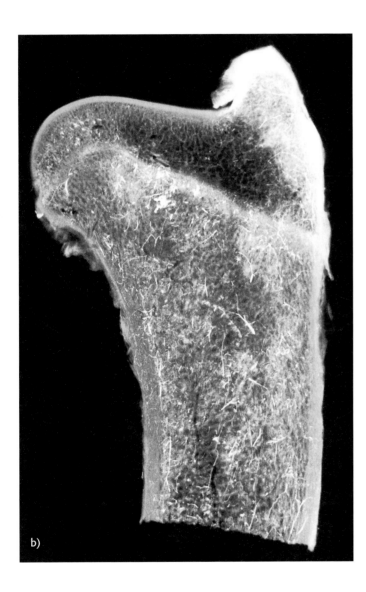

b)

enter marrow sinusoids. Arterioles supplying the cortex seldom branch. They radiate from the nutrient artery within the medullary cavity and enter the cortex singly or in bundles. Within the cortex these arterioles divide to supply the vessels of the haversian canals. Occasionally, arterioles traverse the cortex and anastomose with the periosteal network of vessels.

The periosteal vasculature is extensive in immature bones; it is only a vestige in mature bones. Arteries, when present, appear to be oriented in either a longitudinal or ring system [103]. Over most of the surface of mature long bones, the periosteum is only loosely attached beneath bellies of muscles. In these areas, blood vessels in the periosteum appear principally to be venules and capillaries located within the fibrous layer of the periosteum [103]. Cooper and Cawley found that, in the canine tibia, blood supply to loosely attached periosteum originated from locations distinct from the muscular vascularization [104]. Arterioles entering bone are found only at fascial attachments and at the origins of muscles (**Fig. 2-14**). In these areas there is a free anastomosis between the vessels of the muscle and those of the periosteum [103, 105]. These attachments afford the necessary protection to arteries and arterioles entering the bone. An artery, traversing a muscle belly, would be torn when contraction moved the muscle along the bony surface. Surface distribution of periosteal arterioles is very different from bone to bone because of the marked variations in fascial attachments. Along the femur, they enter only at the fascia aspera (**Fig. 2-15**); in the tibia, all across the posterior cortex. Periosteal vessels, entering the cortex directly beneath these attachments, provide a limited blood supply to the outer cortical layers, which are estimated to be the external 1/4 to 1/3 of the cortical thickness. Terminal branches anastomose in the cortex with terminal branches of the medullary arterial system. The flow within is regulated by the pressure at their ends. Under normal conditions, medullary pressure probably restricts periosteal blood flow to the outer third of the cortex.

Periosteal-medullary anastomosis was found to be unable to replenish the medullary arterial supply when the latter was obliterated by a nail which completely filled the medullary cavity [1]. Using a segmental femoral osteotomy model in the dog, Wilson et al. found that periosteal vessels at the attachment were only able to supply the full thickness of the cortex directly under the attachment [106]. No radial supply to bone adjacent to the attachment was seen, nor was the supply sufficient to re-establish the medullary circulation (**Fig. 2-16**). Cortical bone remained viable only directly under the fascia aspera. The rest of the cortex was devoid of osteocytes.

CROSS-SECTION OF DIAPHYSIS OF A LONG-BONE

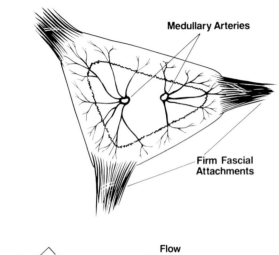

Medullary Arteries

Firm Fascial
Attachments

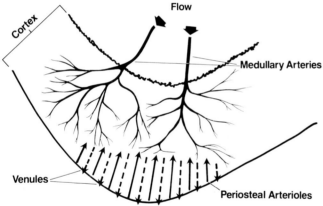

Cortex

Flow

Medullary Arteries

Venules

Periosteal Arterioles

ENLARGEMENT AT FIRM FASCIAL ATTACHMENTS

Fig. 2-14: Cross-sectional drawings of an idealized long bone. Branches of the medullary arteries supply the full-thickness cortex everywhere except at firm fascial attachments. The enlargement demonstrates periosteal arterioles *(solid arrows)* supplying the outer 1/3 of the cortex at these fascial attachments. All venous drainage *(broken arrows)* is to the periosteal surface [119].

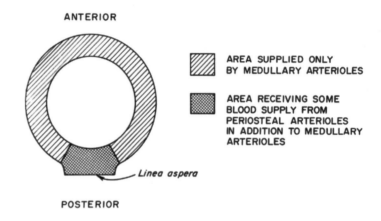

ANTERIOR

AREA SUPPLIED ONLY
BY MEDULLARY ARTERIOLES

AREA RECEIVING SOME
BLOOD SUPPLY FROM
PERIOSTEAL ARTERIOLES
IN ADDITION TO MEDULLARY
ARTERIOLES

Linea aspera

POSTERIOR

Fig. 2-15: Drawing of a cross-section of canine femoral shaft to demonstrate the experimentally observed difference in arterial supply to the medial-anterior-lateral, and to the posterior, portions of the cortex. The indicated limitations of these areas are only approximate, and at their junctions there is undoubtedly overlap and blending of the two types of afferent blood supply [1].

4.2.2 Intermediate vascular system

The intermediate vascular system is the link between the afferent and efferent vascular systems. It is the direct source of nutrition to, and of waste removal from, the cells of bone. In cancellous bone, capillaries are present in the marrow spaces between the trabeculae. In cortical bone, these vessels occupy the bony canals to which the names of Havers and Volkmann have been given (**Fig. 2-17**). Generally, a bony canal contains only one vessel. However, two or even three have been reported. I have observed canals in which one vessel was evidently active at the time of our perfusion and contained barium granules, whereas the other was filled with stagnant erythrocytes and was evidently inactive. The vessels within cortical bone are thin-walled structures, similar to the usual capillary; however, neither a basement membrane nor fenestrations have been demonstrated, but transcapillary clefts have been seen.

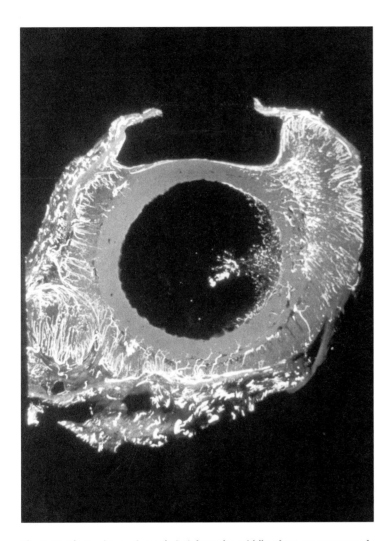

Fig. 2-16: Photomicroangiograph (x5) from the middle of a 4-cm segment of midfemoral canine diaphysis with fascia aspera, at the right, preserved. The cortex directly under the fascia aspera attachment has Micropaque-filled vessels. The remaining cortex is avascular. Position of the plate can be seen above.

Fig. 2-17: Diagram showing the basic structure of compact bone. Note the vascular channels and canaliculi. The indicated distribution of efferent vessels into marrow is incorrect [295].

The only route of molecular transport to bone, and sustenance to the osteocyte, is by way of minute channels called canaliculi. Cell processes of the osteocyte can be seen within the canaliculi [107]. Osteocytes appear to communicate with osteocytes in adjacent lacunae and with osteoblasts on the bone surface at specialized gap junctions between processes within these canaliculi [108–110]. There is evidence to suggest that canaliculi also contain a unique extravascular, extracellular tissue fluid [111, 112]. Water-soluble solutes appear to transfer across the vessels, and eventually to bone, by the process of passive free diffusion. The extravascular bone-tissue fluid space has been measured and found to be quite large. Serum albumin is present throughout this tissue-fluid region [113, 114]. Studies suggest there might be four fluid compart-

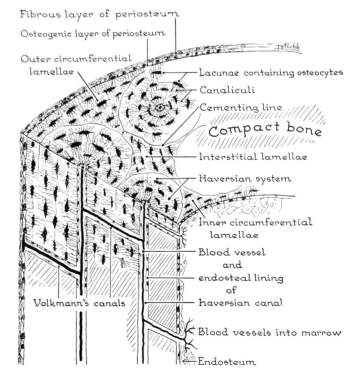

Fibrous layer of periosteum

Osteogenic layer of periosteum

Outer circumferential lamellae

Lacunae containing osteocytes

Canaliculi

Cementing line

Compact bone

Interstitial lamellae

Haversian system

Inner circumferential lamellae

Blood vessel and endosteal lining of haversian canal

Volkmann's canals

Blood vessels into marrow

Endosteum

ments in bone corresponding to a vascular space, the bone crystal, and two separate extravascular fluid spaces [115]. The physical characteristics of bone require a very specialized intermediate vascular system, which, by the very nature of bone, is very susceptible to alteration or damage.

4.2.3 Efferent vascular system

The efferent vascular system provides the drainage of blood from bone. It is abundant and free-flowing and it requires retrograde infusion for delineation of its component parts [75]. Drainage of all portions of the metaphysis is via the multiple metaphyseal veins that accompany the metaphyseal arteries (vena comitans). In the diaphysis, cortex and marrow are drained separately. Cortex supplied by medullary arteries is drained almost entirely by vessels at the periosteal surface of the bone. Cortex supplied by periosteal arterioles is also drained at the periosteal surface, specifically by accompanying periosteal veins. Medullary arterioles supplying the marrow cavity empty into a dense network of sinusoids, then into collecting sinusoids, and eventually into a large central medullary sinus. This system appears to contain no valves [18, 116]. Venous return to the general circulation is by emissary veins traversing cortex directly and by the nutrient vein. Venous return can also occur through venous vessels that travel in the same canals in which radially flowing cortical arterioles are located. These venous vessels join the periosteal network, as do the emissary veins. Leriche and Policard described the flow through cortex as being very sluggish [117]. This is in keeping with our observations on the escape of blood from the surface of the femur after periosteal stripping.

The system appears able to shunt venous effluent past externally applied tourniquets by bypassing the tourniquet through communicating medullary veins [118]. Surgical stripping of loosely attached periosteum causes no vascular problem. Free punctate bleeding results. Application of a tight plate or band to the periosteal surface has been incriminated to cause temporary suppression of active arterial supply to the underlying cortex [106, 119]. Since normal cortical flow is centrifugal, and cortical vessels appear to have limited branches, blocking the efflux would theoretically suppress the influx [119]. Kirby and Wilson placed metal and nylon bands of varying widths around the femoral diaphysis of dogs in an attempt to infer the extent of arborization of cortical vessels [120]. Regardless of size or type of band applied, there was no evidence of complete obstruction of cortical blood flow. Numerous examples were seen of vessels traversing the entire thickness of the cortex, even directly beneath the 10-mm-wide bands. Direct count of cortical osteocytes did not suggest impairment of viability related to placement of the bands. Apparently, when normal periosteal efflux is blocked, cortical venous flow is directed back to the endosteal surface and then to the periosteal surface, along adjacent venous channels.

4.3 Blood flow to bones

Brookes has suggested that approximately 25% of the cardiac output passes to the human skeleton at a mean flow of 20 mL/min/100g for mixed bone tissue [75]. Aalto and Slatis estimated the percentage of microsphere-measured cardiac output to the rabbit skeleton to be 6.7% [121]. Using microspheres and sampled portions of bone, Gross et al. estimated that 11% of the cardiac output was directed to the canine skeleton [48] whereas Morris and Kelly estimated 9.6% [50]. Also using microspheres, but with whole skeletal tracer counts, Tothill and MacPherson calculated the percentage of cardiac output to the total skeleton for the dog to be 7.5%, for the rabbit 4.2%, and for the rat 4.5% [51]. The same investigators found a wide range of flow per unit mass in different parts of the skeleton. Flows to flat bones were, in general, greater than flows to long bones, and flows in proximal long bones were greater than in distal long bones. They suggested that wide variation in individual bone flow rates made total body flow estimates based on sampled portions of bone inaccurate. However, in 1988 Wooton [122] found that boiling the carcass, as Tothill and MacPherson [51] did to obtain bones free of soft tissues for measurement, caused a substantial reduction in the microsphere content of the bone. Wooton suggested that actual total flow to the skeleton may be as much as 60% higher than calculated [122].

Blood flow to flat bones has been calculated to be greater than to other bones of the skeleton, and flow to proximal long bones greater than flow to distal bones [51]. Blood flow to the long bones also varies markedly. In the dog, the highest long-bone flow rates are to the humerus [51, 55]. This was found to be true for the rat, but not the rabbit [51]. The species differences may, in part, be due to the difference in percent of body weight carried by front or rear limbs. Flow to the ends of long bones is greater than flow to the center [85, 101, 123]. Flow to the proximal end of the femur was calculated to be greater than to the distal end [124] and, although not reported, there is probably greater flow to the proximal end of most long bones. In the mature dog, cancellous blood flow of long bones is three or four times higher than that of the cortex [55]. This is probably true in most mammalian species, including man.

Willans and McCarthy found a substantial heterogeneity of blood flow rate within diaphyseal cortex when they used both microspheres and ^{85}Sr clearance to measure blood flow in multiple transverse and quartered sections of canine tibia [125]. They concluded that the regional cortical blood flow rates were not attributable to corresponding changes in capillary density within the cortex and proposed that their results indicate a functional heterogeneity, possibly related to an underlying variation in the physiologic activity in bone.

In immature rats Kirkeby and Berg-Larsen found that ^{85}Sr incorporation rate distribution correlated with the regional distribution of microspheres [85]. Their data demonstrated a close association between blood flow and mineral turnover in the normal rat skeleton. They concluded that blood supply, at least in part, modulates mineral incorporation within bone tissues.

Unfortunately, because the sample of bone measured to obtain flow values and the units of measure used to report flows vary greatly between investigations, it is difficult to compare results and draw conclusions. For example, Morris and Kelly used pooled cortical samples to obtain a cortical bone mean blood flow of 2.5 mL/min/100g [50] whereas Jones et al. used cleaned femoral diaphysis to obtain a cortical bone mean blood flow of 4.67 mL/min/100g [124] and Li et al., using cortical bone pieces, obtained cortical bone mean blood flows to individual long bones ranging from 2.5 mL/min/100g in the

femur to 7.9 mL/min/100g in the humerus [55]. All three studies used microspheres in dogs to measure flow. As another example, Tothill and MacPherson calculated microsphere-measured total flow to the canine tibia to be 0.1% cardiac output [51], and Morris and Kelly found microsphere-measured mean flow to the canine tibia to be approximately 7.75 mL/min/100g [50]. In the ovine tibia, ^{41}Ar-clearance mean blood flow was reported to be 0.2 mL/min/100g [24], whereas microsphere-measured mean flow was reported to be approximately 29 mL/min/100g to the proximal part and 30 mL/min/100g to the diaphysis [63].

5   Physiologic effects on bone blood supply

Exercise, physical training, anesthesia, vasoactive drugs, nerve activity, hormones, and, of course, pathology and injury have all been suggested as having the capability of altering the blood supply to bone. As mentioned in **Section 4.1**, some factors can produce a reversal of the direction of flow through cortex. The effects of these stimuli, and the difference between resting and physiologically altered vasculature and blood flow, are important because in many ways they represent the potential that exists within a bone.

5.1   Effect of anesthesia

Anesthetic agents are known to have vasoactive effects on the body. Potentially, measurement of blood flow rates or representations of vasculature could be drastically altered when evaluated in anesthetized subjects. To avoid these possible effects, Morris and Kelly used conscious dogs in their microsphere measurement of bone blood flow [50]. Unfortunately, no anesthetized dogs were injected; thus quantitative effects were not evaluated. Niv et al. noted that repeated barbiturate injections modified recorded bone blood flow markedly [27]. Jones et al. did evaluate the effects of anesthesia on bone directly [124]. Although flow values were slightly lower in dogs during anesthesia, the flows were not significantly different to values obtained while the dogs were awake and standing immediately prior to anesthesia, or while awake and standing 40 days prior to the day of anesthesia. In contrast, Davis et al. found substantial reduction in microsphere-measured bone blood flow in rabbits during 1 hour of anesthesia using a combination of fentanyl, fluanisone, and midazolam [126]. Using serial microsphere injections McGrory et al. reported a significant fall in bone blood flow over time in the anesthetized dog [56]. The fall occurred in spite of maintenance of vital signs and irrespective of surgical intervention. Anesthetic regime was not reported.

Anesthesia, in and of itself, should not be expected to have a constant or singular effect on bone blood flow. The finding of nerve receptors in bone, the known effect of vasoactive drugs on bone blood flow, and the known variable effect of differing anesthetic regimes on systemic blood pressure and cardiac output would, however, suggest that effects on bone blood flow will vary with the anesthetic regime utilized. Fortunately, many anesthetic regimes exist which have minimal systemic circulatory effects. The recent finding that pressure is the most important factor in determining bone perfusion [73] would suggest that anesthetic regimes with minimal effects on systemic circulation could be expected to have minimal effects on bone perfusion. This hypothesis needs to be corroborated by a comparative study.

5.2 Effect of exercise or physical training

Tondevold and Bulow measured flow using microspheres in tibiae and femora of conscious dogs at rest and during exercise [127]. They found calculated flows in cortical bone to increase slightly, but not significantly, after 1 hour of physical exercise. After 2 hours, cortical flows had significantly increased to almost twice resting flows. This trend held true in cancellous areas except for the femoral neck. They found the hyperemia to be sustained at the 45-minute postexercise measurement.

Maximum cortical mean flow obtained was 2.5 mL/min/100g. After 15 weeks of physical training, Jurvelin et al. found ^{133}Xe measured flow to the femoral bone compartment, and to the marrow compartment, to have increased by approximately 54% [26]. They noted that the increased flow to the bones could be a reflection of either an increased cardiac output or a changed organ distribution. Their control mean flow rate was 11 mL/min/100g. The runner mean flow rate was 17 mL/min/100g. Williams et al. evaluated the effect of treadmill exercise on the microsphere-measured bone blood flow of exercise-trained dogs [128]. They found a decrease in vascular resistance and an increase in blood flow in weight-bearing bones but not in non-weight-bearing bones. The authors compared the exercise data with measured effects from the injection of norepinephrine, angiotensin II, and acetylcholine and suggested that hormonal or neuronal transmitters could account for the selective bone changes in resistance and blood flow. Intrinsic control mechanisms were not looked at, however, and could not be excluded. Jespersen et al. found microsphere-measured blood flow of the axial skeleton to be substantially greater than that of peripheral long bones in exercised minipigs [129]. Axial blood flows were evenly distributed along the vertebral column, and exercise was not found to precipitate ischemia in any of the bony regions studied.

In instrumented, externally-loaded rabbit tibiae McDonald and Pitt Ford reported that following the application of a static load to bone, LDF-measured bone blood flow decreased on the compressive aspect and increased on the tensile aspect [130]. They found a point-in-load above which increases in strain did not affect bone blood flow. Following prolonged periods of load, there seemed to be a reactive hyperemia. Dynamic loads did not appear to influence flow.

A stimulated vascular pattern is illustrated in **Fig. 2-18**. These are serial photomicroangiograms of the normal ulna of a dog which had received an undisplaced fracture of the opposite forelimb 3 weeks previously. The ulna depicted was itself uninjured. The enhanced circulation in this ulna had presumably been stimulated by the fracture of the contralateral extremity or by the increased function which this uninjured limb had to perform.

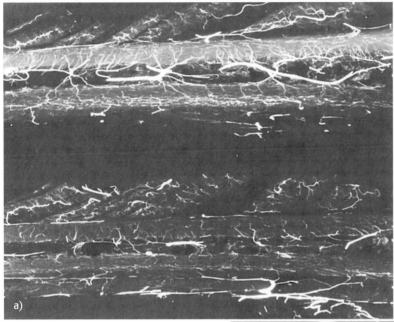

5.3 Effect of immobilization

In addition to measuring the effect of physical training on blood flow, Jurvelin et al. also measured the effect of immobilization [26]. They found no significant effect on femoral-bone hemodynamics following immobilization of the hind leg in a full-leg fiberglass cast for 11 weeks.

In a study to compare mobilization and immobilization on blood flow at a fracture site, Bitz et al. reported no increase in hydrogen washout-measured blood blow with early mobilization of the fractured limb [131]. They concluded that factors other than blood flow are probably responsible for the improved mechanical characteristics observed in their study, and seen in others. In rabbits, casting had no major effect on tibial microsphere-measured blood flow at either 1 or 2 weeks [132].

Fig. 2-18: Normal mature canine ulna with circulation physiologically stimulated by a fracture of the opposite forelimb [185].
a) Photomicroangiograph (×3) of two adjacent 1-mm diaphyseal slices. The major medullary artery curves from one slice to the next.
b) Enlargement (×12) of the upper microangiograph of (a). The full thickness of the superior cortex, beneath loosely attached strands of muscle, and the inner 2/3 of the inferior cortex are supplied by blood vessels from the medulla, while the outer 1/3 of the inferior cortex receives anastomosing arterioles from the firmly attached interosseous membrane.

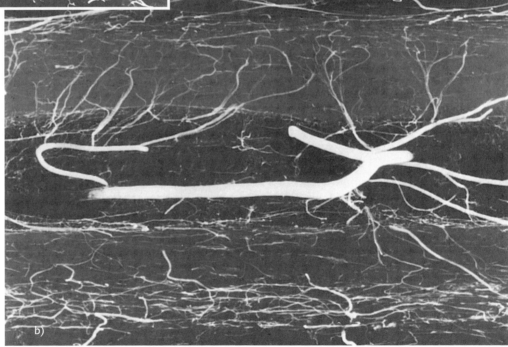

Dynamic loading one week following tibial osteotomy and external fixation in dogs was found to result in greater osteotomy osteoblastic activity and advanced callus remodeling.

5.4 Effect of steroids

A long-known side effect of steroid therapy is osteonecrosis of the femoral head. Kawai et al. found an increase in intraosseous pressure and a decrease in hydrogen washout-measured intraosseous bone flow of the proximal tibia in rabbits treated with steroids [133]. Fatty marrow was noted histologically at the measurement sites. The authors speculated that the vascular changes they observed could be due to aberration of fat metabolism induced by the treatment. In a study comparing osteoporosis induced by steroids and oophorectomy in rabbits, Yoshida et al. noted a decrease in diameter and an increase in number of barium-filled vessels in the steroid-induced-osteoporosis-study animals [134]. They speculated that accelerated skeletal metabolism and, in particular, lipid metabolism might be involved.

5.5 Effect of innervation and neurovascular drugs

Davis et al. found that microsphere-measured mean bone blood flow in the canine femur increased by 24% to 41% following sympathectomy [135]. Higher flow rates were noted in the tibia (37%–59%) and metatarsus (58%–67%). Flows returned to control within 2–6 weeks. They concluded that surgical sympathectomy exerts a significant, yet transient, effect on blood flow in bone and that sympathetic tone is progressively greater distally. Tothill et al. did not confirm this finding and instead noted a reduction in microsphere-measured flow in dogs [101]. They found that although tibial flow was reduced after sympathectomy, the reduction in flow was similar in both the denervated and opposite control side. Takahashi et al. performed cordotomies, hemicordotomies with rhizotomy, and sciatic neurotomies in rats and measured regional blood flow to the proximal tibial metaphyses using hydrogen washout and whole tibial blood flow using microspheres [136]. They found that regional tibial metaphyseal bone blood flows increased in the denervated tibia following cordotomy and hemicordotomy with rhizotomy, but did not change following sciatic neurotomy. Takahashi et al. concluded that the spinal nervous system contributes to the control of bone blood flow and concurred with Davis et al. that surgical transection causes a significant transient effect on blood flow in the denervated limb. Buma et al. used calcitonin-gene-related peptide antibodies to identify neural fibers in bone [137]. They found small, free-running neural fibers associated with the blood vessels that entered bone through Volkmann's canals. Insertion of an implant which destroyed endosteal blood supply caused concurrent denervation of the bone. Renewed innervation was found to accompany revascularization at 6 weeks after implantation. The concurrence of extensive neural sprouting with revascularization inevitability suggests a possible role of bone nerve fibers in regulation of angiogenesis, bone remodeling, or both.

Bjurholm et al., using immunofluorescent labeling, demonstrated the presence of both noradrenergic and cholinergic sympathetic neurons in the femur and tibia of rats [138]. Nutton et al. noted a marked increase in canine tibial mean blood flow with intra-arterial infusion of ATP and a marked decrease with norepinephrine, compared to a contralateral control [40]. When flows were compared to that of control animals, the decrease in flow with norepinephrine was still evident; however, the increase in flow with ATP was minimal. McCarthy et al. reported that ATP did not produce any direct effect on rat bone [139]. They also reported that both noradrenaline and PGE_2 produced a dose-related decrease of bone blood flow and a related increase in vascular resistance. No change in ^{85}Sr clearance was observed with noradrenaline; however, a significant decrease occurred with infusion of PGE_2. Brinker et al., using an in vivo canine model, found that the bone vascular bed appeared to have adrenergic and cholinergic receptors, which were sensitive to agonistic and antagonistic agents [140]. In harvested canine tibiae, perfusion studies also suggested an interosseous vascular response to alpha[1], alpha[2], and beta blockade [141–143]. Pan et al. found alpha[1] receptors most responsive and concluded that alpha[1]-blocking agents would therefore have the greatest intraosseous vasodilation effect [141]. Later, it was found that the effect of alpha receptors was additive-dependent and dose-dependent [144]. Ye et al. also found that calcium-entry antagonism did not appear to be as important as alpha-subtype blockade in bone vessels [144]. Increased, femoral metaphyseal trabecular mineral apposition rates and an increase in defect callus formation and bone union were identified in propranolol-treated rats at 12 weeks [145].

In an in vivo and in situ-perfused porcine model, Linblad et al. reported that neuropeptide Y was a potent vasoconstrictor of bone blood vessels with a molar efficiency in excess of norepinephrine [146]. Vasoactive intestinal peptide, substance P, and calcitonin-gene-related peptide were found to have a vasodilatory effect in porcine bone in vivo, whereas neuropeptide Y was found to act along with noradrenaline as sympathetic vasoconstrictors [147]. A possible, but unsubstantiated, role for neuropeptides in bone metabolism was suggested [147].

The gene that codes for the synthesis of calcitonin also codes for a peptide called calcitonin-gene-related peptide (CGRP). CGRP is a neuropeptide that elicits vasodilation and certain calcitonin-like effects on bone resorption. Nervous tissues containing CGRP have been identified in bone in areas of high osteogenic activity. Lindblad et al. reported a vasodilatory effect of CGRP in porcine bone, both alone and in interaction with sympathetic neurotransmitters [147, 148]. They speculated that CGRP might function in integrating bone-osteoclast activity and vascular function. Recently Grills et al. evaluated the effect of local application of nerve growth factors on the physical properties of repairing bone [149]. They found that constant treatment of a fracture site with 10 mg of nerve growth factor stimulated osteogenesis. They observed decreased size, increased Young modulus, and increased breaking strain of callus in treated animals. This would support the notion that innervation is an important factor in callus development. In addition to the positive neurotrophic effect, nerve growth factor may also have an effect on fracture vascularity by stimulating angiogenesis, similar to that seen with other neuropeptides.

5.6 Effect of biologic factors

The effect of certain hormones on the number and activity of the cells in bone, and on the mineral content of bone, is better known than the effect hormones may have on the blood flow and vasculature of bone. Parathyroid hormone (PTH) has long been known to have a hypotensive effect. This has been shown to be due to decreased peripheral resistance and increased flow in many soft-tissue organs. A decrease in microsphere-measured bone blood flow has been reported 15 minutes after PTH injection [150]. Flow was noted to return to control values within 240 minutes. The authors concluded that the observed effect was more likely due to systemic hypotension than to local factors.

Transforming growth factor beta, (TGF-β) has been shown to stimulate bone formation. Although changes seen were not marked, a study by Heckman et al. indicated a dose-dependent trend toward increases in mechanical strength and radiographically assessed healing of a defect in the canine radius with rhTGF-1 and a variation in effect dependent upon formulation of the TGF utilized [151]. Also, one study has reported that TGF-β absorbed onto the surface of implants coated with tricalcium phosphate enhanced the mechanical fixation and bone growth into the porous coating after 6 weeks [152]. Sumner et al. suggested that TGF-β acts by enhancing recruitment and proliferation of osteoprogenitor cells and by increasing the ability of committed osteoblasts to synthesize matrix [153]. A stimulation of vascular budding may also be likely since osteoprogenitor recruitment, differentiation into osteoblasts, and vascular ingrowth are linked.

Eppley et al. evaluated the effect of a local infusion of basic fibroblast growth factor (bFGF, a reported mitogen for chondrocytes, osteoblasts, and possibly undifferentiated mesenchymal cells) in autogenic bone-grafted defects in mandibles of rabbits [16]. They noted an increase in the number and depth of penetration of vessels into the grafted defects. Mineral deposition rate was not altered. Cancellous bone plugs impregnated with bFGF and implanted in rats were observed to produce increased bone ingrowth into the graft [154, 155]. Basic FGF appeared to induce neovascularization by promoting proliferation and differentiation of endothelial cells. The response seen is dose dependent and appears to effect amount of ingrowth and type of tissue formed [156–158]. Acidic fibroblast growth factor (aFGF) was found to increase fracture callus by stimulating production of cartilage tissue that had an altered collagen make-up and was mechanically weakened. No direct effect on blood flow was noted [159]. Studies with endochondral ossification models have identified a possible role for plasminogen activator during angiogenesis and vascular invasion [160]. Plasminogen activator is responsible for conversion of the zymogen-plasminogen to plasmin. Plasmin has been shown to activate procollagenase and prostromelysin in cultured fibroblasts; it has also been shown that neutral protease activity may be responsible for degradation of proteo-glycans during growth-plate vascular invasion [161, 162]. Neutral proteases also appear during fracture healing [163] in addition to alkaline phosphatase. Thus, plasminogen activator, plasmin, and proteases may all sequentially play a role in degradation of extracellular matrix macromolecules during endochondral ossification and bone remodeling.

Platelets may play a role in enhancing osteogenesis and angiogenesis by providing a source of insulin-like (IGF-I and IGF-II), platelet-derived (PDGF), and TGF-β growth factors upon degranulation at a site of injury or fracture [164]. Notte-baert et al. studied the effect of local administration of an omental angiogenic lipid fraction on bone healing in a rat model. The substance was found to have a potent angiogenic effect on bone [42]. In addition to positive effects on resultant healed bone stength related to presence of the factor, enhanced bone perfusion and increased vasculature were also identified.

Other substances have been found, or suggested, to be present in the immediate environment of healing fractures and osteotomies. In the future, some of these substances may be found, to some extent, to mediate their effect through their action on vascularity. One substance that has drawn considerable attention is BMP. Although not directly linked to bone vascularity, it has repeatedly been shown to be osteoinductive and to promote bone healing in certain circumstances. Bostrom et al. have recently demonstrated the presence of proteins 2 and 4 within the callus of healing fractures in adult rats [165].

5.7 Effect of ischemia and reperfusion

Kiaer et al. measured intraosseous pressure Po_2, and Pco_2 during periods of hypovolemia in the femoral condyles of rabbits [166]. The measurements revealed a linear relationship between intraosseous pressure and arterial pressure, indicating pressure to be the most important factor in determining bone perfusion. Bone blood flow was not preserved, but did not cease completely, during hypovolemia. The authors concluded that the regulatory mechanisms identified in bone do not appear to preserve bone blood flow during hypovolemic hypotension, nor do they appear to actively decrease bone blood flow, in concert with other systemic mechanisms, to improve central circulation during hypotensive crises.

Settergren et al. found that the responsiveness of bone vascular smooth muscle to norepinephrine remained after prolonged normothermic ischemia and that the time of responsiveness could be extended by mild hypothermia [167]. Davis and Wood reported that acidosis and alkalosis affects the responsiveness of bone blood vessels to norepinephrine and sympathetic nerve stimulation and concluded that H ion concentration may regulate the sensitivity of long-bone vascular resistance and blood flow [168, 169]. Davis et al. reported that alpha^2-mediated vasoconstriction usually sur-vived 96 hours of hypothermic ischemia, whereas the alpha^1-vasoconstriction was often attenuated after 48 hours of hypo-thermic ischemia [170]. It was suggested that circulation, through hypothermically stored free vascularized bone grafts, might be increased with perioperative use of adrenergic antagonists, such as phentolamine. Moran et al. confirmed an increase in bone blood flow with blockade of alpha-adrenergic receptors [171, 172]. They noted that alpha^1 receptors are post-synaptic and thus less important in vascularized (denervated) bone grafts. Alpha^2 blockade would potentially be more useful in vascularized grafts. Hypoxia was found to have no detectable effect on the vasoconstrictive action of norepinephrine or neuropeptide Y on the bone vascular bed [173]. Coessens et al. suggested that acidosis-induced relaxation of canine tibial nutrient artery was endothelium dependent and that the activation of endothelin-A receptors during acidosis was coupled to a release of an endothelium-derived relaxing factor (EDRF) [174].

Dysfunction following restoration of circulation after a period of ischemia, reperfusion injury, is thought to be caused by excessive production of free oxygen radicals (superoxide and hydroxyl ions, and hydrogen peroxide) during ischemia, which, when dispersed after circulation is restored, damage cell membranes. The endothelium of blood vessels synthesizes and secretes EDRF and a prostaglandin, both of which, under normal conditions, can decrease vascular resistance by vascular smooth muscle relaxation. Oxygen radicals are thought to damage endothelial cell membranes by a number of mechanisms, one of which is to block production of EDRF and prostaglandin, resulting in increased vascular resistance, decreased flow, and more free radical production. It has also been suggested that the superoxide anion may combine with EDRF becoming instrumental in the production of an endothelium-derived contracting factor (EDCF) [175].

In an in vivo vascularized bone allograft, Moran et al. found evidence to suggest that an EDCF, dependent on L-arginine, was produced during reperfusion after 24 hours preservation [176]. They suggested the possible role of superoxide radicals in mediating a reperfusion damage in vascularized bone grafts. Weiss et al. had reported that superoxide dismutase appeared to improve overall revascularized bone graft survival [177]. Davis and Wood found secretion of EDRF and prostaglandin from canine tibie after 48 hours of hypothermic ischemia [178, 179]. Vascular resistance and the sensitivity of intraosseous blood vessels to circulating norepinephrine were increased; however, pretreatment with allopurinol or oxypurinol did not ameliorate the hypertension. They could not confirm that xanthine-oxidase-mediated reperfusion injury was an important cause of ischemic-induced changes in intraosseous blood vessels. Acetylcholine attenuated the norepinephrine pressure response [179]. This attenuation was partially abolished by inhibition of prostaglandin synthesis and completely abolished by inhibition of EDRF synthesis [179]. Acetylcholine stimulates the release of EDRF, which results in an increase in blood flow. Using LDF, Swiontkowski and Senft found that release of 6–16 minute occlusions of the femoral artery resulted in a

characteristic "overshoot" increase in bone perfusion [65]. No mechanism or mediators were studied. Bone exhibited a typical hyperemic response to short-term ischemia and thus could be susceptible to reperfusion injury. To their surprise, Kregor et al. found that oxygen-free radical scavengers in fractures retarded or decreased the quality of healing [180]. They indirectly concluded that oxygen-free radicals might be influential in normal fracture healing.

5.8 Influence of electrical current

Studies on the effects of electrical current on osseous healing have focused primarily on bone formation in animal models and the clinical course of injuries in human and animal patients. Collins found that hydrogen washout-measured bone blood flow increased around stimulated electrodes implanted into the femoral medulla of cats [29]. The greatest effect was noted at 2 and 3 weeks following implantation. In canine rib osteotomies, Adams et al. found microsphere-measured blood flow to be significantly increased in electrically stimulated ribs at 2 weeks, and significantly increased in the osteotomy callus at 2 and 4 weeks [181]. Significantly increased mineral content at the osteotomy was found at 2 weeks, but not at 4 and 6 weeks. Nannmark et al. used an optical bone chamber to evaluate vascularity between two implanted electrodes [182]. They reported that blood flow rate did not change during 2.5 hours of electrical stimulation. Over a follow-up time of 11 weeks, they noted an increase in size and number of capillaries, concurrent with an increase in bone formation. Zichner et al. implanted electrodes 13 mm apart through drill holes in the diaphyses of the femora of dogs [183]. After 1 day of stimulation, there was considerable enhancement of the medullary circulation in the vicinity of the active electrodes, in comparison with the unstimulated control. After longer time periods, there was a progressive increase in size and number of vessels and an accompanying increase in new woven bone around the cathode (**Fig. 2-19**). Similar vascular changes and bone formation were not seen in the vicinity of the anode. Bone resorption around the anode was not noted either. It would appear that electrical current can stimulate vascular growth; the optimal conditions and mode of stimulation are, as yet, unsettled.

5.9 Thermal effects

Even when a saw blade or drill bit is sharp, and the kerf in bone is cooled by saline irrigation, thermal necrosis may develop when bone is cut using power-driven equipment [100]. The combination of speed of rotation and rate of feed affects the generation of heat within the bone being cut. Mismatch of speed and feed is more serious than the single effect of either. This is demonstrated in the canine radius 3 weeks after power-driven osteotomy (**Fig. 2-20**). The opposing cortical surfaces at the osteotomy appear glazed. A zone of necrosis, extending 0.8–1.5 mm in from the surface, can be identified by the presence of empty osteocyte lacunae. The osteotomy is being vascularized from the underlying medullary circulation and osteoclasts can be seen removing necrotic cortex. The problem is much less evident in the metaphysis. The thin and well-vascularized cortices are much more resistant to thermal necrosis.

Using scintigraphy in human adult volunteers, Ho et al. reported a slight but consistent decrease in the soft-tissue pool and bone phases as early as 5 minutes following icing [184]. Arterial phase image decreases occurred after 10 minutes and all three phases decreased progressively after up to 25 minutes

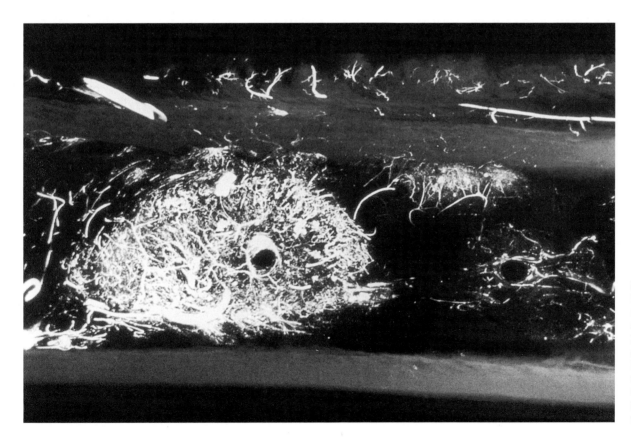

Fig. 2-19:
Photomicroangiograph (×5) of the femur at the site of electrodes after 3 weeks of electrical stimulation. Hypervascularity fills the medullary cavity at the cathode, while at the anode only a few perfused vessels can be seen [296].

post-icing. Thus, application of ice appears to temporally decrease blood flow to superficial, soft-tissue, and bony structures for at least 20–25 minutes.

5.10 Effect of pathology and trauma

A stimulated vascular pattern is illustrated in **Fig. 2-18**. The dog had a 3-week-old fracture of the opposite forelimb. The ulna depicted was itself uninjured [**185**]. This vasodilatory effect of trauma has been seen by others [**186, 187**]. Whereas Wray and Spencer noted an effect in the entire traumatized limb [**186**], Chang et al. observed an increase in microsphere-measured bone blood flow only to the distal ulna following a proximal-third ulnar osteotomy [**187**]. They suggested that this side effect might contribute to the improved union rates of pseudarthroses treated by the Ilizarov technique [**187**].

The specific effects of osteotomy, fracture, surgical intervention, and certain pathological conditions will be treated in subsequent chapters.

6 Blood supply of healing long bones

6.1 General responses to injury

In a discussion of research methodology and results, osteotomy is to be distinguished from fracture. Healing activities may vary between fracture and osteotomy in a given area of a long bone. In experimental studies, osteotomies are generally used because they can be better controlled and, therefore, standardized. Although differences can, and do, exist in healing between osteotomy and fracture, the fundamental processes of repair, and the attendant vascular reactions, are very similar.

The ability of the vasculature to efficiently and effectively vascularize an injury is directly influenced by motion at the site of the injury. A certain measure of fracture stabilization is required to promote the essential vascular responses. The degree of stabilization or motion profoundly effects the type and rate of healing. Variations in blood supply, within the

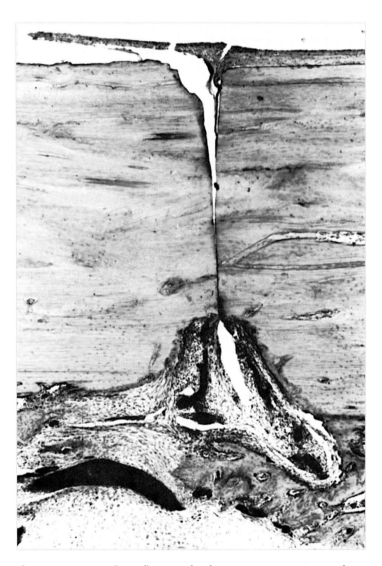

Fig. 2-20: Mature canine radius 3 weeks after transverse osteotomy and fixation with a 4-hole plate and screws: Histological section (H and E stain; ×58.5) showing thermal necrosis of the cortex on both sides of the osteotomy. The plate was above [1].

required total amount, also affect the type and rate of healing. Thus, the two essential factors in fracture healing are blood supply and stabilization. Each factor can affect, and is affected by, the other. Both are needed for bone healing to occur. This consideration is important when selecting appropriate treatment for a specific fracture.

6.2 Extraosseous blood supply

Following injury, the existing components of the normal vasculature become enhanced locally. In some injuries, and following certain methods of fracture repair, this may be the only vascular response seen. However, the ability of the normal vasculature within bone to respond to injury is very limited, and in most circumstances a supplementary blood supply, external to the bone, develops. Although frequently referred to as "periosteal" because of its origin outside the bone, this supplementary blood supply is neither a proliferation of periosteal arterioles nor is it derived from them. The source of this new blood supply is the soft tissues surrounding the bone. Vessels tend to orient perpendicular to the bone and can supply bone at any surface, not just at fascial attachments. It is preferably referred to as the "extraosseous blood supply" [100]. At 1 and 2 weeks after osteotomy, surgical alteration of vascularity, and cast stabilization in rabbits, Triffitt et al. concluded from microsphere measurements of blood flow to bone that early blood supply to healing bone is principally derived from the periosteum and extraosseous tissues [188]. In canine tibial segmental osteotomies, Richards et al. found that microsphere-measured blood flow was marked in the soft tissues of the operated limb at 1 and 3 months after surgery [189]. The extraosseous soft-tissue effect of fracture appeared extensive and prolonged. Schemitsch et al. found no difference in microsphere-measured blood flow to the anterior and posterior canine tibial diaphysis and concluded that clinically and experimentally observed variations in healing properties of the tibial diaphysis relate primarily to the vascularity of surrounding soft tissues, and not to intrinsic vascularity of the tibia [123]. Richards et al. noted that local vascularity to tibial cortex was enhanced by a muscle flap and resulted in augmented

healing of an osteotomy [190, 191]. The enhanced vascularity correlated histologically with increased cortical porosity. Rotation of a muscle flap over a devascularized segmental tibial diaphyseal osteotomy resulted in an increase in segmental microsphere-measured bone blood flow by a factor of 2–5 times that of the control osteotomy 31 days postoperatively in dogs [189]. Rizk et al. reported improved structural strength at 8 weeks in locking-nail stabilized tibias in which a muscle flap was created to cover the fracture site compared to no muscle flap [192]. Strachan et al. found that following osteotomy of canine tibias and ligation of the nutrient artery, marked cortical and osteotomy blood flow was evident 2 weeks postoperatively [193]. They noted that this recruitment of vessels from surrounding soft tissue seemed to be influenced by the osteotomy since reductions in cortical flow of 70% have been reported after nutrient artery ligation in intact tibias.

The extraosseous blood supply starts to develop immediately after injury. It supplies the early periosteal callus and, in so doing, blends with the periosteal arterioles in areas where they are present (**Fig. 2-21**). It revascularizes bone that has been removed from, and can no longer be reached by, the medullary circulation. The extraosseous blood supply is transitory and persists only during healing. As the normal components of the blood supply are re-established, and become sufficient to sustain the bone, this supplemental vasculature subsides. The medullary arterial supply maintains its normal dominance in simple fractures, and returns to its dominant position as soon as possible in complex situations.

6.3 Callus

Callus formation begins when a fracture occurs. Hematoma formation at the fracture site results in a fibrin network laid down between the bone ends. Pluripotential cells of the endosteum and periosteum begin to proliferate within 48 hours. Their numbers increase rapidly during the first few days. Cells in the forming callus may grow faster than their blood supply and differentiate to chondroblasts. The amount of cartilage that forms is dependent on the speed at which callus grows and the rate of vascularization, both of which are

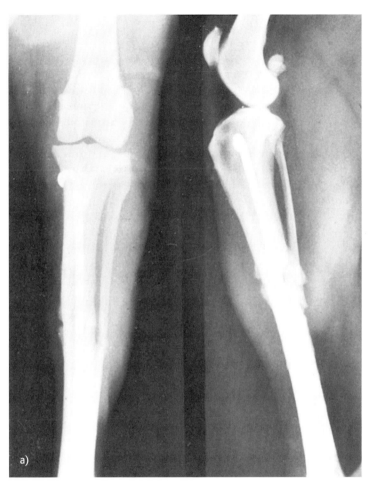

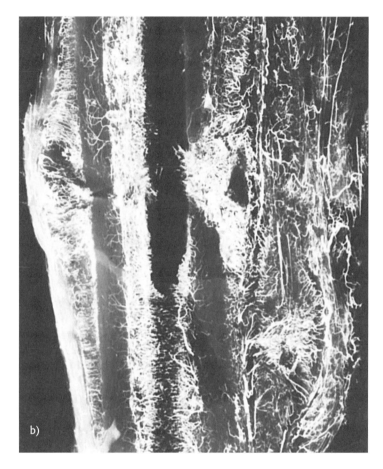

Fig. 2-21: Mature canine tibia 3 weeks after fracture and internal fixation with a loose-fitting medullary rod.
a) Radiograph shows good position of all the components of the fracture. Note the small butterfly fragment posteriorly *(to the right)* [100].
b) Photomicroangiograph (×3) of the area of fracture. The tissue slice of the microangiograph is oblique, containing part of the rod tract *(above)*. The cortex, separated from the rod tract, has maintained blood supply derived from medullary arterioles, whereas the cortex abutting the rod tract *(upper right)* is avascular over its inner 2/3. The outer 1/3 of this area of cortex, where periosteal arterioles enter the tibia, remained vascularized. The posterior detached butterfly-fragment is itself avascular, but arterioles of the extraosseous blood supply have surrounded it. The mass of periosteal callus anteriorly exhibits the typical vascular pattern of extraosseous arterioles approaching the bone surface perpendicularly [213].

effected by the amount of instability at the fracture site. Cartilage proliferation requires O_2 and is a minimally aerobic, not anaerobic, function. Chondrogenesis has been found to be maximal at 15–21% O_2 and is inhibited under hypoxic conditions [194]. Once the reactive hyperemia subsides and the pH becomes alkaline, calcium and phosphorus that were in solution are deposited. When callus calcium content reaches approximately 40% it becomes radiographically apparent. Bony union occurs when the callus of the two fragments meet, grow together, and become calcified. The formed callus then gradually diminishes and is replaced by lamellar bone. The continuity of the medullary cavity is restored. Callus formation is not accelerated by attempts to raise blood calcium by increasing calcium intake.

Three types of osseous callus will be considered in the discussion of blood supply to healing bone (**Fig. 2-22**). Periosteal callus is external and is the callus revealed by standard radiograph. It is initially supplied entirely by the extraosseous blood supply, and as healing progresses, it receives progressively more of its blood supply from the medulla. The size of the callus in fracture healing bears no relationship to the size of the hematoma. Medullary callus is confined to the medullary cavity. It is vascularized only by the medullary arterial supply. Intercortical callus forms between the opposing ends of cortex at the fracture site, and is the framework upon which the injured cortical bone is rebuilt. Its volume depends entirely upon the space available between fragments of cortical bone. It is vascularized entirely from the medulla when the medullary arterial supply is not interrupted [**195**]. If the medullary arterial supply is disrupted or blocked, vascularity comes from the extraosseous supply. As healing progresses and medullary blood supply is re-established, normal medullary-derived centrifugal flow will become dominant.

Production of periosteal callus can be influenced by three conditions in the periosteous environment. Instability at a fracture site can lead to production of callus to counteract motion. Callus is formed subsequent to extraosseous blood supply stimulation in response to massive cortical devascularization. And callus is produced in reaction to inflammation, especially infection of bone.

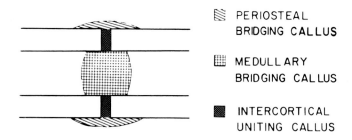

Fig. 2-22: Diagrammatic representation of the three types of osseous callus encountered at sites of bone repair [**119**].

PERIOSTEAL BRIDGING CALLUS

MEDULLARY BRIDGING CALLUS

INTERCORTICAL UNITING CALLUS

6.4 Simple undisplaced closed fractures

The progressive sequence of vascular and cellular events in fracture healing is illustrated from a study of fractures of the radius and ulna which were created by external hydraulic press, stabilized by full leg plaster cast, and evaluated at varying intervals [**196, 197**]. Two types of fractures were created. In one type, there was fracture of the bone without displacement of the fractured ends. This type will be discussed here. In the other, the bone was manipulated after fracture to cause more severe injury to the bone and displacement of the fractured ends. That type will be discussed in the next section.

In fractures in which there was no, or very little, displacement of the fracture ends, the normal afferent blood supply was disturbed but remained intact. Some areas of cortex, close to the main fracture, become avascular and devitalized, not only from the direct effects of trauma but also as a result of microfracture interruption of canaliculi and haversian canals. The amount of this devitalization was directly proportional to the severity of the injury. A uniform 1-mm-zone of completely avascular, devitalized cortical bone did not always develop. The photomicroangiograph in **Fig. 2-23** reveals an active blood vessel in a bone canal 30 µm from the cortical fracture 1 day after fracture. Lockwood and Latta observed a drop in microsphere-measured cortical blood flow at the fracture site and a rise at the opposite ends of the bone in both the proximal and distal segment after midshaft fracture of canine femora 15 minutes after injury [**198**]. They noted that with nutrient artery disruption at the fracture site, distal fragment vascularity was very dependent on metaphyseal arteries. By day five, active production of periosteal callus was seen, supplied by capillaries of the extraosseous circulation. Static-scan scintigraphy counts have been shown to increase at this time as a result of the increase in bone blood flow [**41**]. At 2 weeks, vasculature had increased dramatically under the conditions of minimal displacement and good stabilization (**Fig. 2-24a**). The medullary blood supply was the dominant source of new vessels. Numerous filamentous vessels pervaded the forming medullary and intercortical callus. The importance of stability is emphasized by the fragile, precarious appearance

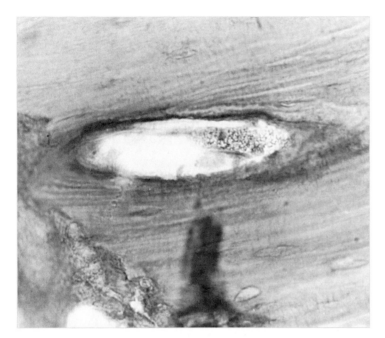

of the advancing vasculature (**Fig. 2-24a–c**). Paradis and Kelly found that bone blood flow reached a maximum on the tenth day after fracture [**199**]. They attributed the increased flow to new vessel recruitment. Mineral deposition during fracture healing was closely related to the increased bone blood flow attributed to these new vessels. Static-scan scintigraphy counts are increased at 14 days [**41**]. The increased uptake of ^{99}Tc detected was attributable, not only to the increased blood flow, but also to uptake by rapidly forming woven bone at the site of injury. A similar peak in blood flow rates, at the second week, was identified by Aalto et al. in a rabbit fracture model [**121**]. As healing progresses, total vascularity to the fracture decreases, and the transitory, extraosseous blood supply

Fig. 2-23: Photomicrograph (H and E stain; ×360) of a canine radius 1 day following fracture, showing granules of barium sulfate in a bone canal very close to the fracture site [**196**].

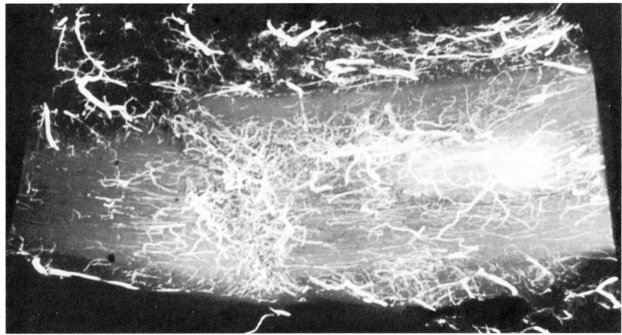

Fig. 2-24a: Mature canine radius 2 weeks after undisplaced closed diaphyseal fracture [**196**].
a) Microangiograph (×3.5) of slightly oblique tissue slice showing a great vascular response in all areas.

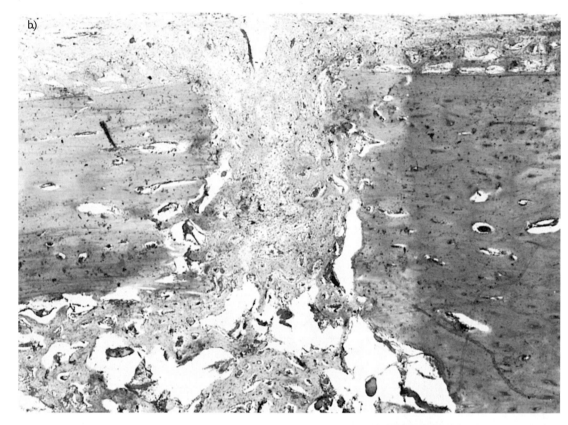

Fig. 2-24b/c: Mature canine radius 2 weeks after undisplaced closed diaphyseal fracture [196].
b) Photomicrograph (H and E stain; ×22) from (a) showing the osseous callus extending from the medullary cavity into the cortical fracture gap.
c) Enlargement (×35) from (a), centered over the fracture of the lower cortex, showing the blood vessels in the intercortical uniting callus. Note that they all occupy a 2-mm tissue slice.

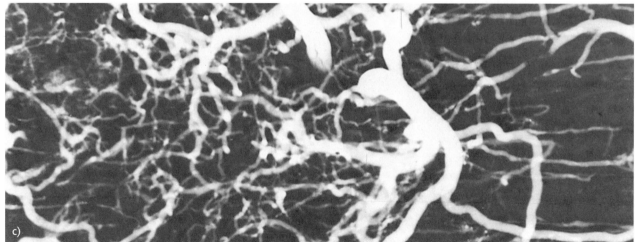

Fig. 2-25: Photomicroangiograph (×7) of a mature canine radius 5 weeks after fracture. Medullary arterioles penetrate full thickness both cortices to supply the external callus that remains. Healing is advanced [196].

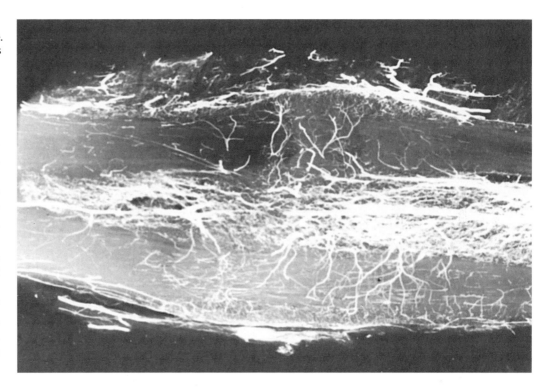

regresses and disappears. There is a parallel progressive decrease in bone blood flow [199]. At 28 days, the static-scan count was found to have decreased to values similar to that at 7 days [41]. At 5 weeks in an undisplaced fracture, the micro-angiogram shows a near normal vascular picture with a dominant medullary derived circulation. Medullary arterioles traverse the cortex full thickness, and even supply the small residual periosteal callus (**Fig. 2-25**). Fracture healing is advanced.

6.5 Displaced closed fractures

In most displaced fractures, the injury to the bone is more severe than in the undisplaced fracture. There is displacement of the fracture ends and complete disruption of the medullary circulation. It has been shown by direct measurement in canine femora that there is a fall in intraosseous pressure, and a decrease in Po_2, immediately following complete osteotomy [23]. An increase in CO_2 follows. The low initial oxygen concentration at the fracture site may induce, or promote, ingrowth of osteoprogenitor cells, capillary buds, and primitive mesenchymal cells into the fracture. Brighton et al. found that low oxygen concentrations (±9%) favor bone cell proliferation in cell culture, whereas higher oxygen concentrations (±13%) favor macromolecular synthesis [200]. Thus, within a fracture, proliferation of osteoprogenitor cells may be promoted by the initial low oxygen concentration. Cell proliferation would then gradually decrease, osteoid deposition would increase, and healing would progress as oxygen concentration at the fracture rises. Microvessels growing into the fracture appear to contribute cells to the pool of large, polymorphic mesenchymal cells that are seen in fracture repair and thus may participate in early bone healing either as osteoprogenitor cells or as regulatory cells [200]. Within budding new vessels the endothelial cells maintain the microvessel lumen and modulate blood delivery, whereas the pericytes are believed to control growth and support the structural integrity of the vessel. It has been suggested that endothelial cells [201] or pericytes [202], or both, may be precursors to the osteoprogenitor cell. Jones et al. found that both endothelial cells and pericytes have a mitogenic effect on osteoblasts that appears to be mediated by soluble factors [203]. The effect of endothelial cells on osteoblasts was found to be nearly twice that of pericytes. A microangiogram at 3 weeks after displaced fracture reveals

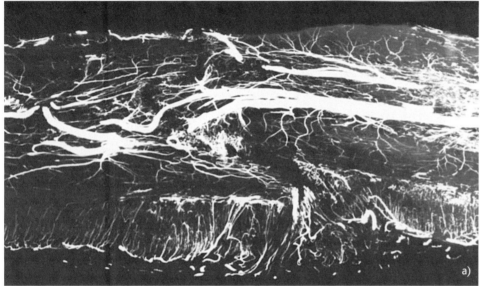

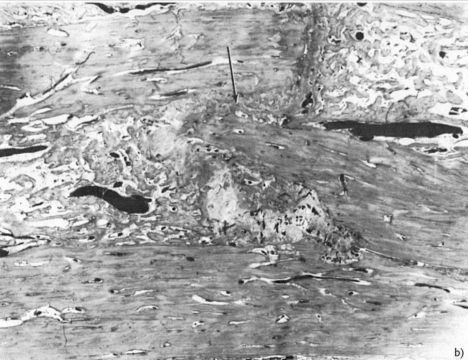

regenerative medullary arteries crossing a thin avascular zone, which is the fracture site (**Fig. 2-26**). The medullary vasculature is the dominant supply to cortex and intercortical callus. There is periosteal callus present, which is supplied by extraosseous vessels. The fracture was obviously stable; the two fracture ends interlocked. Medullary callus had already produced osseous union between this spike and the cortex above it, and fracture healing is well advanced. In contrast, the microangiogram from another displaced fracture at 6 weeks shows no blood vessels crossing between fracture fragments (**Fig. 2-27**). There are large masses of periosteal callus that appear to be attempting to bridge the fracture. The callus is largely avascular and consists of fibrocartilage. Osseous union is obviously in abeyance. The fracture appears to be incompletely stabilized and vascularization to the fracture site is being inhibited.

Motion at the site of fracture delays fracture healing and stimulates production of periosteal callus. Large masses of external callus become visible radiographically, with a prominent radiolucent zone traversing both callus and cortex.

Fig. 2-26: Mature canine radius 3 weeks after fracture and stable fixation in a plaster cast [197].
a) Photomicroangiograph (×4) shows regeneration of large medullary arteries across the fracture site. Periosteal arterioles approach, characteristically, at right angles to the cortical surface.
b) Photomicrograph fragment (H and E stain; ×9) showing osseous union (*arrow*) between the endosteal surface of the left-hand fracture fragment and the impaling cortical spike of the right-hand fracture.

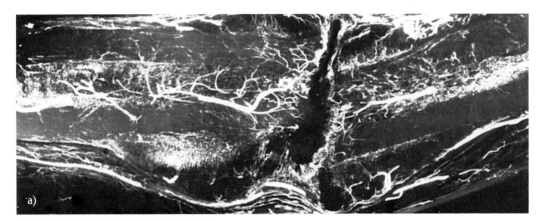

Fig. 2-27: Mature canine radius 3 weeks after fracture and unstable fixation in a plaster cast.
a) Photomicroangiograph (×3) shows blood vessels on all sides of the fracture site, but none traversing it [185].
b) Photomicrograph (H and E stain; ×4.5) shows abundant periosteal cartilaginous callus, but no union across the fracture [100].

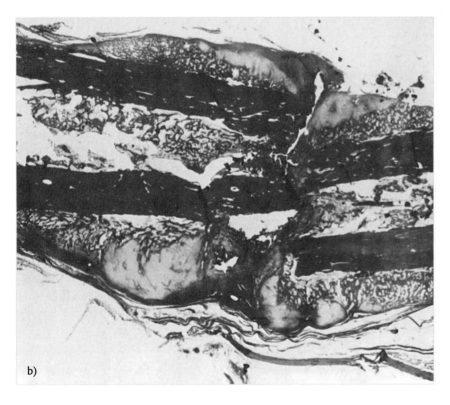

a)

b)

This situation is illustrated in a 6-week displaced fracture of the canine radius and ulna. The radiograph in **Fig. 2-28a** shows excellent alignment of both bones, but large masses of periosteal callus and a wide radiolucent zone crossing both callus and cortex are present. The photomicroangiograph in **Fig. 2-28b** reveals the microvascular situation. The medullary vasculature is increased. Blood supply to the cortex is adequate and is coming from the medullary vasculature. There is proliferation of extraosseous vessels supplying prominent periosteal callus concentrated in the region of the fracture. Brush borders of terminal capillaries face each other across an avascular zone in both the medullary cavity and in the periosteal callus. Stabilization of this fracture was insufficient to permit rapid osseous union. Blood supply was adequate but the abundant capillaries, available for direct osseous repair, were constantly being ruptured by motion at the fracture site. The histological details are shown in **Fig. 2-28c**. An osteogenic front is invading a transverse zone of fibrocartilage, which has been deposited at the fracture site. If external coaptation is maintained, the

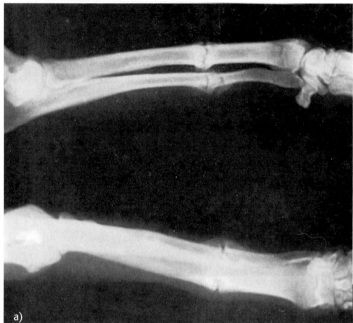

periosteal callus will eventually bridge the fracture region and the bone will heal (**Fig. 2-29**).

These are the microvascular and histological features characteristic of bone healing under conditions of less than totally rigid fixation. It is referred to as "secondary bone healing", "indirect bone healing", "healing with callus", or "fibrocartilaginous bone healing". The production and deposition of fibrocartilage are constant features of this kind of bone healing. Osteoprogenitor cells, found on the endosteal and periosteal surfaces of bone, have the ability to transform to osteoblasts, chondroblasts, or fibroblasts under differing local environmental conditions [204]. Low oxygen tension favors chondroblast transformation. With limited stabilization, revascularization of the fracture site is inhibited by motion and a zone conducive to cartilage formation is produced. If stability

Fig. 2-28a/b: Mature canine radius and ulna 6 weeks after displaced fracture and application of plaster cast.
a) Radiographs show abundant external callus traversed by a zone of radiolucency; the typical picture of fibrocartilaginous delayed union [197].
b) Photomicroangiograph (×4) of the radial fracture shows the avascular zone corresponding to the zone of radiolucency [197].

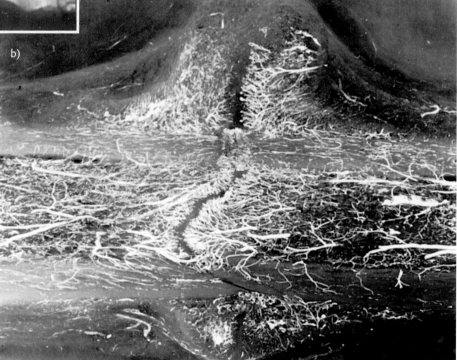

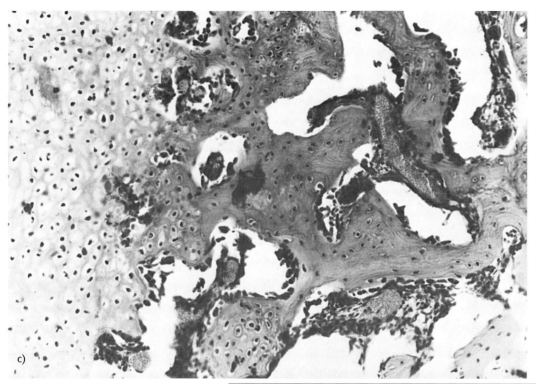

c)

Fig. 2-28c: Mature canine radius and ulna 6 weeks after displaced fracture and application of plaster cast.
c) Photomicrograph (H and E stain; ×125) showing active vascular invasion at the fibrocartilage and replacement by new bone in the external callus [196].

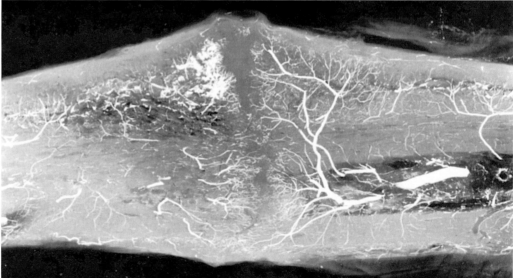

Fig. 2-29: Photomicroangiograph (×6) of mature canine radius 12 weeks after displaced fracture showing complete vascular dominance of the medullary blood supply [197].

increases, mineralization and vascular invasion of the deposited fibrocartilage take place, followed closely by replacement by woven bone. The whole process is very similar to normal endochondral bone formation. Carter et al. have shown in a finite element model that avascularity and/or intermittent compressive dilatational stresses can lead to chondrogenesis and discourage osteogenesis and cartilage ossification [205]. Revascularization is inhibited or prevented in areas subjected to high intermittent hydrostatic compression. The progressive development of fracture callus has been modeled using finite element analyses [206]. The model that fits recognized patterns of callus development was based on relating mechanical-loading history and vascular changes to the differentiation of mesenchymal tissue.

The geometric and organizational changes that take place in periosteal callus play an important role in changing the mechanical properties at the fracture site. As periosteal callus expands, the fractured bone's resistance to bending increases proportionally to the third power of the diameter of the callus measured from the center of the fracture. In addition, the expanding callus has a progressively increasing area moment of inertia. Both properties contribute to a progressively in-creasing rigidity of the fracture site. As motion at the fracture site decreases, the fibrocartilaginous callus begins to mineralize, vascularize, and be replaced by woven bone. The trans-formation to bone results in further increase in rigidity. Early in healing, the increase in vasculature and blood flow is directed in support of the expanding periosteal callus. As stability increases, the focus in vasculature and blood flow shifts to the medullary cavity. Chidgey et al. found periosteal-callus microsphere-measured blood flow to be 1,100% that of normal controls 3 weeks following osteotomy [8]. At 6 weeks, periosteal callus flow had decreased to only 160% of normal, while medullary flow was 350% of normal. The change in measured flows correlated with vasculature changes observed in India-ink-injected specimens. It has also been reported that fracture callus does generate a significant electrical signal in response to mechanical deformation or stress [207]. These stress-generated potentials may be an important physiological mechanism through which controlled weight bearing enhances bone healing. If motion at the fracture site is decreased by the

mechanical properties of the expanding periosteal callus or by intervention by the orthopedic surgeon, then indirect bone healing will proceed to osseous union.

Recently, a surgical philosophy of planned, or at least allowed, partial fracture motion has resurfaced as a method to encourage callus formation and promote healing. Increasing interfragmentary movement by flexible fixation can induce increased callus formation [208]. However, as noted by Claes et al., fracture-gap size greatly degrades quality and rate of healing when there is interfragmentary motion [208].

6.6 Rigid fixation

The great regenerative power of the medullary arterial supply of the diaphysis is demonstrated in a microangiogram of a canine radius 1 week after transverse osteotomy and fixation with a 4-hole neutralization plate and screws (**Fig. 2-30**). Medullary arterioles and capillaries can be seen crossing the osteotomy site. Rigid fixation provides a degree of stability conducive to near-maximal proliferation of medullary vessels across the fracture site. Under these conditions, medullary vasculature can take an early dominant role in fracture healing.

If the distance, or gap, between the ends of the bone is small, a unique variation of bone healing can occur. The microangiogram in **Fig. 2-31a** is of the radius of a dog 4 weeks after plate and screw fixation [100]. The gap at the osteotomy site is less than 1 mm in width. A medullary derived arteriole can be seen oriented perpendicular within the gap. Bone can be seen being deposited on the two opposing surfaces (**Fig. 2-31b**). Fibrocartilage has not filled the gap prior to bone deposition. The type of bone deposited is not randomly oriented woven bone, but is mature lamellar bone. This is "gap healing". Under conditions of rigid fixation, arterioles may enter minimal fracture gaps and deposit haversian bone directly. This direct osteon deposition of haversian bone within the fracture gap can be likened to a solder weld of the two fracture ends.

If the fracture is compressed, the gap can be eliminated and the opposing bone surfaces brought into contact. This is the condition most commonly associated with compression fixa-tion in conjunction with application of bone plates. The

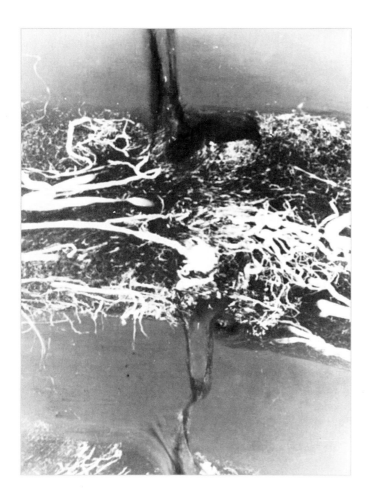

Fig. 2-30: Mature canine radius 1 week after osteotomy and internal fixation with a standard 4-hole plate and screws. Photomicroangiograph (×22.5) shows the arterioles and capillaries of the medullary supply already reconstituted in the medullary bridging callus across the osteotomy site [185, 188].

vascular and histological sequence of bone healing can be seen in a series of canine radial osteotomies repaired with a "compression plate" [209]. At 2 weeks, medullary callus can be seen starting to bridge the osteotomy site (**Fig. 2-32**). The osteotomy gap in the cortices has been eliminated and the bone surfaces are in contact. At 4 weeks, histologically the osteotomy site shows mature medullary callus and advanced healing within the cortex. A microangiogram reveals several cortical blood vessels crossing the osteotomy (**Fig. 2-33a**). A histological section, including one of these vessels, shows clearly that these are osteons depositing new haversian bone directly across the osteotomy (**Fig. 2-33b**). At 8 weeks, bony union is advanced, with large arterioles and many cutter heads seen crossing the osteotomy (**Fig. 2-34**). Fracture healing by osteons has been termed "primary healing", "contact healing" or "haversian healing" [210]. Gap healing and haversian healing can be collectively referred to as modes of direct bone healing.

The process of haversian healing can be likened to a progressive increase in spot welds at the fracture ends. The rate at which these welds occur is directly influenced by the limitations of recruitment, linear growth, and bone deposition that have been identified with osteon or haversian remodeling of bone. This is unlike indirect bone healing, in which an intermediate material, fibrocartilage or woven bone, is deposited at an accelerated rate at the fracture site. Since the rate of haversian remodeling decreases with advancing age, one should expect the rate at which haversian bone healing occurs to decrease also.

Swiontkowski et al. studied the effect of femoral neck osteotomy on femoral head blood flow utilizing LDF [211]. They found that femoral neck osteotomy appeared to decrease femoral head blood flow, at least in part, by venous occlusion, a type of "intraosseous compartment syndrome". Revascularization after 4–5 weeks produced trabecular mechanical weakening and femoral head collapse. Immediate internal fixation improved femoral head blood flow and the authors suggested that compression fixation enhanced healing.

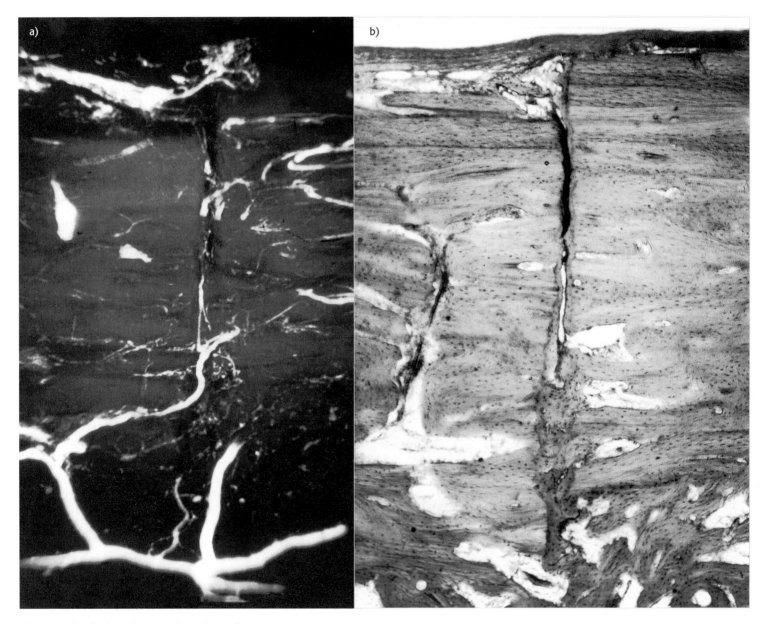

Fig. 2-31: The diaphyseal cortex of a canine radius
4 weeks after osteotomy and rigid fixation.
a) Photomicroangiograph (×15) shows a medullary-derived perpen-
dicularly-oriented arteriole within a small gap at the osteotomy site [100].

b) Corresponding photomicrograph (H and E stain; ×15) shows mature
lamellar bone being deposited within the fracture gap identical in
appearance to that deposited within secondary osteons [100].

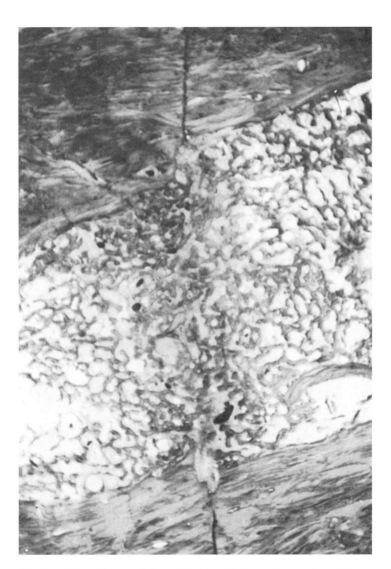

Fig. 2-32: Photomicrograph (H and E stain; ×5) of a mature canine radius, 2 weeks after transverse osteotomy and compression-plate fixation. There is direct osseous union by medullary-bridging callus without a cartilage stage [119].

6.7   Bone fragments and segmental fractures

It had long been believed that fragments or segments of bone, deprived of blood supply, would "die" and become "necrotic". These fragments were thought not to enter into the process of bone healing and had to be revascularized, removed, and replaced. Wilson et al. followed the healing of 4-cm segmental osteotomies in the canine femoral diaphysis under neutralization plate fixation [106]. Segments in which all blood supply had been removed healed in a similar manner, and at a similar rate, to segments in which the fascias aspera had been carefully preserved. Examples of haversian healing under conditions of surface contact, and of gap healing in areas of minimal gap, could be seen in both preparations. New bone was deposited directly onto surfaces of the devascularized segment. Wilson and Hoefle reported on the correlated microradiographic, microangiographic, and histological appearance of a 4-cm diaphyseal cortical allograft, 8 years after implantation in a dog [5]. The graft had persisted and was easily identified. The cortical bone had not been completely revascularized; acellular bone remained, active resorption was not evident, and new bone had been deposited directly on the surfaces of the transplanted bone (see **Section 9.3**). The graft had become an integral part of the repaired femur. Olerud and Danckwardt-Lilliestrom evaluated the healing of a much smaller intermediate fragment under compression plate fixation [212]. They observed rapid revascularization of the medullary cavity, and examples of both haversian and gap healing, after 4 weeks. They noted rapid vascularization and rebuilding of the fragment without any collapse. Clearly, size of fragment and degree of stability affect the fate of bone fragments and segments. Resorption and replacement is not the fate of all devascularized bone. Rigid fixation favors incorporation. The adjectives "dead" and "necrotic" imply connotations that are inappropriate for bone that is merely devascularized or devoid of osteocytes.

The revascularization and/or incorporation of bone fragments and segments take three routes. As noted by Olerud and Danckwardt-Lilliestrom and Wilson et al., areas of a fragment close to intact medullary vessels are vascularized by the

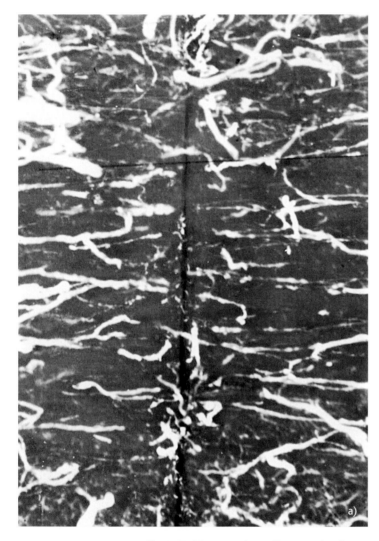

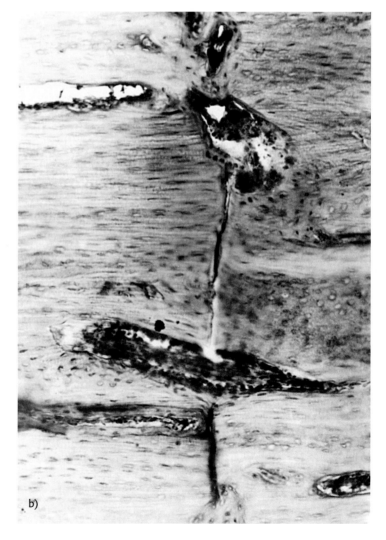

Fig. 2-33: Mature canine radius 4 weeks after transverse osteotomy and compression-plate fixation [1].
a) Photomicroangiograph (×40) centered at the cortical osteotomy shows injected blood vessels crossing the osteotomy crevice.
b) Photomicrograph (H and E stain; ×180) with a longitudinally oriented osteon crossing the compressed osteotomy and other active cutter heads approaching the site from both sides.

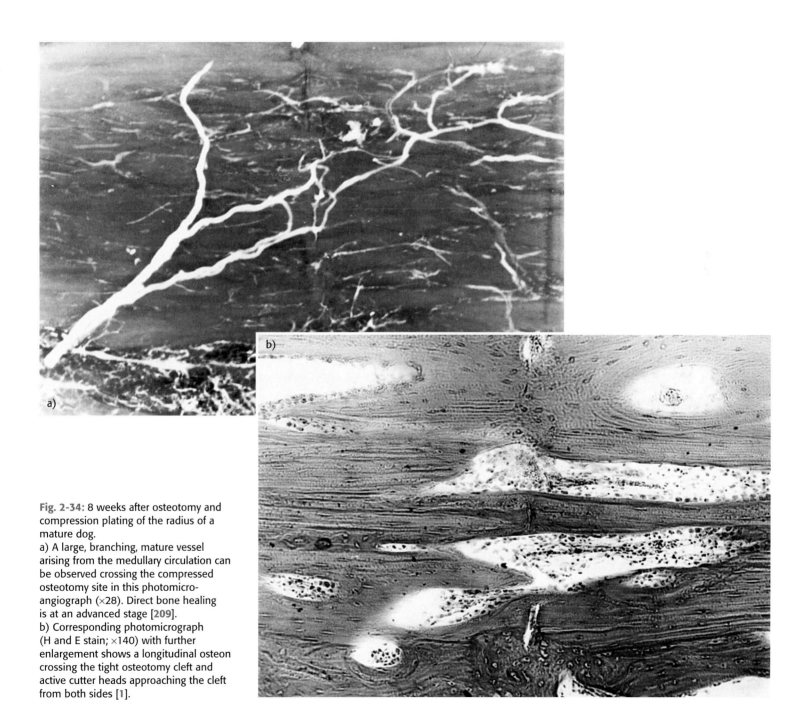

a)

b)

Fig. 2-34: 8 weeks after osteotomy and compression plating of the radius of a mature dog.

a) A large, branching, mature vessel arising from the medullary circulation can be observed crossing the compressed osteotomy site in this photomicro-angiograph (×28). Direct bone healing is at an advanced stage [209].

b) Corresponding photomicrograph (H and E stain; ×140) with further enlargement shows a longitudinal osteon crossing the tight osteotomy cleft and active cutter heads approaching the cleft from both sides [1].

medullary circulation [106, 212]. Wilson et al. found that the segments in which the fascias aspera had been preserved were largely avascular [106]. Only cortical bone, directly under the fascial attachment, was seen to have blood supply. Micro-angiograms showed functional vessels within the full thickness cortex, confirming the suspected anastomosis of periosteal and medullary vasculature within cortical bone under these attachments. The existing channels in bone appeared insufficient, however, to supply the medullary cavity or adjacent cortical bone (see Fig. 2-16). Osteocytes were seen only in cortex directly under the fascial attachment. Lacunae else-

where were vacant. Thus, preserved fascial attachments are able to preserve viability of cortical bone only in limited areas and they are not able to supplement blood supply to adjacent areas. In microangiograms at 10 weeks, large arterioles, which originated from the surrounding soft tissues, were seen penetrating full thickness the avascular bone (Fig. 2-35). These large extraosseous vessels were termed "neonutrient arteries". They directly penetrated the cortex without giving off cortical branches. Once within the medulla, they arborized to re-establish a medullary circulation. The vessels appeared, and were functioning, as new nutrient arteries. After longer time

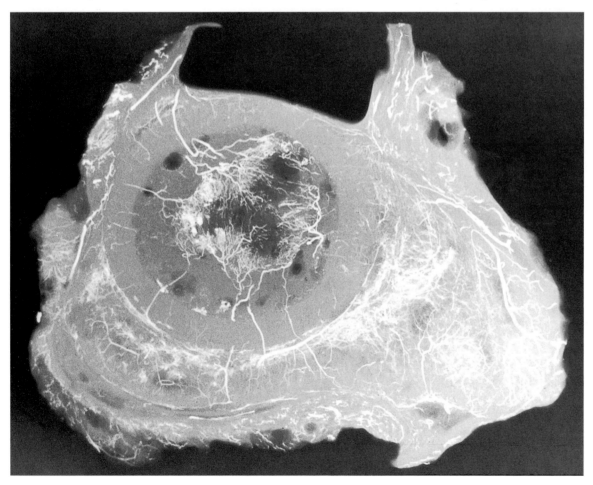

Fig. 2-35:
Photomicroangiograph (×5) from the mid section of a large avascular segment of midshaft mature canine femoral cortex rigidly stabilized under a neutralization plate. Large arterioles, originating from the surrounding soft tissues can be observed penetrating the cortical bone and arborizing within the medulla. These vessels appear similar to nutrient arteries and are re-establishing the medullary circulation.

periods, vessels originating from this reconstituted medullary circulation were seen to penetrate and arborize within the cortex.

As with all bone healing, stability and blood supply are important and are paired factors which influence the course and fate of segments and fragments of bone at a fracture site. Stability favors incorporation of the fragment into the repair process. There is a propensity toward re-establishment of medullary circulation to the fragment by extension of medullary arterioles and by extraosseous neonutrient arteries. Preserved fascial attachments may supply limited areas of the fragment but do not appear to substantially supplement revascularization.

a mature dog with a non-union of at least 4 years' duration at the time of study. High-resolution radiograph of the excised femur showed a distinct radiolucent gap at the fracture site, mature inactive callus, and a sclerotic rounding of the fracture ends. The enlarged fracture ends have a bulbous appearance and the medullary cavity has expanded and is filled with trabecular bone (**Fig. 2-37a**). There is a thin layer of dense bone juxtaposed to, and lining, the fracture gap. The extraosseous blood supply is inactive, and the nutrient medullary vasculature has arborized to supply the fracture ends (**Fig. 2-37b**). The vasculature appears to have a low, steady flow. In general, the fracture ends have taken on the appearance and structure of a mature metaphysis. Histologically, the bone ends of the old

7 Fibrous non-union and pseudarthrosis

Non-union may be the sequel to fracture regardless of method of repair or type of bone healing induced. There are distinct histological and vascular characteristics that distinguish it from healing bone. The development of non-union can be seen in **Fig. 2-36**. Six weeks after osteotomy of the radius, the 4-hole neutralization plate has loosened and the fracture has become unstable [213]. A microangiogram of the fracture site reveals an irregular mass of blood vessels within the original osteotomy site, rather than the neat alignment of capillaries along an avascular zone, as observed with secondary bone healing. Histologically, there is no evidence of fibrocartilage. Instead, the site is infiltrated with irregularly arranged fibrous tissue, detritus, and fragments of acellular bone. Fibrous tissue is not a precursor to bone formation. It does not undergo transformation to bone in any manner similar to that of fibrocartilage. It is not a component of endochondral bone formation. The fibrous tissue needs to be eliminated in order to provide a suitable environment for bone formation. This is the early histological picture of fibrous non-union.

Persistent non-union may progress to a state known as pseudarthrosis, or "false joint". The following case history is of

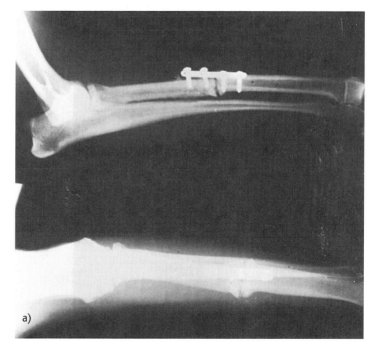

a)

Fig. 2-36a: Mature canine radius 6 weeks after osteotomy and fixation with a standard 4-hole plate and screws.
a) Standard radiograph shows loosening of the two proximal screws with elevation of the plate. The osteotomy site is radiolucent and is bordered by small mounds of external callus [119].

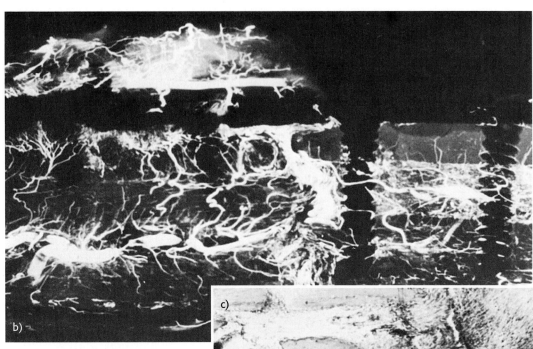

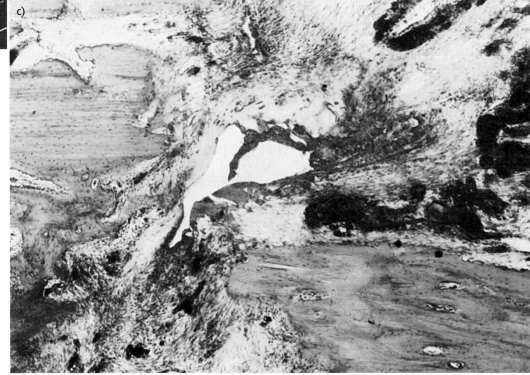

Fig. 2-36b/c: Mature canine radius 6 weeks after osteotomy and fixation with a standard 4-hole plate and screws.

b) Microangiograph (×5) from (a) shows excellent blood supply in cortex beneath the loosened plate, whereas cortex beneath the tight portion of the plate, on the right, contains only a few small vessels coming from the medulla. Vessels in the osteotomy site are a congested mass [1].

c) Photomicrographic enlargement (H and E stain; ×52.5) at the osteotomy site shows debris and fibrous tissue adjacent to the mass of disorganized blood vessels [1].

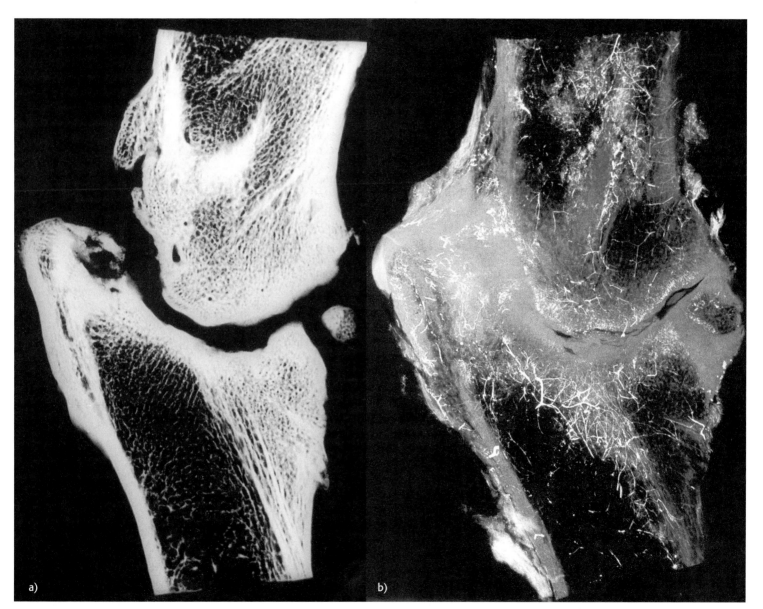

a)

b)

Fig. 2-37a/b: a) The site of pseudarthrosis in the femur of a mature dog is clearly visible in this longitudinal photomicroradiograph (×5). The opposing bulbous ends of the old fracture site are filled with trabecular bone similar to that seen in the metaphyseal end of a long bone. Dense sclerotic bone lines the two opposing surfaces [297].

b) Photomicroangiograph (×5) from a section adjacent to that shown in the preceding figure. Vasculature is reminiscent of that seen in a mature metaphysis.

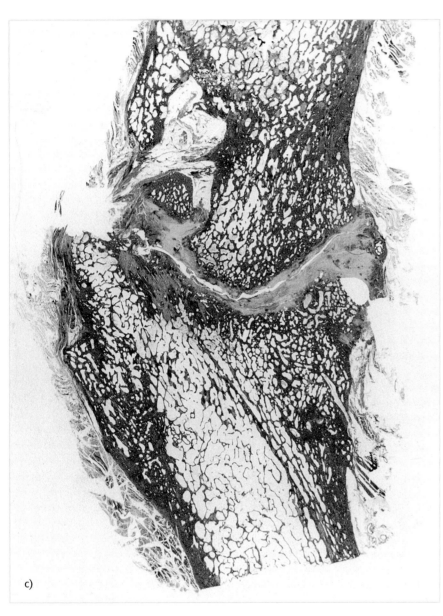

c)

fracture surfaces have become covered with a
poorly differentiated fibrocartilage that stains
unevenly with safranin O and with other stains
specific for fibrous tissue (**Fig. 2-37c**). The opposing
surfaces are separated by a fluid-filled space and
are surrounded by a fibrous capsule. The general
appearance is similar to that of a very poorly differentiated diarthrodial joint. Hence the name
"false joint".

8 Effects of fixation on bone blood supply

8.1 Intramedullary fixation

Intramedullary rods and nails have a permanent
place in the orthopedic surgeon's fracture armamentarium. They act primarily as an internal
splint that shares loading with the bone and
maintains alignment of the fracture from within.
The once simple rod, or bar, has evolved into an
array of devices that vary in cross-sectional
geometry, length, and shape. They can be inserted
after open or closed reduction of the fracture,
with or without reaming of the medullary canal,
and can be "locking" or not. The mechanical
properties inherent in each nail, and the effect
each has on fracture stability, varies between
nails and methods of use. In vitro and in vivo
mechanical tests have shown nails to constitute a
less rigid method of fracture fixation than bone
plates. Intramedullary nailing reduces fragment
motion but does not abolish it completely. Consequently, healing with periosteal callus is a

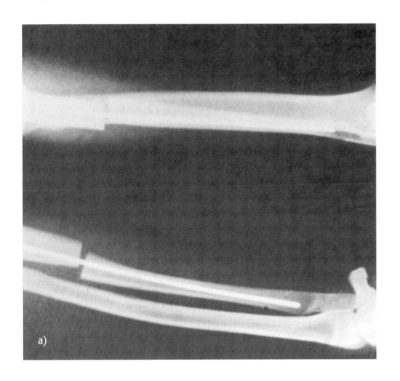

a)

constant feature following fracture repair. Insertion of a nail into the medullary canal certainly must damage medullary circulation. And, most likely, the effects on the bone and on bone healing will be influenced by the geometry of the nail and the method of insertion.

8.1.1 Loose-fitting rods

Fig. 2-38a depicts a case 1 week after insertion of a rod that was about 1/2 the diameter of the medullary cavity of the bone [1, 185, 213, 214]. The pin tract within the medullary cavity is readily visible in the microangiogram in **Fig. 2-38b**. The medullary circulation appears to have recovered from the damage caused by insertion of the rod. Observe that the cortex has no active vessels where the medullary rod lies in tight contact with the endosteal surface. Medullary arteriole access has been blocked by the rod. Elsewhere, the cortex is vascular. The small round rod contacted the endosteal cortical surface minimally. The situation with a loose-fitting medullary rod at 3 weeks is shown in **Fig. 2-21**. Persistent lack of vessels is seen in cortex where the rod abutted the endosteal surface. If this

Fig. 2-38: Mature canine radius 1 week after osteotomy and internal fixation with a loose-fitting medullary rod [119].
a) Radiograph showing areas of the endosteal surface, where the rod makes contact and where it does not.
b) Photomicroangiograph (×6) showing absence of injected blood vessels in cortex where the medullary rod was in contact. Where the tract of the rod is separated from cortex, the intervening medullary space is well vascularized and furnishes a normal cortical blood supply.

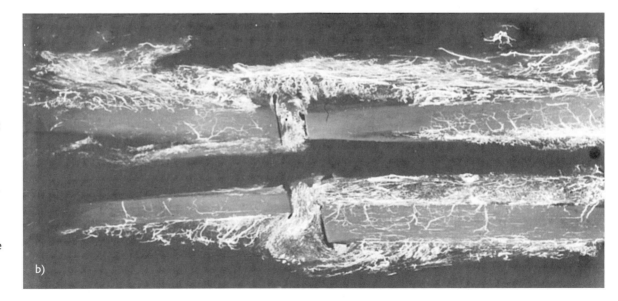

b)

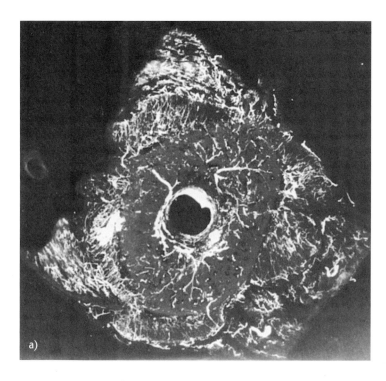

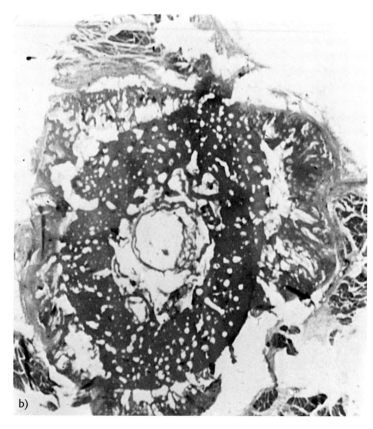

Fig. 2-39: a) Photomicroangiograph (×6) of a mature canine radius, 7 weeks after osteotomy and internal fixation with a loose-fitting medullary rod. The rod is centrally placed, with normal blood supply to all areas of the surrounding cortex [1].
b) Corresponding photomicrograph (H and E stain; ×6). The porosity, indicative of enhanced blood supply, is equal in all areas of the cortex [1].

was at a place in which there were soft-tissue attachments to the bone, the lack of vessels was within the inner 2/3. The outer 1/3 retained vascularity from the periosteal arterioles. In areas of no fascial attachment to bone, the entire full thickness of cortex was avascular. Periosteal callus is evident at the osteotomy site and is being supplied by vessels of the extra-osseous blood supply as expected. The dominance and great regenerative ability of the medullary arterial supply are emphasized in **Fig. 2-39a**. This cross-sectional microangiogram at 7 weeks shows an area near the osteotomy site. The fixation rod was situated centrally, with open medullary space all around it. Despite probable disruption of blood supply when the rod was passed, the entire cortex visualized here is well vascularized by arterioles radiating from large medullary trunks that surround the nail tract. Histologically, the porosity of the cortex is consistent with the stage of fracture repair and is similar all around the circumference in **Fig. 2-39b**. No part of this cortex was deprived of blood supply for any marked period.

The experiments with loose-fitting medullary rods clearly demonstrate that the supply of arterial blood to diaphyseal cortex is suppressed where the intramedullary rod abuts the endosteal surface. Elsewhere medullary circulation is dominant, extraosseous blood supply is stimulated, and bone healing occurs with fibrocartilaginous callus.

8.1.2 Intramedullary reaming and tight-fitting nails

The strength of fixation of intramedullary nailed fractures is greatly influenced by the amount and type of contact between the bone and the nail. The grip of bone to nail effects resistance to torsion and/or collapse of the fracture. Grip is increased by increasing total nail/bone contact and by distributing the contact over as long a section of bone as possible. Reaming the medullary cavity to a more uniform diameter allows for a closer match of nail to medullary cavity and a tighter fit, and provides for increased contact over a longer working length. Many nailing "systems" in use today have in common medullary reaming before nail insertion. However, it can be easily seen that increased strength of fixation would seem to be at the expense of the blood supply to the bone.

Two types of tight-fitting medullary nails were compared in experiments on canine femora: "the cloverleaf" nail or Küntscher nail, and the 4-fluted Schneider nail [1, 214]. A standard transverse midshaft osteotomy was made with a guided Gigli saw. The medullary cavity was reamed, proximally and distally, to a diameter appropriate for the size of the femur. The osteotomy was reduced, with care to maintain correct rotation, and the nail was passed normograde from the trochanteric fossa. A mechanical expander was made, which was inserted into the Küntscher nail's interior after insertion, to ensure a uniform tight fit of the nail within the reamed cavity. Schneider nails were oriented before insertion so that one of the flutes centered posteriorly. The size of each nail used was 1 mm larger than the diameter of the last reamer passed. Thus, the Küntscher nail fit snugly, and the broaching cutters of the Schneider nail made grooves 0.5 mm deep into the cortex.

Cloverleaf nails

Medullary blood supply was totally obliterated by reaming. At 4 weeks with Küntscher nails, where the nail tightly fit the medullary cavity, medullary blood vessels were observed only in the small spaces provided by the shallow grooves along the nail's external surface. Medullary arterioles also appeared in spaces where the smooth surface of the nail did not completely match the reamed endosteal surface. The hollow interior of the nail was occupied by blood vessels only at the most distal tip, and then only in a limited area by local blood vessels. The nail was not traversed longitudinally by medullary arteries.

A prominent feature of the histological situation was the lack of osteocytes and the presence of empty lacunae (**Fig. 2-40**). Only the caudal cortex, underlying the fascies aspera, contained viable osteocytes. Here, periosteal arterioles, undamaged by the reamer, supplied the cortex. However, as noted earlier (**Sections 4.2.1** and **6.7**), the cortex which the periosteal vessels can supply is limited to that area directly under the soft-tissue attachment. There were no osteocytes in the cranial, medial, and lateral cortex. No reversal of blood flow to cortex occurred from the periosteum through existing cortical vascular channels. On the endosteal surface, many osteoclasts and Howship lacunae could be identified.

From 4–8 weeks after Küntscher nailing, there was a progressive increase in amount of extraosseous blood supply and periosteal callus (**Fig. 2-41**). Large longitudinal arteries could be seen on the periphery of the periosteal callus. Perpendicular branches supplied the callus. Large "neonutrient" arteries traversed the callus, perforated the underlying cortex, and arborized within the medulla, presumably in endosteal resorption cavities created by osteoclastic activity observed at earlier time periods. These are similar arteries to those described in the process of revascularization of bone fragments (**Section 6.7**).

At 12 weeks the medullary cavity had enlarged through endosteal resorption and the nail had become surrounded by a highly vascular fibrous membrane (**Fig. 2-42**). Blood supply to this fibrovascular tissue came from neonutrient arteries and from regenerative branches of the nutrient artery. The femoral cortex had become far more porous due to extensive resorption along newly established vascular channels. Remodeling to a more compact bone was beginning.

At the osteotomy site, a typical microvascular and histological appearance of indirect bone healing could be seen. There was periosteal callus focusing at the osteotomy site. There were mounds of woven bone proximally and distally, and a vascular front advancing on a zone of fibrocartilage. As medullary circulation returned and motion decreased, extra-

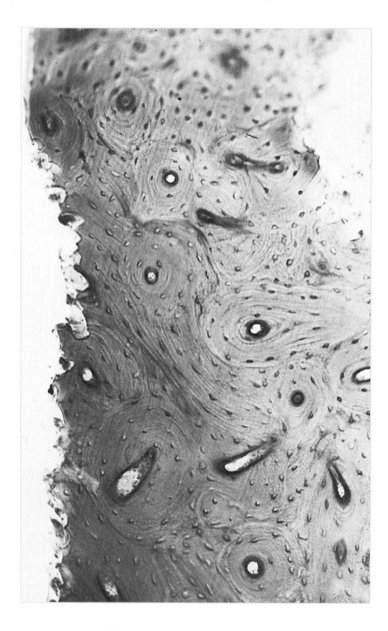

Fig. 2-40: Photomicrograph (H and E stain; ×180) of a mature canine femur 6 weeks after transverse midshaft osteotomy, reaming and internal fixation with a cloverleaf nail. The proximal diaphyseal cortex bordering the nail tract is devoid of osteocytes and shows active osteoclasia [1].

osseous vascularity subsided, periosteal callus regressed, and healing at the osteotomy site progressed. In a separate study in which canine femora were reamed only and followed up, the regenerative ability of the multiple metaphyseal arteries distally was seen to be greater than that of the single nutrient artery proximally. Presumably then, initial blood supply to these osteotomies followed that same course.

Browner et al. found similar results in femoral fractures in sheep after reaming and insertion of a tight-fitting Küntscher nail. In areas near the isthmus, where the nail fit tightly against cortical bone, there was devascularization and loss of osteocytes of the inner cortex [215]. In areas more proximal or distal, where the endosteal diameter was greater than at the isthmus, and there was a separation between nail and cortex, this was not seen (Fig. 2-43). All fractures healed with abundant periosteal callus. Also in sheep, Turchin et al. reported that overall cortical porosity was greater with reamed nails than with unreamed nails at 12 weeks [216]. Fluorochrome labels indicated similar new bone formation between groups. They commented that unreamed nailing might have an advantage initially in cases of severe vascular compromise but also that not reaming had little effect on new bone formation.

In a study with tight-fitting nails in the reamed tibia of dogs, Rand et al. found that ^{85}Sr-measured whole bone blood flow peaked 14 days following nailing (16.29 mL/min/100g) [217]. Blood flows at the fracture site were highest between 2 and 6 weeks and reached a rate of 20.23 mL/min/100 g. All fractures healed with periosteal callus. Bone blood flow reached higher rates and remained elevated longer in fractures fixed with rods than in similar fractures fixed with plates. O'Sullivan et al. reported that prior to any fixation, blood flow at an osteotomy site in the canine tibia decreased to 50% of normal immediately after osteotomy and further decreased to 1.78 mL/min/100 g at 4 hours [218]. Reaming the tibia and inserting a tight-fitting nail reduced diaphyseal blood flow to 1.15 mL/min/100g. Unfortunately, measurement of blood flow was apparently only confined to the fracture site and the general effect on the bone was not noted.

In sheep, Reichert et al. noted that intramedullary reaming alone of the intact tibia did not result in a significant decrease of LDF-measured bone blood flow [219]. Osteotomy significantly reduced cortical flux with subsequent reaming having no further significant effect. Their measurements were taken from the periosteal cortex, and they attributed their findings to a reduced capacity of the periosteum to contribute to cortical perfusion after longitudinal disruption. It is more likely that their findings reflect the limited capacity of LDF to measure blood flows and poor choice of probe position. Reichert et al. found no decrease in cortical microsphere-measured blood flow in intact ovine tibia following reaming but did find increased periosteal flow [220]. It is possible that the 10-mm reamer used did not totally disrupt medullary vasculature as intended. The periosteal reaction seen could indicate stimulation of immature bone still forming primary osteons rather than "compensatory, periosteal blood flow in the acute phase following reaming".

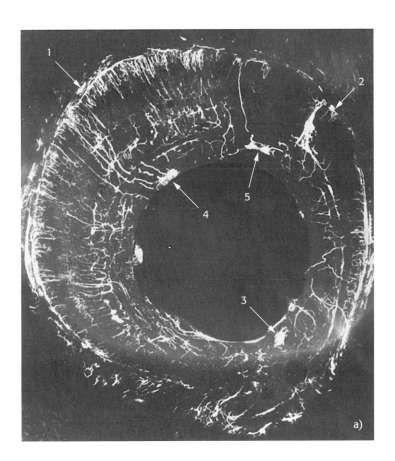

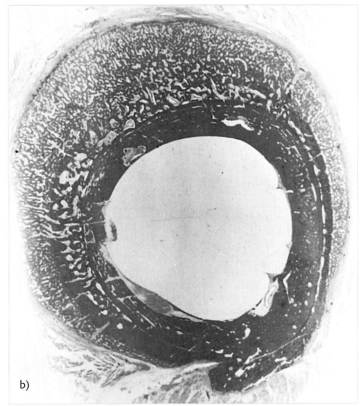

Fig. 2-41: Mature canine femur 8 weeks after transverse midshaft osteotomy, reaming, and internal fixation with a cloverleaf nail.
a) Photomicroangiograph (×7) from the proximal diaphyseal cortex, showing large arteries (arrows 1 and 2) lying just outside the external callus of the anterior-lateral sector of the femur, and the nutrient artery (*arrow 3*) in its cortical canal. *Arrows 4* and *5* point to well-vascularized cavities in the old anterior cortex [1].
b) Photomicrograph (H and E stain; ×7) of histological section from tissue slice adjoining that of (a) shows the nutrient artery as it was turned back into the cortex by the presence of the medullary nail and extraosseous arteries and the cortical cavities, which are designated by arrows in the photomicroangiograph [214].

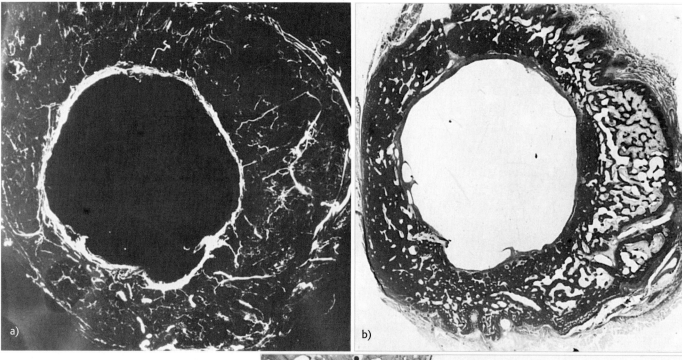

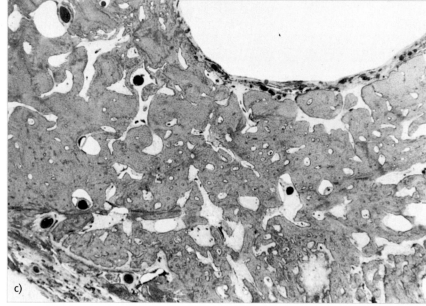

Fig. 2-42: Mature canine femur 12 weeks after transverse midshaft osteotomy, reaming, and internal fixation with a cloverleaf nail [1].
a) Photomicroangiograph of the proximal diaphysis shows a regenerative, highly vascular membrane completely surrounding the nail tract at the endosteal surface. The posterior cortex contains short arterial segments derived from the nutrient artery (×7).
b) Corresponding photomicrograph showing the thick endosteal membrane (H and E stain; ×7).
c) Photomicrograph of histologic enlargement from b), to demonstrate details of the posterior femoral cortex. Observe the arterioles of the endosteal membrane and the intracortical arterial trunks. grater magnification (not shown) reveals more definitely the muscular coat of these arteries (H and E stain; ×14).

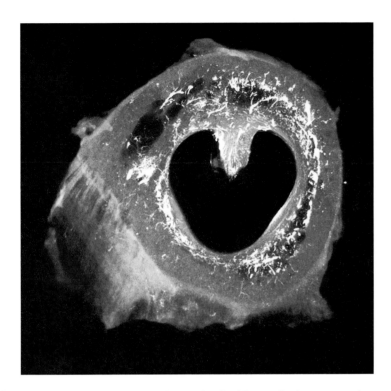

Fig. 2-43: Photomicroangiograph from the distal femur of a sheep, 12 weeks after osteotomy, reaming, and insertion of a cloverleaf nail. The nail does not completely fill the medullary cavity. Vessels fill the unoccupied medullary cavity, pervade the slot in the nail, and enter the cortex circumferentially (×2.5).

Fluted nails

The self-broaching, 4-fluted nail cuts shallow grooves in the endosteal cortex, during insertion, into which the four fillets of the nail ride. This locking of the nail into the endosteal surface of the bone provides resistance to torsion of the bone around the nail. At 4 weeks proximal to the osteotomy, the large spaces in the medullary cavity, corresponding to the four flutes along the nail, could be seen to provide a channel for medullary revascularization. Branches of the nutrient artery could be seen entering the posterior channel whereas the medial and lateral channels were only partially vascularized.

The cortex facing these vascularized channels contained injected blood vessels. The anterior channel and adjacent cortex showed no injected blood vessels. Distal to the osteotomy, all four channels were well vascularized. This is in accord with the experiment described above, in which regeneration of the arterial supply, after simple reaming, was found to be more pervasive when derived from the distal metaphyseal arteries.

At 12 weeks, all four channels around the nail tract were well vascularized, even in the proximal diaphysis. The large spaces provided by the flutes purveyed medullary blood supply from all sources (**Fig. 2-44a**). The corresponding histological section shows medullary callus in the four channels. There was much less periosteal callus than would have developed with the Küntscher nails (**Fig. 2-44b**).

In a canine fracture model comparing a tightly fitted, fluted intramedullary rod, placed following medullary reaming, with a compression plate and an external fixator, Smith et al. found that microsphere-measured bone blood flow was lowest in rod-stabilized fractures at all time periods [221]. Fracture callus was exuberant in eight out of ten rod-stabilized fractures. However, bone formation and porosity in transverse section of 90-day fractures was not significantly different between the three modes of repair. They concluded, as have others, that reaming of the medullary cavity and insertion of the rod initially damaged the perfusion of cortical bone adjacent to the fracture site. They found that this effect was overcome within 90 days and suggested, as has been shown above, that this was perhaps by collateralization of vessels to the endosteal cortex.

8.1.3 Locking nails

Other than the added feature of enhanced fixation, locking of a nail with proximal and distal screws would have no vascular advantage unless locking allowed use of a smaller nail, or a nail configuration that spared medullary vasculature and promoted optimal fracture revascularization. In fact, results identical to those summarized in the previous section, comparing reamed and unreamed cloverleaf nails were reported in a comparison of reamed and unreamed locked intramedullary nails [222].

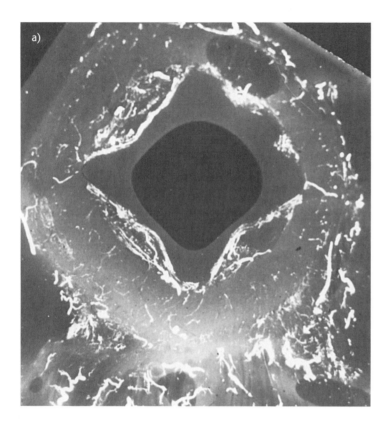

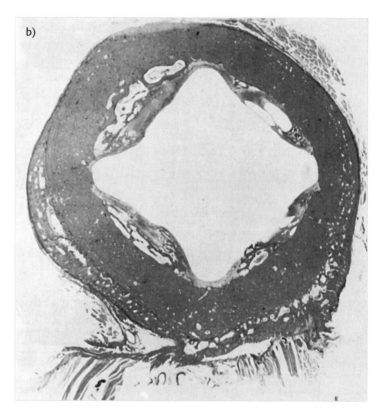

Fig. 2-44: Mature canine femur 12 weeks after transverse midshaft osteotomy, reaming, and fixation with a 4-fluted nail [284].
a) Photomicroangiograph of the proximal diaphysis showing vascularization
in the channels of all flutes (×8).
b) Corresponding photomicrograph showing medullary callus in all the
flutes, and minimal periosteal callus (H and E stain; ×8).

Reaming and insertion caused significant endosteal devascularization, which was more than unreamed nail insertion.
Reaming did not retard callus blood supply and, although not
commented on, data presented appeared to confirm callus
stimulation with reaming. In a subsequent publication Schemitsch et al. reported that Doppler-measured blood flow to
healing callus was similar at 2, 6, and 12 weeks, whether
medullary cavities were reamed prior to nail insertion or not
[223]. The final bending strength and stiffness at 12 weeks

were also similar. A similar comparison between reamed and
unreamed interlocking nail by Runkel et al. found the unreamed callus to exceed that of reamed callus at 4 weeks, but
not at later time periods [224]. Damage to cortical circulation
was significantly greater in reamed tibia. They recommended
unreamed nailing in open, comminuted, or tissue-damaged
fractures.

8.1.4 Multiple nails

Browner et al. followed the healing of midshaft femoral
fractures in sheep stabilized with multiple Ender nails [215].
They found that insertion of multiple small nails destroyed
medullary circulation, devitalized diaphyseal cortex, and
impeded medullary revascularization similar to that after

reaming and Küntscher nailing. Insertion of multiple small nails resulted in many areas of nail-endosteal contact. Where ever a nail contacted cortex there was devitalization. Fractures healed with abundant periosteal callus. The spaces in the medullary cavity between the multiple nails rapidly filled with fibrovascular tissue (**Fig. 2-45**). Although blood flow was not measured, microangiograms indicated a greater number and size of medullary vessels, suggestive of a greater medullary flow than in Küntscher-nailed femora. Chidgey et al. noted the correlation and accuracy of microangiogram prediction of flow differences [**8**].

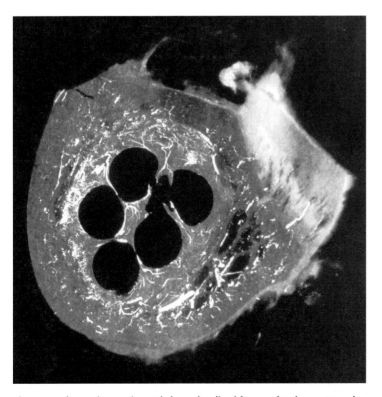

Fig. 2-45: Photomicroangiograph from the distal femur of a sheep, 4 weeks after osteotomy and insertion of Ender nails. The cortex is vascular and vessels fill the medullary cavity in and around the nails (×2.5).

8.1.5   Summary

Insertion of an intramedullary rod or nail disrupts medullary vasculature. The larger the nail, in comparison with the medullary cavity, the greater the damage. Reaming totally destroys normal medullary circulation and devitalizes the cortex. Only cortical bone directly under fascial attachments is spared. Revascularization of the medullary cavity takes place by regeneration of nutrient and metaphyseal vessels, and, at least in the canine femur, is more pervasive from the distal metaphysis. The cross-sectional size and configuration of an intramedullary nail controls the course and rapidity of re-generation of the medullary arterial circulation. If cortical damage is extensive and if regeneration of the medullary circulation is blocked, extraosseous neonutrient arteries will form. Periosteal callus is common, due to the less than rigid mode of fixation, and/or due to the generalized extraosseous response to cortical devitalization if reaming is performed. Whole bone and fracture-site blood flows are greater and remain at high rates longer than similar fractures stabilized with rigid plates.

8.2   Wire loops and wide bands

Repair of long-bone fractures with encircling wires is probably the oldest documented form of internal fixation [**225**]. The encircling wires or bands, and the method of use, are referred to as "cerclage", which originates from the French word for encircling hoops placed around barrel staves. Use of cerclage fell into disrepute early because the crude wires used quickly corroded and broke. With development of biocompatible materials, cerclage was re-introduced [**226**]. Failures occurred. Cerclage was once again decried. This time it was thought to strangle underlying cortical bone and prevent extension of periosteal callus along the area of repair [**227, 228**].

Numerous studies have since refuted the detrimental effect of cerclage on cortical bone and on bone healing [**119, 185, 229–234**]. The arterial supply to the diaphysis of a mature long bone cannot be suppressed by an encircling wire because no afferent vessels run longitudinally in the periosteum. The major blood supply to all areas is medullary. A minor blood supply, confined to the outer 1/3 of the cortex at fascial attachments, comes from periosteal arterioles, which are not blocked by small encircling wires. Furthermore, venous efflux at the periosteal surface is not interfered with by round wires since they contact bone minimally (**Sections 2** and **4**).

During growth, large longitudinally-oriented arterioles can be found in the periosteum. These vessels support active periosteal bone deposition, which increases bone girth. Wilson et al. evaluated the effect of three sizes of wires placed circumferentially around the mid-diaphyses of 22-week-old puppies [**232**]. No blockage of blood supply was noted, even when the wires were placed directly over the periosteum (**Fig. 2-46**). At

8 weeks after placement, continued appositional bone deposition on the periosteal surface had resulted in the wires becoming embedded within the enlarging cortex.

Under conditions of bone healing, there is still no interference with vascularization by wire loops. The arterioles of periosteal callus, components of the transitory extraosseous blood supply, approach the external cortical surface perpendicularly. **Fig. 2-47a** shows vascularized callus surrounding the tracts of six wire loops at 4 weeks after fracture fixation. The area of the second loop from the left is magnified histologically (**Fig. 2-47b**). The wire is in firm contact with bone and is closely surrounded by osseous callus. Today, cerclage failure is known to be due to errors in application, and not to adverse biologic

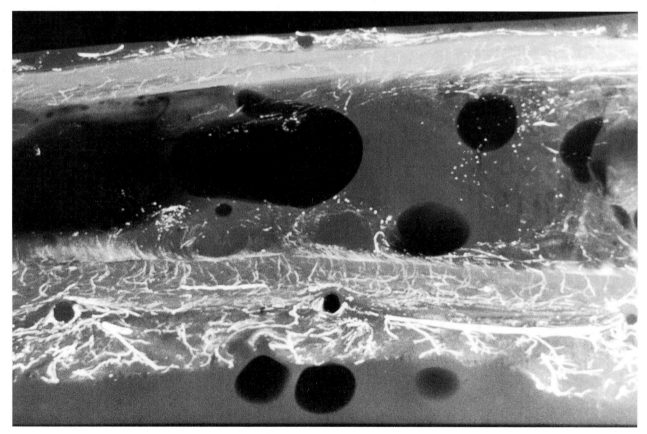

Fig. 2-46: Photomicroangiograph from the femur of a 22-week-old dog, 3 weeks after cerclage wires were placed circumferentially over the periosteum. Micropaque-filled vessels can be seen in the cortex beneath all wires and in the periosteum between and around all wires (×5).

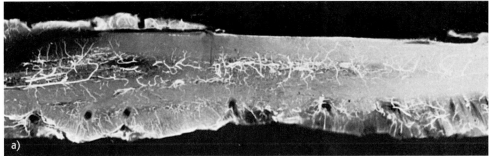

Fig. 2-47: Mature canine radius 4 weeks after internal fixation of an oblique osteotomy by six circumferential wire loops.
a) Photomicroangiograph showing periosteal callus closely investing the small round tracts of the wires (×5.5) [103].
b) Greatly enlarged histological photomicrograph centered over the tract of a wire in (a). There has been no erosion of bone or formation of fibrous tissue. Periosteal callus has closely invested the wire (H and E stain; ×40.5) [188].

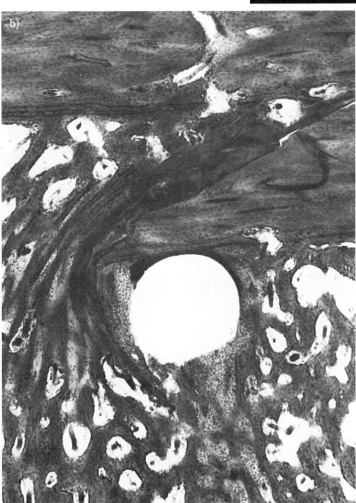

effects [235–238]. Using a finite element model, Serina and Mote reported that cerclage application can produce cortical pressures sufficient to reduce crack widths to less than 100 μm (±1.0 MPa) and optimal for bone healing (1.0–2.5 MPa) [239].

Parham and Martin introduced broad metal bands for circumferential application to long oblique fractures [240]. Because these bands are flat and wide, failures were attributed to disruption of cortical blood flow by blockade of the venous efflux at the periosteal surface [185, 241]. Nylon bands with "bumps" on the undersurface were introduced by Partridge [242, 243], and recommended for fixation of fractures in elderly patients with osteoporotic bone [244]. The bumps are there to circumvent the disruption of circulation thought to be associated with flat bands. Although some fractures healed with these nylon bands, others did not. Cortical erosion by the lock mechanism and non-union associated with use of these nylon bands were attributed to local vascular complications [245]. However, Wilson found that the knot slip resistance of metal bands was significantly weaker than twist-knotted 1.2-mm wire [246]. The physical fact that fewer bands than wires could be placed over a given diaphyseal distance suggested that metal band failures were probably due to mechanical weakness, not to biologic disturbance. In 1989 Kirby and Wilson reported that the knot slip resistance of the three smaller sizes of nylon bands was actually less than that of twist-knotted 0.8-mm wire [247]. Autoclaving and a 24-hour-soak in saline reduced knot slip resistance of all sizes of nylon bands significantly. After saline soaking even the 9.0-mm-wide nylon band was weaker than twist-knotted 1.2-mm wire.

In 1990, Nyrop et al. reported on the microangiographic and correlated histological effect of 0.8-mm wires, 5.0-mm Parham-Martin bands, and 7.9-mm Florio-Circumferential Partial Contact bands placed around radii of mature ponies [234]. They observed no loss of bone vascularity beneath any of the cerclage devices, even the Parham-Martin bands, and suggested that equine cortical bone may have greater radial blood flow than either human or canine bone. When double-loop cerclage, conventional single-loop cerclage, and a Parham-Martin band were applied to midfemoral diaphyses of mature greyhound dogs, Blass et al. also found no loss of underlying cortical viability regardless of type of cerclage, position of the cerclage either over or under the periosteum, or duration of placement [233]. Kirby and Wilson placed both metal and nylon bands of varying widths around the femoral diaphyses of dogs [120]. Regardless of size or type of band applied, there was no evidence of complete obstruction of cortical blood flow.

Numerous examples were seen of vessels traversing the entire thickness of the cortex, even directly beneath the 10-mm-wide bands (**Fig. 2-48**). Direct count of cortical osteocytes did not suggest impairment of viability related to placement of the bands.

Apparently, when normal periosteal efflux is blocked, cortical venous flow can be directed along alternate or secondary routes. This secondary flow is suspected to be back toward the endosteal surface and then to the periosteal surface along adjacent venous channels [120, 234]. Thus, cerclage devices, even when flat and wide, do not disrupt normal cortical vascularity. However, in healing fractures, wide bands may block extraosseous arterioles as they approach the cortical surface perpendicularly and thereby reduce extraosseous supply to developing callus and neonutrient artery augmentation of medullary circulation. For this reason, and because of the inherent weakness of both metal and nylon bands, potential use for bands in fracture management is limited.

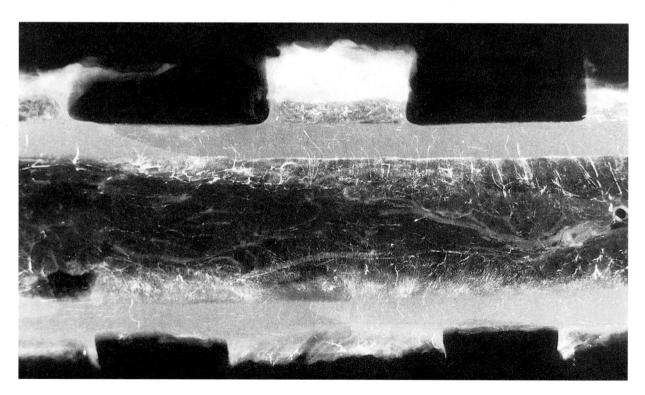

Fig. 2-48: Photomicroangiograph of a longitudinal section of femur from a dog 7 days following subperiosteal placement of 316L stainless-steel bands. Numerous filled vessels can be seen in the cortex beneath all bands, including the largest which measures 10.0 mm in width (×5).

8.3   Plates and screws

The great advantage provided by plate fixation is the excellent fracture stability that can be obtained. Early limb function allows early use of joints and muscles and would seem to accelerate fracture healing. If the separation between fracture surfaces is less than 1 mm in width, haversian bone may be deposited directly in the gap. This direct osteon deposition of haversian bone, within the fracture gap, can be likened to a solder weld of the two fracture ends. It is a mode of direct bone healing referred to as "gap healing". If the fracture is compressed, the gap can be eliminated and the opposing bone surfaces brought into contact. This is the condition most commonly associated with compression fixation in conjunction with bone plates. Under these conditions, osteons can cross the fracture directly and new haversian bone can be deposited. Fracture healing by osteons is a mode of direct bone healing

referred to as "haversian bone-healing". It can be likened to a progressive increase in spot welds at the fracture ends.

It has been shown that medullary arterioles and capillaries can be seen crossing an osteotomy site within the first week following plate fixation. They can be seen filling minimal gaps and crossing contact sites as early as the fourth week (Section 6.6). Lewallen et al. found that technetium and [85]Sr-measured blood flow to the canine tibia was less in an osteotomy stabilized with a plate than in an osteotomy stabilized with an external fixator [34]. The greater periosteal callus in the externally fixed fracture could account for this difference. Endosteal new bone formation, however, was greater on the plated side. When healing was compared between fixation with or without compression, Hart et al. found no significant difference in [85]Sr clearance-measured blood flow to the healing osteotomies and no difference in histological healing patterns at 90 days [35]. Plate fixation fosters direct bone healing of fractures by providing excellent stability and contact of fracture surfaces or diminution of gaps.

In 1965, Rhinelander noted that cortical bone directly beneath a tight bone plate did not perfuse with injected contrast media (Fig. 2-49) [213]. The explanation for this devascularization appeared to be that blockage of the efflux of blood at the periosteal surface prevented any influx from the medulla [1, 185].

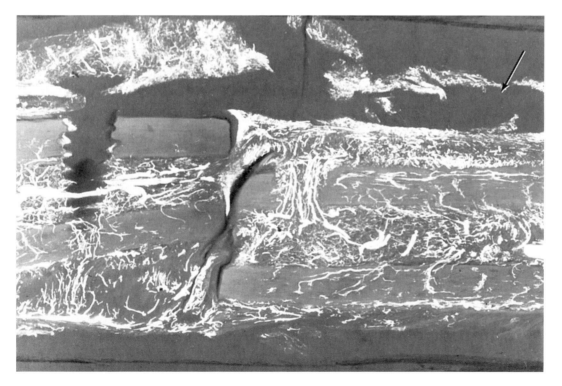

Fig. 2-49: Photomicroangiograph from a mature canine radius at 3 weeks after osteotomy and internal fixation with a plate. One end of the plate has loosened *(arrow)* and blood vessels stream through the space provided by a loosened screw. Note the vascularity of cortex beneath the loose portion of the plate and the avascularity beneath the tight portion (×3.5) [216].

Since a plate is applied longitudinally, the site of devascularization and the effect of plate application were thought to be confined to a small sector of the circumference, and osseous healing around the remainder of the circumference was fostered by the plate's stabilizing effect. Furthermore, the lack of blood supply beneath the plate was thought to be short-lived. Also at this same time, the early 1970s, cortical osteopenia in association with rigid internal fixation became recognized [248–251]. An increase in intracortical porosity was seen soon after plating, with cortical thinning caused by endosteal bone resorption seen later. Much of the recent work on the effect of plates on bone has focused on the mechanical effect of fixation on cortical bone and bone healing—so-called stress protection or stress shielding. The bone is protected from its normal loading by the implant, and remodeling is effected by the lesser stresses resulting in a weaker bone. It has been shown that bone strength decreases immediately after plate removal [252], and many orthopedists have recommended supplemental protection following plate removal for a variable period of time.

In 1979, Wilson et al. suggested that the porosity under plates could be accounted for by a revascularization process, in response to the devascularization observed following placement of the plate [106]. Beginning at the fourth week, an increase in vessels directed toward the cortex under the plate was seen (**Fig. 2-50**). This vasculature increased progressively through the 12th week (end of time period evaluated). Accompanying the vascular increase was a histological increase in cortical porosity. The changes were attributed to a response to cortical devitalization induced by the presence of the plate.

Luethi and Rahn stated that normally contact between a plate and the underlying bone amounts to about 30% of the total plate undersurface area [253]. Recently, a technique was devised whereby the contact between bone and plate is increased by luting the interface between the bone and the plate with polymethylmethacrylate cement [254, 255]. Plate luting is thought to increase the interfacial shear strength between bone and plate, sparing the screws from excessive shear, and thus increasing the strength of the bone-plate unit. This technique has been used clinically in fracture repair of equine long bones [254]. Roush and Wilson used the luting

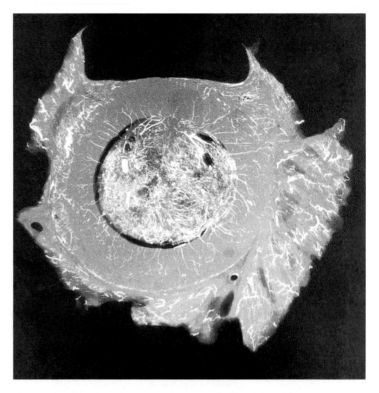

Fig. 2-50: Photomicroangiograph of a transverse section of femur from a mature dog, 6 weeks after placement of a neutralization plate. The cortex at the 12 o'clock position, which was directly under the plate, is devoid of arterioles, whereas the remainder of the cortex is vascular and viable (×6).

technique to evaluate the effect of plate contact area on the underlying cortex [256]. At the fifth week, cortex beneath luted plates had a greater porosity and fewer osteocyte-filled lacunae than cortex beneath non-luted plates. When compared to normal non-operated femoral cortex, filled lacunae were significantly decreased in number throughout the entire cortex, and empty lacunae were significantly increased in the outer 1/3 of the cortex. Beneath non-luted plates, the numbers of filled and empty lacunae were different from normal, but not significantly. Microangiograms showed a decrease in vasculature in the outer 1/3 and a normal-to-increased vascularity in the inner 2/3 of cortex beneath luted plates (**Fig. 2-51**). At the tenth week, vasculature had increased throughout the cortex beneath luted plates. There was no difference in the number of filled lacunae in cortex beneath either mode of plating; however, there was a significantly increased number of empty lacunae in the middle 1/3 of cortex beneath luted plates. In the non-luted plate the percentage of empty cortical lacunae had increased. The progressive increase in porosity and vascularity beneath plates seemed to be related to the amount of contact between plate and underlying bone; however, the amount of devascularization and devitalization, seen at the fifth week, was not as marked as was expected for a potential threefold increase in area of bone contact over that of normal plate placement. In the light of the fact that Kirby and Wilson

found that loss of osteocytes in outer cortical strata was more related to surgical exposure than presence of encircling bands [122], changes are even less remarkable.

In a related experiment, 1.0-mm circumferential cerclage wires were placed (by the author) between screws and under 6-hole dynamic compression plates placed on the lateral surface of non-osteotomized femora in mature dogs. This raised the plate off the surface of the bone by 1 mm and reduced the plate–bone contact to less than 3% as measured by pressure sensitive film. There was minimal change in vascularity in the cortex under elevated plates at 5 weeks when compared to normal femora, but markedly less vascularity when compared to normal plate placement after 5 weeks. At 10 weeks, cortical

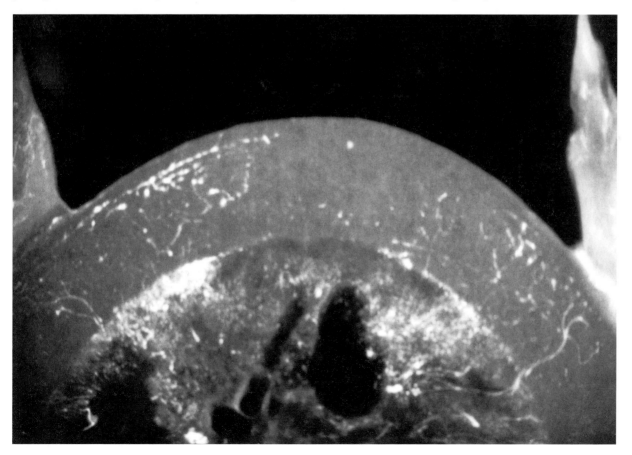

Fig. 2-51:
Photomicroangiograph of a transverse section of femur beneath a luted plate from a mature dog at the 5th week. There is a decrease in vasculature in the outer 1/3 and a normal to increased vascularity in the inner 2/3 of cortex beneath the luted plate. The cortex had a greater porosity and fewer osteocyte-filled lacunae than cortex beneath non-luted plates (×6).

vascularity under the elevated plate had increased to slightly greater than that seen in normal femora and no greater than in normally placed plates after the same time period. Elevating the plate with wires correlated with significantly less porosity under the plate at both 5 and 10 weeks than porosity under comparatively normally placed plates. These differences would suggest that elevating the plate away from the bone and reducing plate–bone contact was beneficial. However, at 5 weeks there were significantly fewer viable osteocytes and more empty lacunae in the cortices under elevated plates than in cortices under normally placed plates or in normal femora, which were not significantly different. This difference in numbers of viable osteocytes and empty lacunae between groups disappeared at 10 weeks. Thus cortical viability did not seem to be spared by elevating the plate and reducing plate–bone contact. The findings seem to be contradictory. Also when considering that in this comparison there was potentially a 30× difference in plate–bone contact between groups, the magnitude of difference seemed inconsequential although statistically significant.

The apparent poor correlation between area of bone contact beneath a plate and plate-associated vascular changes has been seen by others. Luethi et al. evaluated the vascular effect of plate application in ovine tibiae utilizing disulfine blue [257]. They found a decrease in dye staining in the cortex beneath the plates, but noted that the defect was wider than the contact area of the plates studied and wider than the actual width of the plates. The defect was not related to contact dimensions of the plates nor to the applied force of the plate. In 1986, Gautier et al. evaluated the effect of altering plate–bone contact area and plate stiffness in ovine tibiae, also utilizing disulfine blue [258]. They found that an 80% decrease in plate contact did not significantly improve dye staining at 4 weeks after plating compared to the standard plate design. Intracortical remodeling was similar between plates with different bending stiffness and different contact areas.

Smith et al. noted no difference, up to 14 days, in microsphere-measured blood flow to the anteromedial cortex (sub-plate region) between compression-plated canine fractures and fractures stabilized with tight-fitting fluted rods following medullary reaming [221]. They concluded that the application

of a plate might cause only a small local interference with blood flow to the anteromedial cortex. They also suggested that studies, using disulfine blue, which demonstrated lack of staining under plates, were recording interstitial fluid flow which is driven by hydrostatic pressure, and not blood flow. This is in agreement with the conclusions of the author of this chapter.

Daum et al. found a fivefold increase in the ^{85}Sr-measured blood flow of non-osteotomized femurs following compression plating at 1 month, and a fourfold increase following neutralization plating [36]. This investigation also included two study groups with drill holes, with and without screws. They reported that, following a crossed comparison, the only consistent change in bone blood flow was associated with application of screws, with or without plates. Following an additional study, it was concluded that an increase in ^{85}Sr-measured bone blood flow seen in the early postoperative period, which occurs in the entire segment beneath the plate, was due principally to the trauma of drilling screw holes [37]. A continued elevation in bone blood flow seemed to correlate best with presence of screws, 1 or 2 months later. And at 6 months, whole-bone blood flow increased related to screw application with a rigid plate. Also at 6 months, presence of the rigid plate produced a regional bone blood flow increase in the midshaft, directly under the center of the plate. When compared with intact control animals, the plated-bone animals showed a relative redistribution of femoral bone blood flow toward the midshaft. Histologically, at the 6th month, cortical thinning and increased cortical porosity were seen [259]. However, the histological changes, although associated with the increase in blood flow at the midshaft, were not statistically correlated with the increased ^{85}Sr clearance. It was suggested that the development of plate-induced osteopenia involves disparate histomorphometric time constants, rather than lack of any association.

The effect on blood supply of screws crossing the medullary cavity is shown in **Fig. 2-52**, from a 6-week experiment on osteotomy and fixation with a 6-hole plate. Blood vessels circumvent the screw tracts in close contact. New bone, of the medullary bridging callus, had grown fully into the screw threads. Obviously, screws traversing the diaphysis cause no impairment of blood supply.

Fig. 2-52:
a) Photomicroangiograph from a mature canine radius 6 weeks after osteotomy and secure internal fixation with a standard 6-hole plate and screws. Medullary arteries and arterioles pass closely around the screws (×5) [121].
b) Photomicrograph of screw hole and osteotomy site shows progression of healing at the osteotomy site, medullary callus surrounding screw threads, and no cortical resorption (H and E stain; ×3) [121].

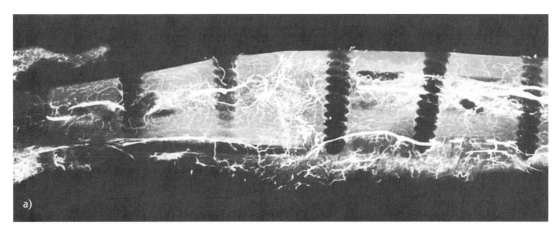

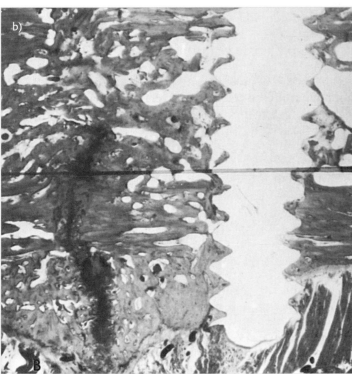

It would thus appear that the drilling of holes, placement of screws, application of a rigid plate, and the amount of contact between the undersurface of the plate and the underlying cortex all affect bone to which a plate is affixed. This effect can be lessened but not abolished by modification in plate placement or design of plate–bone contact area. I now believe that in addition to the mechanical effects of plate presence, the biologic effect to the surface of bone directly under a plate is not cortical devascularization by venous blockade, but is alteration in sub-plate cortical blood flow. Normal vascular drainage may be diverted from the periosteal surface in cortex beneath a plate back toward the endosteum where adjacent connecting vessels could provide an alternate drainage conduit to the periosteal surface. The altered flow may in turn result in a change in electrical streaming potentials in the cortical bone beneath a plate. This could alter the microenvironment in cortical bone beneath plates, inducing vascular ingrowth and bone resorption. Experiments to study this are underway.

8.4 External fixators

External fixators provide many of the attributes of plate fixation but without the need for extensive surgical exposure. As a non-operative technique, they provide more stability than casts and allow more movement of adjacent joints. They do not disturb medullary circulation as do intramedullary rods and nails. However, if they are too stable, stress shielding develops, and if they are not stable enough, delayed union or non-union develops. They also add new complications: pin tract infection and osteomyelitis.

Aalto and Slatis found microsphere-measured tibial bone flow in rabbit osteotomies stabilized with external fixators to be greater than in control bones [121]. Highest blood flows were found at 18 days. Court-Brown found that microsphere-measured tibial blood flow in leporine osteotomies was less in legs stabilized with external fixators than in legs stabilized with casts [260]. Both osteotomies healed with periosteal callus. Cast-treated osteotomies had more marked periosteal callus, whereas osteotomies treated with external fixators showed relatively more medullary callus. He concluded that use of external fixators decreased the periosteal response but seemed to enhance both the endochondral ossification of callus and medullary ossification. When compared to compression plating, Lewallen et al. found increased ^{85}Sr clearance-measured tibial blood flow at 120 days in canine osteotomies stabilized with external fixators [34]. Intracortical new bone was greater in plate-fixed osteotomies. External-fixator osteotomies had greater bone turnover and increased porosity. Hart et al. found that ^{85}Sr clearance-measured tibial blood flow at 90 days was similar in canine osteotomies fixed with external fixators applied with and without compression [35]. No differences in histological healing patterns were seen between the two methods. Examples of both haversian and gap healing were seen with each method. Smith et al., using microspheres, found less changes in blood flow to canine fractures stabilized with external fixators than in fractures with either reamed fluted intramedullary nails or compression plates [221]. When all soft tissues were separated from the bone by interposition of a silicone sleeve around the diaphysis, Wallace et al. found that little healing occurred at 14 days and concluded that extraosseous blood supply was of primary importance in bone healing in which external fixators were utilized [261]. Park et al. evaluated external fixators of varying rigidity on closed fractures in rabbits [262]. They found that, at 2 weeks, intermittent shear motion resulted in greater callus volume with lower fracture strength than a more rigid fixation. However at 4 weeks, mineralization of the greater callus resulted in fracture strength equal to or greater than more rigid forms of fixation. They concluded that shear motion at a fracture site is not necessarily detrimental to fracture healing.

External fixators are utilized in distraction osteogenesis for bone lengthening, a technique popularly known by the name of one of its original proponents, Ilizarov. Kojimoto et al. reported that following osteotomy, bone lengthening by callus distraction was successful as long as the periosteum was preserved [263]. Revascularization occurred during the waiting period prior to distraction. Lengthening failed at a distraction rate of 1 mm/12 hours. The usefulness of scintigraphy and quantitative CT to evaluate distraction osteosynthesis was evaluated by Aronson et al. [264]. They detected increased bone blood flow and decreased mineralization at the distraction site as expected.

Thus, the mode of healing in fractures repaired with external fixators is related to the rigidity provided. More rigid external fixators provide conditions conducive to direct bone healing, whereas fractures repaired with frames of lower rigidity heal by fibrocartilaginous bone healing. Bone and fracture vascularity and blood flow correspond to the mode of healing.

8.5 Secondary internal fixation

Karlstrom and Olerud evaluated the effect of revision of internal fixation on ultimate healing of leporine tibial osteotomies [265]. In one group of rabbits primary plate fixation was revised after 3 or 6 weeks by intramedullary reaming and nailing, and the reverse was performed in another group. Animals were evaluated using Spalteholz and fluorochromes. They found that secondary internal fixation did not affect the microcirculation or healing, nor were the risks of cortical necrosis, infection, and delayed union increased. A prompt revascularization was generally seen after the secondary operation. It is of interest that the authors commented that intramedullary nails gave a more reliable secondary fixation than plates.

9 Vascularization of bone grafts

9.1 Inlay cortical grafts

Inlay grafts of diaphyseal cortex were interchanged between the right and left radii of a series of mature dogs [100]. Full-thickness segments of cortex, 0.4 cm × 2.0 cm in size, were removed subperiosteally and transferred immediately, with the same orientation. Thermal necrosis at the kerf was carefully avoided. The grafts fit snugly into their recipient sites and were held in position by closure of the periosteum and overlying soft tissues.

Ingrowth of blood vessels into the grafts was obvious at 2 weeks. Revascularization of old cortical channels appeared likely but could not be definitely determined. Osteoclasis was not observed histologically. The microangiographic picture at 6 weeks is seen in **Fig. 2-53**. The number and size of injected blood vessels is much greater in the graft than in the neighboring cortex, indicative of supernormal blood supply in the graft. Corresponding histological sections showed greater porosity of the graft than of adjacent bone, consistent with the greater vascularity. Advanced osseous union at each end of the graft had developed in the 6-week period. After 12 weeks, this type of graft appeared to be fully incorporated into host bone.

In these experiments, the major vascularization of the grafts did not come from the extraosseous blood supply, as will be seen with cancellous chip grafts, but rather from the normal medullary arterial supply of the recipient site, as if the graft comprised some of the original cortex. Also, the inlay bone was incorporated directly into the recipient site, not resorbed and used as a scaffold for new bone.

9.2 Grafts of small particle size

The vascularization of cancellous chip grafts in dogs was evaluated in a standardized incomplete defect in the proximal tibial metaphysis and in a standardized complete defect in the proximal 1/3 of the ulnar diaphysis. The ulna was utilized because the adjacent intact radius would support the defect and help exclude instability as a variable in comparisons of graft incorporation. Cancellous chip grafts, of approximately match-head size, obtained from the iliac crest or the proximal tibia were packed firmly into the recipient site, filling it completely. Free blood in the recipient site mixed thoroughly with the chips, forming a spongy mass. The experimental periods were for 1–12 weeks. A comparison was made between fresh autogenous, frozen homogenous, and processed heterogenous grafts [1, 4, 100, 266].

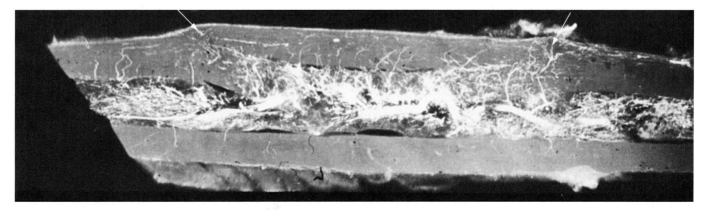

Fig. 2-53: Photomicroangiograph of a mature canine radial diaphysis, 6 weeks after insertion of a cortical inlay autograft taken from the hetero-lateral radius showing thorough vascularization of the graft from the medulla. The arrows indicate the two ends of the graft (×55) [103].

In the incomplete defects, the autogenous chips were vascularized the most rapidly. Vascularization of the homogenous chips was satisfactory, but was at least 3 weeks slower than vascularization of the autogenous chips. The heterogenous chips of immature calf bone (Boplant) were totally unsatisfactory.

In the experiments on complete long-bone defects, an inert Teflon spacer was inserted for 3 weeks before grafting to establish conditions similar to those that exist in a non-union. A small medullary pin was used to hold the spacer in position and was maintained when the grafts were introduced. At the time of grafting, the spacer was removed, the ends of the defect were debrided, the pin was reinserted, and the graft material to be studied was inserted.

The vascular situation at 1 week, after grafting with fresh autogenous cancellous chips, is shown in **Fig. 2-54a**. Note the tremendous invasion of the entire grafted area by blood vessels. New bone abundantly developed in contact with the chips, as shown clearly in the histological section (**Fig. 2-54b**).

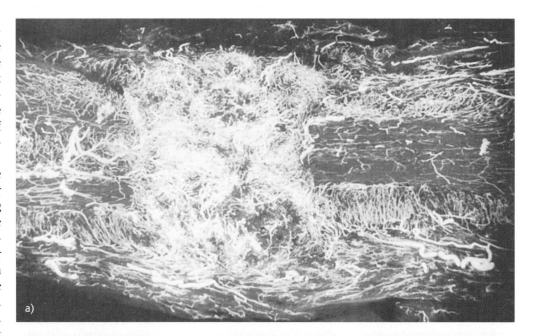

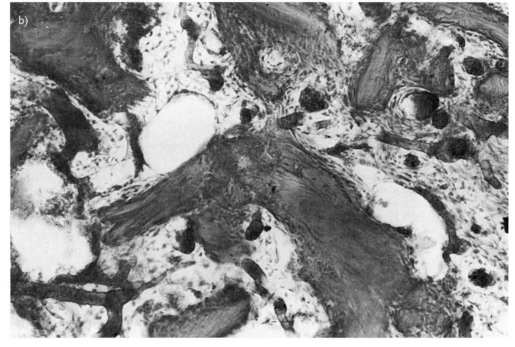

Fig. 2-54:
Mature canine ulnar diaphysis 1 week after insertion of fresh autogenous iliac cancellous chip grafts into a 1-cm complete defect:
a) Photomicroangiograph shows active vascularization of the entire recipient site (×5.5) [103].
b) Corresponding photomicrograph shows new bone formation along the surfaces of the chip grafts. Many capillaries are in the spaces between the portions of graft (H and E stain; ×200) [121].

During the ensuing weeks the local blood supply decreased progressively, as the need for intense vascularization declined, and new bone developed to occupy most of the space between the chips. At 12 weeks, the vascular pattern in the grafted area (**Fig. 2-55a/b**) approached that of the adjacent host bone. Histologically, the new bone is seen to be well developed and solidly united to recipient cortical bone. The radiograph (**Fig. 2-55c**) shows excellent repair of the 1.5-cm ulnar defect. In these experiments, the major vascularization of the grafts came from the extra-osseous blood supply and was similar to that which occurs in ordinary fracture healing.

Freeze-dried allograft is clinically widely used due to certain advantages over fresh-frozen allo-

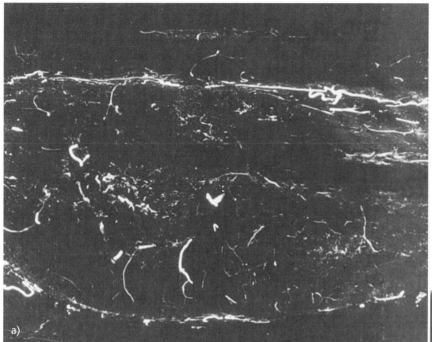

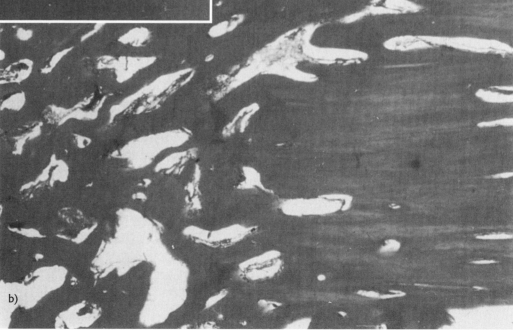

Fig. 2-55a/b: Mature canine ulnar diaphysis 12 weeks after insertion of fresh autogenous cancellous iliac chip grafts into a 1-cm complete defect:
a) Photomicroangiograph shows marked recession in vascularization of the grafted area and surrounding host bone, in comparison with 1 week (×6) [1].
b) Corresponding photomicrograph showing advanced new bone formation in the grafted area and secure union with the host cortex, on the right (H and E stain; ×50) [103].

Fig. 2-55c: Mature canine ulnar diaphysis 12 weeks after insertion of fresh autogenous cancellous iliac chip grafts into a 1-cm complete defect:
c) Radiograph of illustrated radius and ulna shows advanced healing of the discontinuity. After removal of the pin, only viable host tissue will remain [103].

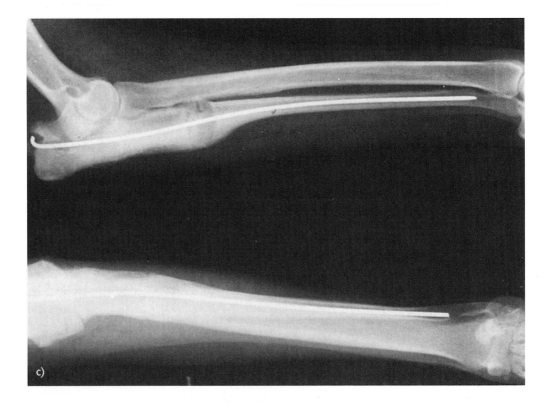

graft, including the ability to be stored almost indefinitely at room temperature and to be easily sterilized secondarily. Kienapfel et al. found fresh autogenous bone to be far superior to freeze-dried allograft due to its superior osteogenic capability [267]. Freeze-dried bone was found to have little actual effect in their model.

Addition of autogenous cancellous chips would seem appropriate to augment the production and maturation of periosteal callus in the situation where indirect bone healing will occur and be slow or retarded. Autogenous cancellous chips would seem well suited as a trellis to augment production and bridging of medullary callus with all modes of bone healing. They would also seem ideal as a material to fill gaps in a fracture, thereby providing a bridging trellis upon which intercortical uniting callus could be deposited. With rigid stabilization, in which direct bone healing is expected, there

seems little point in applying an autogenous cancellous graft around the outside of a fracture [268]. Periosteal callus and extraosseous blood supply are inhibited in rigidly stabilized fractures. It would seem to be of little purpose to augment a process that will not be a prominent factor in fracture healing or that should not occur at all.

9.3 Segmental diaphyseal grafts

To look at the vascular response to transplantation of large segments of diaphyseal cortex we can first turn to the study of plate-stabilized segmental osteotomies by Wilson et al. (**Section 6.7**) [106]. The segment, freed of all attachments, can be considered to be an orthotopic autograft. Haversian healing was seen in areas of surface contact and gap healing in areas of minimal gap, at junctions between graft and femur. In larger defects, bridging intercortical callus was seen. Fibrocartilaginous periosteal callus was seen at sites of partial instability. New bone was deposited directly onto the surface of the avascular nonviable autograft. Revascularization of the autograft took two courses. Autograft near intact medullary vessels was directly vascularized by the femoral medullary circulation. Near the center of the graft, large arterioles originating from the surrounding soft tissue penetrated the nonviable bone (see **Fig. 2-35**). These neonutrient arteries directly traversed the cortical bone without giving off branches. Once within the medulla they arborized to re-establish a medullary circulation within the interior of the graft. Incorporation, not resorption, was the prominent feature of healing of these ideal diaphyseal grafts. There appeared to be little inducement for the body to replace the nonviable segment.

Data on the fate of nonvascular bone segments can be found indirectly by evaluation of the controls used in studies on the fate of vascular pedicle bone transfers. Siegert and Wood found that after 2 weeks, microsphere-measured blood flow to conventional (avascular) and vascularized transfers were similar to, or even exceeded, the blood flow values in undisturbed control bone [269]. In four of the eight conventional grafts blood flow was greater than that in the vascularized bone transfers.

For comparison, we now turn to a report by Wilson and Hoefle in which a similar, but allogeneic, 4-cm-segment was evaluated 8 years after implantation in the femur of an adult dog [5]. Much of the transplanted bone remained after 8 years. Transverse microradiographs, from the center of the grafted area, showed dense transplanted bone surrounded by a porous irregular envelope of recipient bone (**Fig. 2-56**). Microangiograms of this area revealed the dense inner bone to be avascular, whereas the outer envelope was richly supplied with vessels (**Fig. 2-57**). The junction between graft and recipient bone could be identified on longitudinal microradiographs and microangiograms by a transition from normal cortex to double-layered bone (**Fig. 2-58**). When longitudinal and transverse sections were compared, it could be seen that the outer recipient osseous envelope was supplied by extraosseous vessels. The dense inner bone consisted of compact haversian

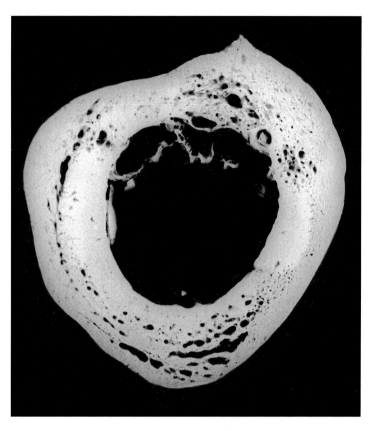

Fig. 2-56: Photomicroradiograph of a transverse slice through the center of an allograft, 8 years after insertion into a canine femur. There is a double-layered appearance to the cortex; dense bone inside and more porous bone outside (×6) [5].

bone. All lacunae were devoid of osteocytes. The outer envelope consisted of a mixture of lamellar and haversian bone. It was more porous, and osteocytes were prominent and numerous. It was concluded that the inner acellular bone must be the original diaphyseal allograft. Viable bone juxtaposed, and was indistinguishable from, nonviable transplant, except for the presence or absence of osteocytes. Acellular haversian bone lay next to viable osteons. Osteons could be seen penetrating several areas of the transplant. In some areas, a thin

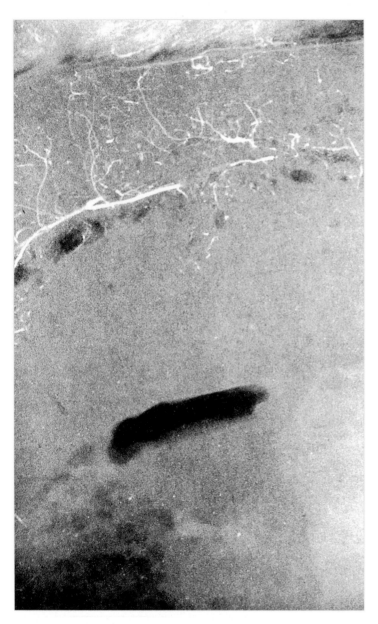

Fig. 2-57: Interface between outer and inner cortex of the allograft shown in **Fig. 2-56** is shown in a enlarged photomicroangiograph. Vessels run circumferentially within the vascular outer bone, but seldom cross into the avascular region (×35) [5].

layer of viable endosteal bone, one to three cell layers thick could be seen covering the inner surface of the transplanted bone. Inflammatory cells were not seen. Very few osteoclasts were seen, and those seen were not inordinately associated with the surface of the transplanted bone.

We may conclude that transplanted diaphyseal segments may remain relatively intact long after transplantation and may never vascularize or be replaced. It appears that resorption and replacement are not the eventual fate of all transplanted bone. So-called "creeping substitution" may not be the slow, relentless process it is often portrayed to be. Transplanted bone may serve as a scaffold for new bone formation and, as such, become an integral component of the healed bone. The allograft in the dog remained structurally intact and served functionally for 8 years. Thus, an excellent long-term clinical result may be achieved without complete replacement of the transplanted bone.

Straw et al. reported on the comparative effect of filling the medullary cavity of an intercalary graft with polymethyl-methacrylate to enhance screw holding within the graft and thus improve fracture healing [270]. Little difference was noted in evaluated biologic and mechanical characteristics between filled and non-filled bones at 9 months.

9.4 Vascular bone transfers

Refer also to information presented in **Sections 5.5** and **5.7**. The time-dependent effects of room temperature and hypothermic storage on endothelial integrity was evaluated by Roorda and Wood using EDRF release as a measure of eccrine function [271]. At room temperature EDRF-measured function deteriorated after 24 hours and was absent by 48 hours. At 4°C eccrine function appeared unimpaired for 72 hours, deteriorated from 96–192 hours, and was absent at 216 hours. Normothermic, continuous perfusion of a canine tibial vascular graft with oxygenated Krebs-Ringer solution preserved normal vascular endothelial function for only 1 hour, with reduced but demonstrable function for up to 4 hours only [272]. Variable in vitro preservation was found by Moran et al. using differing protocols with the University of Wisconsin Cold Storage

Solution (UWCSS) [273]. Endothelial eccrine function was preserved for up to 5 days by washout with UWCSS and cold storage without continuous perfusion. Bone vascular integrity, however, was maximally maintained for only 24 hours utilizing washout with UWCSS and simple cold storage, and by washout with mannitol followed by continuous hypothermic microperfusion with UWCSS. However, in a later animal experiment, Moran et al. concluded that UWCSS did not preserve normal endothelial function in the microcirculation of bone in vivo [176]. They found no evidence that the endothelium was producing EDRF in vivo after 24 hours of preservation.

Endothelins are strong vasoactive paracrine hormones with at least three isoforms. Endothelin-1 seems to be the only one produced by vascular endothelium. Two subtypes of endothelin receptors are suspected. Endothelin-A receptors, found on the vascular smooth muscle cells, have a high affinity for endothelin-1 and are thought to mediate vascular smooth muscle contraction. Endothelin-B receptors are located on vascular endothelial cells and are thought to mediate a vascular dilatory action. It has been suggested that endothelial-B receptors may not be present in the intraosseous vessels of the canine tibia [274]. In a follow-up study Coessens et al. concluded that endothelin-B receptors do not contribute to the control of

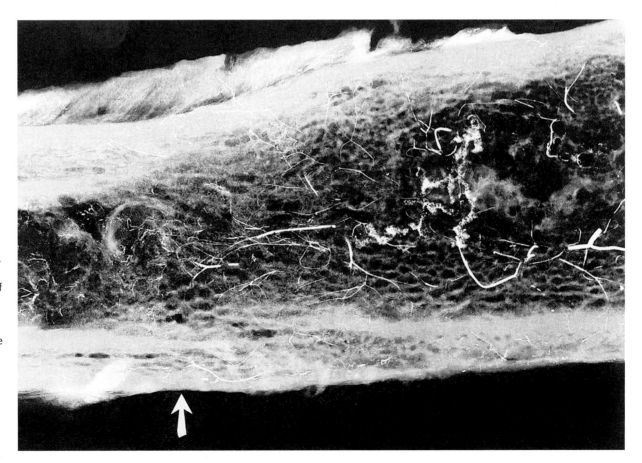

Fig. 2-58: Longitudinal-section photomicrograph of the junction of recipient and grafted bone seen in **Fig. 2-56** and **Fig. 2-57**. Viable and nonviable bone are juxtaposed, and indistinguishable, except for the presence, or absence, of osteocytes. Acellular osteons lie next to viable, cellular osteons (H and E stain; ×6) [5].

vascular resistance in bone, that the preponderance of receptors are endothelin-A, and that the effect of endothelin-1 is exerted through bone vascular smooth muscle endothelin-A receptors [275]. Coessens et al. demonstrated an increase in the response mediated by endothelin-A receptors in canine bone blood vessels after 24 hours of cold ischemia [274]. The authors suggested that the increased response might be due to either an increased sensitivity or intracellular change in the endothelin-A receptors. Use of UWCSS did not inhibit the endothelin-A response. Whether the degradation of the endothelin-A receptors was related to ischemia, lack of adequate substrate restoration by the UWCSS perfusate, or reperfusion injury, or simply associated with the conditions of the model were not determined. Increased endothelial-A-receptor response coupled with possible increased endothelial-A production in ischemia would seem to provide conditions for severe, sustained vasospasm and may contribute to the no-reflow state following transplantation.

CGRP has potent vasodilatory action. Allen et al. found that post ischemic infusion of CGRP significantly improved reperfusion blood flow in skeletal muscle [276]. Since Buma et al. used calcitonin-gene-related peptide antibodies to identify neural fibers in bone, it is possible that CGRP may have use in prevention of no-reflow phenomenon in vascular bone transfers [137].

9.5   Other graft materials

Many biologics, synthetics, and chemicals have been formulated and utilized to stimulate, enhance, or augment bone production. The majority of investigations reported have evaluated the end mechanical strength of a grafted defect or quantified the amount of new bone produced, as a test of the usefulness of the graft material. Few studies have focused on vascular responses. Oral surgeons advocate use of hemostatic agents to stimulate bone formation in oral defects. The effect of packing a hemostatic gelatin sponge, on bone formation in a defect within the proximal humeral metaphysis, was evaluated by Howard et al. [277]. Unpacked defects had filled with new trabeculae of variable thickness by the 4th month, whereas in packed defects no regeneration of cancellous bone

was seen. The original defect was clearly visible microradiographically (Fig. 2-59a). In histological sections, the gelatin sponge was easily distinguished. In some places, the interface between bone and sponge contained a thin layer of fibrous tissue, and in other areas normal bone marrow elements and cancellous trabeculae abutted the sponge directly (Fig. 2-59b). Inflammatory cells were not seen.

In contrast to studies with implantation into the oral cavity, the gelatin sponge remained in this sterile defect and blocked cancellous bone regeneration. Howard et al. concluded that oral implantation results in contamination of the sponge, inflammation, and elimination of the sponge, rather than incorporation of the sponge within the defect, or any stimulatory effect of implantation of the sponge upon the surrounding bone. Similar results were seen when granules or blocks of polyglycolic acid were implanted in humeral defects [278]. Thus, it can be clearly seen that site and environment both effect the response to implanted materials.

10   Bone blood supply in relation to various biomaterials

10.1   Metals

All metals are more or less corrosive in bodily tissues. The so-called surgical metals are the least reactive and are used in the fabrication of devices for temporary or permanent implantation. The interface between metal and bone is the critical area. A membrane was seen to form when disks of stainless steel and wrought Vitallium were implanted into slots cut in the proximal tibial metaphysis of dogs [279]. All implants were unstressed and lay in well-vascularized cancellous bone. In other experiments, stainless-steel screws (see Fig. 2-52) and stainless-steel wire loops (see Figs. 2-46 to 2-48) did not produce a membrane at the metal–bone interface. These implants were tight, completely stable, and lay against living bone. There was no need for new blood supply to be brought in at the interface, and there was no bone resorption. In contrast, when an intramedullary nail was placed in tight contact with the endosteal surface, the overlying cortex became deprived of its medullary blood supply. Growth of a vascular membrane was requisite to convey regenerative medullary arterioles to the devitalized cortex (see **Fig. 2-42**). Some implants, with intentionally porous surfaces, are conducive to fibrous tissue and bone ingrowth. Internal vascularity is evidently excellent, otherwise the observed widespread pervasion by tissue would not occur. Thus, the vascular response of bone to metals is dependent chiefly upon the site of placement, the effects of implantation upon normal blood supply, the stability of the implant, its surface characteristics, and its continued function.

10.2   Ceramics

Aluminum oxide ceramics can be totally inert in osseous tissue under the same unstressed conditions that cause encapsulation of implants of the surgical metals [280]. The ceramic was porous, but with an average pore size of only 18 μm; too small for invasion by osseous tissue. It has been shown that a pore size of at least 100 μm is required for the growth of bone into a compatible implant. A ceramic implant with interconnecting pores may become totally invaded by bone [281]. Internal vascularization must therefore be excellent.

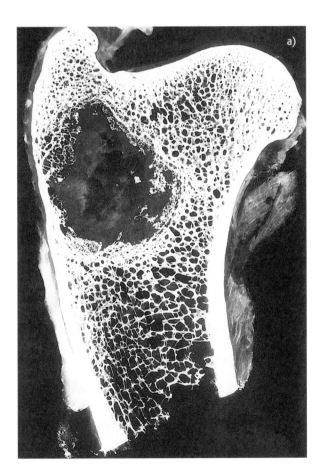

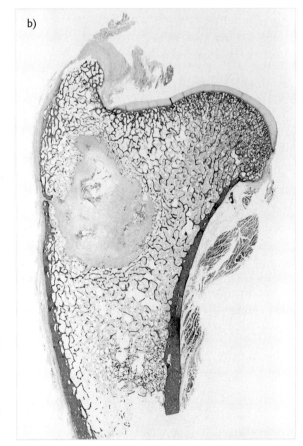

Fig. 2-59:
Proximal canine humerus 4 months after implantation of a gelatin sponge into a metaphyseal defect [281].
a) Original defect can be distinguished easily on photomicroradiograph (×4).
b) and on photomicrograph (Goldner's stain; ×4).

10.3 Polymeric and composite materials

Polymeric materials produce no specific vascular effects. The physical form of the material and the site of placement affect bone blood supply. A highly porous and resilient composite of polytetrafluoroethylene (Teflon) and pyrolytic graphite, known commercially as Proplast, was studied extensively in our laboratory [280, 282, 283]. Implants of Proplast in long bones were readily and completely invaded by vessels and connective tissue, and by osseous tissue marginally. The lack of deep invasion of the Proplast by osseous tissue was considered an asset because the resiliency of the raw Proplast was preserved.

In a preliminary test of a medullary implant with four flutes and a coating of Proplast in the flutes, we found that the Proplast was fully invaded by fibrous tissue, and marginally invaded by bone [283]. Medullary arterioles were observed within the Proplast coating (**Fig. 2-60**). Push-out tests showed good fixation. It was believed that the slight residual flexibility of the Proplast coating might produce a desirable situation around a prosthesis stem, functionally analogous to the shock-absorbing periodontal membrane around the root of a tooth.

10.4 Acrylic cement

Acrylic cement has been used very successfully as a grouting material following reaming to assist the internal fixation of hip prostheses [284]. As has been addressed earlier in discussion of tight-fitting medullary nailing, reaming destroys medullary circulation, devascularizes overlying cortex, and devitalizes bone (**Section 8.1.2**, "Cloverleaf nails"). In canine experiments simulating hip arthroplasty, full recovery by the osseous tissue of the femur was not observed until 6 months after reaming [282]. When reaming was followed immediately by insertion of acrylic cement, devitalization persisted for longer (**Fig. 2-61**) [285]. The cement was tight, but not under weight-bearing stress. Nevertheless, the cement became separated from the inner surface of the reamed cortex by a membrane bringing in regenerative medullary vessels to the devitalized cortex

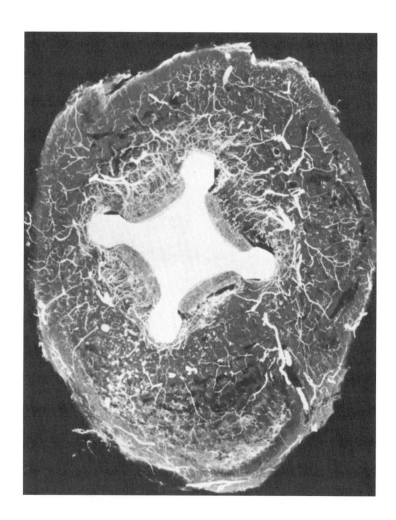

Fig. 2-60: Mature canine femur 14 weeks after transverse osteotomy, medullary reaming and fixation with a 4-fluted nail, with Proplast coating the depths of the flutes. Photomicroangiograph of a transverse section proximal to the osteotomy showing vascular invasion in the Proplast. A moderate amount of periosteal callus, derived from the healing osteotomy, is present externally (×8).

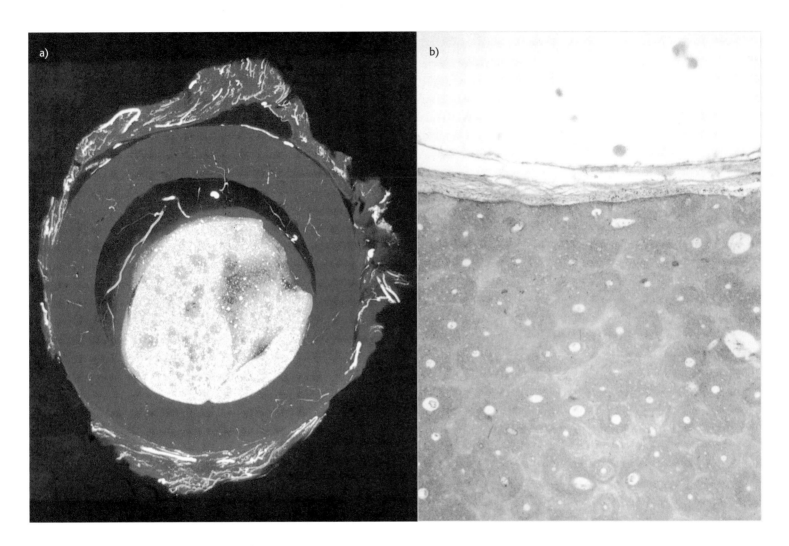

Fig. 2-61: Canine proximal femur 6 months after reaming and insertion of acrylic cement.

a) Photomicroangiograph distal to the tip of the prosthesis. Above, a thick membrane separates the cement from the open medullary space containing blood vessels. Below, the cement is in close contact with the cortex. Medullary blood vessels enter the cortex except where blocked by the cement (×10) [284].

b) Photomicrographic enlargement of the endosteal cortex where the acrylic cement was in tight contact. The intervening membrane is thin, and all the cortex is devoid of osteocytes (H and E stain; ×120) [288].

(**Fig. 2-61b**). The fibrovascular membrane was analogous to what we had observed after Küntscher medullary nailing (**Section 8.1.2**, "Cloverleaf nails"). Revitalization of the cortex was not complete in the canine femur even after a year. The presence of a membrane, where cement and cortex had originally been in tight contact, produced a situation favorable for loosening of the prosthesis.

Vascular studies with Simplex cement in canine femora demonstrated the lack of thermal or toxic reaction. The persistent cortical devitalization was due entirely to the physical presence of the cement, blocking return of the medullary blood supply destroyed by the preliminary reaming. This problem existed only in the diaphysis. The cancellous bone of the femoral metaphysis retained vascularization derived from the multiple metaphyseal arteries.

For a longer lasting, biologic fixation of prostheses within bone, orthopedists have turned to cementless prostheses, which have a surface conducive to bone ingrowth. de Waal Malefijt et al. compared the vascular changes up to 6 weeks following hip arthroplasty with and without cementing in African pygmy goats [286]. Cortical devascularization and de-vitalization were seen with the cemented hips. Endosteal revascularization was first seen at the 5th postoperative week, with very gradual progression in the 6th week. In cementless hips, metaphyseal trabecular bone remained richly vascular. Small incongruities, between the press-fit prosthesis and adjacent bone, were vascularized at 3 weeks, with progressive regeneration of the medullary circulation through these gaps to the 6th week. LDF red-cell flux changes have been reported following intramedullary reaming and cement implantation [287]. The greatest insult from reaming occurred to cortical red-cell flux. The greater blood supply seemed to diminish the effects of reaming to the metaphysis. However, with cement implantation, metaphyseal red-cell flux was significantly re-duced. The marked increases in intramedullary pressure and physical obstruction to vascular shunting that occurs with cement implantation caused the metaphyseal red-cell flux to diminish to the levels seen in the cortex following reaming. Supposedly, a similar situation occurs with many of the non-cemented arthroplasty systems, although few studies have included actual evaluation of vascularity.

Ischemia resulting from vascular interruption is not the only side-effect seen with reaming, and with reaming and implantation of acrylic cements. Danckwardt-Lilliestrom [288] demonstrated that intracortical bone-marrow embolisms could be an important complication to reaming. Also, Olerud et al. found massive fat embolism in the femoral vein after reaming lapine tibiae [289]. Danckwardt-Lilliestrom et al. later reported mortality due to pulmonary fat emboli of 11% in reamed animals with clinical signs of embolism in an additional 10%

[290]. The correlation between high intramedullary pressure during reaming and implantation of acrylic and pulmonary fat-embolism has also been reported clinically. Postmortems on patients who had acute cardiac arrest during a total hip or knee arthroplasty or hemiarthroplasty have revealed massive pul-monary fat embolism and bone-marrow embolism [291, 292].

10.5 Other materials

Polylactide-polyglycolide has recently been shown to delay neo-osteogenesis around and into a bone chamber containing the copolymer [293]. The authors suggested that the observed delay in angiogenesis and osteogenesis was a consequence of a macrophage response to slowly eroding poly-L-lactide crystal nano-particles. Vessel ingrowth slowed down and vessels matured prematurely, resulting in vessel caliper exceeding the diameter for optimum oxygen and nutrient exchange. Osteogenesis was thus impaired due to reduced oxygen supply and reduced nutrient exchange in the area of the implant.

11 Compendium on the blood supply to bone

Bone must be alive for any of its physiologic processes to function, and that requires an adequate blood supply. The blood supply of a long bone is best considered in terms of vascular systems. The afferent vascular system carries arterial blood and is derived chiefly from the principal nutrient artery, supplemented through its anastomoses with metaphyseal arteries. It goes principally to the interior of a long bone where the intravascular pressure is highest. The direction of blood flow through the cortex is normally centrifugal, from medulla to periosteum. The periosteal arterioles are a minor component of the afferent system: they supply the outer layers of cortex only in the vicinity of firm fascial attachments (Fig. 2-62).

The efferent vascular system drains venous effluent from all portions of a long bone. Medullary cavity and cortex are drained separately. Normally, the cortex appears to be drained principally from the periosteal surface, in keeping with the centrifugal direction of blood flow (**Fig. 2-62**). Under perturbed conditions, the direction of blood flow through cortex may follow alternate channels. Drainage of the marrow contents is through veins which traverse the full cortical thickness.

The intermediate vascular system, composed of thin-walled vessels of fixed size in the cortical canals of Havers and Volkmann, is the link between the afferent and efferent systems in compact bone. Bone tissue fluid within the lacunae and canaliculi of bone appears to comprise a distinct and separate fluid compartment. Cell processes within the canaliculi convey nutrients from the vessels of the bone canals to the osteocytes.

Vessels do not cross the active physeal plate; thus, during growth, the epiphysis and metaphysis have separate vascular supplies. An extensive longitudinal vasculature supplies the periosteum in support of appositional bone deposition to increase bone girth. Blood flow is greater than in mature bones and is centered on areas of active growth. At maturity, vessels cross the growth plate, the metaphyseal and epiphyseal vasculature becomes one, and the periosteal vasculature atrophies to only a vestige.

The flow of blood in cortical bone canals has a resting level and a stimulated level. The difference represents bone's potential for increased functional blood supply. At a site of bone repair, the afferent vascular components increase in functional activity. When required, supplemental blood supply can be derived from periosteous soft tissues. It is preferably referred to as the "extraosseous blood supply". It is variable, transitory, and distinct from the normal component comprising

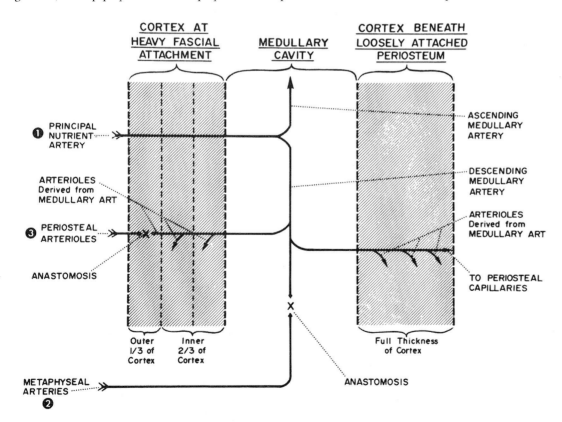

Fig. 2-62: Diagram showing the distribution of the afferent vascular system to a mature long bone. Components 1, 2, and 3 are its source of blood from the general arterial circulation. The arrows indicate the direction of blood flow.

the periosteal arterioles. The new extraosseous supply furnishes blood to detached bone fragments, to periosteal callus, and to cortex, which has been devascularized by trauma or surgical intervention. As the normal components of the bone's blood supply are re-established, the extraosseous vasculature subsides. The process of bone healing is directed toward regeneration of the normal pattern of blood supply to the bone. Its regenerative powers are rapid and enormous.

The two essential factors in fracture healing are blood supply and stabilization. Each may be partially compromised, but both must be present to an adequate degree for healing to occur. If not, non-union and eventual pseudarthrosis may result. The various methods of fixation available provide a varying amount of the stabilization necessary for fracture healing. However, each method compromises the blood supply to bone to some degree, and it is this compromise that must be considered when selecting appropriate treatment for a specific fracture (**Fig. 2-63**).

Fractures stabilized with intramedullary nails or rods heal with bridging fibrocartilaginous callus. Insertion of an intramedullary rod or nail disrupts medullary vasculature. The larger the nail is, in comparison with the medullary cavity, the greater the damage. Reaming totally destroys normal medullary circulation and devitalizes the cortex. The cross-sectional size and configuration of an intramedullary nail control the course and rapidity of regeneration of the medullary arterial circulation.

Cerclage devices, even when flat and wide, do not disrupt normal cortical vascularity. Bands have been found to be inherently weaker than wires and, for this reason alone, have limited use in fracture management. Wire loops do not interfere with appositional bone deposition in growing bone, even when placed directly over the periosteum. During bone healing there is still no interference with vascularization by wire loops. Wide bands, however, may block extraosseous arterioles as they approach the cortical surface perpendicularly and

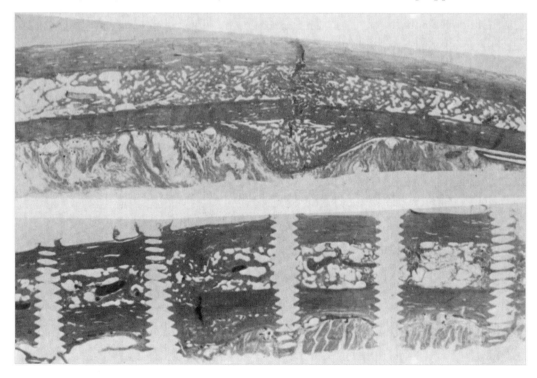

Fig. 2-63: Photomicrographs of paired radii of a mature dog, 8 weeks after osteotomy and internal fixation with different degrees of stabilization, shows the production of osseous callus with respect to the stabilization achieved (H and E stain; ×3.5) [1].

thereby reduce extraosseous supply to developing callus and neonutrient-artery augmentation of medullary circulation.

The use of strong plates, and screws, in fracture repair has led to: more anatomical repairs, more rapid ambulation, improved joint use, and in certain circumstances augmented bone healing. We now recognize that, in addition to the direct effect on fracture healing, the drilling of holes, placement of screws, plate application, and long-term presence of the plate all play a role in development of osteopenia of the bone, to varying degrees and at differing times. Much of this effect can be attributed to alteration in blood flow to bone beneath the plate.

The vascular response, and degree of incorporation of bone grafts, are dependent on site of implantation, stability of the grafted site, and, of course, the type of graft material. Vascularization to the graft may come from medullary blood supply, as with inlay cortical grafts, or may be chiefly by the extraosseous blood supply, as with cancellous chips. As the grafted defect fills, medullary-derived blood supply becomes dominant. Transplanted diaphyseal segments may remain relatively intact long after transplantation and may never completely vascularize or be replaced. Transplanted bone may serve as a scaffold for new bone formation and, as such, become an integral component of the healed bone. An excellent long-term clinical result may be achieved without complete replacement of transplanted bone.

The vascular response of bone to all implants of biocompatible materials is chiefly dependent upon: the site of placement; the effect of implantation upon normal blood supply; the stability of the implant and its surface characteristics, as well as its continued function. Bone physiology should be foremost in the consideration of the bioengineer who designs implants, and of the surgeon who inserts them [294].

12 Bibliography

Blue references indicate links to abstracts of articles available online:
http://www.aopublishing.org/BONE/2.htm

1. **Rhinelander FW** (1972) Circulation in bone. In: Bourne GD, editor. *The Biochemistry and Physiology of Bone.* 2nd ed. New York: Academic Press, 1.

2. **Eitel F, Seiler H, Schweiberer L** (1981) [Morphological examination of animal-experiment results: comparison with regeneration of the human bone-structure. II. Research results (author's transl)]. *Unfallheilkunde;* 84 (6):255–264.

3. **Rhinelander FW, Stewart CL, Wilson JW** (1979) Bone vascular supply. In: Simmons DL, Kunin AS, editors. *Skeletal Research.* New York: Academic Press, 367.

4. **Wilson JW, Rhinelander FW, Stewart CL** (1985) Vascularization of cancellous chip bone grafts. *Am J Vet Res;* 46 (8):1691–1699.

5. **Wilson JW, Hoefle WD** (1990) Diaphyseal allograft: Eight year evaluation in a dog. *Vet Comp Orthop Traumatol;* 3:74.

6. **Trueta J, Barclay AE, Daniel PM, et al.** (1947) *Studies of the Renal Circulation.* Oxford: Blackwell Scientific Publications.

7. **Barclay AE** (1951) *Microangiography and Other Radiological Techniques Employed in Biological Research.* Oxford: Blackwell Scientific Publications.

8. **Chidgey L, Chakkalakal D, Blotcky A, et al.** (1986) Vascular reorganization and return of rigidity in fracture healing. *J Orthop Res;* 4 (2):173–179.

9. **Wilson JW, Arighi M** (1999) A proposed method of quantifying microangiograms. *Vet Comp Orthop Traumatol;* 12:227.

10. **Spalteholz KW** (1911) *Über das Durchsichtigmachen von menschlichen und tiereschen Präparaten nebst Anhang: Über Knochenfärbung.* Leipzig: S Hirzel Verlag.

11. **Pinard A** (1952) *Structure et vaisseauz de la diaphyse des os longs chez le foetus humain* [Diss]. Basel.

12. **Novak V** (1959) Arrangement of vessels in the periosteum of long bones in the newborn. *Cesk Morf;* 7:353.

13. **Irving MH** (1965) The blood supply of the growth cartilage and metaphysis in rachitic rats. *J Pathol Bacteriol;* 89:461.

14. **Brookes M, Helal B** (1968) Primary osteoarthritis, venous engorement and osteogenesis. *J Bone Joint Surg [Br];* 50 (3):493–504.

15. **Day B, Shim SS, Leung G** (1984) Effect of the high femoral osteotomy upon the vascularity and blood supply of the hip joint. *Surg Gynecol Obstet;* 158 (5):443–449.

16. **Eppley BL, Doucet M, Connolly DT, et al.** (1988) Enhancement of angiogenesis by bFGF in mandibular bone graft healing in the rabbit. *J Oral Maxillofac Surg;* 46 (5):391–398.

17. **Eitel FM, Seibold RC, Schmid HC** (1986) Progress in microangiography by modification of the Spalteholz technique. *Proc 32nd Ann Mtg Orthop Res Soc;* 11:189.

18. **deMarneffe R** (1951) Recherches morphologiques et experimentales sur la vascularisation osseuse. *Acta Chir Belg;* 50:469.

19. **Wray JB, Lynch CJ** (1959) The vascular response to fracture of the tibia in the rat. *J Bone Joint Surg [Am];* 41:1143.

20. **Arsenault AL** (1987) Microvascular organization at the epiphyseal-metaphyseal junction of growing rats. *J Bone Miner Res;* 2 (2):143–149.

21. **Zamboni L, Pease DC** (1961) The vascular bed of red bone marrow. *J Ultrastruct Res;* 5:65.

22. **Kelly PJ** (1973) Comparison of marrow and cortical bone blood flow by 125 I-labeled 4-iodoantipyrine (I-Ap) washout. *J Lab Clin Med;* 81 (4): 497–505.

23. **Kofoed H, Sjontoft E, Siemssen SO, et al.** (1985) Bone marrow circulation after osteotomy. Blood flow, Po_2, Pco_2, and pressure studied in dogs. *Acta Orthop Scand;* 56 (5):400–403.

24. **Rosenthal MS, DeLuca PM, Pearson DW, et al.** (1987) An in vivo technique for the measurement of bone blood flow in animals. *Phys Med Biol;* 32 (4):453–462.

25. **Oberg PA, Tenland T, Nilsson GE** (1984) Laser-Doppler flowmetry—a non-invasive and continuous method for blood flow evaluation in microvascular studies. *Acta Med Scand Suppl;* 687:17–24.

26. **Jurvelin J, Lahtinen T, Kiviranta I, et al.** (1988) Blood flow, histomorphology and elemental composition of the canine femur after physical training or immobilization. *Acta Physiol Scand;* 132 (3):385–389.

27. **Niv AI, Hungerford DS, Jones LC** (1980) Simultaneous bone blood flow measurements in dogs utilizing radioactive tracer microspheres and hydrogen washout. *Proc 26th Ann Mtg Orthop Res Soc;* 5:156.

28. **Jones LC, Weiland AJ, Berggren A** (1981) Microcirculation in cortical bone as measured by the hydrogen washout technique. *Proc 27th Ann Mtg Orthop Res Soc;* 6:256.

29. **Collins PC** (1982) The relationship of electrically stimulated bone growth and juxta-electrode blood flow. *Proc Inst Med Chic;* 35 (3):74–76.

30. **Schoenecker PL, Lesker PA, Ogata K** (1984) A dynamic canine model of experimental hip dysplasia. Gross and histological pathology, and the effect of position of immobilization on capital femoral epiphyseal blood flow. *J Bone Joint Surg [Am];* 66 (8):1281–1288.

31. **Zdeblick TA, Shaffer JW, Field GA** (1988) The healing of canine vascularized segmental tibial osteotomies. The effect of retained endosteal circulation. *Clin Orthop;* (236):296–302.

32. **Kiaer T, Gronlund J, Jensen B, et al.** (1990) Effects of variation in systemic blood pressure on intraosseous pressure, Po_2, and Pco_2. *J Orthop Res;* 8 (4):618–622.

33. **Weinman DT, Kelly PJ, Owen CA, et al.** (1963) Skeletal clearance of [47]Ca and [85]Sr and skeletal blood flow in dogs. *Proc Staff Mtg Mayo Clin;* 38:559.

34. **Lewallen DG, Chao EY, Kasman RA, et al.** (1984) Comparison of the effects of compression plates and external fixators on early bone-healing. *J Bone Joint Surg [Am];* 66 (7):1084–1091.

35. **Hart MB, Wu JJ, Chao EY, et al.** (1985) External skeletal fixation of canine tibial osteotomies. Compression compared with no compression. *J Bone Joint Surg [Am];* 67 (4):598–605.

36. **Daum WJ, Simmons DJ, Chang SL, et al.** (1985) Effect of fixation devices on radiostrontium clearance in the intact canine femur. *Clin Orthop;* (194):306–312.

37. **Daum WJ, Simmons DJ, Calhoun JH, et al.** (1988) Regional alterations in long bone produced by internal fixation devices. Part I. [85]Sr clearance. *J Orthop Trauma;* 2 (3):241–244.

38. **Riggs SA, Wood MB, Cooney WP, et al.** (1984) Blood flow and bone uptake of 99mTc-labeled methylene diphosphonate. *J Orthop Res;* 1 (3): 236–243.

39. **Tothill P, Hooper G** (1984) Invalidity of single-passage measurements of the extraction of bone-seeking tracers in rats and rabbits. *J Orthop Res;* 2 (1):75–79.

40. **Nutton RW, Fitzgerald RH, Brown ML, et al.** (1984) Dynamic radioisotope bone imaging as a non-invasive indicator of canine tibial blood flow. *J Orthop Res;* 2 (1):67–74.

41. **Nutton RW, Fitzgerald RH, Kelly PJ** (1985) Early dynamic bone-imaging as an indicator of osseous blood flow and factors affecting the uptake of ^{99m}Tc hydroxymethylene diphosphonate in healing bone. *J Bone Joint Surg [Am];* 67 (5):763–770.

42. **Nottebaert M, Lane JM, Juhn A, et al.** (1989) Omental angiogenic lipid fraction and bone repair. An experimental study in the rat. *J Orthop Res;* 7 (2):157–169.

43. **Einhorn TA, Vigorita VJ, Aaron A** (1986) Localization of technetium-99m methylene diphosphonate in bone using microautoradiography. *J Orthop Res;* 4 (2):180–187.

44. **Prinzmetal M, Simkin B, Bergman HC, et al.** (1947) Studies on the coronary circulation—II. The collateral circulation of the normal human heart by coronary perfusion with radioactive erythrocytes and glass spheres. *Am Heart J;* 33:420.

45. **Kane WJ, Grim E** (1969) Blood flow to canine hind-limb bone, muscle, and skin. A quantitative method and its validation. *J Bone Joint Surg [Am];* 51 (2):309–322.

46. **Lunde PK, Michelsen K** (1970) Determination of cortical blood flow in rabbit femur by radioactive microspheres. *Acta Physiol Scand;* 80 (1):39–44.

47. **Maki Y, Breidenbach WC, Firrell JC** (1993) Evaluation of a local microsphere injection method for measurement of blood flow in the rabbit lower extremity. *J Orthop Res;* 11 (1):20–27.

48. **Gross PM, Heistad DD, Marcus ML** (1979) Neurohumoral regulation of blood flow to bones and marrow. *Am J Physiol;* 237 (4):H440–448.

49. **Triffitt PD, Gregg PJ** (1990) Measurement of blood flow to the tibial diaphysis using 11-microns radioactive microspheres. A comparative study in the adult rabbit. *J Orthop Res;* 8 (5):642–645.

50. **Morris MA, Kelly PJ** (1980) Use of tracer microspheres to measure bone blood flow in conscious dogs. *Calcif Tissue Int;* 32 (1):69–76.

51. **Tothill P, MacPherson JN** (1986) The distribution of blood flow to the whole skeleton in dogs, rabbits and rats measured with microspheres. *Clin Phys Physiol Meas;* 7 (2):117–123.

52. **Tothill P, Hooper G, Hughes SP, et al.** (1987) Bone blood flow measured with microspheres: the problem of non-entrapment. *Clin Phys Physiol Meas;* 8 (1):51–55.

53. **Robertson WW, Janssen HF, Walker RN** (1985) Passive movement of radioactive microspheres from bone and soft tissue in an extremity. *J Orthop Res;* 3 (4):405–411.

54. **Buckberg GD, Luck JC, Payne DB, et al.** (1971) Some sources of error in measuring regional blood flow with radioactive microspheres. *J Appl Physiol;* 31 (4):598–604.

55. **Li G, Bronk JT, Kelly PJ** (1989) Canine bone blood flow estimated with microspheres. *J Orthop Res;* 7 (1):61–67.

56. **McGrory BJ, Moran CG, Bronk JT, et al.** (1993) Canine blood flow measurements using serial microsphere injections. *Proc 39th Ann Mtg Orthop Res Soc;* 18:250.

57. **Hansen ES, Soballe K, Kjolseth D, et al.** (1990) Uneven distribution of microspheres and soluble tracers in bone: Microvascular skimming or arteriovenous shunting? *Proc 36th Ann Mtg Orthop Res Soc;* 15:285.

58. **McCarthy ID** (1994) An alternative to microspheres for the measurement of bone blood flow. *Proc 40th Ann Mtg Orthop Res Soc;* 19:789.

59. **Bray RC, Butterwick DJ, Doschak MR, et al.** (1996) Coloured microsphere assessment of blood flow to knee ligaments in adult rabbits: effects of injury. *J Orthop Res;* 14 (4): 618–625.

60. **Notzli HP, Swiontkowski MF, Thaxter ST, et al.** (1989) Laser Doppler flowmetry for bone blood flow measurements: helium-neon laser light attenuation and depth of perfusion assessment. *J Orthop Res;* 7 (3):413–424.

61. **Lausten GS, Kiaer T, Dahl B** (1993) Laser Doppler flowmetry for estimation of bone blood flow: studies of reproducibility and correlation with microsphere technique. *J Orthop Res;* 11 (4):573–580.

62. **Swiontkowski MF, Tepic S, Perren SM, et al.** (1986) Laser Doppler flowmetry for bone blood flow measurement: correlation with microsphere estimates and evaluation of the effect of intracapsular pressure on femoral head blood flow. *J Orthop Res;* 4 (3):362–371.

63. **Swiontkowski MF, Schlehr F, Collins JC, et al.** (1988) Comparison of two laser Doppler flowmetry systems for bone blood flow analysis. *Calcif Tissue Int;* 43 (2):103–107.

64. **Swiontkowski MF, Senft D** (1990) Ischemic and flow variable influences on cortical bone microperfusion. *Proc 36th Ann Mtg Orthop Res Soc;* 15:588.

65. **Swiontkowski MF, Senft D** (1992) Cortical bone microperfusion: response to ischemia and changes in major arterial blood flow. *J Orthop Res;* 10 (3):337–343.

66. **Schemitsch EH, Kowalski MJ, Swiontkowski MF** (1994) Evaluation of a laser Doppler flowmetry implantable fiber system for determination of threshold thickness for flow detection in bone. *Proc 40th Ann Mtg Orthop Res Soc;* 19:787.

67. **Fukuoka S, Hotokebuchi R, Terada K, et al.** (1995) Experimental studies on a measurement of subchondral bone blood flow by the laser speckle method. *Proc 41st Ann Mtg Orthop Res Soc;* 20:787.

68. **Lewallen DG, Wikenheiser MA, Chao EYS, et al.** (1990) MRI assessment of the canine femoral head after subcapital osteotomy with correlation to bone blood flow changes. *Proc 36th Ann Mtg Orthop Res Soc;* 15:266.

69. **Neff B, Jones L, Cova M, et al.** (1990) A new MRI technique to detect changes in bone blood flow. *Proc 36th Ann Mtg Orthop Res Soc;* 15:586.

70. **Martiat P, Ferrant A, Cogneau M, et al.** (1987) Assessment of bone marrow blood flow using positron emission tomography: no relationship with bone marrow cellularity. *Br J Haematol;* 66 (3):307–310.

71. **Kimori K, Iwanami H, Kubo T** (1994) The study of the vascular bed volume distribution in femoral heads of healthy adult males by positron emission tomography. *Proc 40th Ann Mtg Orthop Res Soc;* 19:794.

72. **Kubo T, Kimori K, Iwanami H, et al.** (1994) Measurement of blood flow and volume in the femoral head by positron emission tomography. *Proc 40th Ann Mtg Orthop Res Soc;* 19:212.

73. **Kiaer T, Dahl B, Lausten G** (1992) Partial pressures of oxygen and carbon dioxide in bone and their correlation with bone-blood flow: effect of decreased arterial supply and venous congestion on intraosseous oxygen and carbon dioxide in an animal model. *J Orthop Res;* 10 (6): 807–812.

74. **Ganey TM, Love SM, Ogden JA** (1992) Development of vascularization in the chondroepiphysis of the rabbit. *J Orthop Res;* 10 (4):496–510.

75. **Brookes M** (1971) *The Blood Supply of Bone.* London: Butterworth.

76. **Hulse DA, Abdelbaki YZ, Wilson JW** (1981) Revascularization of femoral capital physeal fractures following surgical fixation. *J Vet Orthop;* 2:50.

77. **Johnson CE, Wang GJ, Croft BY, et al.** (1980) The circulatory anatomy of the distal femoral epiphysis in the dog. *Proc 26th Ann Mtg Orthop Res Soc;* 5:263.

78. **Naito M, Ogata K, Emoto G, et al.** (1994) The effects of surgical procedures on the blood supply to the greater trochanter. *Proc 40th Ann Mtg Orthop Res Soc;* 19:793.

79. **Firth EC, Poulos PW** (1982) Blood vessels in the developing growth plate of the equine distal radius and metacarpus. *Res Vet Sci;* 33 (2):159–166.

80. **Firth EC, Poulos PW** (1983) Microangiographic studies of metaphyseal vessels in young foals. *Res Vet Sci;* 34 (2):231–235.

81. **Arighi M, Wilson JW** (1990) Effects of periosteal stripping on bone growth (Abstr). *Vet Surg;* 19:56.

82. **Hill MA, Ruth GR, Bagent JK, et al.** (1985) Angiomicrographic investigation of the vessels associated with physes in young pigs. *Res Vet Sci;* 38 (2):151–159.

83. **Oki S, Matsuda Y, Itoh T, et al.** (1994) Scanning electron microscopic observations of the vascular structure of vertebral end-plates in rabbits. *J Orthop Res;* 12 (3):447–449.

84. **Nakano T, Thompson JR, Christopherson RJ, et al.** (1986) Blood flow distribution in hind limb bones and joint cartilage from young growing pigs. *Can J Vet Res;* 50 (1): 96–100.

85. **Kirkeby OJ, Berg-Larsen T** (1991) Regional blood flow and strontium-85 incorporation rate in the rat hindlimb skeleton. *J Orthop Res;* 9 (6): 862–868.

86. **Light T, McKinstry M, Schnitzer J, et al.** (1981) Regional osseous flow determination in neonatal, immature, and mature canines. *Proc 27th Ann Mtg Orthop Res Soc;* 6:218.

87. **Roush JK, Howard PE, Wilson JW** (1989) Normal blood supply to the canine mandible and mandibular teeth. *Am J Vet Res;* 50 (6):904–907.

88. **Roush JK, Wilson JW** (1989) Healing of mandibular body osteotomies after plate and intramedullary pin fixation. *Vet Surg;* 18 (3):190–196.

89. **Rischen CG, Wilson JW, Swain CA** (1987) Effect of application of polyvinilidine plates on the dorsal spinous processes of dogs. *Vet Surg;* 16 (4): 294–298.

90. **Brookes M, Harrison RG** (1957) The vascularization of the rabbit femur and tibiofibula. *J Anat;* 91:61.

91. **MacNab I** (1957) Blood supply of the tibia. *J Bone Joint Surg [Br];* 39:799.

92. **MacNab I** (1958) Blood supply of tubular and cancellous bone. *J Bone Joint Surg [Am];* 40:1433.

93. **MacAuley GO** (1958) The blood supply of the rat's femur in relation to the repair of cortical defects. *J Anat;* 92:665.

94. **Jackson RW, MacNab I** (1959) Fractures of the shaft of the tibia: A clinical and experimental study. *Am J Surg;* 97:543.

95. **Nelson GG, Kelly PJ, Lowell FA, et al.** (1960) Blood supply of the human tibia. *J Bone Joint Surg [Am];* 42:625.

96. **Brookes M** (1964) The blood supply of bone. In: Clark JMP, editor. *Modern Trends in Orthopaedics.* London: Butterworth, 91.

97. **Brookes M** (1967) The osseous circulation. *Biomed Eng;* 2:294.

98. **Bauer MS, Walker TL** (1988) Intramedullary pressure in canine long bones. *Am J Vet Res;* 49 (3): 425–427.

99. **Branemark P-I** (1959) Vital microscopy of bone marrow in rabbits. *Scand J Clin Lab Invest;* 38S:5.

100. **Rhinelander FW** (1974) Tibial blood supply in relation to fracture healing. *Clin Orthop;* 105 (0):34–81.

101. **Tothill P, Hooper G, McCarthy ID, et al.** (1987) The pattern of distribution of blood flow in dog limb bones measured using microspheres. *Clin Phys Physiol Meas;* 8 (3):239–247.

102. **Shim SS, Copp DH, Patterson FP** (1968) Measurement of the rate and distribution of the nutrient and other arterial blood supply in long bones of the rabbit. A study of the relative con-tribution of the three arterial systems. *J Bone Joint Surg [Br];* 50 (1): 178–183.

103. **Simpson AH** (1985) The blood supply of the periosteum. *J Anat;* 140 (Pt 4):697–704.

104. **Cooper RC, Cawley AJ** (1988) Blood supply to the periosteum of the canine tibia. *Am J Vet Res;* 49 (8): 1419–1423.

105. **Whiteside LA, Schoenecker PL** (1980) The effect of experimental subperiosteal and extraperiosteal dissection on the blood supply of the periostem. *Proc 26th Ann Mtg Orthop Res Soc;* 5:200.

106. **Wilson JW, Stewart CL, Rhinelander FW** (1980) A microangiographic and correlated histologic investigation of healing canine segmental osteotomies. *Proc 26th Ann Mtg Orthop Res Soc;* 5:203.

107. **Robinson RA, Cameron DA** (1958) Electron microscopy of the primary spongiosa of the metaphysis at the distal end of the femur in the newborn infant. *J Bone Joint Surg [Am];* 40:687.

108. **Holtrop ME** (1975) The ultra-structure of bone. *Ann Clin Lab Sci;* 5 (4):264–271.

109. **Doty SB** (1981) Morphological evidence of gap junctions between bone cells. *Calcif Tissue Int;* 33 (5): 509–512.

110. **Palumbo C, Palazzini S, Marotti G** (1990) Morphological study of inter-cellular junctions during osteocyte differentiation. *Bone;* 11 (6):401–406.

111. **Hughes S, Davies R, Khan R, et al.** (1978) Fluid space in bone. *Clin Orthop;* (134):332–341.

112. **Jowsey JD** (1978) Personal communication.

113. **Triffitt JT, Terepka AR, Neuman WF** (1968) A comparative study of the exchange in vivo of major constituents of bone mineral. *Calcif Tissue Res;* 2 (2):165–176.

114. **Owen M, Trifitt JT, Melick RP** (1973) Albumin in bone. In: Elliott K, Fitzsimmons DW, editors. *Hard Tissue Growth, Repair and Mineralization. Ciba Foundation Symposium 11.* Amsterdam: Elsevier, 263.

115. **Hughes SP, McCarthy ID, Hooper G** (1986) The vascular system in bone. Its importance and relevance to clinical practice. *Clin Orthop;* (210): 31–36.

116. **Tilling G** (1958) The vascular anatomy of long bones: A radiological and histological study. *Acta Radio-logica;* 161S:12.

117. **Leriche R, Policard A** (1926) *Les Problemes de la Physiologie Normale et Pathologique de IO's.* Paris: Masson.

118. **Janssen HF, Culbertson MC, Williams CD, et al.** (1988) Anatomy of venous drainage from the femur of dogs and Rhesus monkeys. *Proc 34th Ann Mtg Orthop Res Soc;* 13:417.

119. **Rhinelander FW, Wilson JW** (1982) Blood supply to developing, mature, and healing bone. In: Sumner-Smith G, editor. *Bone in Clinical Orthopaedics.* 1st ed. Philadelphia: W. B. Saunders Co., 81.

120. **Kirby BM, Wilson JW** (1991) Effect of circumferential bands on cortical vascularity and viability. *J Orthop Res;* 9 (2):174–179.

121. **Aalto K, Slatis P** (1984) Blood flow in rabbit osteotomies studied with radioactive microspheres. *Acta Orthop Scand;* 55 (6):637–639.

122. **Wooton R** (1988) Errors in bone blood flow measured with microspheres due to sample preparation technique. *Clin Phys Physiol Meas;* 9:273.

123. **Schemitsch EH, Richards RR, Bertoia JT** (1988) A quantitative evaluation of regional bone blood flow in the normal canine tibial diaphysis. *Proc 34th Ann Mtg Orthop Res Soc;* 13:413.

124. **Jones LC, Niv AI, Davis RF, et al.** (1982) Bone blood flow in the femora of anesthetized and conscious dogs in a chronic preparation, using the radioactive tracer microsphere method. *Clin Orthop;* (170):286–295.

125. **Willans SM, McCarthy ID** (1991) Heterogeneity of blood flow in tibial cortical bone: an experimental investigation using microspheres. *J Orthop Res;* 9 (2):168–173.

126. **Davis TR, Holloway I, Pooley J** (1990) The effect of anaesthesia on the bone blood flow of the rabbit. *J Orthop Res;* 8 (4):479–484.

127. **Tondevold E, Bulow J** (1983) Bone blood flow in conscious dogs at rest and during exercise. *Acta Orthop Scand;* 54 (1):53–57.

128. **Williams CD, Homan JA, Lust RM, et al.** (1989) Comparison of bone blood flow alterations produced by exercise and vasoactive compounds. *Proc 35th Ann Mtg Orthop Res Soc;* 14:517.

129. **Jesperson SM, Hoy K, Christensen KO** (1994) Axial and peripheral skeletal blood flow at rest and during exercise. *Proc 40th Ann Mtg Orthop Res Soc;* 19:293.

130. **McDonald F, Pitt Ford TR** (1993) Blood flow changes in the tibia during external loading. *J Orthop Res;* 11 (1):36–48.

131. **Bitz DM, Lux PS, Whiteside LA** (1980) The effects of early mobilization and casting on blood flow and mechanical properties of fracture healing. *Proc 26th Ann Mtg Orthop Res Soc;* 5:199.

132. **Triffitt PD, Cieslak CA, Gregg PJ** (1992) Cast immobilization and tibial diaphyseal blood flow: an initial study. *J Orthop Res;* 10 (6):784–788.

133. **Kawai K, Hirose T, Kita K, et al.** (1989) Changes of intraosseous blood flow and pressure in steroid treated rabbits. *Proc 35th Ann Mtg Orthop Res Soc;* 14:74.

134. **Yoshida M, Wang GJ, Fechner RE** (1993) Microangiographic approach to osteoporosis: A comparative study of vascular changes between postmeno-pausal and steroid-induced osteo-porosis. *Proc 39th Ann Mtg Orthop Res Soc;* 18:556.

135. **Davis RF, Jones LC, Hungerford DS** (1987) The effect of sympathectomy on blood flow in bone. Regional distribu-tion and effect over time. *J Bone Joint Surg [Am];* 69 (9):1384–1390.

136. **Takahashi H, Yamamuro T, Okumura H, et al.** (1990) Bone blood flow after spinal paralysis in the rat. *J Orthop Res;* 8 (3):393–400.

137. **Buma P, Elmans L, Oestreicher AB** (1995) Changes in innervation of long bones after insertion of an implant: immunocytochemical study in goats with antibodies to calcitonin gene-related peptide and B-50/GAP-43. *J Orthop Res;* 13 (4):570–577.

138. **Bjurholm A, Kreicbergs A, Terenius L, et al.** (1988) Neuro-peptide Y-, tyrosine hydroxylase- and vasoactive intestinal polypeptide-immunoreactive nerves in bone and surrounding tissues. *J Auton Nerv Syst;* 25 (2-3):119–125.

139. **McCarthy ID, Cochrane E, Hughes SPF** (1990) The effects of vaso-active substances and calcium regulating hormones on bone blood flow and strontium clearance. *Proc 36th Ann Mtg Orthop Res Soc;* 15:288.

140. **Brinker MR, Lippton HL, Cook SD, et al.** (1990) Pharmacological regulation of the circulation of bone. *J Bone Joint Surg [Am];* 72 (7):964–975.

141. **Pan Y, Wood MB, Vanhoutte PM** (1989) Influence of alpha 1 and alpha 2 adrenergic receptor blockage on canine intraosseous vascular smooth muscle tone. *Proc 35th Ann Mtg Orthop Res Soc;* 14:419.

142. **Dean MT, Wood MB, Vanhoutte PM** (1990) Effect of antagonist drugs on bone vascular smooth muscle. *Proc 36th Ann Mtg Orthop Res Soc;* 15:287.

143. **Dean MT, Wood MB, Vanhoutte PM** (1992) Antagonist drugs and bone vascular smooth muscle. *J Orthop Res;* 10 (1):104–111.

144. **Ye Z, Wood MB, Vanhoutte PM** (1990) Cumulative alpha subtype and calcium entry antagonism and bone vascular smooth muscle. *Proc 36th Ann Mtg Orthop Res Soc;* 15:286.

145. **Minkowitz B, Boskey AL, Lane JM, et al.** (1991) Effects of propranolol on bone metabolism in the rat. *J Orthop Res;* 9 (6):869–875.

146. **Lindblad BE, Nielsen LB, Bjurholm A, et al.** (1993) Vasoconstrictive action of neuropeptide Y in bone. *Proc 39th Ann Mtg Orthop Res Soc;* 18:249.

147. **Lindblad BE, Nielsen LB, Bjurholm A, et al.** (1995) Vasodilatory action of vasoactive intestinal peptide and substance P in bone. *Proc 41st Ann Mtg Orthop Res Soc;* 20:791.

148. **Lindblad NE, Nielsen LN, Bjurholm A, et al.** (1994) Vasodilatory action of calcitonin gene-related peptide in bone. *Proc 40th Ann Mtg Orthop Res Soc;* 19:792.

149. **Grills BL, Schuijers JA, Ward AR** (1997) Topical application of nerve growth factor improves fracture healing in rats. *J Orthop Res;* 15 (2): 235–242.

150. **Brindley GW, Williams EA, Bronk JT, et al.** (1988) Parathyroid hormone effects on skeletal exchange-able calcium and bone blood flow. *Am J Physiol;* 255 (1 Pt2):H94–100.

151. **Heckman JD, Aufdemorte TB, Athanasiou KA, et al.** (1995) Treatment of acute ostectomy defects in the dog radius with rhTGF-1. *Proc 41st Ann Mtg Orthop Res Soc;* 20:590.

152. **Lind M, Overgaard S, Soballe K, et al.** (1996) Transforming growth factor-beta 1 enhances bone healing to unloaded tricalcium phosphate coated implants: an experimental study in dogs. *J Orthop Res;* 14 (3): 343–350.

153. **Sumner DR, Turner TR, Purchio AF, et al.** (1996) Transforming growth factor beta enhances gap healing and bone ingrowth. *Proc 41st Ann Mtg Orthop Res Soc;* 20:191.

154. **Aspenberg P, Wang JS** (1994) Basic fibroblast growth factor increases new bone ingrowth into bone allografts. *Proc 40th Ann Mtg Orthop Res Soc;* 19:181.

155. **Wang JS, Aspenberg P** (1994) Basic fibroblast growth factor increases allograft incorporation. Bone chamber study in rats. *Acta Orthop Scand;* 65 (1):27–31.

156. **Aspenberg P, Thorngren KG, Lohmander LS** (1991) Dose-dependent stimulation of bone induction by basic fibroblast growth factor in rats. *Acta Orthop Scand;* 62 (5):481–484.

157. **Wang JS, Aspenberg P** (1993) Basic fibroblast growth factor and bone induction in rats. *Acta Orthop Scand;* 64 (5):557–561.

158. Wang JS, Aspenberg P (1996) Basic fibroblast growth factor enhances bone-graft incorporation: dose and time dependence in rats. *J Orthop Res;* 14 (2):316–323.

159. Jingushi S, Heydemann A, Kana SK, et al. (1990) Acidic fibroblast growth factor (aFGF) injection stimulates cartilage enlargement and inhibits cartilage gene expression in rat fracture healing. *J Orthop Res;* 8 (3):364-371.

160. DeSimone DP, Reddi AH (1992) Vascularization and endochondral bone development: changes in plasminogen activator activity. *J Orthop Res;* 10 (3):320–324.

161. Ehrlich MG, Armstrong AL, Mankin HJ (1984) Partial purification and characterization of a proteoglycan-degrading neutral protease from bovine epiphyseal cartilage. *J Orthop Res;* 2 (2):126–133.

162. Ehrlich MG, Armstrong AL, Mankin HJ (1984) Partial purification and characterization of a proteoglycan degradation by a neutral protease from human growth plate epiphyseal. *J Bone Joint Surg [Am];* 64:1350.

163. Einhorn TA, Hirschman A, Kaplan C, et al. (1989) Neutral protein-degrading enzymes in experimental fracture callus: a preliminary report. *J Orthop Res;* 7 (6):792–805.

164. Slater M, Patava J, Kingham K, et al. (1995) Involvement of platelets in stimulating osteogenic activity. *J Orthop Res;* 13 (5):655–663.

165. Bostrom MP, Lane JM, Berberian WS, et al. (1995) Immunolocalization and expression of bone morphogenetic proteins 2 and 4 in fracture healing. *J Orthop Res;* 13 (3): 357–367.

166. Kiaer T, Dahl B, Lausten GS (1993) The relationship between inert gas wash-out and radioactive tracer microspheres in measurement of bone blood flow: effect of decreased arterial supply and venous congestion on bone blood flow in an animal model. *J Orthop Res;* 11 (1): 28–35.

167. Settergren CR, Wood MB, Vanhoutte PM (1989) The effects of progressive normothermic and hypothermic ischemia on bone vascular smooth muscle: An ex vivo study. *Proc 35th Ann Mtg Orthop Res Soc;* 14:418.

168. Davis TRC, Wood MB (1991) The direct effects of hydrogen ion concentration on long bone vascular resistance. *Proc 37th Ann Mtg Orthop Res Soc;* 16:674.

169. Davis TR, Wood MB (1993) The effects of acidosis and alkalosis on long bone vascular resistance. *J Orthop Res;* 11 (6):834–839.

170. Davis TR, Wood MB, Vanhoutte PM (1992) The effect of hypothermic ischemia on the alpha-adrenergic mechanisms of the canine tibia vascular bed. *J Orthop Res;* 10 (1): 149–155.

171. Moran CG, McGrory BJ, Roorda J, et al. (1993) Adrenergic control mechanisms of bone blood flow in a vascularized canine allograft. *Proc 39th Ann Mtg Orthop Res Soc;* 18:251.

172. Moran CG, McGrory BJ, Roorda J, et al. (1993) Adrenergic control mechanisms of blood flow in a vascularized canine tibial allograft. *J Orthop Res;* 11 (3):429–437.

173. Bundgaard-Nielsen L, Lindblad BE, Gjedsted J, et al. (1995) Vasoactivity of the sympathetic transmitters norepinephrine and neuropeptide Y during local ischemia in bone. *Proc 41st Ann Mtg Orthop Res Soc;* 20:184.

174. Coessens BC, Miller VM, Wood MB (1996) Endothelin-A receptors mediate vascular smooth-muscle response to moderate acidosis in the canine tibial nutrient artery. *J Orthop Res;* 14 (5):818–822.

175. Pearson PJ, Lin PJ, Schaff HV (1991) Production of endothelium-derived contracting factor is enhanced after coronary reperfusion. *Ann Thorac Surg;* 51:788.

176. Moran CG, McGrory BJ, Bronk JT, et al. (1995) Reperfusion injury in vascularized bone allografts. *J Orthop Res;* 13 (3):368–374.

177. Weiss APC, Wang ESJ, Moore JR, et al. (1986) The role of oxygen free radicals in the reperfusion injury of ischemic revascularized bone grafts. *Proc 32nd Ann Mtg Orthop Res Soc;* 11:195.

178. Davis TR, Wood MB (1991) The effects of ischemia on long bone vascular resistance. *J Orthop Res;* 9 (6):883–889.

179. Davis TR, Wood MB (1992) Endothelial control of long bone vascular resistance. *J Orthop Res;* 10 (3):344–349.

180. Kregor PJ, Simonian PT, Bain S, et al. (1994) Oxygen free radicals in fracture healing. *Proc 40th Ann Mtg Orthop Res Soc;* 19:510.

181. Adams E, Bradford DS, Einzig S, et al. (1989) The change in fracture blood flow and the mineral content after electrical stimulation. *Proc 35th Ann Mtg Orthop Res Soc;* 14:471.

182. Nannmark U, Buch F, Albrektsson T (1988) Influence of direct currents on bone vascular supply. *Scand J Plast Reconstr Surg Hand Surg;* 22 (2):113–115.

183. Zichner L, Rhinelander FW, Nelson CL, et al. (1977) Electrical stimulation of bone formation—a microangiographic study. *Ortho Transact J Bone Joint Surg;* 1:225.

184. **Ho SSW, Illgen R, Meyer R, et al.** (1993) The effect of ice on skeletal blood flow and metabolism over time. *Proc 39th Ann Mtg Orthop Res Soc;* 18:298.

185. **Rhinelander FW** (1968) The normal microcirculation of diaphyseal cortex and its response to fracture. *J Bone Joint Surg [Am];* 50 (4):784–800.

186. **Wray JB, Spencer MP** (1960) The vasodilatory response to skeletal trauma. *ACS Surg Forum;* 11:444.

187. **Chang MC, Briggs PJ, Wood MB** (1994) Investigation of the acute effect of proximal osteotomy on regional blood flow changes in the canine ulna. *Proc 40th Ann Mtg Orthop Res Soc;* 19:791.

188. **Triffitt PD, Cieslak CA, Gregg PJ** (1993) A quantitative study of the routes of blood flow to the tibial diaphysis after an osteotomy. *J Orthop Res;* 11 (1):49–57.

189. **Richards RR, Anderson GI, Schemitsch E, et al.** (1990) Soft tissue blood flow after tibial osteotomy: A canine investigaion using cerium 41. *Proc 36th Ann Mtg Orthop Res Soc;* 15:290.

190. **Richards RR, Schemitsch EH, McKee MD** (1989) The relationship of bone blood flow to reparative activity in devascularized tibial cortex: An experimental investigation in the dog. *Proc 35th Ann Mtg Orthop Res Soc;* 14:420.

191. **Richards RR, Schemitsch EH** (1989) Effect of muscle flap coverage on bone blood flow following devascularization of a segment of tibia: an experimental investigation in the dog. *J Orthop Res;* 7 (4):550–558.

192. **Rizk WS, Levin LS, Glisson RR, et al.** (1995) The effect of rotational flap coverage on open fracture healing in a canine model. *Proc 41st Ann Mtg Orthop Res Soc;* 20:254.

193. **Strachan RK, Levin LS, Glisson RR, et al.** (1988) Microsphere estimation of bone blood flow in the osteotomized canine tibia and the role of the tibial nutrient artery. *Proc 34th Ann Mtg Orthop Res Soc;* 20:254.

194. **O'Driscoll SW, Fitzsimmons JS, Commisso CN** (1994) *In vitro* response of periosteum to variations in oxygen tension. *Proc 40th Ann Mtg Orthop Res Soc;* 19:353.

195. **Gothman L** (1961) Vascular reactions in experimental fractures. *Acta Chir Scand;* 284S.

196. **Rhinelander FW, Phillips RS, Steel WM, et al.** (1962) Microangiography in bone healing. I. Undisplaced closed fractures. *J Bone Joint Surg [Am];* 44:1273.

197. **Rhinelander FW, Phillips RS, Steel WM, et al.** (1968) Microangiography in bone healing. II. Displaced closed fractures. *J Bone Joint Surg [Am];* 50 (4):643–662 passim.

198. **Lockwood R, Latta LL** (1980) Bone blood flow changes with diaphyseal fracture. *Proc 26th Ann Mtg Orthop Res Soc;* 5:158.

199. **Paradis GR, Kelly PJ** (1975) Blood flow and mineral deposition in canine tibial fractures. *J Bone Joint Surg [Am];* 57 (2):220–226.

200. **Brighton CT, Schaffer JL, Shapiro DB, et al.** (1991) Proliferation and macromolecular synthesis by rat calvarial bone cells grown in various oxygen tensions. *J Orthop Res;* 9 (6): 847–854.

201. **Burwell BG** (1964) The fresh composite homograft-autograft of cancellous bone: An analysis of factors leading to osteogenesis in marrow transplants and in marrow-containing bone grafts. *J Bone Joint Surg [Br];* 46:110.

202. **Diaz-Flores L, Gutierrez R, Lopez-Alonso A, et al.** (1992) Pericytes as a supplementary source of osteoblasts in periosteal osteogenesis. *Clin Orthop;* (275):280–286.

203. **Jones AR, Clark CC, Brighton CT** (1995) Microvessel endothelial cells and pericytes increase proliferation and repress osteoblast phenotypic markers in rat calvarial bone cell cultures. *J Orthop Res;* 13 (4): 553–561.

204. **Bassett CAL, Herrman I** (1961) Influence of oxygen concentration and mechanical factors on differentiation of connective tissues in vitro. *Nature;* 190:460.

205. **Carter DR, Blenman PR, Beaupre GS** (1987) Mechanical stress and vascular influence on fracture healing. *Proc 33rd Ann Mtg Orthop Res Soc;* 12 :99.

206. **Blenman PR, Carter DR, Beaupre GS** (1989) Role of mechanical loading in the progressive ossification of a fracture callus. *J Orthop Res;* 7 (3):398–407.

207. **Steinberg ME, Lyet JP, Pollack SR** (1980) Stress-generated potentials (SGPs) in fracture callus. *Proc 26th Ann Mtg Orthop Res Soc;* 5:115.

208. **Claes L, Wilke H-J, Augat P, et al.** (1994) The influence of fracture gap size and stability on bone healing. *Proc 40th Ann Mtg Orthop Res Soc;* 19:203.

209. **Milner JC, Rhinelander FW** (1968) Compression fixation and primary bone healing. *Surg Forum;* 19:453–456.

210. **Schenk R, Willenegger H** (1965) Fluoreszenzmikroskopische Untersuchungen zur Heilung von Schaftfrakturen nach stabiler Osteosynthese am Hund. *Proc 2nd Eur Symp Calcif Tiss Collect Colloq;* Univ Liege :125.

211. **Swiontkowski MF, Tepic S, Rahn BA** (1987) The effect of femoral neck fracture on femoral head blood flow. *Proc 33rd Ann Mtg Orthhop Res Soc;* 12:255.

212. **Olerud S, Danckwardt-Lilliestrom G** (1971) Fracture healing in compression osteosynthesis. An experimental study in dogs with an avascular, diaphyseal, intermediate fragment. *Acta Orthop Scand Suppl;* 137:1–44.

213. **Rhinelander FW** (1965) Some aspects of the microcirculation of healing bone. *Clin Orthop;* 40:12.
214. **Rhinelander FW** (1973) Effects of medullary nailing on the normal blood supply of diaphyseal cortex. *Amer Acad Orthop Surg Instr Course Lect.* St Louis: C. V. Mosby, 161.
215. **Browner BD, Wilson JW, Sitter TC, et al.** (1987) Comparative biologic characteristics of ovine femoral osteotomies stabilized with Kuntscher and Ender medullary nails. *Proc 33rd Ann Mtg Orthop Res Soc;* 12:381.
216. **Turchin D, Schemitsch E, Kowalski M, et al.** (1995) Cortical porosity and new bone formation following reamed and unreamed intramedullary nailing of the fractured sheep tibia. *Proc 41st Ann Mtg Orthop Res Soc;* 20:586.
217. **Rand JA, An KN, Chao EY, et al.** (1981) A comparison of the effect of open intramedullary nailing and compression plate fixation on fracture-site blood flow and fracture union. *J Bone Joint Surg [Am];* 63 (3): 427–442.
218. **O'Sullivan ME, Chao EY, Kelly PJ** (1989) The effects of fixation on fracture-healing. *J Bone Joint Surg [Am];* 71 (2):306–310.
219. **Reichert ILH, McCarthy ID, Hughes SPF** (1995) Regional hemodynamics of intramedullary reaming on the intact and osteotomized ovine tibia. *Proc 41st Ann Mtg Orthop Res Soc;* 20:185.
220. **Reichert ILH, McCarthy ID, Hughes SPF** (1995) Regional hemodynamics of intramedullary reaming in the ovine tibia-evaluation of the acute response. *Proc 41st Ann Mtg Orthop Res Soc;* 20:797.
221. **Smith SR, Bronk JT, Kelly PJ** (1990) Effect of fracture fixation on cortical bone blood flow. *J Orthop Res;* 8 (4):471–478.

222. **Schemitsch EH, Kowalski MJ, Swiontkowski MF, et al.** (1994) A comparison of the effect of reamed and unreamed locked intramedullary nailing on callus blood flow and strength of union following fracture of the sheep tibia. *Proc 40th Ann Mtg Orthop Res Soc;* 19:534.
223. **Schemitsch EH, Kowalski MJ, Swiontkowski MF, et al.** (1995) Comparison of the effect of reamed and unreamed locked intramedullary nailing on blood flow in the callus and strength of union following fracture of the sheep tibia. *J Orthop Res;* 13 (3):382–389.
224. **Runkel M, Wenda K, Rudig L, et al.** (1995) Unreamed versus reamed nailing: Remodelling and bone regeneration. *Proc 41st Ann Mtg Orthop Res Soc;* 20:581.
225. **Evans PE** (1983) Cerclage fixation of a fractured humerus in 1775. Fact or fiction? *Clin Orthop;* (174):138–142.
226. **Goetz O** (1933) Subkutane Drahtnaht bei Tibia-Schrägfrakturen. *Arch Klin Chir;* 177:445.
227. **Charnley J** (1957) *The Closed Treatment of Common Fractures.* 2nd ed. Edinburgh London: E & S Livingstone.
228. **Newton CD, Hohn RB** (1974) Fracture nonunion resulting from Cerclage appliances. *J Am Vet Med Assoc;* 164 (5):503–508.
229. **Rhinelander FW, Brahms MA** (1961) Internal fixation of bone fragments with flexible wire and pins. *J Bone Joint Surg [Am];* 43:599.
230. **Gothman L** (1962) Local arterial changes caused by surgical exposure and the application of encircling wires (cerclage) on the rabbit's tibia: A microangiographic study. *Acta Chir Scand;* 123:9.

231. **Gothman L** (1962) Local arterial changes associated with experimental fractures of the rabbit's tibia treated with encircling wires (cerclage): A microangiographic study. *Acta Chir Scand;* 123:17.
232. **Wilson JW, Rhinelander FW, Stewart CL** (1985) Microvascular and histologic effect of circumferential wire on appositional bone growth in immature dogs. *J Orthop Res;* 3 (4):412–417.
233. **Blass CE, vanEe RT, Wilson JW** (1991) Microvascular and histologic effect on cortical bone of applied double loop cerclage. *J Am Anim Hosp Assoc;* 27:432.
234. **Nyrop KA, DeBowes RM, Ferguson HR, et al.** (1990) Vascular response of the equine radius to cerclage devices. *Vet Surg;* 19 (4): 249–253.
235. **Hinko PJ, Rhinelander FW** (1975) Effective use of cerclage in the treat-ment of long-bone fractures in dogs. *J Am Vet Med Assoc;* 166 (5):520–524.
236. **Rooks RL, Tarvin GB, Pijankowski GJ, et al.** (1982) *In vitro* cerclage wiring analysis. *Vet Surg;* 11:39.
237. **Wilson JW, Belloli DM, Robbins T** (1985) Resistance of cerclage to knot failure. *J Am Vet Med Assoc;* 187 (4): 389–391.
238. **Blass CE, Piermattei DL, Withrow SJ, et al.** (1986) Static and dynamic cerclage wire analysis. *Vet Surg;* 15:181.
239. **Serina ER, Mote CD** (1994) Intra-operative femoral fractures treated with cerclage fixation: A finite element stress analysis. *Proc 40th Ann Mtg Orthop Res Soc;* 19:543.
240. **Parham FW, Martin ED** (1913) A new device for the treatment of fractures. *New Orl Med Surg J;* 16:451.

241. **Trueta J** (1974) Blood supply and the rate of healing of tibial fractures. *Clin Orthop;* 105 (0):11–26.

242. **Partridge A** (1976) Nylon straps for internal fixation of bone. *Lancet;* 2 (7997):1252.

243. **Partridge A** (1977) Nylon plates and straps for internal fixation of osteoporotic bone. *Lancet;* 1 (8015):808.

244. **Partridge AJ, Evans PE** (1982) The treatment of fractions of the shaft of the femur using nylon cerclage. *J Bone Joint Surg [Br];* 64 (2):210–214.

245. **Jones DG** (1986) Bone erosion beneath partridge bands. *J Bone Joint Surg [Br];* 68 (3):476–477.

246. **Wilson JW** (1988) Knot strength of cerclage bands and wires. *Acta Orthop Scand;* 59 (5):545–547.

247. **Kirby BM, Wilson JW** (1989) Knot strength of nylon-band cerclage. *Acta Orthop Scand;* 60 (5):696–698.

248. **Uhthoff HK, Dubuc FL** (1971) Bone structure changes in the dog under rigid internal fixation. *Clin Orthop;* 81:165–170.

249. **Braden TD, Brinker WO, Little RW, et al.** (1973) Comparative biomechanical evaluation of bone healing in the dog. *J Am Vet Med Assoc;* 163 (1):65–69.

250. **Akeson WH, Woo SL, Coutts RD, et al.** (1975) Quantitative histological evaluation of early fracture healing of cortical bones immobilized by stainless steel and composite plates. *Calcif Tissue Res;* 19 (1):27–37.

251. **Akeson WH, Woo SL, Rutherford L, et al.** (1976) The effects of rigidity of internal fixation plates on long bone remodeling. A biomechanical and quantitative histological study. *Acta Orthop Scand;* 47 (3):241–249.

252. **Nunamaker DM, Hayes WC, Schein S, et al.** (1982) Mechanical properties of healing fractures following removal of compression plate fixation. *Proc 28th Ann Mtg Orthop Res Soc;* 7:200.

253. **Luethi UK, Rahn BA** (1980) Kontaktfläche zwischen Osteosyntheseplatten und Knochen. *Aktuel Traumatol;* 10:131.

254. **Nunamaker DM, Bowman KF, Richardson DW, et al.** (1986) Plate luting: A preliminary report of its use in horses. *Vet Surg;* 15:289.

255. **Nunamaker DM, Richardson DW, Butterweck DM** (1988) Mechanical effects of plate luting. *Proc 34th Ann Mtg Orthop Res Soc;* 13:305.

256. **Roush JK, Wilson JW** (1990) Effects of plate luting on cortical vascularity and development of cortical porosity in canine femurs. *Vet Surg;* 19 (3):208–214.

257. **Luethi UK, Rahn BA, Perren SM** (1982) Implants and intracortical vascular disturbance. *Proc 28th Ann Mtg Orthop Res Soc;* 7:337.

258. **Gautier E, Rahn BA, Perren SM** (1986) Effect of different plates on internal and external remodelling of intact long bones. *Proc 32nd Ann Mtg Orthop Res Soc;* 11:322.

259. **Simmons DJ, Daum WJ, Calhoun JH** (1988) Regional alterations in long bone ^{85}Sr clearance produced by internal fixation devices. Part II. Histomorphometry. *J Orthop Trauma;* 2 (3):245–249.

260. **Court-Brown CM** (1985) The effect of external skeletal fixation on bone healing and bone blood supply. An experimental study. *Clin Orthop;* (201):278–289.

261. **Wallace AL, Draper ER, Strachan RK, et al.** (1991) The effect of devascularisation upon early bone healing in dynamic external fixation. *J Bone Joint Surg [Br];* 73 (5):819–825.

262. **Park SH, McKellop H, Sarmiento A** (1995) Comparison of healing rates of transverse and oblique tibial fractures in the rabbit, with and without free motion. *Proc 41st Ann Mtg Orthop Res Soc;* 20:256.

263. **Kojimoto H, Yasui N, Sasaki K, et al.** (1989) Blood supply during experimental bone lengthening by callus distraction—a microangiographic study. *Proc 35th Ann Mtg Orthop Res Soc;* 14:564.

264. **Aronson J, Harp JH, Walker CW, et al.** (1990) Blood flow, bone formation and mineralization during distraction oteosynthesis. *Proc 36th Ann Mtg Orthop Res Soc;* 15:589.

265. **Karlstrom G, Olerud S** (1977) Secondary internal fixation: Studies on revascularization and healing in osteotomized rabbit tibias. *Proc 23rd Ann Mtg Orthop Res Soc;* 2:131.

266. **Rhinelander FW** (1966) Observations on the microcirculation of experimental bone grafts. *Proc 10th Congr Int Chir Orthop Traumatol;* SICOT Xe Congr:636.

267. **Kienapfel H, Sumner DR, Turner TM, et al.** (1992) Efficacy of autograft and freeze-dried allograft to enhance fixation of porous coated implants in the presence of interface gaps. *J Orthop Res;* 10 (3):423–433.

268. **McKibbin B** (1978) The biology of fracture healing in long bones. *J Bone Joint Surg [Br];* 60-B (2):150–162.

269. **Siegert JJ, Wood MB** (1990) Blood flow evaluation of vascularized bone transfers in a canine model. *J Orthop Res;* 8 (2):291–296.

270. **Straw RC, Powers BE, Withrow SJ, et al.** (1992) The effect of intramedullary polymethylmethacrylate on healing of intercalary cortical allografts in a canine model. *J Orthop Res;* 10 (3):434–439.

271. **Roorda J, Wood MB** (1993) Effect of ischemic storage on endothelium in canine bone. *J Orthop Res;* 11 (5): 648–654.

272. **Moran CG, Wood MB** (1992) Failure of perfusion with oxygenated Krebs-Ringer solution to preserve the eccrine function of the vascular endothelium in bone. *J Orthop Res;* 10 (6):813–817.

273. **Moran CG, Adams ML, Wood MB** (1993) Preservation of bone graft vascularity with the University of Wisconsin cold storage solution. *J Orthop Res;* 11 (6):840–848.

274. **Coessens BC, Adams ML, Wood MB** (1995) Evaluation of influence of 24-hour cold preservation on endothelin production and on endothelin receptors in the bone vasculature. *J Orthop Res;* 13 (5):725–732.

275. **Coessens BC, Miller VM, Wood MB** (1996) Endothelin induces vasoconstriction in the bone vasculature in vitro: an effect mediated by a single receptor population. *J Orthop Res;* 14 (4):611–617.

276. **Allen DM, Chen LE, Seaber AV, et al.** (1997) Calcitonin gene-related peptide and reperfusion injury. *J Orthop Res;* 15 (2):243–248.

277. **Howard PE, Wilson JW, Ribble GA** (1988) Effects of gelatin sponge implantation in cancellous bone defects in dogs. *J Am Vet Med Assoc;* 192 (5):633–637.

278. **Howard PE** (1989) Unpublished data.

279. **Rhinelander FW, Rouweyha M, Milner JC** (1971) Microvascular and histogenic responses to implantation of a porous ceramic into bone. *J Biomed Mater Res;* 5 (1):81–112.

280. **Rhinelander FW** (1977) A flexible composite as a coating for metallic implants—microvascular and histological studies. *Int Orthop;* 1:77.

281. **Klawitter JJ, Hulbert SF** (1971) Application of porous ceramics for the attachment of load-bearing internal orthopaedic appliances. *J Biomed Mat Res (Symposium);* 2:161.

282. **Rhinelander FW, Nelson CL** (1974) Experimental implantation of porous materials into bone. Proplast for low modulus fixation of prostheses. *Acta Orthop Belg;* 40 (5–6):771–798.

283. **Rhinelander FW, Stewart CL, Wilson JW, et al.** (1982) Growth of tissue into a porous, low modulus coating on intramedullary nails: an experimental study. *Clin Orthop;* (164):293–305.

284. **Charnley J** (1972) *Acrylic Cement in Orthopaedic Surgery.* Edinburgh London: Churchill Livingstone.

285. **Rhinelander FW, Nelson CL, Stewart RD, et al.** (1979) Experimental reaming of the proximal femur and acrylic cement implantation: vascular and histologic effects. *Clin Orthop;* (141):74–89.

286. **de Waal Malefijt J, Slooff TJ, Huiskes R, et al.** (1988) Vascular changes following hip arthroplasty. The femur in goats studied with and without cementation. *Acta Orthop Scand;* 59 (6):643–649.

287. **Humeniuk B, Anderson GI, Richards RR, et al.** (1993) Femoral red cell flux changes after reaming and implant placement: A canine study using laser Doppler flowmetry. *Proc 39th Ann Mtg Orthop Res Soc;* 18:252.

288. **Danckwardt-Lilliestrom G** (1969) Reaming of the medullary cavity and its effect on diaphyseal bone. A fluorochromic, microangiographic and histologic study on the rabbit tibia and dog femur. *Acta Orthop Scand Suppl;* 128:1–153.

289. **Olerud S, Danckwardt-Lilliestrom G, Lorenzi GL** (1969) Do medullary components appear in the femoral vein during the reaming of the tibia? *Europ Surg Res;* 1:243.

290. **Danckwardt-Lilliestrom G, Lorenzi GL, Olerud S** (1970) Intramedullary nailing after reaming. An investigation on the healing process in osteotomized rabbit tibias. *Acta Orthop Scand Suppl;* 134:1–78.

291. **Milne IS** (1973) Hazards of acrylic bone cement. A report of two cases. *Anaesthesia;* 28 (5):538–543.

292. **Herndon JH, Bechtold CO, Crickenberger DP** (1962) Fat embolism during total hip replacement: A prospective study. *J Bone Joint Surg [Am];* 56:1350.

293. **Winet H, Hollinger JO, Stevanovic M** (1995) Incorporation of polylactide-polyglycolide in a cortical defect: neoangiogenesis and blood supply in a bone chamber. *J Orthop Res;* 13 (5):679–689.

294. **Rhinelander FW** (1974) The normal circulation of bone and its response to surgical intervention. *J Biomed Mater Res;* 8 (1):87–90.

295. **Ham AW, Cormack DH** (1979) *Histology.* 8th ed. Philadelphia: JB Lippincott.

296. **Rhinelander FW** (1980) The blood supply of the limb bones. In: Owen R, Goodfellow J, Bullough P, editors. *Scientific Foundations of Orthopaedics and Traumatology.* London: William Heineman Medical Books, 126.

297. **Wilson JW** (1991) Vascular supply to normal bone and healing fractures. *Semin Vet Med Surg (Small Anim);* 6 (1): 26–38.

3 Morphology and physiology of the growth cartilage under normal and pathologic conditions

Sten-Erik Olsson & Stina Ekman

1 Normal morphology and physiology

1.1 Bone and cartilage: two interrelated components of the growing skeleton

1.1.1 Bone

Cartilage is a precursor of bone in most parts of the skeleton and it plays an important role in the process of growth from fetal life to maturity. In the adult skeleton, all cartilage except the joint cartilage has been replaced by the more unyielding substance of bone, which is better suited for the more strenuous supportive and protective function of the skeleton in the mature individual. Bone has a high tensile and compressive strength combined with some elasticity and relatively light weight (see **Chapter 8**), but it is more dependent upon a well-developed blood supply than cartilage (see **Chapter 2**). Bone is constantly renewed and reconstructed and is very responsive to mechanical stimuli and to metabolic, nutritional, and endocrine influences. Bone can grow only by surface apposition, a process in which some of the bone forming cells, the osteoblasts, become enclosed in the mineralized matrix and turn into bone cells called osteocytes. These cells in their lacunae are rather uniformly spaced throughout the matrix, which is rich in collagen type I fibrils and also contains a number of other matrix proteins [1]. The osteocytes have numerous slender processes that extend into canaliculi in the mineralized matrix. The processes are in contact through gap junctions with the processes of neighboring osteocytes. While the active osteoblast has the structure expected of a cell actively engaged in protein synthesis, such as extensive endoplasmic reticulum, many ribosomes and lysosomes, and a well-developed Golgi apparatus, the osteocyte deep in the bone shows regression of these organelles. It is believed, however, that the osteocyte is not metabolically inactive. It is possible that it can modify the surrounding matrix and dissolve and resorb some bone mineral in a process called osteolysis. The third bone cell, of as equal importance as the osteoblast and the osteocyte, is the multinucleated osteoclast, which is actively involved in resorption of bone. This cell also digests calcified cartilage and when found doing so is called chondroclast. Its origin and mode of action will be discussed under resorption of cartilage.

1.1.2 Cartilage

Cartilage is a strong, slightly pliable and resilient tissue with its cells, the chondrocytes, and its extracellular fibers embedded in an amorphous matrix. Cartilage can either be hyaline, elastic, or fibrous in nature, with hyaline cartilage being the most common type. Cartilage is either void of blood vessels or is sparsely vascularized, and the colloidal properties of its matrix are therefore important to its nutrition. The capacity of cartilage for both rapid interstitial and appositional growth and its relative firmness make it an excellent tissue material for the rapidly growing skeleton of the fetus.

The cartilage cell, the chondrocyte, lies within its lacuna encompassed by its extracellular matrix. The chondrocyte usually conforms to the shape of the lacuna which is usually elliptical or semicircular. In routine histologic section the cells appear stellate because fixation and dehydration have retracted them from the wall of the lacunae (**Fig. 3-1**). The cells are often clustered in small groups, each group containing isogenic cells (progeny of one cell) in one lacuna. The chondrocyte has a large round or oval nucleus with one to several nucleoli. The cytoplasm contains elongated mitochondria, lipid droplets, and some glycogen. In cells of growing cartilage the Golgi complex is prominent, a granular endoplasmic reticulum is well developed, and many cytoplasmic dense bodies are present (**Fig. 3-2** and **Fig. 3-3**).

The hyaline matrix appears homogeneous under the microscope and is deeply colored with the periodic acid-Schiff reaction for glycosaminoglycans. It also has an affinity for basic dyes and stains metachromatically with toluidine blue. The principal constituents of cartilage matrix are water, collagen [**2**], and many noncollagenous macromolecules of which proteoglycans [**3**] are the most common. About 70% of the

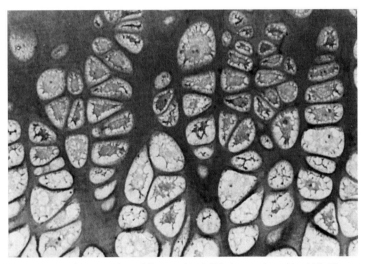

Fig. 3-1: Histologic section of the proximal tibia in a 9-day-old rabbit. The section was taken from the growth cartilage between the cartilaginous epiphysis and the metaphysis. This cartilage is responsible for longitudinal growth and, after ossification of the epiphysis, is called the metaphyseal growth plate. The upper half of this picture shows transitional cells and the lower half hypertrophying cells, of which some are disintegrating. (Toluidine blue stain; ×500.)

weight of the matrix is water and the remaining 30% is made up of collagen, several proteoglycans, and a number of other noncollagenous proteins [**4, 5**].

Up to 40% of the dry weight of cartilage is composed of collagen in an interlacing fabric of fine fibrils. Collagen type II is the most abundant collagen molecule of hyaline cartilage. The chondrocytes synthesize and secrete procollagen, formed by three polypeptide chains. Tropocollagen is formed outside the cell by enzymatic cleaving of the terminal peptides of the procollagen. The three polypeptide chains are stabilized by hydroxyproline residues forming hydrogen bonds between its polypeptide chains. Collagen type II fibrils and the orientation of these fibrils are responsible for the tensile strength of cartilage [**6, 7**].

There are several minor collagens in cartilage (collagen VI, IX, X, and XI). Collagens IX and XI, together with collagen II, participate in the formation of the striated fibrils of cartilage. Collagen type X has been found in the hypertrophic region of the growth cartilage [**8, 9**] and in the superficial layer of the articular cartilage [**10**]. Beside collagen, the most prominent component of the cartilage matrix is a large proteoglycan (aggrecan). There are also three types of small proteoglycans (PG-SI, decorin, and fibromodulin). The large proteoglycan molecule provides the joint cartilage with a low friction surface in the joint. Many properties of cartilage depend on the combined functions of the fibril-forming collagen II and the large aggregating proteoglycan. The collagen fibrils have great tensile strength and reinforce the mechanically weak proteoglycan gel. This gel has a high fixed-charge density leading to a large osmotic swelling pressure. The proteoglycan aggregates are hydrophilic, polyanionic, and they occupy a large domain in solution. In free solution the proteoglycan occupies about five times the volume it has in the tissue. In the matrix the swelling is counteracted by the collagen fibrils. The interaction between collagen and proteoglycan gives the cartilage great tensile and compressive strength [**5**]. According to these authors, the major proteoglycan in cartilage represents some 5–10% of the matrix wet weight. It has a protein core with glycosaminoglycans (GAGs) covalently attached (**Fig. 3-4**). The protein core has an aminoterminal part: a globular domain (Gl) that allows specific interaction with hyaluronate, a GAG

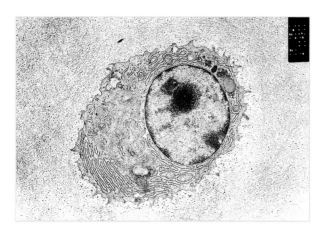

Fig. 3-2: Transmission electron micrograph of a chondrocyte with surrounding matrix in the resting region of the epiphyseal growth cartilage from a 4-week-old minipig. The rounded chondrocyte has the characteristic features of a metabolic active cell, with an extensive reticulum, well-developed Golgi complex, aggregates of glycogen and lipid droplets. Short cellular processes are present. (Conventional fixation; ×7,300.)

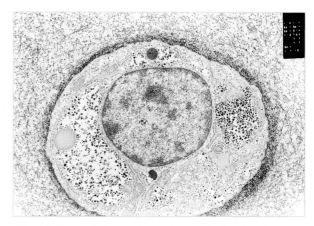

Fig. 3-3: Transmission electron micrograph of a chondrocyte in the resting region of the epiphyseal growth cartilage from a 10-week-old commercial pig. Ruthenium Hexamine Trichloride (RHT) fixation. Here a close attachment between the cell membrane and the pericellular matrix is seen. (×9,500.)

consisting of several thousand repeat disaccharide units. Many proteoglycan molecules can thus bind to a single hyaluronate molecule. The binding is stabilized by a distinct molecule, the link protein that binds to the hyaluronate-binding region of the proteoglycan molecule. The most striking feature of the large proteoglycan is the large number of negatively charged glycosaminoglycan side chains. There are some 100 chondroitin sulfate chains, each with about 100 negatively charged carboxyl and sulfate groups responsible for the resilience of the cartilage.

A large number of noncollagenous proteins in cartilage have been uncovered [5, 11]. The function of many of these proteins is not yet understood. As seen in **Fig. 3-5**, in the matrix adjacent to the chondrocyte are besides collagens and proteoglycans, ancorin, 36 kd protein [12], 58 kd protein, fibronectin, 148 kd protein (CMP), cartilage oligomeric matrix protein (COMP) [13], and 21 kd protein [14]. In addition, there are C-propeptide II (chondrocalcin) [15] and chondronectin [16].

1.2   Growth and ossification

1.2.1   Endochondral and intramembranous ossification

Most of the bones of the skeleton are first made of cartilage which is gradually turned into bone by a process called endochondral ossification (see **Fig. 3-15**). Only some flat bones of the skull are not formed via a cartilage model. Their mode of formation is intramembranous ossification, which means that bone is formed directly in connective tissue (see **Fig. 3-15**).

At a certain stage of fetal development, usually before midterm, a primary ossification center appears in the hyaline cartilage at the midshaft of the long bones (**Fig. 3-6**). Specific changes take place in the cartilage before ossification begins. The cartilage cells enlarge and become vacuolated. The matrix is reduced and begins to calcify, a process known as provisional calcification. The chondrocytes disintegrate when vessels grow into the spaces of the opened chondrocyte lacunae and multinucleated chondroclasts [17], morphologically identical to

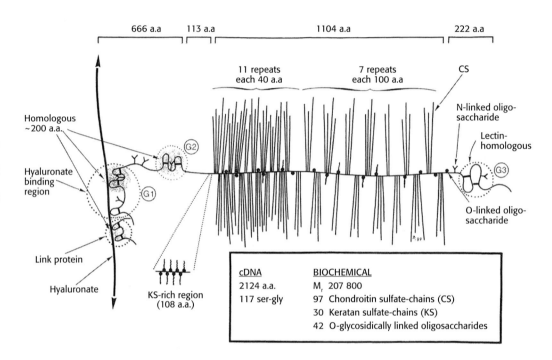

Fig. 3-4: Schematic presentation of cartilage proteoglycans and link protein. The central protein core with three globular domains is substituted with a large number of negatively charged chondroitin sulfate chains (CS), keratan sulfate (KS), and oligosaccharides (for reference, see Heinegård and Sommarin, 1987). The number of amino acids corresponding to the various domains are shown at the top as identified in rat chondrosarcoma proteoglycans. The keratan-sulfate-rich region found in bovine cartilage proteoglycans (P. Antonsson, Å. Oldberg, and D. Heinegård, unpublished results) is illustrated in insert. A corresponding structure is found by chemical means in cartilage proteoglycans from several sources, eg, human and pig (for reference, see Heinegård and Sommarin, 1987). The Ser-Gly structures correspond to the putative attachment sites for the CS side chains. The biochemical data are derived from studies of bovine nasal proteoglycans (for reference, see Heinegård and Sommarin, 1987) (Courtesy FASEB Journal, vol 3, p. 2043, 1989; Heinegård and Oldberg [5]).

osteoclasts, resorb the calcified cartilage matrix. Osteoprogenitor cells, which are turned into osteoblasts, accompany the vessels. These cells begin to lay down bone on remnants of the calcified cartilage. The whole process—chondrocyte differentiation, matrix calcification, vascular invasion, and ossification—is called endochondral ossification.

1.2.2 Development of the growth plates and the joint cartilage

At the time when the primary ossification center appears at midshaft in the cartilage model of a long bone of a fetus, the perichondrium, the connective tissue sheath surrounding the cartilage model, starts laying down bone called woven bone in a cortical collar around the midportion of the diaphysis (**Fig. 3-6**). The bone formed by endochondral ossification inside the

cortical collar consists of a trabecular three-dimensional network, interspersed by cavities filled by bone marrow (**Fig. 3-6**). The perichondral bone, which is the first compact bone of the fetus, has a different appearance. In most laboratory animals and in birds the newly formed cortical bone is loosely meshed, with large haversian spaces. In the larger domestic animals and in man, this bone consists of circumferential lamellae with numerous circumferential and radial vascular channels. The trabecular network, the spongy bone, at midshaft is rapidly resorbed and replaced by a second generation of trabecular bone as the fetus grows.

At the time of birth, the trabecular bone at the midshaft has been resorbed and entirely replaced by bone marrow. At each end of the marrow cavity there is spongy bone, which is called the metaphysis (**Fig. 3-7**). Peripheral to the metaphysis is the epiphysis which, early in life, is cartilaginous (**Fig. 3-7**). Between the metaphysis and the epiphysis is the growth plate (**Fig. 3-7**). When birds such as turkeys and chickens are hatched, their

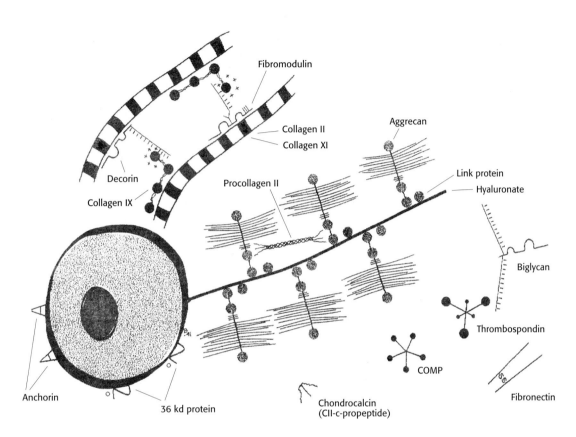

Fibromodulin

Collagen II
Collagen XI

Aggrecan

Decorin

Procollagen II

Link protein

Hyaluronate

Collagen IX

Biglycan

Thrombospondin

Anchorin

COMP

Fibronectin

36 kd protein

Chondrocalcin
(CII-c-propeptide)

Fig. 3-5: Schematic illustration of cartilage matrix also indicating suggested interactions. The shorter side chains in aggrecan represent keratan sulfate, and the longer chains represent chondroitin sulfate. (Courtesy Articular Cartilage and Osteoarthritis, eds Kuettner, K.E., Schleyerbach, R., Peyron, J.G., Hascall, V.C. Raven Press, New York, 1992; Heinegård and Pimental, "Cartilage Matrix Proteins" p. 96.)

bones have not reached the same degree of development as have the bones of mammals at the time of birth.

In the literature, the cartilage growth plate is usually called the epiphyseal growth plate but, in the present text, the name metaphyseal growth plate is being used because it is the growth plate of the metaphysis, not of the epiphysis. Most bones have two epiphyses but the metacarpal, metatarsal, and phalangeal bones have only one epiphysis and thus only one metaphyseal growth plate.

The metaphyseal growth plates are unipolar, which means that growth takes place in one direction—for example, proximal or distal in the extremities, cranial or caudal in the vertebral bodies. The growth plates of the various apophyses, such as the olecranon, anconeal process, iliac crest, and tibial crest are also of the unipolar type. In the pelvis three bones, the ilium, pubis, and ischium, together form the acetabulum

with the aid of a bipolar growth plate of triradiate shape. In this growth plate a fourth bone, the acetabular Y-shaped bone, is formed, thereby turning the bipolar triradiate growth plate into two unipolar growth plates. All four bones then unite [18].

At certain times after birth, secondary ossification centers appear in the epiphyses (**Fig. 3-7**). They are formed in a similar manner as the primary ossification centers, beginning with hypertrophy of the chondrocytes accompanied by calcification of the longitudinal septal matrix, invasion of vessels, partial resorption, and subsequent ossification. In most domestic animals and in man rapid ossification of the calcified cartilage of the epiphysis is facilitated by the presence of vascular channels in the preformed cartilage model (**Fig. 3-7**). From these vascular channels, vessels invade the calcifying cartilage, indicating that the period between the beginning of calcification and ossification is very short. Because of the close

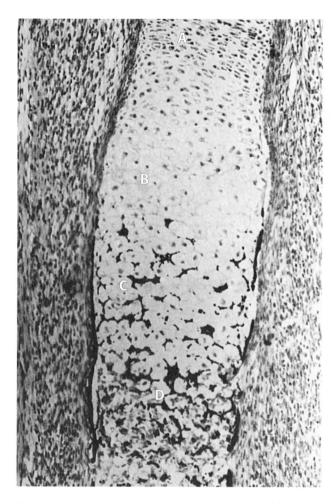

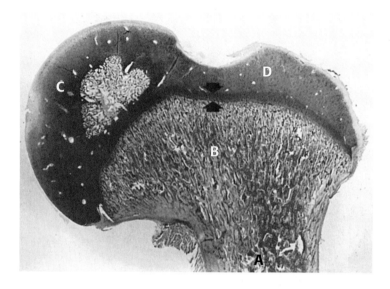

Fig. 3-7: Histologic section from the proximal femur of a German shepherd dog, 4 weeks old. The most proximal part of the diaphysis (A), the metaphysis (B), the metaphyseal growth plate (between arrows), and the epiphysis of the femoral head (C) and that of the greater trochanter (D) are seen. The metaphyseal growth plate is slightly darker-stained than the epiphyseal cartilage. The two cartilaginous epiphyses are penetrated by a large number of vascular channels. In the epiphysis of the femoral head, a large ossification center has already been formed. (H and E stain; ×8.) (From Gustafsson et al., 1975 [71].)

Fig. 3-6: Histologic section of the proximal 1/2 of the tibia of a midterm rabbit fetus. In the most proximal part of the diaphysis (A) the chondrocytes are arranged in columns as an indication of active longitudinal growth. Chondrocyte hypertrophy (B) and matrix calcification (C), as well as formation of trabecular bone (D) and bone marrow, are seen. A collar of bone has been formed at mid-diaphysis. (von Kossa's stain; ×125.)

chronological relationship between calcification and ossification, both in the epiphysis and in the growth plate, the biochemical processes involved in cartilage calcification are difficult to separate from those involved in ossification. The femoral head of young rats is an exception to the rule that cartilage calcification and ossification are closely related in time (**Fig. 3-8**). Calcification of the cartilage matrix of the femoral head of the rat starts at the age of 3 weeks, and because there are no vascular channels in the femoral head, ossification does not begin until 3 weeks later when vessels from the outside begin invading [19].

At varying times, depending upon the species, ossification advances to the point that the metaphyseal growth plates and the immature joint cartilage (the latter is also called articular-epiphyseal cartilage complex [20]) are the only cartilage structures in the long bones.

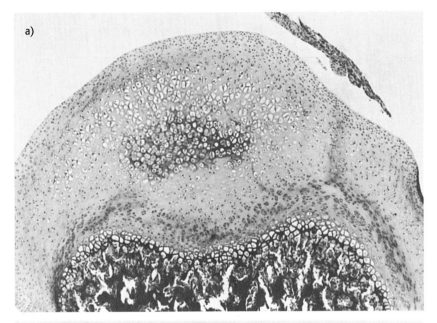

a)

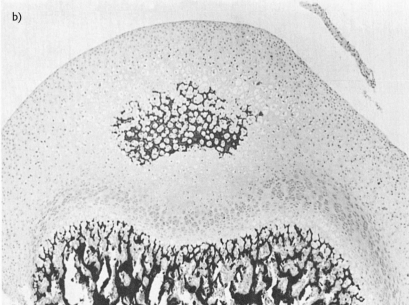

b)

Fig. 3-8: Undecalcified histologic section from the proximal femur of a 25-day-old rat. The cartilage femoral head, the metaphyseal growth plate, and the most proximal part of the metaphysis are seen.
a) The chondrocytes in the center of the femoral head are hypertrophying and some have a markedly basophilic matrix. In contrast to the femoral head of the dog, in **Fig. 3-7**, there are no vascular channels in the femoral-head epiphysis of the rat. (H and E stain; ×40.)
b) The center of the femoral head is calcified (dark in color) but, because of lack of vessels, ossification has not begun. Only after penetration of vessels from the outside will ossification take place. (von Kossa's stain; ×40.)

1.2.3 Histology and function of the metaphyseal growth plate and the immature joint cartilage (articular-epiphyseal cartilage complex)

The cartilage of the metaphyseal growth plate is highly specialized. The chondrocytes are arranged in a more or less distinct longitudinal columnar pattern (**Fig. 3-9**). In the domestic pig, the columnar arrangement of the cells is less obvious than in its wild counterpart, the wild hog. The same difference in arrangement of the chondrocytes is seen when the growth plates of the fast-growing broiler and the more slow-growing Leghorn chicken are compared. Both the domestic pig and the broiler grow very rapidly and this seems to be correlated with some derangement of the growth plates.

In domestic mammals, the cells in the columns of the metaphyseal growth plate are separated by thin transverse septa (territorial matrix), while the columns are separated by rather thick bars of matrix (interterritorial matrix) (**Fig. 3-9** and **Fig. 3-10**). Mitotic division of the chondrocytes takes place on the epiphyseal side of the growth cartilage, while

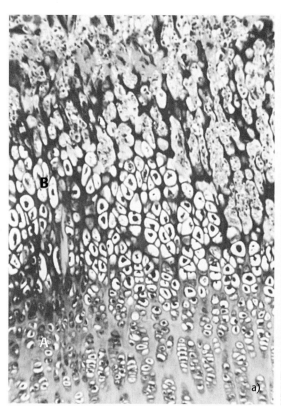

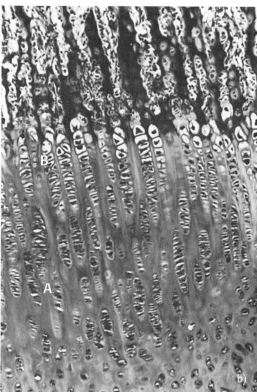

Fig. 3-9: Histologic section from the costochondral junction of the seventh rib from a 7-month-old Landrace pig (a) and from a wild hog of the same age (b). In comparison to the wild hog, the Landrace pig has a less well-organized zone of proliferating cells (A) and a more irregular and wider zone of hypertrophying (vacuolated) cells (B). (H and E stain; ×125.)

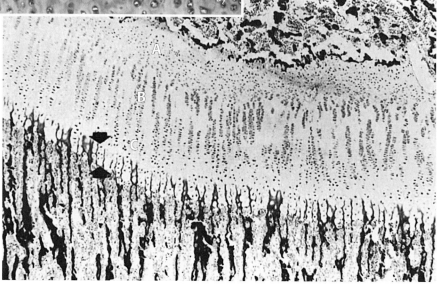

Fig. 3-10: Undecalcified histologic section of the proximal tibial metaphyseal growth plate with part of the epiphysis (*above*) and the metaphysis (*below*) from a 9-day-old rabbit. In the growth plate, the zone of germinal cells (A), proliferating cells (B), transitional cells (C), and hyper-trophying cells (*between arrows*) are seen. The matrix in the longitudinal zone of the hypertrophying cells is calcified. (von Kossa's stain; ×50.)

ossification progresses from the diaphysis toward the epiphysis. The chondrocytes undergo the same sequence of changes described previously for the primary ossification center. However, the sequence of changes now occurs in a much more orderly fashion.

The growth plate has several fairly distinct zones which are characterized by changes in the morphology of the chondrocytes and the composition of the extracellular matrix. Closest to the epiphysis is the zone of resting cells (**Fig. 3-10**). This zone has also been called the zone of the germinal cells, since these cells initiate the process of mitotic division upon which postfetal growth is dependent. The zone of resting (germinal) cells is distinct in certain species (**Fig. 3-10**) and inconspicuous in others (**Fig. 3-11**). After the resting cells comes the zone of

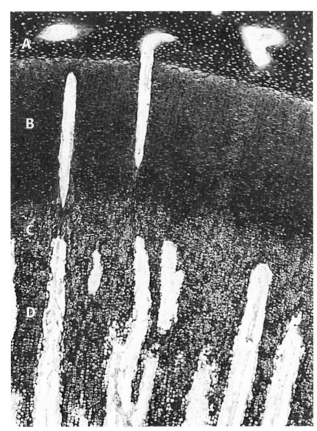

Fig. 3-11: Histologic section of the proximal tibia from a 4-week-old Leghorn chicken. The epiphysis (A), the zone of proliferating cells (B), the zone of transitional cells of the metaphyseal growth plate (C), and the metaphysis (D) can be recognized. There are vascular channels in the epiphysis, some of which penetrate deep into the growth plate. In the metaphysis, which contains a large amount of cartilage with vacuolated cells, the vascular channels reach the zone of transitional cells of the growth plate. (Toluidine blue stain; ×50.)

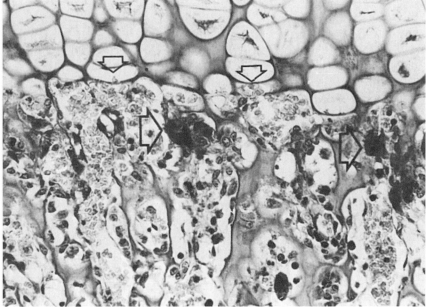

Fig. 3-12: Histologic section of the junction between the proximal tibial metaphyseal growth plate (*above*) and the metaphysis (*below*) in a newborn puppy. The picture illustrates how the horizontal bars of the cartilage matrix are eroded by vascular sprouts (*small arrows*) and how chondroclasts (*large arrows*) are resorbing calcified matrix in the longitudinal bars. (H and E stain; ×250.)

Fig. 3-13:
Histologic section of part of the metaphysis from a 4-week-old Leghorn chicken. Chondroclasts are resorbing calcified cartilage *(short straight arrow)* and osteoblasts are laying down bone *(curved arrow)* on the thick columns of calcified cartilage found deep in the metaphysis. (Toluidine blue stain; ×125.)

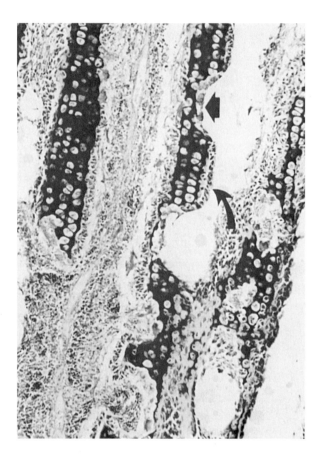

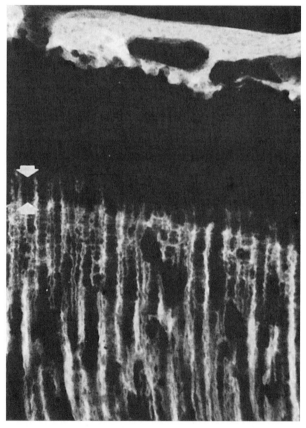

proliferating cells. It is characterized by the division of small flattened chondrocytes, which provide for elongation of the columns (**Fig. 3-9** and **Fig. 3-10**).

Next to the zone of proliferating cells is the zone of maturating (transitional) cells (see **Fig. 3-10** and **Fig. 3-23**). The cells are larger and have ceased to divide. Closest to the metaphysis is the zone of hypertrophying vacuolated cells, which are large and vacuolated. The hypertrophic chondrocytes are viable cells that produce a unique matrix [21–23] that undergoes provisional calcification (**Figs. 3-10, 3-11, 3-12,** and **3-14**).

The matrix in the longitudinal septa calcifies and osteoprogenitor cells begin to invade the cartilage. Endothelial cells from capillary loops enter the empty lacunae through the

Fig. 3-14: Microradiograph of the metaphyseal growth plate of the proximal tibia from a 4-month-old Shetland sheepdog showing the bony plate of the epiphysis *(above)* and the metaphysis *(below)*. The largest part of the metaphyseal growth plate, which is not calcified, can only be seen as a dark area between the epiphysis and the metaphysis. The only part of the growth plate with enough density to be seen on the microradiograph is the zone of calcified longitudinal bars *(between arrows)* adjacent to the metaphysis. Compare with **Figs. 3-10** and **3-22**. (×125.)

Fig. 3-15: Histologic section of the proximal ulna from a 3-week-old mongrel dog. The picture shows the base of the coronoid process (*above*) and the part of the ulna just below it (*below*). The growth zone of the cartilaginous coronoid process is actively engaged in endochondral ossification, and a dark-stained cartilage core is seen in all the newly-formed bone trabecular. The perichondrium of the coronoid process blends with the periosteum of the bone distal to the process. The periosteum is here actively engaged in intramembranous bone formation. The difference between the resulting thick trabeculae of woven bone and the ones formed by endochondral ossification is striking. (H and E stain; ×50.)

horizontal bars of noncalcified matrix, while multinucleated chondroclasts erode and resorb the calcified cartilage matrix (**Fig. 3-12**). The osteoprogenitor cells are thought to originate from the cells of the marrow spaces of the metaphysis, but there are also studies indicating that hypertrophic chondrocytes may modulate to osteoprogenitor cells [**24**]. Osteoprogenitor cells differentiate into osteoblasts, which congregate on the surface of longitudinal irregular remnants of the calcified cartilage (**Figs. 3-9, 3-12,** and **3-13**).

A thin layer of bone matrix, the osteoid seam, is laid down by these osteoblasts on the remnants of calcified cartilage (**Fig. 3-13**). The bone matrix soon begins to mineralize as apposition of new, unmineralized matrix continues. The ensuing, more or less longitudinally-oriented irregular bone

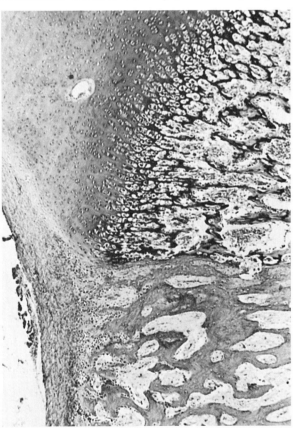

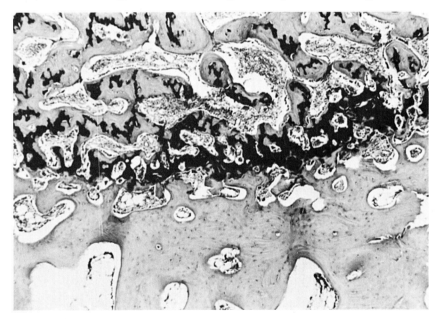

Fig. 3-16: Histologic section of the distal humerus from an 8-month-old Labrador retriever dog. Growth has almost ceased, as the growth plate is about to close. The marrow spaces of the metaphysis (*above*) and the epiphysis (*below*) are confluent at certain sites. The calcified cartilage (dark-stained) within the bone trabeculae of the metaphysis are not oriented in the same direction as the trabeculae. This indicates that a substantial remodeling of the bone has taken place since the trabeculae were originally formed. On the other hand, all bone trabeculae contain some cartilage, which is a sign that at least some parts of the original trabeculae formed by endochondral ossification are maintained. (H and E stain; ×50.)

lamellae thus contain a cartilaginous core (**Figs. 3-14, 3-15,** and **3-16**). When the bone grows longer, the diaphyseal ends of the primary bone trabeculae are eroded by the osteoclasts at the same rate as new bone is being formed on the epiphyseal side of the metaphysis. In this way the metaphysis remains relatively constant in thickness, as measured from the diaphysis to the growth plate. Until the time when growth of the bone begins to slow down and then ceases (**Fig. 3-16**), the metaphyseal growth plate also remains approximately constant in thickness, as measured from epiphysis to metaphysis. The reason for this is that the resorption of cartilage and the formation of bone on the metaphyseal side of the growth plate keep pace with the proliferation of chondrocytes on the epiphyseal side.

The growth cartilage of the immature joint cartilage is arranged in similar zones to the growth plate, with chondrocytes undergoing the same sequence of changes. However, the proliferative and hypertrophic zones occupy a smaller area with groups of chondrocytes without columnar formation (see **Fig. 3-7** and **Fig. 3-21**). The main part of the immature joint cartilage of most domestic animals consists of a vascular epiphyseal cartilage covered by an avascular articular cartilage [**25, 26**] (see **Fig. 3-7** and **Fig. 3-21**). However, the vascularization of the immature joint cartilage differs between species. For example, the rabbit and the rat have an avascular epiphyseal cartilage (see **Fig. 3-8** and **Fig. 3-20**).

1.2.4   Cartilage calcification and resorption

Endochondral bone formation cannot occur without provisional calcification and vascular invasion of the cartilage. Calcification and vascular invasion are interdependent, at least in the metaphyseal growth plate. It has been shown experimentally, for example, that calcification of the metaphyseal growth plate does not take place if the blood supply to the metaphysis is disturbed [**27–29**]. Likewise, if the calcification of the growth plate does not occur because of experimentally induced rickets, vascular invasion will not occur [**30**].

As mentioned previously, this close relationship between calcification and vascular invasion is not seen in the cartilage of the femoral head epiphyses of the growing rat. In this

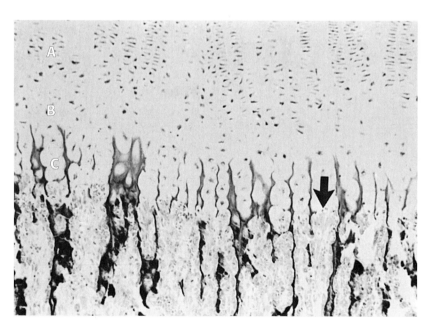

Fig. 3-17: Undecalcified histologic section from the proximal tibia of a 9-day-old rabbit. Part of the metaphyseal growth plate *(above)* and part of the metaphysis *(below)* with the advancing front of vascular invasion *(arrow)* are shown. The zone of proliferating cells (A), the zone of transitional cells (B), and the zone of hypertrophying cells (C) with calcification (dark stain) of the longitudinal bars of matrix can be identified. It is noteworthy that calcification precedes vascular invasion. In the metaphysis, which is very rich in vessels, only thin, longitudinally oriented remnants of cartilage are left. Bone is laid down by osteoblasts on these remnants. Compare with **Fig. 3-16.** (von Kossa's stain; ×125.)

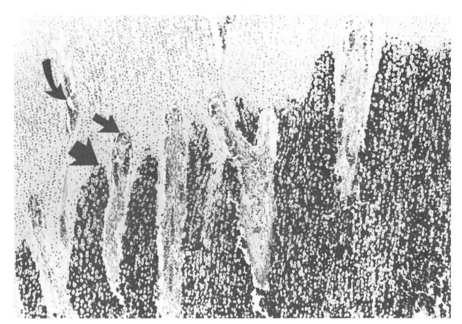

Fig. 3-18: Undecalcified histologic section of part of the metaphyseal growth plate *(above)* and the metaphysis *(below)* of the proximal tibia from a 3-week-old broiler chicken. The calcified cartilage is dark in color. The vascular channels containing vessels of diaphyseal origin *(thin straight arrow)* are invading the noncalcified cartilage of the growth plate in advance of the calcification front *(thick straight arrow)*. There are fewer vessels in the metaphysis than in that of mammals (compare with **Fig. 3-17**). In the growth plate are two retracting vessels of epiphyseal origin, of which one is indicated with a *curved arrow*. (von Kossa's stain; ×50.)

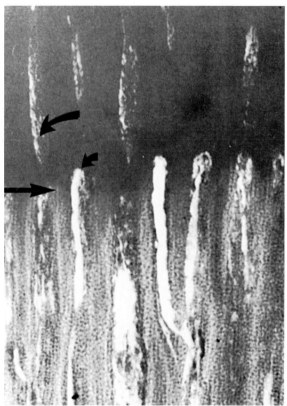

Fig. 3-19: Undecalcified microangiogram of part of the proximal tibial growth plate *(above)* and part of the metaphysis *(below)* from an 11-day-old turkey. The picture demonstrates how the vascular channels with their contrast-medium-filled diaphyseal vessels *(short curved arrow)* invade the growth plate in advance of the calcification front *(straight arrow)*. There is more calcified cartilage than vessels in the metaphysis. Several epiphyseal vessels are seen *(long curved arrow)*. They reach deep into the growth plate, but do not anastomose with the diaphyseal vessels. (×50.)

cartilage, extensive calcification takes place without the presence of vessels. Not until 3 weeks after the beginning of calcification do vessels invade from the lateral side, thereby paving the way for ossification [19].

There are some striking differences between the metaphyseal growth plate of domestic mammals and that of domestic birds. In mammals, calcification precedes vascular invasion at the junction of the growth plate and metaphysis (**Fig. 3-17**), while the opposite is found in birds (**Fig. 3-18** and **Fig. 3-19**). In the very young rapidly growing mammals only thin remnants of calcified cartilage are left as a framework for the bone laid down by the osteoblasts, while in the birds thick columns of calcified cartilage remain rather intact, even deep in the metaphysis. The number of vessels per square unit invading the growth plate from the metaphyseal side is also greater in mammals than in birds (**Figs. 3-11, 3-12, 3-17,** and **3-18**).

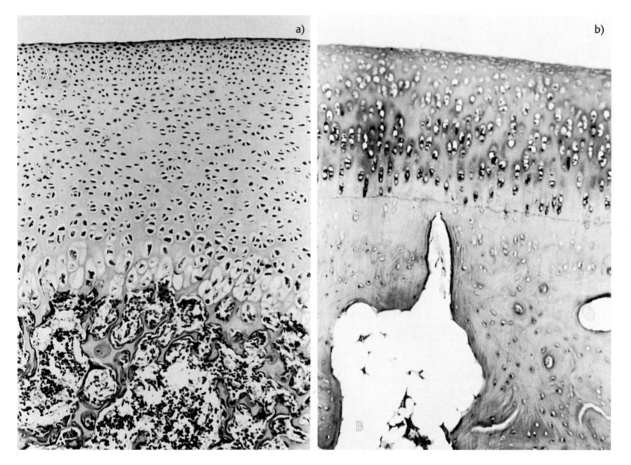

Fig. 3-20: Histologic section: a) of articular cartilage from the proximal humerus of a 9-day-old rabbit; and b) from the proximal tibia of a 2-year-old rabbit. The immature joint cartilage of the young rabbit is the active growth cartilage of the epiphysis with the zone of germinal cells (A) located about four or five cell layers away from the joint surface. Deeper in the cartilage is the zone of proliferating cells (B) and the zone of hypertrophying cells (C), where the cartilage is invaded by vessels, which are paving the way for ossification. In the old rabbit, there is a distinct border tidemark between the noncalcified and calcified joint cartilage. The subchondral bone is thick, and growth is completed. (H and E stain; ×50.)

The process by which cartilage matrix is calcified is not fully understood, but in recent years electron microscopical observations, as well as histochemical and biochemical investigations, have considerably increased our knowledge about this mechanism [25, 31]. There seems to be general agreement that certain components acting as nucleators play an important role in matrix calcification. The nucleators' identity has been debated and some scientists are convinced that the so-called matrix vesicles act as nucleators [32]. In 1967, Bonucci [33] found particles that he called osmophilic bodies in the cartilage matrix. Anderson [34] named these bodies "matrix vesicles" and he found that there were needle-shaped apatite crystals in close connection with them. Ali et al. [35] made the observation that

the matrix vesicles were seen mostly in the longitudinal septa of the growth plates and that the mineral content of the matrix vesicles increased gradually as they approached the calcified septa region. The matrix-vesicle hypothesis of mineralization states that biological calcification occurs in two phases. During the first phase the first crystals of hydroxyapatite form within vesicles in close association with the membrane. In this phase, calcium is concentrated by its affinity for vesicle phospholipids and phosphate is localized by the action of phosphatases [36]. The second phase begins with the exposure of preformed apatite crystals to the extracellular fluid, which in a normal animal contains adequate concentrations of calcium and phosphate ions to support apatite crystal proliferation by a process of homogenous nucleation. Anderson [37] makes the statement that matrix vesicles are the initial site of calcification in all growing skeletal tissues (for review see Sela et al [38]).

This postulate has, however, been questioned by Hunziker et al. [39], who suggested that early mineral crystal seen in various structures, with the aid of electron microscopy, could be the result of overprojection and the so-called truncation phenomena. A decrease in the number of large matrix vesicles during calcification in the growth cartilage from rats were described [40], and this at least suggests that matrix vesicles are involved in calcification.

The extracellular matrix proteins are also put forward as the crucial nucleators [41, 42]. Proteoglycans may play a role in cartilage calcification, by having an inhibitory effect on calcification [43], and a decrease in proteoglycan aggregate size is probably a step in lowering the inhibitory effect. The large hydrodynamic size of the proteoglycan aggregates and the negatively charged sulfate and carboxyl groups in the chondroitin sulfate can bind calcium ions and hide them as they are spread out in a large volume. This will cause an increase of the local concentration of calcium ions in the cartilage. Just preceding the onset of calcification, the proteoglycans have a lower glycosaminoglycan content, are smaller, and contain a larger proportion of molecules that are not capable of interacting with hyaluronic acid [44]. This change of proteoglycan structure, without a net loss of proteoglycans [23], could be sufficient for the initiation of calcification.

Other factors that could be of importance for calcification may be the presence of specific macromolecules in the hypertrophic region, such as the 21 kd protein, and collagen type X. Also, the C-propeptide of collagen type II (chondrocalcin), which binds to hydroxyapatite crystals, is more prominent in the hypertrophic region [45]. The key role of the growth plate chondrocytes in longitudinal bone growth has been emphasized by many authors [25, 31], and the importance of the chondrocytes in cartilage metabolism and cartilage calcification is not questioned.

The vascular invasion of the cartilage and the simultaneous resorption of part of the calcified matrix have been the subject of many investigations, and there is now a relatively clear picture of the events. For example, the matrix of the meta-physeal growth plate of rats and rabbits is calcified in the bars that separate the cell columns (interterritorial matrix), while the transverse cartilaginous walls between the chondrocytes (territorial matrix) remain unmineralized (**Fig. 3-17**). At the resorption zone, perivascular cells and endothelial cells of the vascular sprouts seem to lyse the unmineralized transverse cartilaginous walls (**Fig. 3-12**). Hydrolytic enzymes released from the hypertrophic chondrocytes and/or from capillary sprouts may participate in the process. Resorption of the mineralized longitudinal septa is mediated by the chondroclasts, with their ruffled border in contact with the calcified matrix (**Fig. 3-12**).

It should be pointed out that this depiction is true for mammals but not for birds, which have more matrix that is calcified all around the chondrocytes. This indicates that chondroclastic resorption plays a greater role in birds than in mammals, something that is easily demonstrated in histologic sections (**Fig. 3-13**).

1.3   Bone formation and remodeling

1.3.1   Endochondral bone formation in the metaphysis and epiphysis

Vascular invasion of the growth cartilage precedes bone formation, which takes place on the remnants of the calcified cartilage. Osteoprogenitor cells accompany the capillary sprouts, which invade the metaphyseal cartilage from the diaphyseal side [46]. Osteoblasts and osteocytes are derived from these cells. The osteoclasts belong to the hematopoietic cell line and are not derived from any cell type of the osteogenic line [47]. According to Vaes [48], the osteoclast progenitor cells are first found in the hematopoietic tissues. They are then disseminated and turned into resting osteoclasts that are activated to become osteoclasts at the contact with mineralized tissues. In bone the osteoblasts appear to control this activation by exposing the mineral to osteoclasts and by mediating hormones, cytokines, and growth factors that serve as enhancing or inhibitory stimuli [49–51].

The osteoblasts, which are responsible for formation of bone matrix, are arranged in an epithelioid layer (**Fig. 3-13**). The cells are cuboidal or low columnar in shape and are connected to one another by short processes. They first form a thin osteoid seam on the remnants of the calcified cartilage. This osteoid seam is soon mineralized as new osteoid is laid down on top of it, leaving an occasional osteoblast to be enclosed by osteoid and turned into an osteocyte. The nucleus of the osteocyte, which usually has one single prominent nucleolus, is often found at the end of the cell, farthest away from the bone surface. In electron micrographs the osteoblasts are seen to have the structure expected of cells actively engaged in protein synthesis, such as an abundance of endoplasmic reticulum, and their membranes are studded with ribosomes.

The primary spongy bone, which consists of bone trabeculae formed on remnants of calcified cartilage, is rapidly replaced by new trabeculae. Osteoclasts and chondroclasts are therefore at work almost immediately after the primary bone trabeculae have been formed.

1.3.2 Importance of skeletal remodeling during growth

The epiphyses are wider than the diaphysis. Hence, the meta-physeal part of the diaphysis is bent outward and, as the metaphysis is moving centrifugally when the skeleton is growing, the thin metaphyseal cortex must be resorbed. On the periosteal side osteoclasts are active, while bone is added by appositional growth on the endosteal side. This cortical remo-deling at the metaphyseal level is different than the remodeling at mid-diaphysis, where bone is formed by the periosteum while bone is resorbed on the endosteal side.

Around the metaphyseal growth plate and the most recently formed endochondral bone of the metaphysis there is a cartilaginous ring, the so-called perichondrial ring of Ranvier's ossification groove. This cartilage ring remains in contact with, and is at the same level as, the metaphyseal growth plate during the whole growth process, which means that the ring is growing on the epiphyseal side and is being resorbed on the diaphyseal side. The fact that the most rapid growth is found in the metaphyseal growth plate of the long bones should not let us forget that every part of a bone in a growing individual is involved in the growth process (**Fig. 3-15**), in which bone resorption is almost as important as bone formation. This may sound contradictory, but when one considers that growth must take place with only little change of the preformed shape of a bone, it is easier to appreciate the importance of resorption. If a bone were to grow in length only, it would soon become disproportionately thin, and, if growth in the width of the shaft took place by periosteal apposition without corresponding endosteal resorption, the cortex would be too thick and the bone marrow cavity too narrow. Considering this, it is easy to understand that remodeling—that is, balanced addition and resorption of bone—is a very important process in skeletal growth. However, remodeling does not only mean addition and removal of bone from the periosteal and endosteal sur-faces, or peripheral addition and central removal of bone from the metaphysis. Remodeling is also resorption and formation of bone trabeculae within the metaphysis and the epiphysis, or resorption and formation of both lamellar and osteonic bone of the cortex. This type of internal remodeling, bone turnover, is triggered both by mechanical forces acting on the skeleton and by the necessity of keeping calcium, phosphorus, and magnesium levels in the body fluids within certain boundaries. Bone resorption and formation is also influenced by circulating hormones and local cytokines and growth factors [**52, 53**].

Growth in the length of a bone is not an exclusive matter for the metaphyseal growth plates, although they are respon-sible both for the entire metaphyseal growth and for some of the very early growth of the epiphysis. The immature joint cartilage is always responsible for a small portion of the longitudinal growth.

The vascular reserve zone cartilage, also termed the epi-physeal growth cartilage, which represents part of the cartila-ginous anlage in the immature joint cartilage, is located close to the joint surface (see **Fig. 3-7** and **Fig. 3-21**). The growth of the epiphysis is the result of interstitial growth of the immature joint cartilage and of perichondrial appositional growth in Ranvier's ossification groove. There is a difference between species in the time when the vascular epiphyseal cartilage disappears. Many vascular channels are still present in the 16-week-old pig (**Fig. 3-21**), but there are no vascular channels in the 9-day-old rat (**Fig. 3-20**).

In case there is no epiphysis at one end of a bone, the growth of the immature joint cartilage and the subsequent endochondral ossification is the only mechanism by which longitudinal growth can be accomplished without a growth plate.

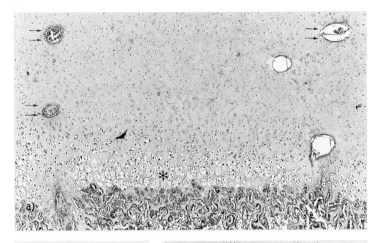

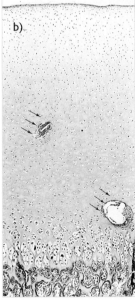
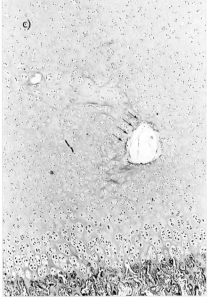

1.4 Blood supply to the metaphyseal growth plate and the epiphyseal growth cartilage

It is often stated that cartilage has no blood vessels of its own. This may be true for the articular cartilage and tracheal rings, but there are vascular channels in the cartilage of the epiphysis of most domestic animals (**Fig. 3-7**). In turkeys and chickens, vessels from the epiphysis penetrate the metaphyseal growth plate as deep as to the zone of transitional cells (**Figs. 3-11, 3-18, and 3-19**). The germinal cells (resting zone) of the metaphyseal growth plates of man, guinea pig, rabbit, and rat and of the larger domestic animals are in close contact with vessels from the epiphysis. Arteries pass through channels in the epiphyseal bone plate, which borders the growth plate. These vessels then divide and form a number of smaller convoluted vessels which end near the cells of the resting zone (**Fig. 3-22**). The veins carry the blood back to the epiphysis through the same channels in the bone plate as used by the arteries. Each of the end arteries from the epiphyseal side seems to vascularize the germinal cells responsible for the growth of five or six columns of proliferating cells.

It should be pointed out that there are no anastomoses between the epiphyseal vessels which supply the growth plate and the metaphyseal vessels which invade the calcified cartilage, although it may seem so on histologic section of growth plates of turkeys and chickens. In these birds there are large vascular channels from the epiphysis, which sometimes seem

Fig. 3-21: Transverse histological sections from the lateral femoral condyles.
a) An 8-week-old LYC (Swedish Landrace × Yorkshire crossbred) pig. Note the blood-filled vascular channels (*arrows*). The basal layer has proliferative (*arrowhead*) and hyperplastic chondrocytes (*asterisk*). Active ossification is present. (H and E stain; ×50.)
b) 16-week-old LYC pig. The growth cartilage with a darker matrix occupies about 2/3 of the joint cartilage. Blood-filled vascular channels are present (*arrows*). (H and E stain; ×18.)
c) 9-week-old LYC pig. An empty vascular channel undergoing chondrification can be seen (arrows). (H and E stain; ×50.) (Courtesy Acta Anatomica, vol 139, p. 241, 1990; Ekman, Rodriguez-Martinez and Plöen.)

to go right through the growth plate and down into the metaphysis (see **Fig. 3-27**). A closer look using higher power reveals, however, that there is no direct connection between the tip of an epiphyseal and that of a metaphyseal vessel (**Fig. 3-22**). A thin eosinophilic fibrous strand separates the two vascular channels (**Fig. 3-23**).

Because of proliferation of cartilage cells on the epiphyseal side of the growth plate and the advance of metaphyseal bone on the other side, the vessels from the epiphysis retract centrifugally and are followed closely by the advancing metaphyseal vessels. However, it should be noted that in the tibia of very young birds less than 4 days old, when most of the tibia

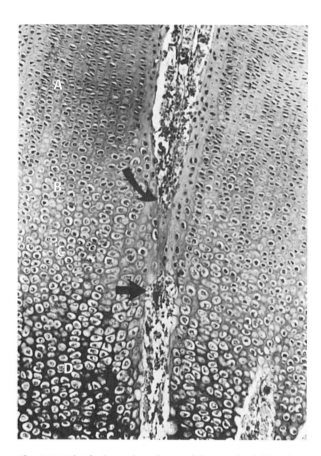

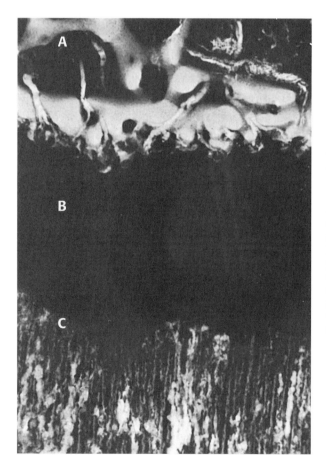

Fig. 3-22: Undecalcified microangiogram of part of the epiphysis (A), the metaphyseal growth plate (B), and part of the metaphysis (C) of the proximal tibia from a 30-day-old rabbit. Through channels in the epiphyseal bony plate, contrast-medium-filled vessels are reaching the zone of the germinal cells of the growth plate. None of these vessels proceeds deeper into the growth plate. On the metaphyseal side, calcification and vascular invasion are seen. (×50.)

Fig. 3-23: Histologic section of part of the proximal tibia of a 4-day-old Leghorn chicken. From top to bottom of the picture are the zones of proliferating cells (A), the zone of transitional cells (B), and the zone of hypertrophying cells (C). Wide columns of cartilage extend into the metaphysis (D). The marked basophilic staining of the cartilage matrix in the columns is an indication of calcification. One vascular channel containing vessels of diaphyseal origin *(straight arrow)* reaches almost to the tip of the vascular channel containing epiphyseal vessels *(curved arrows)*. A thin eosinophilic strand separates the two vascular channels. It seems obvious that the diaphyseal vascular channel is advancing in the path of the retracting epiphyseal vascular channel. (H and E stain; ×125.)

is made of cartilage, most of the cartilage, even deep in the diaphysis, seems to be vascularized mainly by the epiphyseal arteries [54]. The immature joint cartilage and the growth plate of many species contain channels harboring blood vessels and pluripotential mesenchymal cells [55–58] (Fig. 3-21). The larger channels contain one venule and one arteriole as well as many capillaries. The smaller non-branching channels consist of capillary glomeruli [59]. All the vascular channels will undergo chondrification and disappear well before maturation [60]. These channels could aid in distributing nutrients, oxygen, and different growth factors as well as removing waste products. Lufti [61] showed that when the blood supply to avian growth cartilage was interrupted, the connective cells of the vascular channels either degenerated or transformed into chondrocytes. The chondrocytes surrounding the vascular channels, however, survived despite the loss of blood supply.

1.5   Hormonal regulation of skeletal growth

Most data on the effects of hormones on the growth cartilage have been obtained from experiments with small laboratory animals. There are reasons to believe that this basic data is, at least to some extent, applicable also to large domestic animals and to man. There are, however, some obvious species differences.

Growth can be measured in different ways. In animals, it has been customary to measure growth either by repeated weighing or by measuring the difference in length of one specific long bone on radiographs taken at various intervals. The most accurate method of measuring growth rate seems, however, to be to measure the distance between two "horizontal" bone-seeking fluorochrome lines in the metaphyseal bone [62]. Knowing the time intervals between the administration of the fluorochromes to the growing animal, the growth in length per time unit can be determined (Fig. 3-24).

Growth in length of a bone depends upon an increase in cell number, cell size, or both in the growth cartilage. The most important increase is the multiplication of the chondrocytes in the germinal layer, leading to an increase of the pool size of proliferating chondrocytes, the second is stimulation of the chondrocytes in the zone of proliferating cells and enlargement of the hypertrophying cells [63, 64]. The thickness of the growth plate is not a true indicator of growth, since decrease or increase in thickness may mean only that the advancing front of the metaphyseal bone is not keeping pace evenly with the growth of the cartilage.

Within the genetic framework, normal growth is influenced by nutritional [65] and humeral endocrinologic factors [53]. Growth hormone from the pituitary is necessary for normal growth after birth and acts directly on the chondroprogenitor cells by stimulating a multiplication and differentiation of the cells. This leads to a local secretion of insulin-like growth factors (IGF-I) with an autocrine and paracrine action. IGF-I stimulates the proliferating cells by increased number of cell divisions (clonal expansion). However, the liver is the major site for the production of IGF-I, which, bound to carrier proteins, will reach the growth plate and act on the growth hormone-stimulated chondrocytes. The secretion of IGF-I is not only stimulated by growth hormone but also by thyroid hormones [66] and nutritional factors [67]. The release of growth hormone is regulated by inhibitory (somatostatin-SRIF) and stimulatory (GRH) hypothalamic factors [68, 69].

It is well known that hypophysectomy of immature animals leads to marked retardation of growth. Growth hormone administered to hypophysectomized animals stimulates longitudinal bone growth, the effect being dependent upon dose and length of administration [70]. Both mitotic division of the cells of the metaphyseal growth plate, as measured by the uptake of tritiated thymidine, and an increase in cell size (due to increased matrix synthesis), as measured by the thickness of the growth plate, are stimulated by growth hormone [71]. Of the other pituitary hormones, only thyroid-stimulating hormone (TSH), through the production of thyroxine, and prolactin stimulate growth.

Like hypophysectomy, thyroidectomy severely hampers growth in rats. Growth hormone given to hypophysectomized and thyroidectomized rats induces cartilage proliferation in the metaphyseal growth plates, with substantial plate thickening.

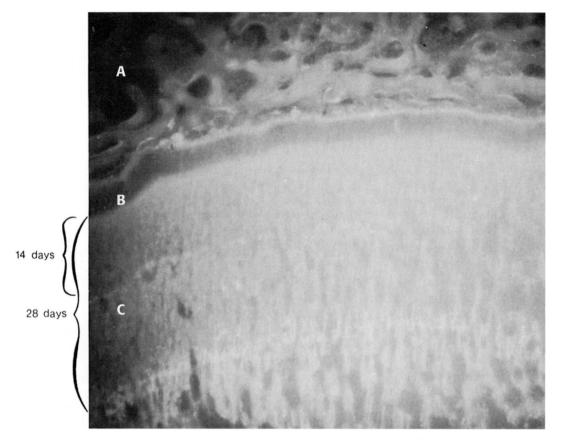

14 days

28 days

Fig. 3-24: Micrograph in transmitted ultraviolet light of an undecalcified ground section of the proximal humerus from a 4-month-old pig. The epiphysis (A), the growth plate (B), and the metaphysis (C) are seen. The animal was injected with oxytetracycline hydrochloride on day 28, with 2,4-bis-N,N'-di(carboxymethy)aminomethyl fluorescein on day 14 and with sodium alizarinsulfonate on day 1 before slaughter. The original color figure is produced here in black and white. Three colored bands are seen in the metaphysis, of which two (the yellow and the green) each have a rather distinct proximal line. The distance from the yellow line to the growth plate represents longitudinal growth during 28 days and the distance from the green line to the growth plate represents longitudinal growth during 14 days. (×25.)

If growth hormone is given together with thyroxine, the growth-stimulating effect is augmented. Thyroxine given alone under similar circumstances induces no cell proliferation and plate thickening. Rather, it causes plate thinning, eventually resulting in disappearance of the plate. It seems paradoxical that when two hormones, having opposite actions on the target, are given simultaneously, the result is marked augmentation of the growth effect.

Asling et al [72] found that thyroid augmentation of growth hormone is manifested by increased maturational changes of the more distal cells in the chondrocyte sequence, and perhaps also by promoted activity of chondrocyte progenitors. Both effects more nearly approximate the changes characterizing normal endochondral osteogenesis than was evident with growth hormone alone, and both are consistent with the known influence of the thyroid hormone on differentiation. By measuring bone growth in hypophysectomized rats with the tetracycline labeling technique, Thorngren et al [73] were able to confirm the finding that thyroxine stimulates longitudinal bone growth and that a combination of thyroxine and growth hormone given to such rats has a potentiating synergistic effect on growth. A direct effect of thyroid hormones on IGF-I production in the liver has been suggested [74]. Stimulation of local IGF-I production may contribute to the in vivo effects of thyroid hormones on bone formation [75].

The steroid hormones, estrogens, androgens, and corticosteroids have an effect on growth which is basically antagonistic to that of growth hormone [76]. All studies on the effect of sex hormones on growth have shown that the effect depends decisively upon age, species, sex, and dose, as well as upon the route and duration of administration. The often apparently contradictory results of various investigators may be explained by differences in these parameters. The reason for the rather opposing effects of androgens and estrogens may be found in their different effects on protein metabolism. The effect of sex steroids may solely be caused by variations in growth-hormone secretion, but could also be a direct action on the cartilage cells. A direct effect of sex-steroid hormones on in vitro rabbit cartilage cell [77] and rat cartilage cell proliferation [78] has been found.

It has been shown that estrogens not only suppress the action of growth hormone, but also directly decrease mitosis of the chondrocytes in the growth plate [71]. Estrogens also enhance maturation of the chondrocytes and promote calcification of the matrix [79]. Castration of young female rats therefore accelerates growth, but castration of young male rats has the opposite effect. This leads to a lag in growth [80], which seems strange since androgens, like estrogens, promote maturation of cartilage. However, in suitable doses, their anabolic effect is apparently stronger; they therefore promote growth more than they retard it. However, with high doses of androgens, increase in body weight is slowed down.

In humans, testosterone accelerates longitudinal growth and bone maturation synchronously while castration delays skeletal maturation. The metaphyseal growth plates close with delay, or not at all, after castration, and, in contrast to what occurs in rats, over-length of the extremities is induced [80].

Cortisone counteracts the effect of growth hormone. Prolonged cortisone treatment leads to stunted growth. Even a single dose of cortisone given to rats at the time of hypophysectomy has been shown to cause lasting depression of growth [81]. In young mice, administration of corticosteroids significantly retarded the proliferative activity of the chondro-progenitor cells, concomitant with an acceleration of the maturational process of the chondrocytes [82]. A suppression of the chondrocyte-proteoglycan production together with a degradation of the proteoglycans already present in the cartilage matrix have been reported [83, 84].

The mechanism by which growth is physiologically slowed down and brought to an end by closure of the growth plates (**Fig. 3-16**) is not completely understood. It is assumed that in man the many alterations occurring during puberty, including closure of the growth plates, are elicited by the male and female sex hormones. During sexual maturation the anabolic effect of androgens prevails, whereas for estrogens the strong maturation-promoting effect dominates. In dogs cessation of growth cannot be explained by an increase of circulatory estrogens, since the peripheral plasma level of estradiol does not increase with age. In a study of female dogs from 17 weeks of age until the first heat period, increase in circulating estradiol was found only a few weeks prior to the first estrus, at an age when growth had already ceased [85].

1.6 Nervous regulation of growth

It is obvious that the growth cartilage, as an integral part of the musculoskeletal system, should be dependent upon a normal musculoskeletal function. Most of our knowledge about the nervous and vascular influences on growth is derived from experimental studies on small laboratory animals, and by clinical observations. For example, it was shown in rabbits that peripheral nerve sectioning leads to a significant acceleration in growth of an extremity followed by a later retardation of growth: the end result being retardation. This effect is seen clinically in young human patients with an extremity paralyzed by poliomyelitis. The same effect on growth of an extremity was found after the sectioning of the anterior (ventral) roots in rabbits. After sensory denervation, or lumbosacral ganglion-ectomy, no significant effect on growth of the involved extremity was observed in rabbits [86]. Many studies appear to agree that little or no bone gross growth changes are associated with denervations, but there is evidence that muscle activity contributes to the form and growth of a long bone, with indirect evidence of interaction between the activity of the growth plate and periosteal tension [87].

1.7 Closure of the growth plate

By the time the growth period is approaching its end, the growth plates are becoming thinner (**Fig. 3-16**). The cartilage ceases to grow and is resorbed and replaced by bone. This is a gradual process and, before the whole growth plate has disappeared, tiny bony bridges uniting the epiphysis and metaphysis are found. It should be noted that in some species, for example, the rat, the growth plates persist for a long time after completion of growth. It is not unusual to find that the growth plates remain open during the entire life span of the animal, with fusion occurring only in senile specimens. Hence, the metaphyseal growth plate of the rat remains as a "resting cartilage" with a certain potential to resume growth.

2 Pathology and pathophysiology of the growth cartilage

2.1 Endocrine disorders

Hyperpituitarism is a condition in which there is excessive secretion of growth hormone by the acidophilic cells of the anterior pituitary lobe. If hyperpituitarism begins well before closure of the growth plates, the condition is characterized by longitudinal overgrowth, resulting in a proportional giant. If overproduction of the growth hormone continues after closure of the growth plates, longitudinal growth is only a little affected, since only the joint cartilage can continue to grow. There is, however, excessive growth of cartilage and bone from the perichondrium and periosteum, leading to distortion of the normal configuration of many bones. The condition is called acromegaly. In man, typical changes in acromegaly are gigantism, with enlarged hands and feet, and coarse facial features; similar changes may also be seen in animals with acromegaly.

True hyperpituitarism is rare in animals. Almost as rare is hypopituitarism, in which there is too little secretion of growth hormone. Congenital or early developing hypopituitarism results in a pituitary dwarf. This has been described in German shepherd dogs [88] and in a family of giant schnauzers [89]. The skeletal proportions present at the onset of growth hormone deficiency will persist, meaning that a pituitary dwarf usually has a relatively large head. The metaphyseal growth plates and the immature joint cartilage are inactive in hypopituitarism but, because of lack of resorption of the metaphyseal growth plates, they persist longer than normal.

As stated earlier (**Section 1.5**), thyroxine acts synergistically with growth hormone on the metaphyseal growth plates. Hypothyroidism, which begins early in life, is called cretinism. It leads to stunted growth, mental retardation, and sexual underdevelopment. Cartilage proliferation, calcification, and bone formation in the metaphyseal growth plates slow down or cease. Cretinism in animals is rare and, like hyperpituitarism and hypopituitarism, is of little or no clinical importance.

Of more clinical and general medical interest than the rare occurrence of endocrine disorders in individual animals is the often overlooked fact that man, through selective breeding of some species of domestic animals, has preserved and even increased certain pathologic features. Many of these features are such that they must be the result of an endocrine imbalance. An example is gigantism with and without signs of acromegaly and dwarfism, proportionate or disproportionate (**Section 2.2.1**).

2.2 Congenital developmental disturbances

There are a number of congenital developmental disturbances which affect the growth plates. However, with the exception of achondroplasia, they are very rare and are therefore of limited clinical interest. Those with particular interest in these lesions are referred to textbooks on bone pathology.

2.2.1 Achondroplasia

True achondroplasia, also called chondrodystrophy, is relatively rare in animals. It is of clinical interest mainly because several breeds of dogs and cattle have some of the characteristics of achondroplasia.

Because of retardation and premature cessation of the whole process of endochondral ossification, the most characteristic feature of achondroplasia is disturbance of growth of those parts of the skeleton that possess the greatest growth capacity: the long bones. The resulting dwarfism is mainly caused by the extremities being abnormally short, while the head and the trunk are of comparatively normal size.

In the metaphyseal growth plate, the proliferating cells lack the usual columnar arrangement. The differentiation of the chondrocytes is disturbed to the point of complete disorganization, leading to a very irregular calcification of the cartilage. There is also irregular penetration by vessels and a scanty, irregular ossification [90].

As mentioned, some features typical for endocrine disorders may be seen as breed characteristics in many species. This is true also for achondroplasia. In the dog, there are, for example, proportional giants and dwarfs with features characteristic of hyperpituitarism and hypopituitarism, respectively. Examples may be seen in the schnauzer breeds; the giant schnauzer represents a proportional giant while the miniature schnauzer is a proportional dwarf. In St. Bernards and some other large heavy breeds, there are definitely some acromegalic traits. Other breeds have traits of achondroplasia, such as short curved legs and a relatively proportional head and body. A typical example is the dachshund, in which there is strong histologic evidence of an achondroplastic body constitution [91].

There are also some breeds of cattle, such as the Aberdeen Angus and Hereford, which have achondroplastic traits. Certain acromegalic traits, such as inferior prognathism and plump long bones, are common in the fast-growing domestic pig. It has also been shown that certain boar lines of the Landrace pig have an increased amount of circulating growth hormone and somatomedin [92].

Skeletal dysplasia within certain bovine and canine breeds may be used as a possible biomedical model for certain aspects of human dwarfism. This warrants an adequate classification of true dwarfism within these breeds. Many examples can be found in the literature such as: achondrogenesis type II dwarfism in the Holstein breed [93]; chondrodysplasia of the rhizomelic type in Japanese Brown cattle [94]; pseudoachondroplasia in the Scottish deerhound [95]; chondrodysplasia in Great Pyrénéens [96]; metaphyseal dysplasia in Alaskan Malamutes [97]; and ocular chondrodysplasia in Labrador retriever dogs [98].

2.3 Nutritionally induced conditions of the growth cartilage

Manifest endocrine disorders in animals are rare, but nutritional problems, which in one way or the other may influence growth, are frequent. Deficiency conditions used to be the most common, but the last 40 years have seen an increase in problems associated with overnutrition and rapid growth.

2.3.1 Rickets and nutritional secondary hyperparathyroidism

A classic deficiency disease is rickets, caused by lack of vitamin D. It should, however, be pointed out that feed exclusively deficient in vitamin D is not often given to animals. Feed low in vitamin D given to herbivores is, for example, often also low in calcium. Highly concentrated fodder and little hay, with no supplementation of vitamins and minerals, is an example of such a feed. If it is given to fast-growing bulls kept indoors, skeletal problems of a complex nature are bound to occur. Before the era of commercial feed it was not uncommon to give omnivores and carnivores a feed low in calcium and high in phosphorous, but vitamin D supplementation was usually adequate. The ensuing clinical problems were nevertheless often grouped together under the diagnosis of rickets. With the knowledge we have today it can emphatically be stated that true rickets has been and is a rare disease in animals. When it is seen, it is usually only part of a complex nutritional problem in rapidly growing individuals.

It should be remembered that there are a number of forms of vitamin D, but only two of practical importance. Vitamin D2, also known as calciferol (ergocalciferol), is derived from the provitamin ergosterol in plants. Vitamin D3, also known as cholecalciferol, is derived from the provitamin 7-dehydrocholesterol in the skin. The transformation of these provitamins to vitamins is a photochemical reaction requiring ultraviolet light of an appropriate wavelength. This means that animals exposed to sunlight may not develop rickets even if they are on a feed low in vitamin D.

Vitamin D is metabolized first in the liver then in the kidney. The metabolites of vitamin D, particularly the active hormone, 1,25-dihydroxycholecalciferol (1,25-$(OH)_2D_3$, calcitriol), are involved in the long-term regulation of the blood calcium level. There are a number of important interactions. 1,25-$(OH)_2D_3$ or some other metabolite is necessary for the action of parathyroid hormone (PTH) on bone, while PTH activates the hydroxylase in the kidneys, which synthesize 1,25-$(OH)_2D_3$. Thus, hypocalcemia, which stimulates secretion of parathyroid hormone, will also increase 1,25-$(OH)_2D_3$ and thus increase calcium absorption from the gut and mobilization from bone. There is also evidence that 1,25-$(OH)_2D_3$ induces osteoblasts to produce a factor that stimulates osteoclastic bone resorption [99].

The role of calcitonin in calcium metabolism is less clear, but Martin [52] states that "calcitonin acts directly upon osteoclasts to decrease their activity". However, calcitonin receptors have been found both on osteoclasts and osteoblasts in the rat [100]. In growing mammals it helps to stabilize the plasma calcium level and the balance between bone resorption and formation.

The main histologic features in rickets, as seen in rats given a vitamin-D-deficient, low-phosphorus diet, and in rare clinical cases, are loss of the normal columnar arrangement of the cartilage cells in the growth plate, decreased ability to calcify the matrix of the zone of hypertrophied cells, and a decrease in the rate of vascular invasion. Another characteristic of rickets is also a difficulty in mineralization of the osseous tissue formed by the osteoblasts. These changes make the growth plate thicker (**Fig. 3-25**) and, because large buds of uncalcified cartilage protrude into the metaphysis, the growth plate also develops a serrated appearance toward the metaphysis.

The bone trabeculae that are eventually formed in a rachitic animal are deficient in mineral; that is, the osteoid seam is much wider than normal. The protruding cartilage buds of the growth plate are usually found in various stages of degeneration, or in a state of regressive transformation into a fibrous tissue. The metaphyseal marrow is often rather fibrous and has thick, irregular osseous trabeculae (**Fig. 3-26**). In advanced rickets, the bone is soft and bowing of the extremities may

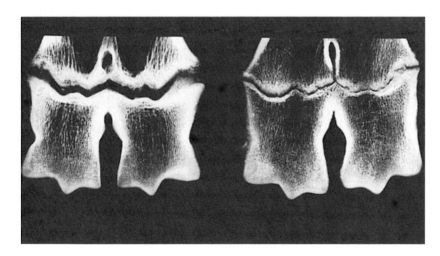

Fig. 3-25: Radiograph of two 5-mm-thick sections, each from the distal metacarpus of a young bull. To the left is a section from a 1-year-old bull which had been on a high-calorie, low-vitamin-D, and low-calcium diet. To the *right* is a section from a 1-year-old bull which had been on a balanced diet. The metaphyseal growth plate in the specimen to the left is irregular and thickened, and the growth plate in the specimen to the *right* is normal. (From Jonsson et al., 1972 [101].)

occur. The metaphyseal areas, particularly of the long bones and the costochondral junctions, are widened because of proliferation of cartilage by the perichondrium.

In most domestic animals the effect of low vitamin-D intake is usually enhanced by a low-calcium content in the feed. The risk of vitamin D and calcium deficiency in animals today is rather small, since most animals are given commercial feed to which sufficient amounts of both vitamin D and calcium have been added. However, in fast-growing bulls fed mainly grain, a feed high in phosphorus, and given only a little hay and no extra vitamin D and/or calcium, a condition was found that had characteristics of rickets (**Fig. 3-26**) and/or nutritional secondary hyperparathyroidism [**101**]. Changes typical for the latter condition were found to dominate in those animals given the most calcium-deficient feed. While rickets affects mainly the growth plate, nutritional secondary hyperparathyroidism has bone as the main target. Because of increased function of the parathyroid glands, triggered by the low serum-calcium level, bone resorption exceeds bone formation and a picture of osteitis fibrosa is established. Bone trabeculae are rapidly formed, but they are soon resorbed and replaced by fibrous tissue [**102**]. Nutritional secondary hyperparathyroidism in its most advanced form is best seen in kittens fed a high-phosphorus and low-calcium diet, such as liver and muscle meat [**103**]. The animals fed such a diet rapidly develop very thin bones which easily fracture, because bone apposition cannot keep pace with bone resorption. In contrast to rickets, the growth plates are not particularly involved in this deficiency.

A rickets-like condition has been reported in growing pigs with experimental hypophosphatemia [**104**]. An increased width of the growth plate and an increased deposition of a poorly mineralized osteoid was described.

a)
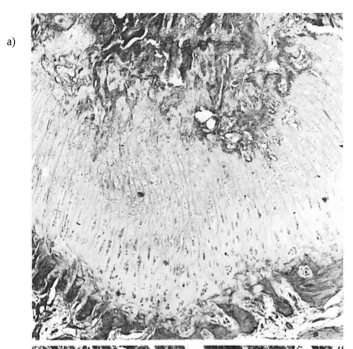

b)
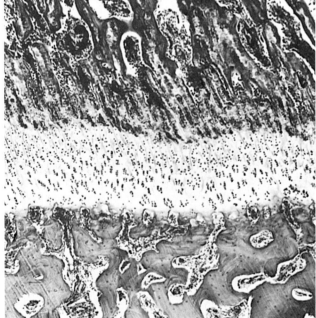

Fig. 3-26: a) Histologic section of the metaphyseal growth plate of the metacarpus from a 9-month-old bull, which had been on a high-calorie, low-calcium, and low-vitamin-D diet.
b) Histologic section of the same area in a bull of the same age which had been on a balanced diet. The growth plate in the bull on the diet low in vitamin D and calcium is thicker than normal and very irregular, and the bone trabeculae, which are formed in the metaphysis, are irregular and interspersed by fibrous tissue and retained cartilage. The growth plate of the bull which had been on the balanced diet is normal.
(From Jonsson et al., 1972 [**101**].)

2.3.2 Other nutritionally induced disturbances of growth

Hypervitaminosis D, caused by an over-ambitious supplementation of this vitamin, may be seen occasionally. The main toxic effect is soft-tissue calcification, but retardation of growth may also occur.

Hypovitaminosis A causes proliferation and differentiation of the cartilage cells to cease and the growth plate to narrow. The cells which have reached the hypertrophying state undergo normal provisional calcification, and the end result of hypovitaminosis A is severe retardation of growth.

Hypervitaminosis A may initially enhance growth, but premature closure of the growth plate seems to be the dominating effect. This is apparently caused by rapid provisional calcification of even the layers of the cartilage which normally do not calcify.

Hypovitaminosis C, which among other things leads to retardation of growth, may occur in man, monkeys, and guinea pigs. Vitamin C is synthesized in domestic animals and in other laboratory animals, and hypovitaminosis C has not been demonstrated in these animals.

Starvation, due to low caloric intake, low protein intake, or both, gives rise to stunted growth. Both the thyroid and pituitary are inactivated, particularly by protein starvation.

2.4 Osteochondrosis

Today, overnutrition is as common in the industrialized countries as is undernutrition or even starvation in many parts of the Third World. Overnutrition of young animals leads to a maximum growth rate, within the genetic framework. Because rapid growth is an important economic factor in animal husbandry, there has, for many years, been a genetic selection for individuals with rapid growth, particularly in pigs, turkeys, and broilers, and to some extent also in beef cattle. The economic gains have been considerable, but an increasing incidence of a disease called osteochondrosis [105], which has been shown to be correlated with rapid growth [106, 107], has begun to make a negative impact. Lameness, mating problems, and leg weakness because of painful joints are the main clinical problems encountered in osteochondrosis.

The basic pathology of osteochondrosis is a multifocal, deficient endochondral ossification of the growth cartilage, both in the metaphyseal growth plates (**Fig. 3-27** and **Fig. 3-28**) and in the epiphyseal growth cartilage (immature joint cartilage, **Fig. 3-29**) [108]. Cartilage growth is rapid but the chondrocyte differentiation is disturbed, with subsequent loss of the prerequisites for bone formation, provisional calcification, and vascular invasion. Hence, cartilage is retained and bone is not formed (**Fig. 3-27**) [105, 109].

In pigs, turkeys, and broilers, the fastest growing of the domestic animals, osteochondrosis is always a generalized condition, histologically and often also macroscopically. On the microscopic level, osteochondrosis has certain features in common with rickets (**Fig. 3-26** and **Fig. 3-28**), but etiologically the two diseases are unrelated. It has not been possible to decrease or increase the incidence of osteochondrosis in pigs with a low or high intake of vitamin A, vitamin D, and calcium. However, low intake of calcium can increase the severity of the lesions induced by osteochondrosis [110]. On the other hand, it has been shown that the incidence and severity of osteochondrosis in pigs can be drastically reduced if the animals' growth rate is slowed down, either by nutritional or genetic means [106]. Domestic pigs on a restricted feed have little or no osteochondrosis. In the dog, a general factor of importance seems to be overnutrition combined with a high intake of calcium [111, 112].

There are certain predilection sites for osteochondrosis, usually typical for each animal species. It seems that the changes occur most frequently where cartilage growth is very rapid and where mechanical forces are at play [113–116].

In the epiphyseal growth cartilage (immature joint cartilage), osteochondrosis leads to a condition called osteochondritis dissecans (osteochondrosis dissecans). A fissure that originates in the necrosis of the growth cartilage (**Fig. 3-30** and **Fig. 3-31**) eventually extends along the border between the calcified and non-calcified joint cartilage (the tide mark). The fissure eventually reaches the surface of the joint cartilage and, in this way, a cartilage flap or joint mouse is formed (**Fig. 3-32**).

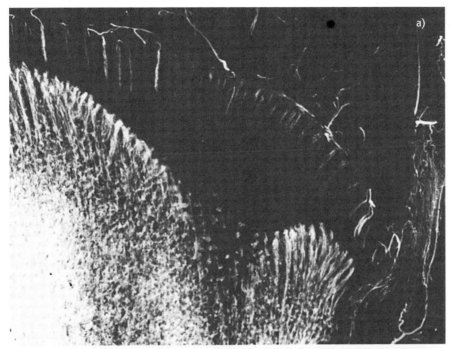

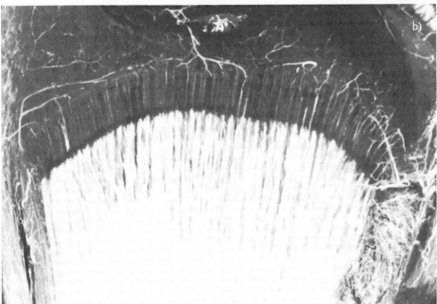

Osteochondrosis has been reported in the dog [115, 117], the pig [105, 118], the horse [119], the turkey [109], the chicken [54], and the rat [120]. The light, microscopic appearance of the affected cartilage has been thoroughly described in these species. Ultrastructural studies of osteochondrosis in the pig, both in the epiphyseal growth cartilage [121, 122] and in the metaphyseal growth plate [123] have shown that the early events in the lesions appear to differ at these two locations.

However, the end result is the same: disturbed focal ossification because of almost complete absence of cartilage calcification and of vascular penetration.

The early lesions in the metaphyseal growth plate of pigs [123, 124] and broilers [125] are characterized by foci of non-maturing hypertrophic chondrocytes that appear to produce an abnormal pericellular matrix. Because of this disturbed ossification, cartilage is retained in the subchondral bone. Chondronecrosis is a later event.

Fig. 3-27:
a) Microangiogram of a decalcified section of the proximal tibia from a 102-day-old turkey with osteo-chondrosis. (×10.)
b) Microangiogram of the proximal tibia of a 32-day-old turkey with a normal growth plate. (×10.) In the turkey with osteochondrosis there are no contrast-medium-filled vessels in the retained portion of the growth plate in spite of an abundance of vessels in the metaphysis. In the bird with the normal growth plate it can be seen that only a very thin zone of the metaphyseal growth plate near the metaphysis is void of vessels. Some of the epiphyseal vessels seem to invade the metaphysis. (From Poulos, 1978 [109].)

Fig. 3-28: Histologic sections of the proximal tibia of a 28-day-old broiler chicken with osteochondrosis.
a) There is retention of cartilage in a large part of the metaphysis. (H and E stain; ×6.)
b) The retained cartilage is not calcified as is seen in this section, in which calcified cartilage and bone are stained dark. (von Kossa's stain; ×6.)
(From Poulos, 1978 [109].)

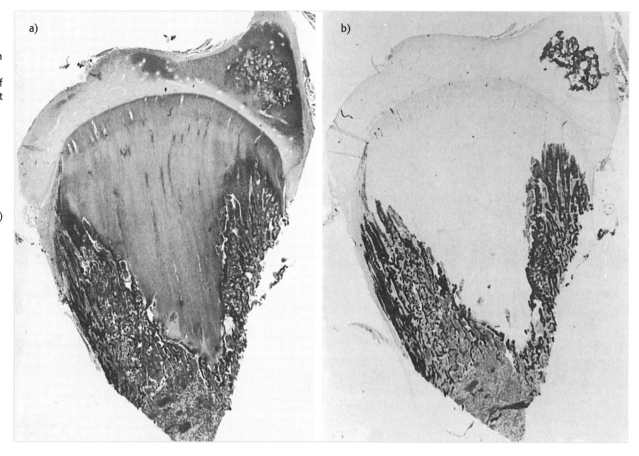

However, the early osteochondrotic lesions in the epiphyseal growth cartilage (immature joint cartilage) are described as chondronecrotic areas in the resting region, with close connection to necrotic vascular channels [126, 127]. Hypoxia caused by vascular necrosis has been suggested as a cause of chondronecrosis in the pig and horse [128–130]. Many microscopic lesions are found in the growth cartilage, but only a few in certain locations will develop into gross lesions. The obvious healing of many of the lesions indicate that additional cartilage damage must occur at the predilection sites. Local ischemia in the cartilage is a key factor and this leads to formation of vulnerable zones of necrotic cartilage secondary to defects in the blood supply. The etiology of osteochondrosis appears to be multifactorial, with trauma, hereditary factors, rapid growth, nutritional factors, and ischemia all having a role in the pathogenesis [131].

When osteochondritis dissecans has developed, healing cannot take place in any other way than by outgrowth of a fibrocartilaginous scar from the floor of the defect in the joint surface. A prerequisite for this is detachment of the cartilage flap that covers the defect. Most of the predilection sites of osteochondritis dissecans are where the joint cartilage during growth is normally thicker than the surrounding cartilage, and where pressure during motion and weight bearing is great.

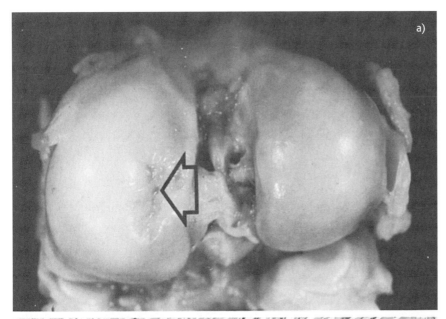

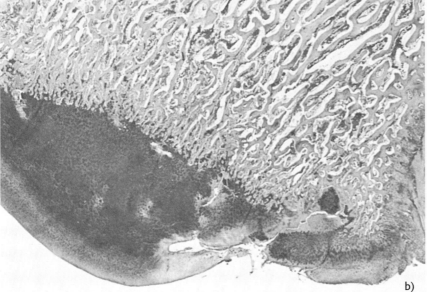

Fig. 3-29: The distal femur from a 4 1/2-month-old German shepherd dog with osteochondrosis.
a) Macrospecimen. There is a collapse of cartilage and a fissure (*arrow*) in the lateral condyle, which is whiter in color than the medial condyle.
b) Histologic section of the lateral condyle. There is large retention of cartilage. This means that endochondral bone formation has not kept pace with the growth of the condyle. On the medial side of the lateral condyle there is widespread necrosis of the partly collapsed cartilage. Several fissures are seen reaching from the subchondral bone to the joint surface. (H and E stain; ×10.)

The role of mechanical factors in the etiology of osteochondrosis has been disputed. Grøndalen [118] and Nakano and Aherne [132] put them relatively high on the etiologic list, while Reiland [105] felt that they were of secondary importance. According to Reiland, this is demonstrated by the fact that osteochondrosis occurs even in places where there is no weight bearing, such as the costochondral junctions. In the dog, it was shown that a combination of general and local factors are at play in the pathogenesis of osteochondrosis [116].

It should be pointed out that in the fastest growing species of domestic animals (e.g., pig, turkey, and broiler), even individuals without osteochondrosis have less well-organized growth plates than their more slowly-growing wild counterparts (Fig. 3-9). This, together with the generalized nature of osteochondrosis and its correlation with rapid growth, speaks in favor of an intrinsic factor as the most important for the occurrence of osteochondrosis.

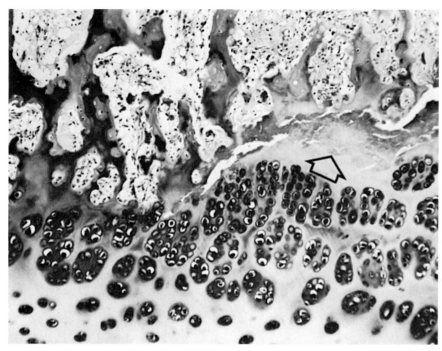

Fig. 3-30: Histologic section of part of the subchondral bone and the basal layers of the joint cartilage from the medial part of the distal talus in a 6-month-old Landrace pig. To the right of the picture the joint cartilage is thickened and necrotic in its deepest layer. As seen by the lack of cartilaginous core of the bone trabeculae to the right, endochondral ossification has ceased in this area. There is a slightly eosinophilic necrotic mass (arrow) that separates the cartilage from the underlying bone. A fissure apparently originates in the necrotic mass. Fibrosis of the bone marrow underlying the fissure is seen. (H and E stain; ×250.) (From Reiland, 1978 [110].)

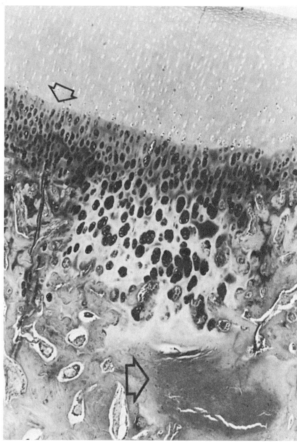

Fig. 3-31: Histologic section of the joint cartilage and subchondral bone of the proximal end of the first phalanx from a 5-month-old horse with clinical signs of osteochondrosis from the age of 2 months. There is a sharp demarcation (small arrow) between the uncalcified joint cartilage (on top) and the calcified cartilage (below). In the center of the picture is retention of cartilage with an abundance of clusters of chondrocytes. Beneath the retained cartilage is an eosinophilic necrotic mass (large arrow), in which a fissure is seen. The changes represent the first stage in the development of osteochondritis dissecans. (H and E stain; ×50.)

Epiphysiolysis is, in addition to osteochondritis dissecans, the most serious complication in osteochondrosis. Because of disturbed endochondral ossification, the metaphyseal growth plate becomes thick and severely weakened. This may lead to fissures in the cartilage and slipping of the epiphysis. The most common example of slipped epiphysis is the one seen in the femoral head epiphysis in man, dogs, and pigs. The ischiatic tuberosity may also slip, particularly in pregnant sows.

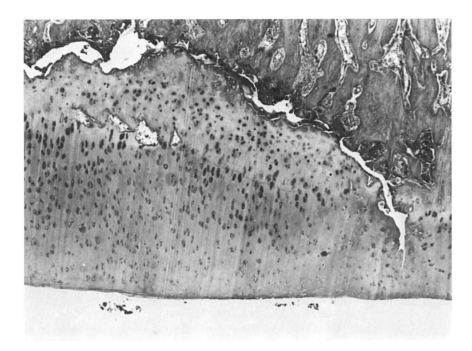

Fig. 3-32: Histologic section of the lateral condyle from a 5-month-old horse with osteochondrosis (the same as in **Fig. 3-31**). The thickened part of the joint cartilage, which is necrotic in its basal layer, is about to form a flap or become detached because the fissure that separates the cartilage from the underlying bone is about to reach the joint surface. (H and E stain; ×50.)

2.5 Premature closure of the growth plates

Premature closure of the growth plates is seen most frequently in the dog. The cause may be traumatic, but in many cases the etiology is unknown. The most serious result of premature closure of the metaphyseal growth plate is seen when the growth plates of the radius and ulna are involved. The distal growth plate of the ulna is responsible for more than 80% of the growth in length of the bone. The radius, on the other hand, has two growth plates which are responsible for longitudinal growth. The distal one is responsible for about 2/3 of the growth in length and the proximal one for about 1/3. If the distal growth plates of both the ulna and radius are injured, premature closure may follow. This means that there will be no more longitudinal growth in the distal ends of the bones. The proximal growth plate of the radius continues, however, to function normally, and the radius becomes proportionately longer than the ulna. This usually leads to bowing of the radius or subluxation of the radial head in the elbow joint. Often, the two deformities are combined. If the distal growth plate of the ulna closes too early for some reason and the two growth plates of the radius remain open, the retardation of ulnar growth leads to even more serious consequences. Usually there will be a very advanced distortion of the leg, characterized by lateral deviation of the peripheral part of the leg, anterior curvature of the radius, lateral dislocation of the radial head in the elbow joint, and change in shape of the anconeal process of the ulna. The anconeal process is damaged because it is pressed against the distal wall of the olecranon fossa of the humerus. This pressure may even lead to non-union of the anconeal process. If only the distal growth plate of the radius is injured, the result will be a pathologic remodeling of the elbow joint because of loss of contact between the lateral humeral condyle and the head of the shortened radius, with a corresponding increase of pressure on the medial condyle and coronoid process of the ulna.

2.6 Hypertrophic osteodystrophy (metaphyseal osteopathy)

Hypertrophic osteodystrophy (metaphyseal osteopathy) is a lesion of the metaphysis, and to some extent of the metaphyseal growth plate, of large, rapidly growing dogs about 3 to 5 months old. The etiology is obscure, but a virus infection (canine distemper virus) has been implicated as a possible etiologic agent both in metaphyseal osteopathy in dogs and in Paget disease of humans [133, 134]. The clinical, radiographic, and histologic pictures of metaphyseal osteopathy in dogs are well known [102, 135]. Baumgärtner et al. [136] experimentally induced metaphyseal bone lesions with canine distemper virus, but these lesions differed in histologic appearance from the naturally occurring disease.

The following histologic features have been described in hypertrophic osteodystrophy: (1) acute inflammation of the osteochondral complexes; (2) a mixed, bizarre picture of the metaphyseal region with apparently deficient resorption of the calcified portion of the growth plate; (3) formation of thick bone trabeculae with a thick cartilage core, necrosis, micro-fractures, and collapse of these trabeculae; (4) fibrosis; (5) osteoclastic resorption; and (6) reparative formation of woven bone (**Figs. 3-33, 3-34,** and **3-35**). In the later stages, periosteal new bone formation is also seen. The lesion often heals spon-taneously after several relapses of the clinical signs, which are severe pain, fever, and swelling of the affected parts of the long bones. In severe cases, persistent deformation of the legs is not an unusual sequel.

2.7 Effect of radiation on the growth cartilage

It has long been known that growing cartilage is relatively radiosensitive. Because of the ease of measuring growth rate and of registering abnormal shape of, for example, the ver-tebrae, the growth cartilage of experimental animals has been used as a target for irradiation of varying doses.

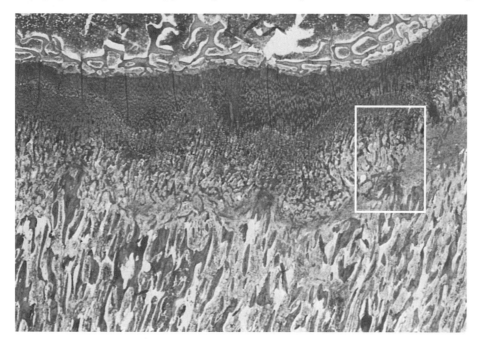

Fig. 3-33: Histologic section of the epiphysis *(above)*, metaphyseal growth plate, and metaphysis of the proximal humerus from a 5-month-old Great Dane dog with the clinical and radiographic signs of hypertrophic osteodystrophy. The growth plate is uneven and the part of the metaphysis which is closest to the growth plate is highly pathological. Thick bone trabeculae with a cartilage core and some retained cartilage have undergone necrosis, fracture, and collapse. There is also extensive bone and cartilage resorption, as well as formation of woven bone and a marked marrow fibrosis. Deeper in the metaphysis the bone trabeculae are rather large and plump and do not have a carti-laginous core. (H and E stain; ×10.)

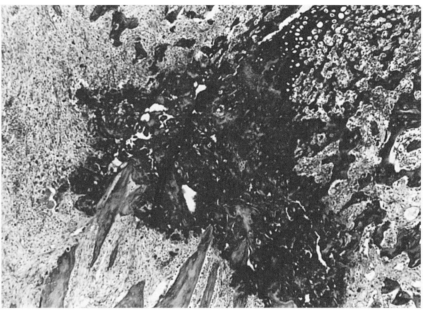

Fig. 3-35: Histologic section of the proximal humerus from a 5-month-old Great Dane dog (the same as in Fig. 3-33 and Fig. 3-34). There is massive necrosis of bone and cartilage in the fibrotic zone that separates the primary bone trabeculae *(upper right)* from the thick and plump older trabeculae deeper in the metaphysis *(lower left)*. (H and E stain; ×50.)

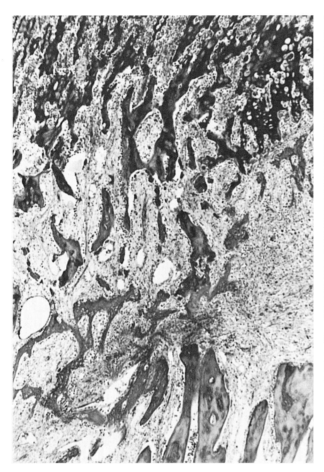

Fig. 3-34: Histologic section at higher magnification of the proximal humerus from the 5-month-old Great Dane dog in Fig. 3-33. (The area shown here is the one within the rectangle in Fig. 3-33.) On top of the picture there are thick primary bone trabeculae and some retained cartilage in fibrotic bone marrow, in which also some trabeculae of woven bone are seen. On the other side of the fibrotic marrow *(below)* are thick bone trabeculae without a cartilaginous core.

There are quantitative dose-time data available for various changes seen in the vertebrae after radiation given to growing animals. The higher the dose and the younger the animal, the more severe are the vertebral changes.

Carrig et al. [137] irradiated the distal growth plate of the ulna to slow down the growth of this bone in order to study the effect on the development of the elbow joint. By giving a 10 Gy depth dose to the center of the growth plate through two opposing fields, a 40–50% retardation of ulnar growth was obtained.

Monkey fetuses receiving 3 Gy at 90 days gestation (60 days before birth) were born stunted but without any congenital defects. Children exposed to atomic bomb radiations at Nagasaki while in utero showed reduction in head circumference, body height, and weight [138].

3 Bibliography

Blue references indicate links to abstracts of articles available online:
http://www.aopublishing.org/BONE/3.htm

1. **Heinegård D, Hultenby K, Oldberg Å, et al.** (1989) Macromolecules in bone matrix. *Connect Tissue Res;* 21 (1–4):3–11.

2. **Bruckner P, van der Rest M** (1994) Structure and function of cartilage collagens. *Microsc Res Tech;* 28 (5): 378–384.

3. **Roughley PJ, Lee ER** (1994) Cartilage proteoglycans: structure and potential functions. *Microsc Res Tech;* 28 (5):385–397.

4. **Heinegård D, Paulsson M** (1984) Structure and metabolism of proteoglycans. In: Piez KA, Reddi AH, editors. *Extracellular Matrix Biochemistry.* New York: Elsevier, 277.

5. **Heinegård D, Oldberg Å** (1989) Structure and biology of cartilage and bone matrix noncollagenous macro-molecules. *Faseb J;* 3 (9):2042–2051.

6. **Kempson GE, Freeman MA, Swanson SA** (1968) Tensile properties of articular cartilage. *Nature;* 220 (172):1127–1128.

7. **Kempson GE, Muir H, Swanson SA, et al.** (1970) Correlations between stiffness and the chemical constituents of cartilage on the human femoral head. *Biochem Biophys Acta;* 215:70.

8. **Gibson GJ, Flint MH** (1985) Type X collagen synthesis by chick sternal cartilage and its relationship to endochondral development. *J Cell Biol;* 101 (1):277–284.

9. **Grant WT, Sussman MD, Balian G** (1985) A disulfide-bonded short chain collagen synthesized by degenerative and calcifying zones of bovine growth plate cartilage. *J Biol Chem;* 260 (6):3798–3803.

10. **Rucklidge GJ, Milne G, Robins SP** (1996) Collagen type X: a component of the surface of normal human, pig, and rat articular cartilage. *Biochem Biophys Res Commun;* 224 (2):297–302.

11. **Heinegård D, Saxne T** (1991) Molecular markers of processes in cartilage in joint disease. *Br J Rheumatol;* 30 (Suppl 1):21–24.

12. **Larsson T, Sommarin Y, Paulsson M, et al.** (1991) Cartilage matrix proteins. A basic 36-kDa protein with a restricted distribution to cartilage and bone. *J Biol Chem;* 266 (30): 20428–20433.

13. **Hedbom E, Antonsson P, Hjerpe A, et al.** (1992) Cartilage matrix proteins. An acidic oligomeric protein (COMP) detected only in cartilage. *J Biol Chem;* 267 (9):6132–6136.

14. **Descalzi Cancedda F, Manduca P, Tacchetti C, et al.** (1988) Developmentally regulated synthesis of a low molecular weight protein (Ch 21) by differentiating chondrocytes. *J Cell Biol;* 107 (6 Pt 1): 2455–2463.

15. **Poole AR, Pidoux I, Reiner A, et al.** (1984) Association of an extracellular protein (chondrocalcin) with the calcification of cartilage in endochondral bone formation. *J Cell Biol;* 98 (1):54–65.

16. **Hewitt AT, Varner HH, Silver MH, et al.** (1982) The isolation and partial characterization of chondronectin, an attachment factor for chondrocytes. *J Biol Chem;* 257 (5):2330–2334.

17. **Nordahl J, Mengarelli-Widholm S, Hultenby K, et al.** (1988) *Ultrastructural morphology of chondro-clasts in long bones of young rats.* In press.

18. **Olsson SE** (1979) Development and pathology of the canine acetabular rim. A study with special reference to hip dysplasia and the radiographic appearance of a separate "ossicle" at the acetabular rim. *Symposium on Osteoarthrosis and Canine Hip Dysplasia;* Helsinki. Aurasen Kirjapaino, Forssa.

19. **Koshino T** (1975) Development of femoral head to the rat from calcification to ossification. *Acta Radiol Suppl;* 344:33–46.

20. **Carlson CS, Hilley HD, Henrikson CK** (1985) Ultrastructure of normal epiphyseal cartilage of the articular- epiphyseal cartilage complex in growing swine. *Am J Vet Res;* 46 (2): 306–313.

21. **Hunziker EB, Herrmann W, Schenk RK, et al.** (1984) Cartilage ultrastructure after high pressure freezing, freeze substitution, and low temperature embedding. I. Chondrocyte ultrastructure—implications for the theories of mineralization and vascular invasion. *J Cell Biol;* 98 (1):267–276.

22. **Farnum CE, Wilsman NJ** (1987) Morphologic stages of the terminal hypertrophic chondrocyte of growth plate cartilage. *Anat Rec;* 219 (3):221–232.

23. **Poole AR, Matsui Y, Hinek A, et al.** (1989) Cartilage macromolecules and the calcification of cartilage matrix. *Anat Rec;* 224 (2):167–179.

24. **Kavumpurath S, Hall BK** (1990) Lack of either chondrocyte hypertrophy or osteogenesis in Meckel's cartilage of the embryonic chick exposed to epithelia and to thyroxine in vitro. *J Craniofac Genet Dev Biol;* 10 (3):263–275.

25. **Hunziker EB** (1994) Mechanism of longitudinal bone growth and its regulation by growth plate chondro-cytes. *Microsc Res Tech;* 28 (6):505–519.

26. **Siffert RS** (1981) Classification of the osteochondroses. *Clin Orthop;* (158):10–18.

27. **Trueta J, Amato VP** (1960) The vascular contribution to osteogenesis III: Changes in the growth cartilage caused by experimentally induced ischaemia. *J Bone Joint Surg [Br];* 42:571.

28. **Trueta J, Little K** (1960) The vascular contribution to osteogenesis II: Studies with the electron microscope. *J Bone Joint Surg [Br];* 42:367.
29. **Trueta J, Morgan JD** (1960) The vascular contribution to osteogenesis I: Studies by the injection method. *J Bone Joint Surg [Br];* 42:97.
30. **Trueta J, Buhr AJ** (1963) The vascular contribution to osteogenesis V: The vasculature supplying the epiphyseal cartilage in rachitic rats. *J Bone Joint Surg [Br];* 45:572.
31. **Engfeldt B, Reinholt PF** (1992) Structure and calcification of epiphyseal growth cartilage. In: Bonucci E, editor. *Calcification in Biological Systems.* Boca Raton: CRC Press, 217.
32. **Bonucci E** (1989) Electron microscope studies of the early stage of the calcification process: Role of matrix vesicles. In: Bonucci E, editor. *Cells and Tissue: A Three-Dimensional Approach by Modern Techniques in Microscopy.* New York: Alan R Liss Inc, 109.
33. **Bonucci E** (1967) Fine structure of early cartilage calcification. *J Ultrastruct Res;* 20 (1):33–50.
34. **Anderson HC** (1969) Vesicles associated with calcification in the matrix of epiphyseal cartilage. *J Cell Biol;* 41 (1):59–72.
35. **Ali SY, Sajdera SW, Anderson HC** (1970) Isolation and characterization of calcifying matrix vesicles from epiphyseal cartilage. *Proc Natl Acad Sci USA;* 67 (3):1513–1520.
36. **Thyberg J, Friberg U** (1978) The lysosomal system in endochondral growth. *Prog Histochem Cytochem;* 10 (4):1–46.
37. **Anderson HC** (1989) Biology of disease: Mechanism of mineral formation in bone. *Lab Invest;* 60:320.
38. **Sela J, Schwartz Z, Swain LD, et al.** (1992) The role of matrix vesicles in calcification. In: Bonucci E, editor. *Calcification in Biological Systems.* Boca Raton: CRC Press, 73.

39. **Hunziker EB, Herrmann W, Cruz-Orive LM, et al.** (1989) Image analysis of electron micrographs relating to mineralization in calcifying cartilage: theoretical considerations. *J Electron Microsc Tech;* 11 (1):9–15.
40. **Reinholt FP, Wernerson A** (1988) Septal distribution and the relationship of matrix vesicle size to cartilage mineralization. *Bone Miner;* 4 (1):63–71.
41. **Landis WJ, Glimcher MJ** (1982) Electron optical and analytical observations of rat growth plate cartilage prepared by ultracryomicrotomy: the failure to detect a mineral phase in matrix vesicles and the identification of heterodispersed particles as the initial solid phase of calcium phosphate deposited in the extracellular matrix. *J Ultrastruct Res;* 78 (3):227–268.
42. **Boskey AL** (1989) Noncollagenous matrix proteins and their role in mineralization. *Bone Miner;* 6 (2):111–123.
43. **Buckwalter JA** (1983) Proteoglycan structure in calcifying cartilage. *Clin Orthop;* (172):207–232.
44. **Franzen A, Heinegard D, Reiland S, et al.** (1982) Proteoglycans and calcification of cartilage in the femoral head epiphysis of the immature rat. *J Bone Joint Surg [Am];* 64 (4):558–566.
45. **Hinek A, Reiner A, Poole AR** (1987) The calcification of cartilage matrix in chondrocyte culture: studies of the C-propeptide of type II collagen (chondrocalcin). *J Cell Biol;* 104 (5):1435–1441.
46. **Jotereau FV, Le Douarin NM** (1978) The development relationship between osteocytes and osteoclasts: a study using the quail-chick nuclear marker in endochondral ossification. *Dev Biol;* 63 (2):253–265.
47. **Eriksson EF, Kassem M** (1992) The cellular basis of bone remodeling. *Sandoz J Med Sci;* 31:45.

48. **Vaes G** (1988) Cellular biology and biochemical mechanism of bone resorption. A review of recent developments on the formation, activation, and mode of action of osteoclasts. *Clin Orthop;* (231):239–271.
49. **Rodan GA, Martin TJ** (1981) Role of osteoblasts in hormonal control of bone resorption—a hypothesis. *Calcif Tissue Int;* 33 (4):349–351.
50. **McSheehy PM, Chambers TJ** (1986) Osteoblastic cells mediate osteoclastic responsiveness to parathyroid hormone. *Endocrinology;* 118 (2):824–828.
51. **Manolagas SC, Jilka RL** (1992) Cytokines, hematopoiesis, osteoclastogenesis, and estrogens. *Calcif Tissue Int;* 50 (3):199–202.
52. **Martin TJ** (1993) Hormones in the coupling of bone resorption and formation. *Osteoporos Int;* 3 (Suppl 1): 121–125.
53. **Nilsson A, Ohlsson C, Isaksson OG, et al.** (1994) Hormonal regulation of longitudinal bone growth. *Eur J Clin Nutr;* 48 (Suppl 1): 150–158; discussion S158–160.
54. **Poulos PW, Reiland S, Elwinger K, et al.** (1978) Skeletal lesions in the broiler, with special reference to dyschondroplasia (osteochondrosis). Pathology, frequency and clinical significance in two strains of birds on high and low energy feed. *Acta Radiol Suppl;* 358:229–275.
55. **Haraldsson S** (1962) The vascular pattern of a growing and full-grown human epiphysis. *Acta Anat;* 48:157.
56. **Lutfi AM** (1970) Mode of growth, fate and functions of cartilage canals. *J Anat;* 106 (1):135–145.
57. **Stockwell RA** (1971) The ultrastructure of cartilage canals and the surrounding cartilage in the sheep fetus. *J Anat;* 109 (3):397–410.

58. **Visco DM, Van Sickle DC, Hill MA, et al.** (1989) The vascular supply of the chondro-epiphyses of the elbow joint in young swine. *J Anat;* 163:215–229.

59. **Wilsman NJ, Van Sickle DC** (1972) Cartilage canals, their morphology and distribution. *Anat Rec;* 173 (1): 79–93.

60. **Haines RW** (1974) The pseudo-epiphysis of the first metacarpal of man. *J Anat;* 117 (1):145–158.

61. **Lutfi AM** (1970) The germinal zone of the growth cartilage at the upper ends of the tibia and fibula in Gallus domesticus. *J Anat;* 106 (3):565–576.

62. **Hansson LI** (1967) Daily growth in length of diaphysis measured by oxytetracycline in rabbit normally and after medullary plugging. *Acta Orthop Scand;* Suppl (101):1.

63. **Isaksson OG, Lindahl A, Nilsson A, et al.** (1987) Mechanism of the stimulatory effect of growth hormone on longitudinal bone growth. *Endocr Rev;* 8 (4):426–438.

64. **Isaksson OG, Nilsson A, Isgaard J, et al.** (1990) Cartilage as a target tissue for growth hormone and insulin-like growth factor I. *Acta Paediatr Scand Suppl;* 367:137–141.

65. **Nap RC, Hazewinkel HA** (1994) Growth and skeletal development in the dog in relation to nutrition; a review. *Vet Q;* 16 (1):50–59.

66. **Ikeda T, Fujiyama K, Takeuchi T, et al.** (1989) Effect of thyroid hormone on somatomedin-C release from perfused rat liver. *Experientia;* 45 (2):170–171.

67. **Isley WL, Underwood LE, Clemmons DR** (1983) Dietary components that regulate serum somatomedin-C concentrations in humans. *J Clin Invest;* 71 (2):175–182.

68. **Brazeau P, Vale W, Burgus R, et al.** (1973) Hypothalamic polypeptide that inhibits the secretion of immunoreactive pituitary growth hormone. *Science;* 179 (68):77–79.

69. **Frohman LA, Jansson JO** (1986) Growth hormone-releasing hormone. *Endocr Rev;* 7 (3):223–253.

70. **Thorngren KG, Hansson LI, Menander-Sellman K, et al.** (1973) Effect of dose and administration period of growth hormone on longitudinal bone growth in the hypophysectomized rat. *Acta Endocrinol (Copenh);* 74 (1):1–23.

71. **Gustafsson PO, Kasstrom H, Lindberg L, et al.** (1975) Growth and mitotic rate of the proximal tibial epiphyseal plate in hypophysectomized rats given estradiol and human growth hormone. *Acta Radiol Suppl;* 344:69–74.

72. **Asling CW, Tse F, Rosenberg LL** (1968) Effects of growth hormone and thyroxine on sequences of chondrogenesis in the epiphyseal cartilage plate. In: Pecile AE, editor. *Growth Hormone.* Amsterdam: Excerpta Medica Foundation, 319.

73. **Thorngren KG, Hansson LI, Menander-Sellman K, et al.** (1973) Effect of hypophysectomy on longitudinal bone growth in the rat. *Calcif Tissue Res;* 11 (4):281–300.

74. **Marek J, Schullerova M, Schreiberova O, et al.** (1981) Effect of thyroid function on serum somatomedin activity. *Acta Endocrinol (Copenh);* 96 (4):491–497.

75. **Stracke H, Rossol S, Schatz H** (1986) Alkaline phosphatase and insulin-like growth factor in fetal rat bone under the influence of thyroid hormones. *Horm Metab Res;* 18 (11): 794.

76. **Silberberg R** (1971) Skeletal growth and aging. *Acta Rheumatol;* 26:1.

77. **Corvol MT, Carrascosa A, Tsagris L, et al.** (1987) Evidence for a direct in vitro action of sex steroids on rabbit cartilage cells during skeletal growth: influence of age and sex. *Endocrinology;* 120 (4):1422–1429.

78. **Somjen D, Weisman Y, Mor Z, et al.** (1991) Regulation of proliferation of rat cartilage and bone by sex steroid hormones. *J Steroid Biochem Mol Biol;* 40 (4-6):717–723.

79. **Koshino T, Olsson SE** (1975) Normal and estradiol induced calcification of the femoral head in rats. *Acta Radiol Suppl;* 344:47–52.

80. **Morscher E** (1968) Strength and morphology of growth cartilage under hormonal influence of puberty. Animal experiments and clinical study on the etiology of local growth disorders during puberty. *Reconstr Surg Traumatol;* 10:3–104.

81. **Thorngren KG, Hansson LI** (1973) Effect of thyroxine and growth hormone on longitudinal bone growth in the hypophysectomized rat. *Acta Endocrinol (Copenh);* 74 (1): 24–40.

82. **Silbermann M, Weiss A, Raz E** (1981) Retardative effects of a cortico-steroid hormone upon chondrocyte growth in the mandibular condyle of neonatal mice. *J Craniofac Genet Dev Biol;* 1 (1): 109–122.

83. **Behrens F, Shepard N, Mitchell N** (1975) Alterations of rabbit articular cartilage by intra-articular injections of glucocorticoids. *J Bone Joint Surg [Am];* 57 (1):70–76.

84. **Mankin HJ, Conger KA** (1966) The acute effects of intra-articular hydrocortisone on articular cartilage in rabbits. *J Bone Joint Surg [Am];* 48 (7):1383–1388.

85. **Edqvist LE, Johansson ED, Kasstrom H, et al.** (1975) Blood plasma levels of progesterone and oestradiol in the dog during the oestrous cycle and pregnancy. *Acta Endocrinol (Copenh);* 78 (3):554–564.

86. **Sunden G** (1967) Some aspects of longitudinal bone growth. An experimental study of the rabbit tibia. *Acta Orthop Scand Suppl;* (103):7.

87. **Dysart PS, Harkness EM, Herbison GP** (1989) Growth of the humerus after denervation. An experimental study in the rat. *J Anat;* 167:147–159.

88. **Eigenmann JE, Zanesco S, Arnold U, et al.** (1984) Growth hormone and insulin-like growth factor I in German shepherd dwarf dogs. *Acta Endocrinol (Copenh);* 105 (3):289–293.

89. **Greco DS, Feldman EC, Peterson ME, et al.** (1991) Congenital hypothyroid dwarfism in a family of giant schnauzers. *J Vet Intern Med;* 5 (2):57–65.

90. **Almlöf J** (1961) On achondroplasia in the dog. *Zentralbl Veterinärmed;* 8:43.

91. **Hansen HJ** (1952) A pathologic-anatomical study on disc degeneration in the dog with special reference to the so-called enchondrosis intervertebralis. *Acta Orthop Scand Suppl;* 11:1.

92. **Ringberg O, Lund-Larsen T, Bakke H** (1975) Growth hormone and somatomedin activities in lines of pigs selected for rate of gain and thickness of backfat. *Acta Agricult Scand;* 25:231.

93. **Jayo MJ, Leipold HW, Dennis SM, et al.** (1987) Bovine dwarfism: clinical, biochemical, radiological and pathological aspects. *Zentralbl Veterinarmed A;* 34 (3):161–177.

94. **Moritomo Y, Ishibashi T, Miyamoto H** (1992) Morphological changes of epiphyseal plate in the long bone of chondrodysplastic dwarfism in Japanese brown cattle. *J Vet Med Sci;* 54 (3):453–459.

95. **Breur GJ, Zerbe CA, Slocombe RF, et al.** (1989) Clinical, radiographic, pathologic, and genetic features of osteochondrodysplasia in Scottish deerhounds. *J Am Vet Med Assoc;* 195 (5):606–612.

96. **Bingel SA, Sande RD** (1994) Chondrodysplasia in five Great Pyrenees. *J Am Vet Med Assoc;* 205 (6): 845–848.

97. **Sande RD, Alexander JE, Spencer GR, et al.** (1982) Dwarfism in Alaskan malamutes: a disease resembling metaphyseal dysplasia in human beings. *Am J Pathol;* 106 (2): 224–236.

98. **Farnum CE, Jones K, Riis R, et al.** (1992) Ocular-chondrodysplasia in labrador retriever dogs: a morphometric and electron microscopical analysis. *Calcif Tissue Int;* 50 (6):564–572.

99. **McSheehy PM, Chambers TJ** (1987) 1,25-Dihydroxyvitamin D3 stimulates rat osteoblastic cells to release a soluble factor that increases osteoclastic bone resorption. *J Clin Invest;* 80 (2):425–429.

100. **Rao LG, Heersche JN, Marchuk LL, et al.** (1981) Immunohisto-chemical demonstration of calcitonin binding to specific cell types in fixed rat bone tissue. *Endocrinology;* 108 (5):1972–1978.

101. **Jonsson G, Jacobsson SO, Stromberg B, et al.** (1972) Rickets and secondary nutritional hyper-parathyroidism. A clinical syndrome in fattening bulls. *Acta Radiol Suppl;* 319:91–105.

102. **Olsson SE** (1972) Radiology in veterinary pathology. A review with special reference to hypertrophic osteodystrophy and secondary hyperparathyroidism in the dog. *Acta Radiol Suppl;* 319:255–270.

103. **Krook L, Barrett LR, Usui K, et al.** (1963) Nutritional secondary hyperparathyroidism in the cat. *Cornell Vet;* 53:224.

104. **Haglin L, Köhler P, Reiland S, et al.** (1993) Osteopenia and hypo-phosphatemic rickets in growing pigs treated with aluminum hydroxide. *Eur J Musculoskel Res;* 2:75.

105. **Reiland S** (1978) Morphology of osteochondrosis and sequelae in pigs. *Acta Radiol Suppl;* 358:45–90.

106. **Reiland S** (1978) The effect of decreased growth rate on frequency and severity of osteochondrosis in pigs. *Acta Radiol Suppl;* 358:107–122.

107. **Carlson CS, Hilley HD, Meuten DJ, et al.** (1988) Effect of reduced growth rate on the prevalence and severity of osteochondrosis in gilts. *Am J Vet Res;* 49 (3):396–402.

108. **Olsson SE, Reiland S** (1978) The nature of osteochondrosis in animals. Summary and conclusions with comparative aspects on osteo-chondritis dissecans in man. *Acta Radiol Suppl;* 358:299–306.

109. **Poulos PW** (1978) Tibial dyschondroplasia (osteochondrosis) in the turkey. A morphologic investigation. *Acta Radiol Suppl;* 358:197–227.

110. **Reiland S** (1978) Effects of vitamin D and A, calcium, phosphorus, and protein on frequency and severity of osteochondrosis in pigs. *Acta Radiol Suppl;* 358:91–105.

111. **Hedhammar A, Wu FM, Krook L, et al.** (1974) Overnutrition and skeletal disease. An experimental study in growing Great Dane dogs. *Cornell Vet;* 64 (2):Suppl 5:5–160.

112. **Hazewinkel HAW, Goedegebuure SA, Poulos PW, et al.** (1985) Influences of chronic calcium excess on the skeletal development of growing Great Danes. *J Am Anim Hosp Assoc;* 21:377.

113. **Olsson SE** (1975) Osteochondritis dissecans in the dog. *Am Anim Hosp Assoc.*

114. **Olsson SE** (1975) Lameness in the dog: A review of lesions causing osteoarthrosis of the shoulder, elbow, hip, stifle, and hock joints. *Am Anim Hosp Assoc;* 1:363.

115. **Olsson SE** (1976) Osteochondrosis–a growing problem to dog breeders. *Gaines Dog Research Center's Seminar for Dog Breeders;* Harrisburg, PA.

116. **Olsson SE** (1987) General and local [corrected] aetiologic factors in canine osteochondrosis. *Vet Q;* 9 (3): 268–278.

117. **Craig PH, Riser WH** (1965) Osteochondritis dissecans in the proximal humerus of the dog. *Am J Vet Rad Soc;* 6:40.

118. **Grøndalen T** (1974) Osteochondrosis and arthrosis in pigs. VII. Relationship to joint shape and exterior conformation. *Acta Vet Scand Suppl;* 46 (0):1–32.

119. **Rejno S, Stromberg B** (1978) Osteochondrosis in the horse. II. Pathology. *Acta Radiol Suppl;* 358:153–178.

120. **Kato M, Onodera T** (1984) Spontaneous osteochondrosis in rats. *Lab Anim;* 18 (2):179–187.

121. **Carlson CS, Hilley HD, Henrikson CK, et al.** (1986) The ultrastructure of osteochondrosis of the articular-epiphyseal cartilage complex in growing swine. *Calcif Tissue Int;* 38 (1):44–51.

122. **Ekman S, Rodriguez-Martinez H, Ploen L** (1990) Morphology of normal and osteochondrotic porcine articular-epiphyseal cartilage. A study in the domestic pig and minipig of wild hog ancestry. *Acta Anat;* 139 (3): 239–253.

123. **Farnum CE, Wilsman NJ, Hilley HD** (1984) An ultrastructural analysis of osteochondritic growth plate cartilage in growing swine. *Vet Pathol;* 21 (2):141–151.

124. **Hill MA, Ruth GR, Hilley HD, et al.** (1985) Dyschondroplasias of growth cartilages (osteochondrosis) in crossbred commercial pigs at one and 15 days of age: radiological, angiomicrographical and histological findings. *Vet Rec;* 116 (2):40–47.

125. **Thorp BH, Farquarson C, Kwan APL, et al.** (1993) Osteochondrosis/dyschondroplasia: A failure of chondrocyte differentiation. *Eq Vet J;* 16:13.

126. **Carlson CS, Hilley HD, Meuten DJ** (1989) Degeneration of cartilage canal vessels associated with lesions of osteochondrosis in swine. *Vet Pathol;* 26 (1):47–54.

127. **Carlson CS, Meuten DJ, Richardson DC** (1991) Ischemic necrosis of cartilage in spontaneous and experimental lesions of osteochondrosis. *J Orthop Res;* 9 (3): 317–329.

128. **Kincaid SA, Allhands RV, Pijanowski GJ** (1985) Chondrolysis associated with cartilage canals of the epiphyseal cartilage of the distal humerus of growing pigs. *Am J Vet Res;* 46 (3):726–732.

129. **Woodard JC, Becker HN, Poulos PW** (1987) Articular cartilage blood vessels in swine osteochondrosis. *Vet Pathol;* 24 (2):118–123.

130. **Carlson CS, Cullins LD, Meuten DJ** (1995) Osteochondrosis of the articular-epiphyseal cartilage complex in young horses: evidence for a defect in cartilage canal blood supply. *Vet Pathol;* 32 (6):641–647.

131. **Ekman S, Carlson CS** (1998) The pathophysiology of osteochondrosis. *Vet Clin North Am Small Anim Pract;* 28 (1):17–32.

132. **Nakano T, Aherne FX** (1988) Involvement of trauma in the pathogenesis of osteochondritis dissecans in swine. *Can J Vet Res;* 52 (1):154–155.

133. **Mee AP, Gordon MT, May C, et al.** (1993) Canine distemper virus transcripts detected in the bone cells of dogs with metaphyseal osteopathy. *Bone;* 14 (1):59–67.

134. **Mee AP, May C, Bennett D, et al.** (1995) Generation of multinucleated osteoclast-like cells from canine bone marrow: effects of canine distemper virus. *Bone;* 17 (1):47–55.

135. **Woodard JC** (1982) Canine hypertrophic osteodystrophy, a study of the spontaneous disease in littermates. *Vet Pathol;* 19 (4):337–354.

136. **Baumgärtner W, Boyce RW, Weisbrode SE, et al.** (1995) Histological and immunocyto-chemical characterization of canine distemper-associated metaphyseal bone lesions in young dogs following experimental infection. *Vet Pathol;* 32:702.

137. **Carrig CB, Pool RR, et al.** (1975) Effects of asynchronous growth of the radius and ulna on the canine elbow joint following experimental retardation of the longitudinal growth of the ulna. *J Am Anim Hosp Assoc;* 11:560.

138. **Rugh R** (1973) Radiology and the human embryo and fetus. In: Dalrymple G, Gaulden M, Kollmorgen G, et al., editors. *Medical Radiation Biology.* Philadelphia: WB Saunders Co., 83.

4 Biomechanics of the growth plate

James Wilson-MacDonald

1 Introduction

The growth plate, like bone, is continually subjected to changes in force and is a living tissue which responds to changes in applied force. It is in a way surprising that the growth plate can continue to grow, despite the constantly changing milieu. The main force applied to the growth plate is compression, and this may be the equivalent to many times the body weight of the individual during, for example, sporting activities. Despite this, growth appears to continue normally in most individuals, and it is predominantly abnormal forces such as torsion or shearing which can damage the growth plate and interfere with normal growth. Indeed it has been suggested that normal growth probably depends upon the growth plate being subjected to alternating forces of compression and possibly also distraction, although this has never been proved scientifically [1–3]. It has been shown that bone responds to intermittent loading by hypertrophy [4], and it appears that the growth plate may be stimulated in a similar way.

However, force only moderates events occurring in the growth plate. For example, it has been shown in in-vivo and in-vitro experiments that the cartilage model forms and grows as a result of the intrinsic cellular characteristics of the cartilage cells [5, 6]. It has been suggested that the cartilage model of bone possesses an inherent capacity to produce a certain amount of bone, and this determines the amount of growth which occurs at any single growth plate [7, 8].

Woolf [9] proposed the "Law of Bone Transformation", which states that the changes in function and shape of a bone produce corresponding and adaptive changes in architectural structure. Although Woolf was primarily studying bone, many of his observations were made on growing bone and he appreciated that it was not only the bone which was responding to normal and abnormal forces, but also the growth plate. Subsequently a "Chondral Modeling Theory" has been proposed which states the following [10]:

1. Pressure greater than physiological pressure on the growth plate will slow growth.
2. Physiological loads stimulate the growth plate.
3. Loads, less than physiological loads, will inhibit the growth plate.
4. A decrease in tension inhibits the growth plate.
5. Normal growth should obey the dictates of mechanical forces; hence small angular deformities should resolve with growth, whereas large deformities should deteriorate.
6. Chondral deformities can be corrected until maturity.
7. Only chondral modeling causes deformity during growth.

These rules attempt to explain the changes which we see at the growth plate in response to deformity, fracture angulation, compression, or distraction of the growth plate, and so on. However, this type of generalization cannot always be correct. Also, when assessing the response of the growth plate to, for example, a deforming force, it must be remembered that it is not only the growth plate and cartilaginous structures which will adapt, but that the metaphysis and diaphysis of the bone will also adapt by remodeling of the bone. This often makes assessment of the site and the amount of correction occurring difficult; particularly as the correction does not usually simply occur in one plane, and thus multi-planar or three-dimensional assessment is necessary.

2 Cellular response to force across the growth plate

The morphology of cells subjected to compression or distraction of the growth plate has been widely studied by many authors, but the biochemical effects of force on the growth plate is less well understood. The effects of compression on the growth plate appear to be widening of the growth plate, probably due to inhibition of mineralization [11], and this effect appears to be enhanced somehow by division of the periosteum [12]. Initially, the cell columns become disorganized with irregular staining of the cells, but the initial widening of the growth plate is followed by gradual narrowing, until blood vessels invade the growth plate and finally the growth plate fuses.

Distraction, on the other hand, causes widening of the growth plate, which persists and which is associated with an increase in both the number of mitoses within the cell columns and an increase in the size of the cells. Kember and Walker have shown that it is these two factors which govern the amount of growth occurring at any one growth plate [6]. It has also been suggested that the size of the cells, within the growth plate, is dependent upon the amount of fluid and stroma within the cells of the growth plate, and that this is how pressure alters growth [13]. This appears to be a rather simplistic theory, and others have found that compression causes the accumulation of matrix at an increased rate, due to a fall in the number of lysosomal enzymes released [14]. The synthesis of lysosomal enzymes appears to be pressure sensitive whereas the synthesis of proteins is not, but whether these changes are the cause, or the result, of decreased growth is not known.

As will be discussed later, the periosteum and the growth plate form a single biometric unit, thus many of the changes affecting the periosteum are likely to affect the growth plate. The periosteum is richly supplied with nerve fibers, and it has been demonstrated that these cells contain sympathetic vaso-active intestinal peptide (VIP), which may mediate bone resorption [15]. Sympathectomy abolishes the VIP within the nerve cells, and this may be one of the mechanisms of bone remodeling. Bubenik et al. have shown that the growth plate in the rabbit can be stimulated by electrical currents, and stimulation of the periosteum of deer antler can result in a 70% increase in the length and a 40% increase in the width of the antler [16]. Thus the periosteum may influence the chondrocytes of the growth plate by a humoral or neurological mechanism. This phenomenon is not yet fully understood. The alternative view is that damage to the periosteum mechanically "unbridles" the growth plate, and thus enhances mechanical growth.

3 Anatomy of the growth plate

The cellular anatomy of the growth plate is fully discussed in **Chapter 3** and will not be reiterated herein. However, the attachments of the growth plate to the surrounding structures are important in determining how the growth plate behaves mechanically (**Fig. 4-1**).

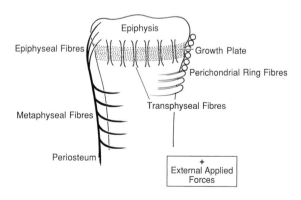

Fig. 4-1: Periosteal and other collagenous attachments of the growth plate. The various attachments of the growth plate to surrounding structures are shown. Because of these attachments, these structures have a mechanical effect on the growth plate in addition to external forces.

3.1   Gross anatomy

The perichondrial growth plate lies around the ossification groove and was first described by Ranvier in 1873. Many authors have studied the cells within the groove, and it is clear that there are different types of cells in different parts of the groove. The cells on the inner surface are almost certainly associated with widening of the growth plate and the proximal metaphysis during growth, while the outer fiber bundles and the fibroblasts on the periphery of the groove are continuous with the periosteum and also have fibers which pass deep into the growth plate. Speer [17] has studied, in great detail, these and other fibers adjacent to the growth plate. Using polarized light, he was able to identify five major groups of collagen fibers in, and around, the growth plate and was able to show that there were fibers traversing the growth plate, from the metaphysis to the epiphysis. Thus, there are strong bonds crossing many anatomical boundaries which interconnect all the important structures adjacent to the growth plate, and it is these which give the growth plate much of its stability. For example it has been shown that division of the periosteum, adjacent to the growth plate, halves the shearing force necessary to fracture the growth plate [18, 19]. The periosteum becomes relatively thin and weak during puberty, and it may be this that eventually causes the failure resulting in a slipped upper femoral epiphysis.

The attachments of the periosteum to the growth plate (see **Fig. 4-1**), and the proximal metaphysis, are extremely strong, while the attachments of the periosteum to the shaft of the bone are relatively weak (**Fig. 4-2**). Similarly, the periosteum itself is very strong in this part of the bone (**Fig. 4-3**), and studies have shown that the force required to rupture the periosteum at the level of the growth plate is 5–15 kg/cm^2 in calves [20]. Although the tension had never been measured, the periosteum is also under considerable tension. It has been suggested that, due to this tension, the periosteum exerts a considerable compression force on the adjacent growth plate, and when the periosteum is divided this compressive force is released; thus growth is stimulated [21]. There is no doubt that division of the periosteum can cause bone overgrowth, but as mentioned in the previous section, the mechanism of growth stimulation may not be entirely mechanical. It is also possible that the tension in the periosteum may be instrumental in the "funneling" of bone which takes place during growth, whereby the wide metaphysis becomes narrower, and ultimately forms the diaphysis, rather like the toothpaste being squeezed out of a toothpaste tube. It has been further suggested that the very strong periosteal fibers, which pass into the metaphysis, may help in the orientation of the bone trabeculae and the growth plate may indirectly stimulate osteogenesis by stretching the periosteum during growth.

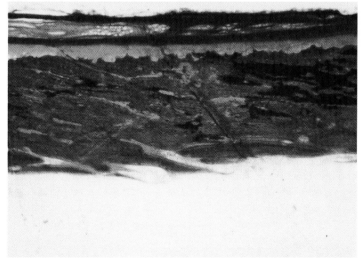

Fig. 4-2: Diaphysis and periosteum.
This figure shows the periosteum in the shaft of the bone (dark-brown staining structure). The bone is stained green, fat and fibrous tissue yellowish-brown. It can be seen that the periosteum is a relatively thin structure, with few attachments to the underlying bone, allowing the periosteum to slide over the surface of the bone. The underlying bone in this case is being resorbed, with lacunae on the periosteal surface of the bone.

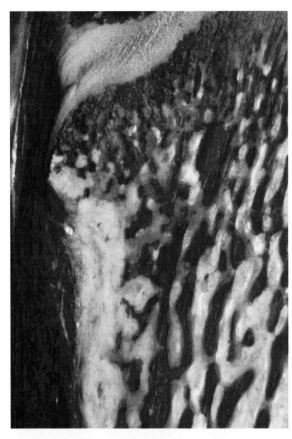

Fig. 4-3: Metaphysis, growth plate, and periosteum.
This figure shows the metaphysis and lateral growth plate of the proximal tibia of a 12-week-old rabbit. The periosteum stains dark brown, the growth plate yellow, and the bone green.

3.2 Vascular anatomy

When assessing mechanics of the growth plate the blood supply of the growth plate is also important. There are three main sources of blood supply to growing bone: the endosteum, the periosteum, and the epiphyseal vessels (**Fig. 4-4**). These different sources of blood supply all communicate with one another, although during growth the epiphyseal and endosteal

circulatory systems do not have a direct connection because the growth plate acts as a barrier. The periosteum has an abundant blood supply [**22, 23**]. There is a rich superficial plexus which communicates directly with muscle and may be important in shunting blood between different muscle groups. Neither stripping of the periosteum by undermining locally or circumferentially, nor cerclage wiring appear to interfere with its blood supply. This suggests that there are numerous anasto-moses around the periosteum.

The endosteal and periosteal circulatory systems, respec-tively, supply a variable amount of the cortex of the bone. The epiphyseal circle of vessels, described in **Chapter 2**, supplies the articular side of the growth plate, and it is this circle of vessels which can be so easily damaged during an operation or by infection, retarding growth at the adjacent growth plate. Trueta and Amato [**24**] showed that the effect of vascular insufficiency on the growth plate was to cause its closure, presumably due to an inability to calcify the cartilage columns of the growth plate. The epiphyseal circle of vessels is connected to the periosteal vessels, and damage to the periosteum may interfere

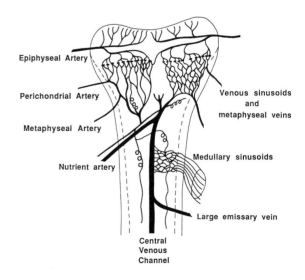

Fig. 4-4: Vascular anatomy of the growth plate.

with these vessels [25, 26]. It should be remembered how easily these vessels can be damaged and, for example, how the simple application of a wire across the bone can stimulate bone growth. Results which are thought to be due to mechanical effects may in fact be due to alteration of the circulation in the region of the growth plate. It is also possible that the mechanical stimuli, in their own right, may interfere with vascularization of the growth plate and, therefore, indirectly with growth.

It should be clear, from study of the anatomy of the growth plate, that it cannot be assessed in isolation and that damage to surrounding structures may interfere either with the biomechanics or the circulation of the growth plate, or both.

4   Compression of the growth plate

Woolf [9] realized that too much pressure on the growth plate could inhibit growth, and Thoma [2] recognized that a surfeit of pressure would eventually stop growth completely. Thoma was probably the first to suggest that alternating pressure was necessary for normal bone growth, and he estimated that the ideal pressure was around 0.6 g/cm². The pressures applied across the growth plate during daily life are probably far in excess of this, but what is important is that the pressure is intermittent. Constant pressure is almost certainly a bad thing for the growth plate, and it has been shown that increasing compression forces cause a proportional decrease in the amount of growth at the compressed growth plate [27]. However, the forces required to stop growth completely are extremely high. For example, Strobino et al. [28] showed that the force required to stop growth in calves, at the proximal tibial growth plate, was nearly 400 kg, but the animals only weighed 150 kg. He suggested that the animals could have lived standing constantly on one leg without interfering with growth, although the evidence of Peruchon et al. [27] would suggest that growth would probably be inhibited to some extent. It has been calculated that the force required to stop growth in children is about 388 kg, enough in many cases to break the staples of an epiphyseodesis [29].

4.1   Epiphyseodesis

Phemister [30] was the first to use epiphyseodesis in clinical practice to inhibit growth of a bone in children. He removed a bone block from the medial and lateral sides of the growth plate, reversed them, and caused a "physiological" epiphyseodesis. Epiphyseodesis has also been widely used in scoliosis surgery in young children. A convex epiphyseodesis can be used, quite successfully, in some children to allow correction of the deformity. However, recent evidence suggests that this is probably most useful in patients with a simple hemivertebra, and that more complex deformities are best treated by other methods [31].

The pioneering experiments of Haas [32], using wire loops around the distal femur, showed that growth could be inhibited by the loop. The loop often broke, demonstrating the enormous power behind growing bone, and release of the wire allowed growth to continue, although not at the normal rate. Blount [29] subsequently used the technique of stapling the growth plate to inhibit growth. The advantage of this technique appeared to be that removal of the staples would allow normal growth to resume and, thus, due to individual variations in growth, correct errors in achieving normal leg length in children. Many authors have suggested that both in animals and in children normal growth can resume after release of the growth plate [11, 33, 34]. Amako and Honda [35] even suggested that growth might be increased after staple removal, but there is little doubt that non-physiological compression of the growth plate does to some extent inhibit subsequent growth [28, 32].

This has also been indirectly demonstrated in children undergoing leg lengthening. Pennecot et al.[36] studied children undergoing leg lengthening by the Wagner technique, where an external fixator is used to lengthen the limb. They showed that the pressures across the growth plate can be as high as 20 kg/cm² for long periods during lengthening. Pouliquen et al. [37] have shown that children in whom lengthening of more than 15% of the bone is achieved are much less likely to resume normal growth than children in whom less lengthening occurs. Similarly, high distraction rates inhibit subsequent growth [38]. The mechanism is probably due to direct damage to the cells within the growth plate, possibly by inhibition of the circulation. It has been suggested that avascular necrosis of the femoral head cartilage can occur due to compression in congenital dislocation of the hip [39], and there is no reason to presume that this cannot occur in the cartilage of the growth plate. However, "physiological" overload of bone does not appear to have any detrimental effect on longitudinal bone growth. For example, Tschantz et al. [40] have shown that removal of the ulna in a dog does not cause inhibition of radial growth, and indeed the width of the bone is increased, presumably due to the overload passing through the bone; a process which stimulates bone formation.

Compression causes widening of the growth plate due to inhibition of calcification of the cartilage columns adjacent to the metaphysis [11, 26] (**Fig. 4-5** and **Fig. 4-6**). The first signs of alteration in the growth plate are disorganization of the cartilage columns and alteration of the staining within the cells. The growth plate then widens and subsequently gradually narrows in width, until finally it is invaded by blood vessels and closes. Release of the compressive force, during the phase of

thickening of the growth plate, results in rapid ossification of the non-ossified cells distant from the resting cells and restoration of a normal thickness of growth plate. Hert and Liskova [13] showed that the cell number in the growth plate decreased with compression, but the cell size increased. Goff [41] studied the changes in the periphery of the growth plate in children 12 months after the time of epiphyseodesis and found that although the growth plate was narrowed, the cell columns were relatively orderly. It was only 36 months after epiphyseodesis that the cell columns became grossly disorganized. The biochemical changes taking place at the same time have been discussed above.

Compression of an individual growth plate will slow growth at that plate. The effect of diminished growth at one end of the bone on growth at the other end (the diametrical growth plate) has not been widely studied. Irradiation has been used experimentally in rabbits as a method of inducing epiphyseodesis [42], and it was found that the predicted amount of shortening was less than would have been expected by the epiphyseodesis. Similarly, epiphyseodesis in children is not predictable in the amount of final shortening. Although this reflects, to some

Fig. 4-5: Normal growth plate.
Normal growth plate of 12-week-old-rabbit, showing the orderly pattern of cells within the cartilage columns and regularity of thickness of the growth plate.

Fig. 4-6: Compressed growth plate.
Compressed growth plate of 12-week-old rabbit, showing disarranged cartilage cell columns, irregularity of growth-plate thickness, and calcification within the growth plate. The overall thickness of the growth plate is increased.

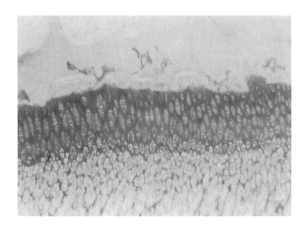

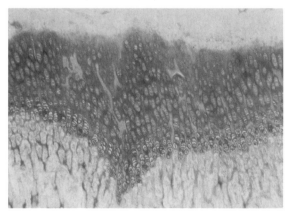

extent, individual variations and differences in the effectiveness of the epiphyseodesis, it seems likely that there is, in fact, some overgrowth of the diametrical growth plate, and this has been shown to occur in the experimental situation [26, 43]. It has been demonstrated that the amount of growth at the two growth plates of the tibia varies almost inversely with one another [12]. Compression, distraction, and division of the periosteum can alter the relationship between the amount of growth occurring at the two growth plates. Lacroix [44] suggested that there was a neutral point on any bone, and that the amount of growth at one or other of the growth plates depended upon the distance of the growth plate from the neutral point. It appears that by dividing the periosteum at a point on the bone, the neutral point can be moved and the ratio of growth at the two growth plates changed. It may be that this is purely a mechanical effect, but the reason for this change is poorly understood.

In summary, compression of a growth plate inhibits growth by causing changes at that plate which are never entirely reversible, and the amount of inhibition is dependent upon the force and duration of the compression. Growth at the diametrical growth plate is inversely related to growth at the compressed growth plate, reducing the expected amount of inhibition of growth.

5 Distraction of the growth plate

Heuter [45] first suggested that reduced pressure on the growth plate would stimulate growth. Ring [46] first described the technique of growth plate distraction but he experienced many complications, including pathological fracture and premature closure of the growth plate. He noted thickening of the growth plate which, as in the compressed growth plate, is due to reduced clearance of the cells from the plate adjacent to the metaphysis, probably caused by ischemia of these cells. Hert [47] showed that in rabbits the increase in length achieved was proportional to the distraction force, but that toward the end of growth virtually all of the increase in length initially

achieved was lost. He concluded that the possible causes of this inhibition of growth, after lengthening, were:
- Premature bridging of the growth plate by bone.
- The growth plate only being capable of a finite amount of growth.
- Loss of functional loading of the limb inhibiting growth.

Hert did not consider that it could be due to inhibition of the diametrical growth plate.

Fishbane and Riley [48] demonstrated that the increase in growth occurred because of a cleavage fracture within the growth plate, and not due to an increased turnover of chondrocytes as had been suggested by others. The cleavage occured at the weakest part of the growth plate, between the hypertrophic zone and the zone of cell degeneration. Spinelli [49] has shown that, at the time of fracture of the growth plate, the gap is filled with hematoma and primitive mesenchymal cells which differentiate into fibroblasts and then become longitudinally oriented. In the third week after epiphysiolysis the mesenchymal cells start forming osteoid and mineralization starts. Histology at 4 weeks shows a trabecular structure of bone with intervening capillaries, and it is only after 1–2 months that true cortical organization of the bone occurs.

Monticelli and Spinelli [50] were among the first to use the technique of epiphysiolysis to induce bone overgrowth in clinical practice. In their experimental results they found that a number of the animals underwent premature growth-plate closure; therefore they only used the technique in children nearing the end of growth. Following his clinical experience, Spinelli [49] reinforced this advice. Eydelshteyn et al. [51] were able to induce growth increments of 4–7 cm in patients with polio, without premature growth-plate closure. Sledge and Noble [52] showed that increased growth could occur without a fracture through the growth plate and that this occurred by increased turnover of the chondrocytes within the growth plate. The mechanism for this phenomenon is not known, although it has been suggested that calcium transport across cell membranes can be altered by pressure applied to the cell, and that this may increase growth.

The amount of lengthening is proportional to the speed of lengthening, but high-rate leg lengthening may inhibit the final length achieved. As mentioned previously, lengthening using the Wagner technique can damage the growth plates, and it is likely that high rates of epiphysiolysis at one growth plate may cause pressure-related damage at the diametrical growth plate, as has been demonstrated experimentally [53].

De Bastiani et al. [54] have reported the use of chondrodiastasis, which, put simply, is distraction of the growth plate without fracture of the plate. It has been shown in rabbits that a 2-kg force will cause epiphysiolysis, whereas a lower force will not [52]. Chondrodiastasis can therefore be achieved either by a reduced but constant force of distraction or by low-rate distraction. Using a rate of 0.25 mm, twice daily, does not appear to damage the growth plate microscopically in experiments on rabbits, and the method has been applied to children with very significant leg-length discrepancies [54]. De Bastiani et al. [54] were able to achieve increases in leg length of up to 36% with few complications and, in particular, no cases of premature growth arrest. In achondroplastic patients it was possible to increase leg length by up to 64.5% without any neurovascular complications. This would therefore appear to be a safe and almost physiological method of leg lengthening. However, Fjeld and Steen [55] found that growth in goat kids is inhibited after the distraction force is removed, suggesting that there is damage to the affected growth plate even with chondrodiastasis. They concluded that the method should only be used toward the end of growth, when growth-plate damage is less important. It has also been demonstrated, experimentally in rabbits, that even after chondrodiastasis there may be some inhibition of growth at the growth plate distant from the site of distraction, with premature closure [12].

6 Periosteum and the growth plate

When discussing distraction or compression of the growth plate, it should be remembered that the growth plate does not lie in isolation but that it is firmly attached to the surrounding structures, especially the periosteum, as discussed previously. As well as nerves and blood vessels, there are many muscles crossing the growth plate. Under normal circumstances, the muscles must apply some compression forces across the growth plate, and during distraction it is likely that all these structures are under considerable tension. It is probably this tension which damages the diametrical growth plate during distraction, causing premature growth-plate closure. It is also this high tensile force on the tissues which causes many of the neurological and vascular complications as well as the joint contractures which arise as a result of leg lengthening [56].

The periosteum is a tubular structure surrounding the whole of the bone apart from the articular part of the bony epiphysis; thus, it probably exerts a compressive force across the growth plate. When the periosteum is divided it retracts some distance, probably due to tension within it. Naturally, the periosteum must grow with the bone, but, unlike bone, it does not grow by appositional growth but rather by interstitial growth throughout its length. Dorfl [57] has carried out some elegant experiments with rabbits; by implanting metal markers in the periosteum and in the bone, he has shown that the periosteum slides over the bone and grows throughout its length. Structures attached to the bone such as tendon insertions, tendons, and ligament insertions move along the bone, by bone remodeling, following the periosteum. These structures are essentially "hitchhikers" on the periosteum. Thus, the muscles, tendons, and ligaments maintain a constant position on the bone during growth, even when the amount of growth at one end of the bone, or the other, is altered. Thus, the periosteum can grow independently of the bone.

Surgery to the periosteum causes a definite increase in growth [12, 21], and studies show that circumferential division and stripping of the periosteum are the most potent methods of stimulating growth experimentally [58]. Circumferential division of the periosteum has been used with some success in stimulating growth in children with minor leg-length discrepancies [59]. It has been suggested that periosteal division releases the normal tension in the periosteum, releasing the growth plate from any inhibition, and that this causes the overgrowth. Experimental studies, in which bone has been transplanted [60] or isolated in a diffusion chamber [61], have demonstrated that division of the periosteum under these circumstances induces overgrowth of the bone, thus reinforcing the idea that this is purely a mechanical effect. It has been shown that combining compression of the growth plate with periosteal division reverses, to some extent, the effects of compression, and that combining distraction of the growth plate with periosteal division enhances the effect of distraction, again suggesting that there may be a mechanical effect [26]. There is some discrepancy between the effects of dividing the periosteum in an isolated bone and dividing the periosteum in a bone that is still functioning in its normal position. The isolated bone will overgrow much more than the functioning one, possibly due to the fact that there are no constraints such as compression from the surrounding muscles or alteration in vascularization of the growth plate.

One might expect that epiphysiolysis and circumferential division of the periosteum may be additive in their effect. However, experiments in rabbits have demonstrated that this combination causes devastation to the metaphyseal region, with irreversible damage to the blood supply and early fusion of the growth plate [62]. In contrast, the combination of chondrodiastasis and periosteal division appears to be much more benign, and the combined effects are to some extent complementary [26], although at the expense of growth at the diametrical growth plate. Thus, although the distracted growth plate overgrows even more with periosteal division, the diametrical growth plate is presumably compressed by the tension in the soft tissues, with the consequent inhibition of growth.

According to some authors, proximal division of the periosteum in the tibia enhances growth more than distal periosteal division [60, 63]. The reasons for this are not clear but, theoretically, dividing the periosteum proximally stimulates the adjacent faster-growing growth plate, and evidence shows that it is this growth plate which is stimulated under normal circumstances. However, there is evidence that it may not always be the proximal growth plate that is being stimulated. Experiments have demonstrated that, after a proximal metaphyseal fracture stimulation of growth occurs at the growth plate distant from the fracture, and that proximal circumferential division of the periosteum under these circumstances causes a further increase in growth, but at the distal growth plate [12]. Thus the effect of periosteal division does not appear to be purely a simple mechanical effect at the adjacent growth plate.

7 Axial deformity and the growth plate

Woolf [9] suggested that deformities of bone could be corrected both by bone remodeling and by differential growth at the growth plate. According to radiological studies by Friberg, following distal radial fractures in children, most of the remodeling of bone occurs by reangulation of the growth plate, presumably by differential growth on the palmar and dorsal sides of the growth plate [64, 65]. Classically it has been taught that, in young children, deformities near to a joint in the plane of movement to the joint will remodel well, whereas deformities in older children, distal from the joint and not in the plane of movement of the joint, will remodel badly. There is probably some truth in all these observations. Certainly very young children have an amazing ability to remodel, but whether the other observations are correct can be debated. There is also doubt about the place where most of the correction of deformity takes place.

In children it is difficult to study bone remodeling because most of the information has to be gathered from sequential radiographs. In this situation it is easy to create errors due to alterations in the angle of the radiographs, and it is difficult to see exactly where new bone is being formed. Also, it is always difficult to study a three-dimensional event in two dimensions. Therefore, much of our knowledge comes from animal experimentation. Under normal conditions there is little angular remodeling of bone, unless there is either an intrinsic abnormality in the bone or an injury. Karaharju et al. [66] studied remodeling of bone after creating a valgus osteotomy of the tibia in dogs where the osteotomy had been fixed with a small plate (following the AO principles). Theoretically, one would expect that this deformity would not remodel well because the fracture was well away from the joint and not in the plane of movement of the joint. They found that 50% of the remodeling took place at the growth plate adjacent to the fracture, but they were unable to decide where the remainder of the correction of angulation took place. Because of disturbance to the soft tissues at the time of the operation and the continued effect of the plate, plating the tibia must considerably alter the pattern of remodeling that takes place. Further studies have been carried out holding a valgus angulated fracture with an external fixator. Following healing of the fracture the fixator was removed and correction of the angulation was studied [12]. It was observed that virtually none of the correction took place at the growth plate itself and that most of the correction took place by remodeling of the bone in the metaphysis and diaphysis of the bone as well as at the fracture site. Zionts and MacEwen [67] have confirmed the experimental evidence that tibial fractures in children with valgus deformity in the metaphysis of the bone remodel well, contrary to previous opinion, but whether the correction takes place at the growth plate or in the shaft of the bone is not clear (Fig. 4-7).

It has been noted that unilateral periosteal division and, in some cases, circumferential periosteal division can cause a valgus deformity of bone [61, 68]. This may be caused by the release of the periosteum: reducing the tension in the periosteum and removing inhibition of the growth plate on the side where the periosteum has been released. Evidence for this is that the growth plate becomes asymmetrical in its shape, reflecting more growth on the convex side of the bone and less growth on the concave side. Deformities created in this way can be subsequently corrected by dividing the periosteum on the opposite side, and this has been used as a technique in veterinary surgery to correct angular long-bone deformities in foals [69, 70]. However, subsequent work looking at the response to remodeling after fracture, and the effect of periosteal division, has shown that damage to the periosteum influences the final correction which takes place. Further, the difference between the different groups with various types of periosteal damage occurs in the shaft of the bone and not at the growth plate. In other words, damage to the periosteum at the time of fracture alters remodeling in the shaft of the bone and does not affect the growth plate [12].

Various theories have been put forward to explain valgus deformity, which may follow a proximal metaphyseal fracture on the medial side of the proximal tibia. This has been recognized as a common cause of late valgus deformity after fracture, and it has been suggested that it may occur because of folding of the periosteum into the fracture. This may prevent healing of the periosteum with resultant release of the medial growth plate [71], which could be corrected by repair of the periosteum. Other theories include: delayed union at the fracture site which could be corrected by compression of the medial side of the fracture; damage to the lateral growth plate at the time of injury; a tension-band effect of the fibula; or alteration of remodeling and bone drift in the metaphysis of the bone caused by periosteal damage [12]. There may be an element of truth in all these suggestions, but this type of problem illustrates the lack of knowledge of the biomechanics of the growth plate.

Potential sites of correction of angulation after angulated fracture

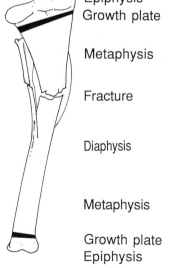

Epiphysis
Growth plate

Metaphysis

Fracture

Diaphysis

Metaphysis

Growth plate
Epiphysis

Fig. 4-7: Potential sites of angular correction of deformity. Shows the possible sites of correction of angulation in long bones. Up to 50% of correction probably takes place at the growth plate, depending upon the circumstances.

To date, periosteal hemicircumferential incision has not been used as a method of correcting long-bone deformities in children, but it may be of some use in deformities such as bilateral *genu varum,* or other angular deformities of long bones. It is a simple procedure provided that the growth-plate circulation is not damaged, and can be repeated until adequate correction is obtained. In horses overcorrection is never seen; it appears to be a self-limiting procedure.

Rotational deformities of the long bones are common in clinical practice and are often associated with other deformities, such as valgus of the long bones. There is clinical evidence that these deformities can improve with time—and yet there has been little research on the subject. Murray et al. [72] demonstrated that, in experimental animals, external rotation deformities could occur in response to valgus deformities of the tibia. They were able to show that the growth plate was growing by torsion and that this resulted in torsion of the limb (**Fig. 4-8**). It seems very likely that torsional deformities can also be corrected by torsional growth of the growth plate. It is highly unlikely that this could occur by any other mechanism, such as bone remodeling.

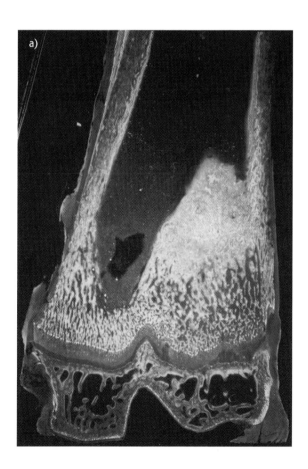

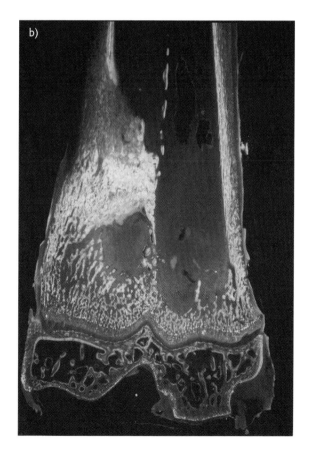

Fig. 4-8: a and b show distal tibial growth plates. The control side shows vertical parallel lines of chondrocytes, whereas on the fractured side the growth plates are sectioned obliquely. This suggests that growth on the side of the fracture is occurring with torsion of the growth plate.
a) Distal tibial growth-plate control.
b) Distal tibial growth plate, fractured side.

8 Fractures and the growth plate

The growth plate is affected by local fractures through or across, as well as fractures distant from, the plate. Fractures of the growth plate and epiphysis comprise about 15% of all childhood fractures, and the classical work of Salter and Harris [73] divided the injuries into five different types with a worsening prognosis from type I to type V. It has subsequently become clear that there are also different fracture patterns and mechanisms which were not covered by Salter and Harris, such as the triplane fracture and the type VI, VII, VIII, and IX fractures proposed by Ogden [74]. The importance of all of these fractures for the growth plate is interruption of the epiphyseal blood supply, compression injury to the growth plate, and healing of the fracture with displacement. All of these problems may lead to premature fusion of either the whole plate or, more commonly, one side of the growth plate. The former leads to simple shortening of the bone, whereas the latter usually leads to angular deformity of the bone, due to asymmetrical growth at the growth plate. The effect on the growth plate is gradual narrowing and eventual closure. Thus, in biomechanical terms this is essentially the same process as occurs with surgical epiphyseodesis and will not be further dealt with here.

Diaphyseal fractures of long bones, on the other hand, behave differently, and overgrowth appears to be a frequent occurrence, after about 90% of fractures; although some believe that overgrowth always occurs to some extent [75]. The amount of overgrowth that occurs does not appear to be predictable. Factors that appear to increase the overgrowth include: oblique fractures; spiral and comminuted fractures; over-riding and displacement of the fracture; youth; the site of the fracture in the bone; and internal fixation. However, there is little agreement on these factors, and there appears to be a considerable discrepancy between the results of different authors. What many of the factors which induce overgrowth appear to have in common is the amount of damage to the periosteum and the vascular supply of the bone. It has been shown that damage to the periosteum, by altering the amount of growth occurring at the growth plate distant from the fracture, does appear to have a direct effect on the amount of

growth which occurs after a particular fracture [12] (Fig. 4-9). This may explain the difficulty in predicting overgrowth after fracture, in the clinical situation.

Fig. 4-9: a and b show distal tibial growth plate and metaphysis of 16-week-old rabbits on the side of proximal metaphyseal fracture (Fig. 4-8b) and on the side without fracture (Fig. 4-8a). Intravenous vital bone markers have been given at 4, 5, 6, and 7 weeks following the fracture, and 1 week before sacrifice (Xylenol Orange, Calcein Blue, Alizarin Complex, Oxytetracycline). This allows accurate assessment of growth on a weekly basis. It can be seen that the width of the lines is greater on the side of the fracture than on the control side. In other words, the growth plate distant from the fracture has been stimulated.

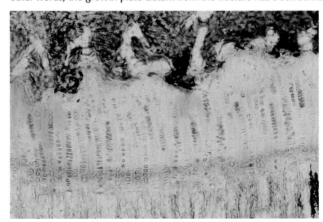

a) Normal distal tibia and growth plate.

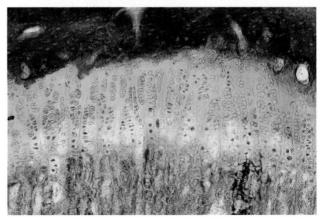

b) Distal tibia and growth plate following fracture.

After a single fracture, overgrowth appears to some extent to be a regional phenomenon, with overgrowth of various long bones in a limb [12, 75] (**Fig. 4-10**). This suggests that it is not only the mechanical effect of damage to the periosteum releasing the growth plates but that there is also some factor which alters the whole limb. The amount of overgrowth in the femur after a tibial fracture is directly related to the amount of overgrowth of the tibia, suggesting that this is not an "all or nothing" response and that there is some measurable factor increasing the growth. The most likely explanation for this is an alteration of the blood supply to the limb as a whole, and thus also to the growth plates. The alternate view is that there might be some humoral factor involved. The vascularity of a limb is increased after a fracture, but it has been shown that the blood supply to bone is not increased experimentally [76]. Wray and Lynch [77] demonstrated that the periosteal vessels dilate within minutes of a fracture occurring and cell division

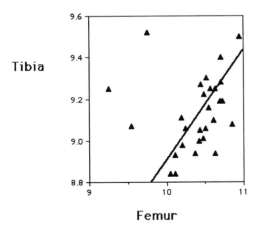

Relationship between femoral and tibial overgrowth following tibial fracture in young rabbits.

Tibia

Femur

(Length of bones in cm, p=0.0146 Kendall Rank Coefficient)

Fig. 4-10: Relationship between femoral and tibial overgrowth following tibial fracture in young rabbits.
It can be seen that the amount of overgrowth in the two bones is related in any one animal, suggesting that a fracture of the tibia induces overgrowth in the femur.

in the growth plate is increased within 16 hours [78]. Alpar [79] has shown that the DNA synthesis is increased in the growth plate after fracture, and that there appears to be some direct effect on the growth plate which causes this. It is most likely not just a single factor that stimulates the growth plate, but probably a combination of mechanical release, alteration in circulation, and hormonal or possibly electrical effects; it is this that makes prediction of overgrowth so difficult at the present time.

9 Abnormal external forces on the growth plate

Delpech [80] was one of the first to appreciate that external force could alter the shape of bones:

"A strong dressing having been used with great diligence, and mutual contact of the deformed areas, in that manner having been carefully prevented, at the end of 16 months...the articular surface having lost its vicious inclination, and the apophysis had grown, and the restoration of the foot was complete and strong; so that the leg which had been shorter had recovered part of its natural length".

In 1934 Appleton [81] described experiments where individual muscle groups in a limb were sectioned, with resulting deformities. In addition he found that the contralateral sound limb often developed rotational deformities of the bones. Most of the deformity was found in the shaft of the bone and he concluded that these rotational deformities were caused by altered growth at the distal growth plate of the bone. The association of various deformities in different bones has been recognized by some authors both experimentally [12], and in clinical practice [82]. For example, it is apparent that particular habits can induce deformities, and that a deformity of one bone can cause a secondary deformity in another bone, presumably due to altered pressures applied to the bone; but these deformities appear to occur as a result of remodeling within the shaft of the bone rather than at the growth plate itself. Similarly, bones respond to pressure under normal circumstances. For example, in infants the tibia is round until walking is started, when it gradually remodels and becomes more angular in shape, probably due to the pressure applied by the surrounding muscles on the bone. Abnormal forces on the growth plate can also cause secondary deformity. For example, young gymnasts can develop reduced radial growth with secondary radial deformity of the forearm [83]. It is thought that this may be due to the abnormal pressures applied to the growth plate during gymnastics, but it is also possible that the disturbance of growth occurs due to microfractures of the subchondral plate, or even the growth plate.

The study of bone changes in paralysis tells us something of the effects of pressure applied to bone. Ring [84] has noted that paralysis of a limb, for example in polio, results in initial increase in growth for about a year, followed by a reduction in the amount of normal growth. The reasons for the initial increase are not clear, but it has been suggested that this may be due to alterations in the blood supply of the bone, with blood initially being shunted from the abnormal muscles into the bone. On the other hand, muscle hypertrophy has been shown to increase bone mass, although there is no increase in the overall length of the bone.

Transplantation experiments have shed some light on bone biomechanics and the effects of external forces on the bone. To some extent, the growth of a particular bone is dependent upon the intrinsic properties of the cells within the growth plate. However, the ultimate shape of the bone can be considerably altered by external forces. Feik and Storey [7] showed that the amount of growth occurring in transplanted bone was not dependent upon vascularization of the bone. In a further experiment they showed that when a bending force was applied to a transplanted bone (rat's tail), the bones became bent with a concave outer surface and a convex inner surface. Meikle [1] has shown that unloaded transplanted bone fails to enlarge by normal periosteal new bone formation, although longitudinal growth continues normally. Harkness and Trotter [60] have contradicted this.

The forces on bone are three-dimensional and thus rather difficult to quantify by two-dimensional assessment. However, transplantation experiments demonstrate that cartilage cells have an inherent ability to grow, which is not dependent upon the recipient site. It has also been shown, by isolating bone and applying different forces to it, that external forces can alter bone shape.

Mente et al. [85] have demonstrated that external angular forces can result in a deformity similar to a scoliosis. By applying an external fixator to a rat's tail they have demonstrated that the initial deformity occurs because of asymmetry at the disks. The vertebrae then become deformed after 6 weeks with gradual wedging of the vertebrae, much as occurs in established scoliosis. The authors suggest that this demonstrates the Heuter-Volkmann law at work. This work would suggest that the severe deformities seen late in scoliosis are occurring secondarily and that there is some underlying abnormality which initiates the early deformity. The secondary severe deformity, with bone wedging, occurs due to the abnormal forces which subsequently occur.

10 Conclusion

The cartilage cells within the growth plate have an inherent ability to divide and enlarge, thus increasing the length of a bone. Bone growth is affected by physiological mechanical changes which occur during normal activities, and this probably stimulates the growth plate. Abnormal external forces also influence growth: compression inhibits growth and distraction enhances growth, and other forces such as shearing or twisting may damage the growth plate. The growth plate is surrounded by different structures which are either directly or indirectly connected to the growth plate mechanically. One such structure is the periosteum. Damage to the periosteum can significantly alter the amount of growth that occurs, in some cases increasing and in other cases decreasing growth, and this may be a simple mechanical effect. However, it is more likely that the mechanical effects are moderated by changes in vascularity, and also possibly by changes in the local hormones and electrical charge. Much work remains to be done before we better understand the mechanics of the growth plate.

11 Bibliography

Blue references indicate links to abstracts of articles available online:
http://www.aopublishing.org/BONE/4.htm

1. **Meikle MC** (1975) The influence of function on chondrogenesis at the epiphyseal cartilage of a growing long bone. *Anat Rec;* 182 (3):387–399.

2. **Thoma R** (1907) Synostosis suturae sagittalis cranis. Ein Beitrag zur Histomechanik des Skelettes und zur Lehre von dem interstitiellen Knochenwachstum. *Virchow's Arch;* 188:248.

3. **Trueta J** (1974) The growth and development of bones and joints: Orthopaedic aspects. *Scientific Foundations of Paediatrics:* Heinemann Medical.

4. **Lanyon LE, Rubin CT** (1985) The effect on bone remodelling of static and graded dynamic loads. *J Bone Joint Surg [Br];* 67:318.

5. **Felts WJL** (1959) Transplantation studies of factors in skeletal organogenesis. I. The subcutaneously implanted immature long bone of the rat and mouse. *Am J Phys Anthrop;* 17:201.

6. **Kember NF, Walker KV** (1971) Control of bone growth in rats. *Nature;* 229 (5284):428–429.

7. **Feik SA, Storey E** (1983) Remodelling of bone and bones: growth of normal and transplanted caudal vertebrae. *J Anat;* 136 (Pt 1): 1–14.

8. **Harkness EM, Trotter WD** (1980) Growth spurt in rat cranial bases transplanted into adult hosts. *J Anat;* 131 (1):39–56.

9. **Woolf J** (1892). *Das Gesetz der Transformation der Knochen.* Berlin: Verlag von August Hirschwald.

10. **Frost HM** (1979) A chondral modeling theory. *Calcif Tissue Int;* 28 (3):181–200.

11. **Trueta J, Trias A** (1961) The vascular contribution to osteogenesis IV. The effect of pressure upon the epiphyseal cartilage of the rabbit. *J Bone Joint Surg [Br];* 43:800.

12. **Wilson-MacDonald J** (1990) *The role of the periosteum in bone growth and bone remodelling.* Thesis: University of Bristol, England.

13. **Hert J, Liskova M** (1964) Proliferation der Epiphysenknorpel-zellen nach Aenderung der Belastung. *Ann Micr Anat Forsch;* 71:185.

14. **Ehrlich MG, Mankin HJ, Treadwell BV** (1972) Biochemical and physiological events during closure of the stapled distal femoral epiphyseal plate in rats. *J Bone Joint Surg [Am];* 54 (2):309–322.

15. **Hohmann EL, Elde RP, Rysavy JA, et al.** (1986) Innervation of periosteum and bone by sympathetic vasoactive intestinal peptide-containing nerve fibers. *Science;* 232 (4752):868–871.

16. **Bubenik GA, Bubenik AB, Stevens ED, et al.** (1982) The effect of neurogenic stimulation on the development and growth of bony tissues. *J Exp Zool;* 219 (2):205–216.

17. **Speer DP** (1982) Collagenous architecture of the growth plate and perichondrial ossification groove. *J Bone Joint Surg [Am];* 64 (3):399–407.

18. **Amamilo SC, Bader DL, Houghton GR** (1985) The periosteum in growth plate failure. *Clin Orthop;* (194):293–305.

19. **Morscher E** (1968) Strength and morphology of growth cartilage under hormonal influence of puberty. Animal experiments and clinical study on the etiology of local growth disorders during puberty. *Reconstr Surg Traumatol;* 10:3–104.

20. **Sebek J, Skalova J, Hert J** (1972) Reaction of bone to mechanical stimuli. 8. Local differences in structure and strength of periosteum. *Folia Morphol;* 20 (1):29–37.

21. **Crilly RG** (1972) Longitudinal overgrowth of chicken radius. *J Anat;* 112 (1):11–18.

22. **Whiteside LA** (1980) The periosteal microvascular anatomy. *Orthop Trans;* 4:271.

23. **Zucman J** (1960) Studies on the vascular connections between periosteum, bone, and muscle. *Brit J Surg;* 48:324.

24. **Trueta J, Amato VP** (1960) The vascular contribution to osteogenesis. Changes in the growth cartilage caused by experimentally induced ischaemia. *J Bone Joint Surg [Br];* 42:571.

25. **Whiteside LA, Lesker PA** (1978) The effects of extraperiosteal and subperiosteal dissection. I. On blood flow in muscle. *J Bone Joint Surg [Am];* 60 (1):23–26.

26. **Wilson-MacDonald J, Houghton GR, Bradley J, et al.** (1990) The relationship between periosteal division and compression or distraction of the growth plate. An experimental study in the rabbit. *J Bone Joint Surg [Br];* 72 (2):303–308.

27. **Peruchon E, Bonnel F, Baldet P, et al.** (1980) Evaluation and control of growth activity of epiphyseal plate. *Med Biol Eng Comput;* 18 (4):396–400.

28. **Strobino LJ, French GO, Colonna PC** (1952) The effect of increasing tensions on the growth of epiphyseal bone. *Surg Gyn Obs;* 95:694.

29. **Blount WP, Clarke GR** (1949) Control of bone growth by epiphyseal stapling. A preliminary report. *J Bone Joint Surg [Am];* 31:464.

30. **Phemister DB** (1933) Operative arrestment of longitudinal growth of bones in the treatment of deformities. *J Bone Joint Surg [Br];* 15:1.

31. **Marks DS, Sayampanathan SR, Thompson AG, et al.** (1995) Long-term results of convex epiphysiodesis for congenital scoliosis. *Eur Spine J;* 4 (5):296–301.

32. **Haas SL** (1945) Retardation of bone growth by a wire loop. *J Bone Joint Surg [Am];* 27:25.

33. **Christensen NO** (1973) Growth arrest by stapling. An experimental study of longitudinal bone growth and morphology of the growth region. *Acta Orthop Scand Suppl;* 3–78.

34. **Sijbrandij S** (1963) Inhibition of growth by means of compression of its proximal epiphyseal disc in the rabbit. *Acta Anat;* 55:278.

35. **Amako T, Honda K** (1957) An experimental study of epiphyseal stapling. *Kyshu J Med Sci;* 8:131.

36. **Pennecot GF, Herman S, Pouliquen JC** (1983) [Effects of progressive lengthening on the growth cartilage. Value of measurement of the torque]. *Rev Chir Orthop Reparatrice Appar Mot;* 69 (8):623–627.

37. **Pouliquen JC, Beneux J, Mener G, et al.** (1979) Etude de la croissance du membre inferieur apres allongement segmentaire chez l'enfant. *Ann Orthop Ouest;* 11:95.

38. **de Pablos J, Villas C, Canadell J** (1986) Bone lengthening by physial distraction. An experimental study. *Int Orthop;* 10 (3):163–170.

39. **Wilkinson JA** (1988) Injury to the growing femoral head. In: Uhtoff HK, Wiley JJ, editors. *Behavior of the Growth Plate.* New York: Raven Press.

40. **Tschantz P, Taillard W, Ditesheim PJ** (1977) Epiphyseal tilt produced by experimental overload. *Clin Orthop;* (123):271–279.

41. **Goff CW** (1967) Histologic arrangements from biopsies of epiphyseal plates of children before and after stapling. Correlated with roentgenographic studies. *Am J Orthop;* 9 (5):87–89.

42. **Reidy JA, Lingley JR, Gall EA, et al.** (1947) The effect of roentgen irradiation on epiphyseal growth. II: Experimental studies on the dog. *J Bone Joint Surg [Am];* 29:853.

43. **Bylander B, Hansson LI, Selvik G** (1983) Pattern of growth retardation after Blount stapling: a roentgen stereophotogrammetric analysis. *J Pediatr Orthop;* 3 (1):63–72.

44. **Lacroix P** (1951). *The Organization of Bones.* London: Churchill.

45. **Heuter C** (1862) Anatomische Studien an den Extremitäten-gelenken von Neugeborenen und Erwachsenen. *Virchow's Arch;* 25:575.

46. **Ring PA** (1958) Experimental bone lengthening by epiphyseal distraction. *Brit J Surg;* 46:169.

47. **Hert J** (1969) Acceleration of the growth after decrease of load on epiphyseal plates by means of spring distractors. *Folia Morphol;* 17 (2):194–203.

48. **Fishbane BM, Riley LH** (1976) Continuous trans-physeal traction: a simple method of bone lengthening. *John Hopkins Med J;* 138 (3):79–81.

49. **Spinelli R** (1988) Bone lengthening through physeal distraction-separation. In: Uhtoff HK, Wiley JJ, editors. *Behavior of the Growth Plate.* New York: Raven Press.

50. **Monticelli G, Spinelli R** (1981) Distraction epiphysiolysis as a method of limb lengthening. III. Clinical applications. *Clin Orthop;* (154):274–285.

51. **Eydelshteyn BM, Udalova NF, Bochkarev GF** (1973) Dynamics of reparative regeneration after lengthening by the method of distraction epiphyseolysis. *Acta Chir Plast;* 15 (3):149–154.

52. **Sledge CB, Noble J** (1978) Experimental limb lengthening by epiphyseal distraction. *Clin Orthop;* (136):111–119.

53. **Pouliquen JC, Chaboche P, Pennecot GF, et al.** (1980) [Consequences of progressive lengthenings on rabbits. Experimental study (author's transl)]. *Chir Pediatr;* 21 (5):363–367.

54. **De Bastiani G, Aldegheri R, Renzi Brivio L, et al.** (1986) Chondro-diatasis-controlled symmetrical distraction of the epiphyseal plate. Limb lengthening in children. *J Bone Joint Surg [Br];* 68 (4):550–556.

55. **Fjeld TO, Steen H** (1988) Limb lengthening by low rate epiphyseal distraction. An experimental study in the caprine tibia. *J Orthop Res;* 6 (3): 360–368.

56. **Moseley C, Mosca V** (1988) Complications of Wagner leg-lengthening. In: Uhtoff HK, Wiley JJ, editors. *Behavior of the Growth Plate.* New York: Raven Press.

57. **Dorfl J** (1980) Migration of tendinous insertions. I. Cause and mechanism. *J Anat;* 131 (1):179–195.

58. **Warrell E, Taylor JF** (1979) The role of periosteal tension in the growth of long bones. *J Anat;* 128 (1): 179–184.

59. **Wilde GP, Baker GC** (1987) Circumferential periosteal release in the treatment of children with leg-length inequality. *J Bone Joint Surg [Br];* 69 (5):817–821.

60. **Harkness EM, Trotter WD** (1978) Growth of transplants of rat humerus following circumferential division of the periosteum. *J Anat;* 126 (2):275–289.

61. **Houghton GR, Rooker GD** (1979) The role of the periosteum in the growth of long bones. An experimental study in the rabbit. *J Bone Joint Surg [Br];* 61 (2):218–220.

62. **Houghton GR, Duriez J** (1980) [Tibial lengthening by transepiphyseal distraction of the proximal growth plate. An experimental study in the rabbit (author's transl)]. *Rev Chir Orthop Reparatrice Appar Mot;* 66 (6):351–356.

63. **Lynch MC, Taylor JF** (1987) Periosteal division and longitudinal growth in the tibia of the rat. *J Bone Joint Surg [Br];* 69 (5):812–816.

64. **Friberg KS** (1979) Remodelling after distal forearm fractures in children. I. The effect of residual angulation on the spatial orientation of the epiphyseal plates. *Acta Orthop Scand;* 50 (5):537–546.

65. **Friberg KS** (1979) Remodelling after distal forearm fractures in children. III. Correction of residual angulation in fractures of the radius. *Acta Orthop Scand;* 50 (6 Pt 2):741–749.

66. **Karaharju EO, Ryoppy SA, Makinen RJ** (1976) Remodelling by asymmetrical epiphysial growth. An experimental study in dogs. *J Bone Joint Surg [Br];* 58 (1):122–126.

67. **Zionts LE, MacEwen GD** (1986) Spontaneous improvement of post-traumatic tibia valga. *J Bone Joint Surg [Am];* 68 (5):680–687.

68. **Carvell JE** (1983) The relationship of the periosteum to angular deformities of long bones. Experimental operations in rabbits. *Clin Orthop;* (173):262–274.

69. **Auer JA, Martens RJ** (1982) Periosteal transection and periosteal stripping for correction of angular limb deformities in foals. *Am J Vet Res;* 43 (9):1530–1534.

70. **Auer JA, Martens RJ, Williams EH** (1982) Periosteal transection for correction of angular limb deformities in foals. *J Am Vet Med Assoc;* 181 (5): 459–466.

71. **Weber BG** (1977) Fibrous inter-position causing valgus deformity after fracture of the upper tibial metaphysis in children. *J Bone Joint Surg [Br];* 59 (3):290–292.

72. **Murray DW, Wilson-MacDonald J, Morscher E, et al.** (1996) Bone growth and remodelling after fracture. *J Bone Joint Surg [Br];* 78 (1): 42–50.

73. **Salter RB, Harris WR** (1963) Injuries involving the epiphyseal plate. *J Bone Joint Surg [Am];* 45:587.

74. **Ogden JA** (1988) Skeletal growth mechanism injury patterns. In: Uhtoff HK, Wiley JJ, editors. *Behavior of the Growth Plate.* New York: Raven Press.

75. **Shapiro F** (1981) Fractures of the femoral shaft in children. The overgrowth phenomenon. *Acta Orthop Scand;* 52 (6):649–655.

76. **Nickodem T, Light T, Bunch W, et al.** (1984) Juxtaphyseal blood flow: Alterations following fracture and overgrowth in immature canines. *Orthop Trans;* 8:242.

77. **Wray JB, Lynch CJ** (1959) The vascular response to fracture of the tibia in the rat. *J Bone Joint Surg [Am];* 41:1143.

78. **Tonna E, Cronkite EP** (1961) Cellular response to fracture studied with tritiated thymidine. *J Bone Joint Surg [Am];* 43:352.

79. **Kaya Alpar E** (1986) Growth plate stimulation by diaphyseal fracture. Autoradiography of DNA synthesis in rats. *Acta Orthop Scand;* 57 (2):135–137.

80. **Delpech JM** (1829). *De l'Orthomorphie, par Rapport de l'Espece Humaine.* Paris: Gabon:301l.

81. **Appleton AB** (1934) Postural deformities and bone growth. An experimental study. *Lancet;* 1:451.

82. **Knight RA** (1954) Developmental deformities of the lower extremities. *J Bone Joint Surg [Am];* 36:521.

83. **DiFiori JP, Puffer JC, Mandelbaum BR, et al.** (1997) Distal radial growth plate injury and positive ulnar variance in nonelite gymnasts. *Am J Sports Med;* 25 (6): 763–768.

84. **Ring PA** (1957) Shortening and paralysis in poliomyelitis. *Lancet;* 2:980.

85. **Mente PL, Stokes IA, Spence H, et al.** (1997) Progression of vertebral wedging in an asymmetrically loaded rat tail model. *Spine;* 22 (12):1292–1296.

5 Radiologic interpretation of bone

Howard Dobson & Lawrence Friedman

1 Introduction

Radiology is indispensable to orthopedics. Over the last two decades, the availability of other diagnostic imaging modalities has become commonplace, and they play an increasingly important role. Nevertheless, plain radiography, on which this chapter is primarily focused, remains the principle initial imaging modality in orthopedic disease.

Radiographic examination is used to either make a diagnosis or assess progression or healing of an abnormality. Each evaluation should include an adequate number of radiographic views. At a minimum, this is two perpendicular projections. Significant diagnoses can be missed if only a single projection is obtained.

2 Imaging modalities

2.1 Radiography

2.1.1 Formation of the radiographic image

The formation of a radiographic image is based on the differential attenuation of the x-ray beam by different tissue types. This is a function of the atomic number, thickness, and density of the attenuating tissue. Five different radiographic opacities can be identified. They are air, fat, soft tissue, bone, and metal [1]. The ability to interpret a radiograph is based on the contrast provided by the differential attenuation of the x-ray beam by different tissue types.

The physical image on the radiographic film is formed by the interaction of the x-ray beam, which emerges from the patient with a film-screen combination. Intensifying screens are located within the cassette and convert the energy of x-rays into light. Radiographic film is much more sensitive to light than it is to x-rays. The use of intensifying screens reduces the amount of radiation required for a given exposure, reducing the patient radiation dose and motion blur. The speed of a given film-screen combination determines how much radiation is required. This is a largely in function of the size of the crystals in both the intensifying screen and the film. Larger crystals give a faster film combination, but at the cost of poorer resolution. Evaluation of subtle orthopedic lesions may require the use of high-detail, slow-speed film-screen combinations.

2.1.2 The radiographic image

Exposure to x-rays causes blackening of the radiographic film. The more x-ray photons the film is exposed to, the greater the degree of film blackening. If tissue attenuates the x-ray beam, a corresponding white area will be present on the film. This white area is known as an opacity. The ability to distinguish separate, but adjacent, organ structures on a radiograph requires that the contiguous structures have a different radiographic opacity. The result of this difference in opacity is known as radiographic contrast. It is defined as the difference between the opacities of the various parts of the body on a radiograph. Contrast depends upon both the type of film used and the patient. Film contrast is generally a constant factor, but subject contrast is variable. Subject contrast as seen on the finished radiograph is due to the differential absorption of x-rays by the various body tissues. Increasing or decreasing the kilovoltage can change the scale of contrast. Decreasing the tube kilovoltage results in decreased penetration of the parts of the body by the x-ray beam and thus a shortened scale of contrast, because the image is more nearly black and white with few shades of intermediate gray. In general, radiographic evaluation of bone requires a relatively low-kilovoltage technique (high contrast) to demonstrate the interfaces between bone and soft tissue [2].

Detail generally refers to image detail or sharpness and may be influenced by a number of factors. Generally, the further the object is from the film, the less distinct it will be. Intensifying screens can also influence detail; the faster the screens, the poorer the detail. A large focal spot in the x-ray tube may result in lack of sharpness. In practice, none of these produce marked loss of detail and, in most instances, none can be detected. By far the most common reason for loss of detail is motion or movement of the object during exposure; this can be minimized by sedation or anesthesia of the patient, or by using a film-screen combination and radiographic technique which allow a short exposure time. When a high-resolution image is required, a detail film-screen combination must be selected and used in circumstances where motion blur is minimized.

2.1.3　Grids

Grids are devices used to reduce the amount of scattered, or secondary, radiation produced when x-rays strike a thick mass of tissue. Scattered radiation is randomly directed. If it strikes the radiographic film, it will add opacities in a random manner, reducing the visible detail. When used, a grid is placed between the patient and the film. It is generally accepted that a grid should be used when the part is 10 cm or more in thickness. Radiographic evaluation of the extremities does not usually require a grid.

2.1.4　Magnification

This technique results in an image considerably larger than would be produced by conventional radiographs. This is particularly helpful in small bones or bone reactions, which are not easily seen by the usual techniques. In this technique, a special x-ray tube with a small focal spot must be used to reduce the blurring of the image which results if an ordinary tube is used.

The object is placed halfway between the film and the x-ray tube. In some instances a conventional radiograph may be enlarged optically (photographically), and the resolution may be as good as that obtained with magnification. The advantage of direct radiographic magnification is that an enlarged image can immediately be obtained, without having to wait for the photographic process.

2.1.5　Subtraction radiography

This method is used primarily to enhance the visualization of contrast studies, particularly when there is considerable overlying bone or soft tissue. A diapositive "mask" is made from a "scout" or plain radiograph; the mask is then superimposed over the contrast radiograph and the subtraction radiograph is produced from these two. This type of radiograph results in bony structures that are reduced in density, thus enabling better visualization of such structures as radiopaque contrasted vessels. The method can also be used to reduce soft-tissue shadows when they interfere with visualization.

2.1.6　Processing

The processing procedure is an important step in the production of a radiograph. The exposed film is first developed in a solution containing a reducing agent; this reduces the exposed grains of silver halide to metallic silver, which is black. The film is next placed in the fixer to remove or dissolve the undeveloped portions of the emulsion. The last two steps are washing and drying the film.

If developing is done manually, the film is placed in a hanger and moved by hand through the various solutions. More commonly, processing is done automatically by a machine that produces a dry finished radiograph in as short a time as 45 seconds. Obviously, automatic processing saves time, but contrast and detail may suffer slightly owing to the higher temperatures and shorter processing times; however, these losses are not usually great.

2.2 Fluoroscopy

Plain radiography uses a very short x-radiation exposure that is detected by a film-screen combination. The technique of fluoroscopy uses a continuous x-ray beam that is detected by an image intensifier. X-rays striking the input phosphor of the image intensifier are converted to visible light and form a very faint image. This image is electronically captured, amplified or intensified, and displayed on a monitor. The result is a real time display of the subject and any movement. The principle uses of fluoroscopy in orthopedic radiology are the closed reduction of some fractures and luxations and guidance of instrument placement, especially biopsy needles.

2.3 Computed tomography

Computed tomographic (CT) images are created by reconstructing an image from multiple projections of the object using thin collimated beams of x-rays. This results in detailed images with higher in-plane resolution of bone and soft-tissue structures in the axial, sagittal, and coronal planes than x-rays. CT also allows accurate measurement of lesions, differentiating between fat, fluid, and calcification with a high degree of accuracy. The ability to scan directly in the sagittal or coronal planes as well as the conventional axial plane in the musculoskeletal system makes CT a far more accurate term than CAT (computerized axial tomography). Since its inception in the early 1970s there have been four generations of scanners. In 4th generation scanners the detectors are fixed and the x-ray tube rotates. The recent introduction of spiral CT represents a major step forward in the evolution of CT scanning. The ability to create a moving focus of x-rays arranged in a ring surrounding the patient has translated into a dramatically improved scanning rate with better contrast utilization, reduced partial-volume artifact, and increased throughput. CT allows accurate assessment of the bony cortex, periosteum, and calcifications. Disadvantages include radiation risk, inability to accurately assess bone marrow, and less in-plane resolution of tendons, muscles, and soft-tissue structures than ultrasound (US) or magnetic resonance imaging (MRI).

2.4 Magnetic resonance imaging

In MRI, images are produced by radiofrequency (RF) pulses interacting with hydrogen nuclei in tissues (containing protons) in the presence of a strong magnetic field. After termination of the RF pulses, the nuclei return to equilibrium and a signal reflecting the spatial nature of the tissues is generated. Contrast is based to a large extent on the relative rates at which stimulated protons in different tissues give off their "energy" or return to equilibrium. The power of MRI lies in the ability to differentiate T1 (longitudinal) and T2 (transverse) relaxation rates of protons in different types of tissues. Recent advances in technology using faster sequences and improved coils have resulted in superior imaging in a shorter time. The advantages of MRI include multiplanar capability, the ability to evaluate bone marrow (not seen by any other modality), and high soft-tissue resolution. These factors make MRI the best modality to assess malignant lesions or bone-marrow disorders. Disadvantages include expense, limited access, and claustrophobia. Patients with ferromagnetic aneurysm clips, cochlea implants, and pacemakers cannot be imaged with this modality.

2.5 Ultrasound

Using high frequencies produced by subjecting a special ceramic material, a piezoelectric crystal or plastic polymer, to slow voltage spikes produces US images. This alters the crystal thickness, producing sound waves. The transducer acts as both a transmitter and receiver. The recent introduction of high-resolution small-parts transducers with frequencies of 7.5–13 or 15 MHz and experimental probes of 20 MHz has revolutionized the US assessment of the musculoskeletal system. This has allowed exquisite detail of the fibrillar pattern of tendons and ligaments, justifying interrogation of joints and muscles in sports-medicine injuries. In addition it has also been shown to be effective in diagnosing subtle occult fractures. Advantages include low cost, easy access, portability, multiplanar capability, dynamic real-time scanning, and high in-plane resolution, exceeding that of CT and equivalent to that of MRI in assessing tendons, ligaments, and some soft-tissue lesions. Disadvantages include operator dependence and a steep learning curve.

2.6 Scintigraphy

The strength of scintigraphy is that it provides physiological data concerning the tissues being evaluated. This is in contrast to the predominantly anatomical data provided by the other imaging modalities. The vast majority of examinations use the isotope Technetium 99m (^{99m}Tc), bound to a carrier molecule. The common carrier molecule used in evaluation of the skeletal system is methylene diphosphonate. The technetium-methylene diphosphonate complex binds to forming bone matrix at sites of active remodeling. The radiopharmaceutical is administered intravenously and its distribution within the body is determined using a gamma camera. Scintillation, and hence scintigraphy, is the conversion of gamma radiation to visible light by certain compounds, in this case a large sodium iodide crystal. The emitted light is electronically converted to an image that is displayed either on a monitor or reproduced on film. The normal background metabolism of bone provides an image of the structure, with areas of pathology demonstrating a more intense uptake. Active growth plates will also demonstrate intense uptake of the radiopharmaceutical. The technique is extremely sensitive for identifying pathology, but its sensitivity for specific pathological diagnoses is much poorer.

2.7 Bone densitometry

Historically, bone density was determined radiographically. However, the proportion of bone lost must be at least 30–50% before it can be recognized radiographically. This is not helpful for the early diagnosis of osteoporosis, as the diagnosis must be made much earlier for helpful intervention to be made. Accurate assessments of bone density and changes in bone density over time are made with various energy absorptiometric methods. These include single-photon absorptiometry, dual-photon absorptiometry, and, more recently, quantitative CT and dual-energy x-ray absorptiometry.

3 Principles of radiographic interpretation

Radiologic interpretation begins before the radiographs are made with consultation between the attending clinician and the radiologist. At the minimum this will include the clinical history and physical examination findings, and a statement of the specific diagnostic questions to be answered. This will allow the radiologist to tailor the examination to the individual case, increasing the diagnostic yield and avoiding unnecessary or inappropriate examinations. It has been clearly demonstrated that in the case of trauma, the lack of an appropriate clinical history leads to suboptimal radiographic interpretation [3].

The examination of the films should take place in a quiet environment without distractions and with appropriate lighting, viewboxes, and a bright light. An inadequate viewbox reduces the detectable spatial resolution and appropriate standards have been proposed [4].

The person examining the radiographs must have an adequate and thorough knowledge of the normal anatomy and its variations. Atlases of the human and animals species are available and are invaluable to both the experienced and inexperienced observer [5–7]. When examining the appendicular skeleton, a radiograph of the contralateral limb may in many cases resolve uncertainties.

The radiographs should then be systematically examined in order to identify the presence or absence of lesions. The precise nature of the examining system is unimportant, as long as it includes each and every part of the skeleton visible on the radiograph and their associated soft tissues. This would include separate evaluation of the epiphysis, physis, metaphysis, diaphysis, trabeculae, cortex, periosteum, endosteum, articular surface, the length of the bone and its tubulation, overall density, texture, and shape. An initial preliminary evaluation is made at a distance of up to a meter from the film. This distant review allows more lesions, particularly subtle lesions, to be identified, than are identified with close scrutiny only. A preliminary examination might involve recognition of the presence of a lesion or lesions, followed by an overall assessment of the number of lesions and the pattern of distribution, followed by close scrutiny of each individual lesion. This will lead to the formation of a list of differential diagnoses which, in consideration of the clinical history and other pertinent data, may result in either a specific diagnosis or a reduction of the list. Where a specific diagnosis cannot be made, a determination of whether the lesion is of an aggressive or benign type should be made.

3.1 Lesion distribution

Bone disorders may be classified as monostotic, involving a single bone (e.g., an osteosarcoma) or polyostotic, involving multiple bones (e.g., multiple myeloma). The symmetry of the distribution of the lesions may provide helpful diagnostic information. For example, osteoporosis and hypertrophic osteoarthropathy are normally bilaterally symmetrical whereas osteomyelitis usually has an asymmetrical distribution.

3.2 Analysis of the lesion

Careful and complete analysis of each individual lesion should take place according to the following criteria. Do not assume that when multiple lesions are present the conclusions reached following scrutiny of one lesion will equally apply to the remainder.

3.2.1 Location

Certain lesions, particularly neoplasms, have a predilection for specific locations. Osteosarcoma has a predilection for the distal femur and proximal tibia in man and the proximal humerus and distal radius in the dog [8, 9]. A predilection for a specific site within a bone is common. Metaphyseal lesions, particularly neoplastic, are the most common because of the prominent vascularity and high metabolic rate of this region. In children and neonatal animals, foci of infection at the metaphyseal side of the physis are common because the peculiarities of the metaphyseal blood supply favor the establishment of foci of infection subsequent to bacteremia or septicemia (**Fig. 5-1**) [10, 11]. In human infants under 1 year of age, vessels commonly cross the physis. As a consequence epiphyseal infection is more common in this age group [12]. Vessels crossing the growth plate in neonatal animals have been described, but appear to be less common than in the human neonate.

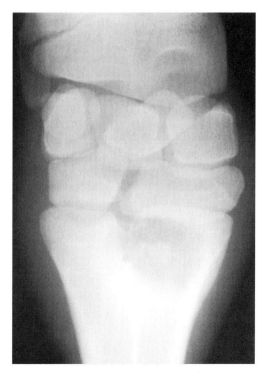

Fig. 5-1: A dorso-palmar projection of the proximal metacarpus of a calf demonstrating a metaphyseal lesion caused by osteomyelitis.

3.2.2 Bone destruction

Bone destruction occurs as a result of the activity of osteoclasts. It is the effect, direct or indirect, of the pathological insult on the osteoclasts which results in the latter's stimulation to activity. The claim of Jaffe that tumor cells directly destroy bone trabeculae is no longer accepted [9, 13, 14]. Under normal circumstances bone destruction is not visible radiographically until 10–14 days following the pathological insult [9]. However, this is a generalization and many exceptions exist.

Radionuclide techniques, however, will identify bone destruction by virtue of the abnormal metabolism and increased blood flow to the site. Osteomyelitis, for example, can be identified within 24 hours of the onset of signs [15].

The visibility of a destructive lesion is dependent on the contrast provided by the adjacent normal bone. The overall greater opacity and more uniform opacity distribution in cortical bone, when compared to the less opaque and uneven distribution of cancellous bone, results in lesions with reduced opacity being more easily detected in cortical bone because of the greater resultant contrast between the normal and abnormal areas. Overall, it is necessary to have a loss of up to 40% of bone mass before it can be identified radiographically [16]. Thus, a small destructive lesion may be considerably more easily identified in dense cortical bone than a larger lesion in osteoporotic cancellous bone. Categorization of a lesion as aggressive or non-aggressive is an important step in the formation of a differential diagnosis. Excessive reliance should not be placed on this differentiation as exceptions do occur. Rather, this criterion should be considered in the context of all the available data. The margination of the lesion or the zone of transition between normal and abnormal bone is an important component of the aggressiveness of a lesion. A non-aggressive lesion typically has a well-defined margin, or a short distance between clearly abnormal bone and clearly normal bone. Usually, peripheral sclerosis of the normal bone will be present. In contrast, an aggressive process has poorly defined margins, without a clear border between normal and abnormal bone. A "punched out" lesion can be associated with either an aggressive or a non-aggressive process. This lesion has a well-defined margin but is without peripheral sclerosis. They occur because the lesion is expanding so rapidly that there is insufficient time for the adjacent normal bone to produce a sclerotic response. Destruction of the cortex is considered to be a feature of an aggressive process. A lesion with clearly defined margins or a short zone of transition is much more easily identified than an ill-defined lesion with a long zone of transition. Early cortical lysis is often identified as a change in texture rather than a focal area of lysis.

A neoplastic process, within the marrow cavity of the diaphysis, may not be completely visible radiographically until it has filled the entire cavity. The earliest radiographic indication of its presence may be endosteal scalloping of the cortex (**Fig. 5-2**).

Patterns of reduced bone density

A pathological insult may modify osteoclast activity, resulting in bone destruction on a generalized, local, regional, or diffuse basis. Descriptive criteria have been developed which relate the appearance of a focal lesion to its rate of growth [14, 17]. Frequently, but by no means invariably, the rate of growth will give an indication of the biology of the primary disease. The three basic patterns of lysis that are recognized are geographic, with a slow rate of growth, moth-eaten, with an intermediate growth rate, and the rapidly changing permeative type (**Fig. 5-3**).

Generalized reduction in bone density

The presence of a generalized reduction in bone density implies the presence of reduced amounts of normal bone [9]. In the strict definition this is best described radiographically by the term osteopenia. In practice, however, osteoporosis, meaning a metabolic disease resulting in osteopenia, is often used synonymously.

Radiographically, a generalized reduction in bone density is recognized by a reduction in the number and width of the bone trabeculae, with the smaller trabeculae being completely lost, resulting in a coarse or lacey appearance. A reduction in width

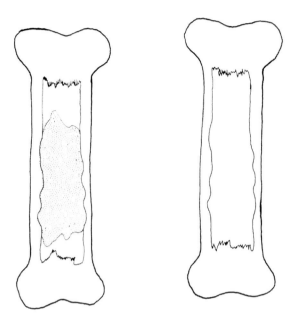

Fig. 5-2: Outline diagram illustrating a mass located in the medullary cavity. The presence of the mass has resulted in reabsorption of areas of the endosteal surface of the cortex. Radiographically the mass is unlikely to be directly visualized. Its presence is recognized indirectly by the endosteal scalloping.

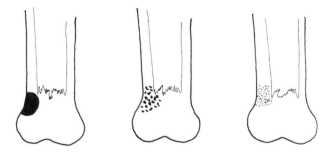

Fig. 5-3: Outline diagram illustrating three patterns of bone lysis. The geographic pattern *(left)* is characterized by the presence of a large area of complete lysis. The moth-eaten pattern *(center)* has multiple discrete areas of lysis, often becoming confluent, which are greater than 2–3 mm in dimension. The permeative pattern *(right)* is identified by the presence of multiple small lysis, less than 2-mm areas of radiolucency.

of the cortices is also present. In some cases, in addition to the reduction in the width of the cortex, there may also be an increased density in the remaining cortex.

A generalized reduction in density may affect a single bone, a limb, or the entire skeleton. Cases involving the latter are typically of a metabolic origin, the classical osteoporosis; whereas involvement of a single limb is more often due to a primary lesion within the limb (**Fig. 5-4**).

Fig. 5-4: a) A lateral projection of a canine tarsus demonstrating a generalized loss of density, especially of the os calcis. The limb had been immobilized in a cast for 3 weeks because of a fracture of the tibia. The periosteal callus associated with healing of the fracture can be identified at the top of the illustration.
b) For comparison, a lateral projection of the normal leg of the same.

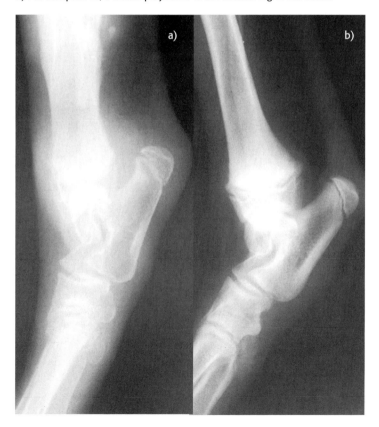

Geographic pattern of bone destruction

The geographic pattern of bone lysis is found predominantly in cancellous bone. The characteristics of the lesion's margin are used for further subdivision of the type. The slowest growing lesions, and the most likely to be benign, have a sclerotic margin. The sclerotic rim represents a layer of lamellar bone that is produced as a mechanical response to the pressure of the primary lesion (**Fig. 5-5**). Frequently the external border is smooth while the internal margin is ill defined. This occurs because the sclerotic rim is being formed by cellular activity on the external surface [**14**], whereas, internally, bone destruction by the primary lesion results in numbers of partially destroyed trabeculae giving a poorly defined margin (**Fig. 5-6**). This pattern of destruction is associated with benign lesions such as bone cysts, enchondroma, or fibrous dysplasia (**Fig. 5-7** and **Fig. 5-8**). However, it has also been associated with both malignant disease, such as plasma cell myeloma, and also with osteomyelitis [**18**]. A sclerotic rim which fades peripherally is typically associated with either chronic osteomyelitis or Brodie

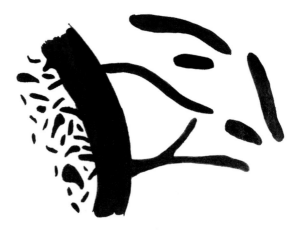

Fig. 5-6: Outline diagram of a part of the wall of a lesion demonstrating a geographic pattern of bone destruction. The broad band in the center represents the sclerotic rim of the lesion. Normal trabeculae can be identified to the right of the sclerotic rim. Remnants of trabeculae that have been destroyed by the primary lesion can be identified to the left of the rim. Radiographically a lesion of this type has a clearly defined outer margin and an ill-defined inner margin.

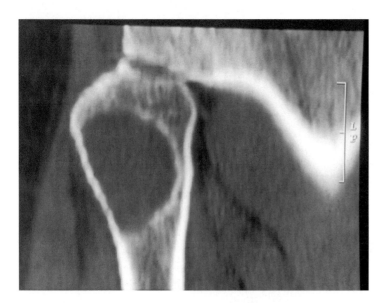

Fig. 5-5: A CT image of a unicameral bone cyst in a 33-year-old woman, demonstrating a geographic pattern of bone destruction with a sclerotic rim.

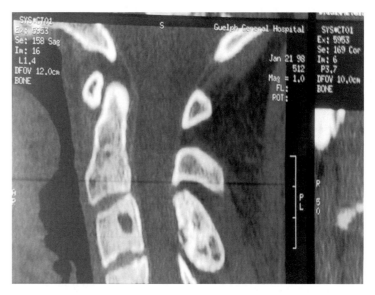

Fig. 5-7: A sagittal CT image of the cervical spine illustrating a geographic pattern of lysis without a sclerotic rim. Compare with **Fig. 5-5**.

abscess [14, 19], a form of chronic osteomyelitis without an acute clinical stage, characteristically identified in the metaphyseal region in young animals and people (**Fig. 5-9**).

In some circumstances a geographic lesion may have a clearly defined margin without sclerosis, known as a "punched out" lesion. Histologically, normal trabeculae can be identified up to the edge of the primary lesion [14]. Examples of this type of lesion would include enchondroma, multiple myeloma, and solitary bone cysts [9, 20].

A more aggressive form is seen where the margins of the lesion are poorly defined. By dint of the lesion's fast growing, aggressive nature, bone destruction is occurring over a wider zone, forming an indistinct margin. Examples of this type of destruction would include primary tumors such as giant cell tumor, osteosarcoma, chondrosarcoma and fibrosarcoma, and secondary tumors (**Figs. 5-10, 5-11,** and **5-12**).

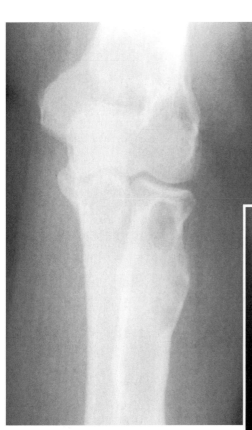

Fig. 5-8: An AP projection of the elbow of a young man demonstrating geographic lesions with poorly defined margins due to fibrous dysplasia.

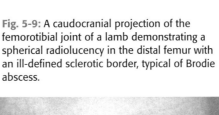

Fig. 5-9: A caudocranial projection of the femorotibial joint of a lamb demonstrating a spherical radiolucency in the distal femur with an ill-defined sclerotic border, typical of Brodie abscess.

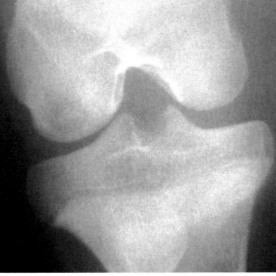

Fig. 5-10: A lateral projection of the proximal tibia of a dog demonstrating a geographic area of bone destruction with poor margination. This feature indicates an aggressive lesion, in this case an osteosarcoma.

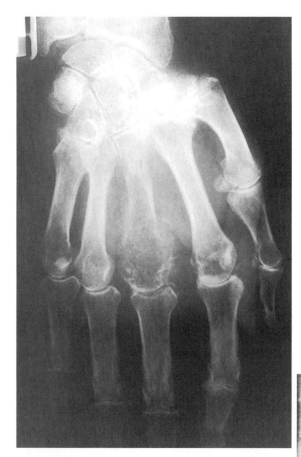

Fig. 5-11: An AP projection of the hand of an elderly man with poorly marginated destructive lesion due to metastatic neoplasia.

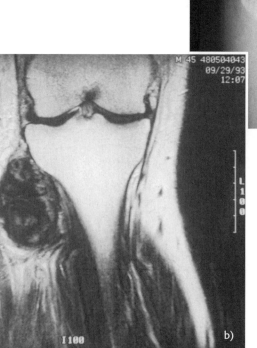

Fig. 5-12: a) An AP projection of the proximal fibula of a 45-year-old male with a giant cell sarcoma. The image demonstrates a fast growing destructive lesion.
b) An equivalent MR image demonstrates a lack of homogeneity in signal intensity in the tumorous mass.

Moth-eaten pattern of bone destruction

This pattern of bone destruction is characterized by the appearance of multiple separate areas of radiolucency with ill-defined margins, usually greater than 2–3 mm in dimension. These lesions represent an infiltrative process where bone destruction is multifocal in nature. At least initially, areas of normal bone can be identified between the lesions, but ultimately coalescence of the lesions may occur. This pattern of abnormality is more easily recognized in the cortex because of the inherent high radiographic contrast, but also occurs in trabecular bone. Typical primary lesions include osteomyelitis and malignant neoplasms such as osteosarcoma, fibrosarcoma, and chondrosarcoma (**Figs. 5-13** to **5-16**). Secondary metastatic lesions may also present a moth-eaten pattern of bone destruction (**Fig. 5-17**). Early lesions can be difficult to identify on plain radiographs. Cross-sectional imaging allows identification of lesions before they become visible radiographically (**Fig. 5-18**).

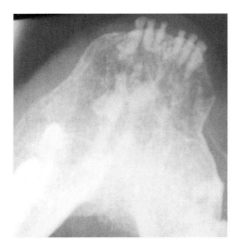

Fig. 5-13: An intra-oral projection of the rostral mandible of a cat, demonstrating a moth-eaten pattern of bone destruction due to osteomyelitis.

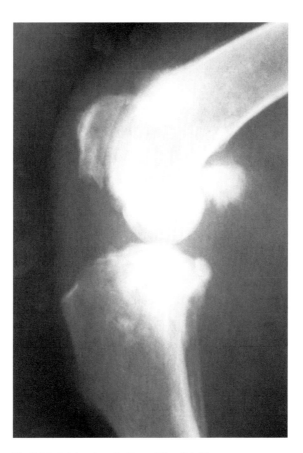

Fig.5-14: A lateral projection of the distal femur and proximal tibia of a dog, demonstrating a moth-eaten pattern of bone destruction due to blastomycosis.

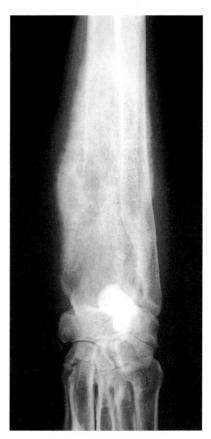

Fig. 5-15: A dorso-palmar projection of the distal radius of a dog, demonstrating a moth-eaten pattern of bone destruction due to osteosarcoma.

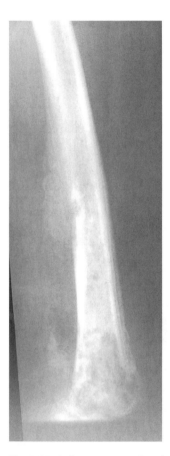

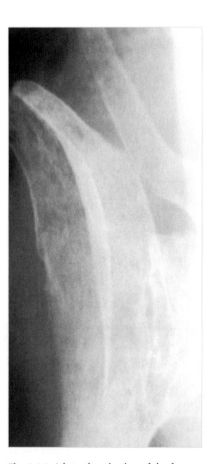

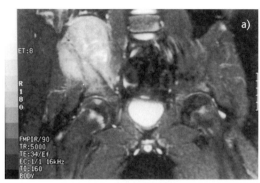

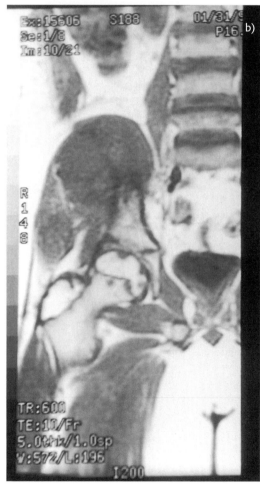

Fig. 5-17: A close-up ventrodorsal projection of the ilium of a dog, demonstrating a moth-eaten pattern of bone destruction due to multiple myeloma.

Fig. 5-16: A lateral projection of the femur, demonstrating a moth-eaten pattern of bone destruction and a lamellated periosteal reaction due to chronic osteo-myelitis in a young woman.

Fig. 5-18: a) MR images of the pelvis of a person with osteosarcoma. The primary lesion involving the ilium is easily identified and was visible radiographically.
b) The secondary lesions involving the femoral head that are visible on the MR image were not visible on radiographs.

Permeative pattern of bone destruction

The permeative pattern of bone destruction presents as uniform, tiny, poorly marginated, longitudinally oriented, oval, or linear radiolucencies. This pattern of radiographic abnormality represents the fastest type of destruction [21]. Pathophysiologically the lesion represents an exaggerated remodeling response with an increased number of "cutting cones", a component of the normal remodeling process being present. Overall, less bone is being laid down than is being absorbed [14].

As originally described, this lesion is primarily recognized in the cortex and represents an aggressive fast-growing lesion [21]. More recently, this pattern of reduced radiodensity of bone has been subdivided on the basis of etiology and radiographic appearance [22]. A pseudopermeative pattern is caused by metabolic disease, such as osteoporosis or thyrotoxicosis, and presents ovoid to elongated radiolucencies which are present throughout the entire width of the cortex. In contrast, a true permeative pattern is an extension of a medullary process, such as osteomyelitis or a round cell tumor, and the radiolucencies are located at the inner endosteal surface only (**Fig. 5-19**).

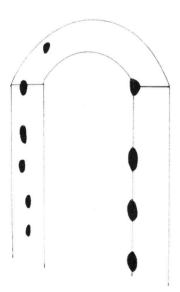

Fig. 5-19: An outline diagram demonstrating the radiolucencies of a permeative pattern of bone destruction located on the endosteal surface *(top),* in contrast to the pseudopermeative pattern where the radiolucencies are located within the cortex *(bottom).*

3.2.3   Increase in bone density

Increased bone density occurs in a wide variety of diseases with varying pathogenesis. Radiographically its presence must be recognized and its distribution and characteristics used to determine its likely etiology and significance. A plethora of congenital conditions have been identified in both man and animals that are characterized by widespread increase in radiodensity. In general, they are the result of incoordination of the roles of the cells responsible for the formation, modeling, and remodeling of bone. The features of these conditions have been described by a number of authors [9, 10]. An extreme example is the widespread involvement of all bones in osteopetrosis with loss of tubulation of the long bones (**Fig. 5-20**).

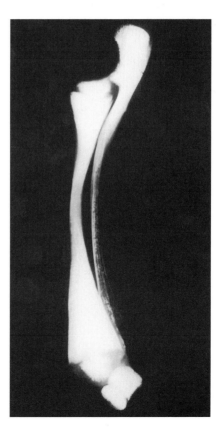

Fig. 5-20: A lateral projection of the radius and ulna of a deer, demonstrating lack of tubulation of both bones.

In the early stages of fluorosis bone density is reduced, but the later stages are characterized by widespread sclerosis of the spine, pelvis, and ribs, and multiple periosteal exostoses [23, 24].

Localized increase in bone density

In regional or localized osteosclerosis, the distribution of the abnormal bone production can have important diagnostic implications. The radiographic features of the new bone production are dependent upon the nature of the matrix within which the mineralization occurs. The matrix can be composed of osteoid, fibrous, or cartilaginous tissue. At its simplest, the increased density may represent reinforcing of the margins of an existing lesion such as a tumor margin or in fracture repair (**Fig. 5-21** and **Fig. 5-22**). In inflammatory disease, both endosteal and trabecular sclerosis may occur, resulting in the ivory-like density seen in chronic osteomyelitis (**Fig. 5-23** and **Fig. 5-24**).

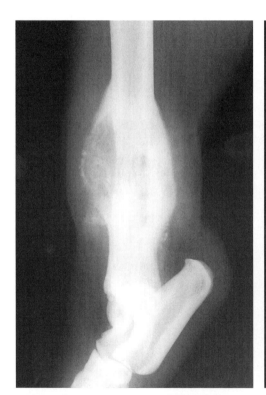

Fig. 5-21: A lateral projection of the tibia of a dog, demonstrating new production on the cortex opposite to a destructive lesion (in this case an osteosarcoma). This has resulted in a change of shape and an increase in density.

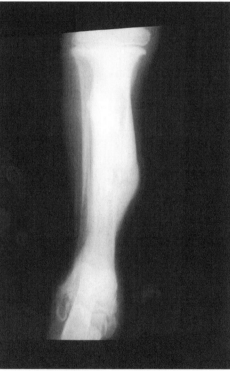

Fig. 5-22: A caudo-cranial projection of the tibia of a dog, demonstrating new bone production on the cortices as a part of the repair process following a fracture. This has both altered the shape of the bone and caused a local increase in density.

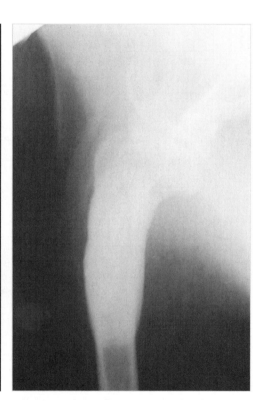

Fig. 5-23: A lateral projection of the humerus of a dog, demonstrating extreme sclerosis of a portion of the proximal metaphysis and diaphysis due to chronic osteomyelitis.

An ivory-like density characterizes complete mineralization of an osteoid matrix. Typically this is seen in osteoma. The definition of osteosarcoma is based on the presence of osteoid. The degree of mineralization of the osteoid matrix within an osteosarcoma is variable. When extensive mineralization of the osteoid is present the tumor has a radiodense appearance (**Fig. 5-25**). Neoplastic lesions metastatic to bone may also present as localized sclerosis (**Fig. 5-26**).

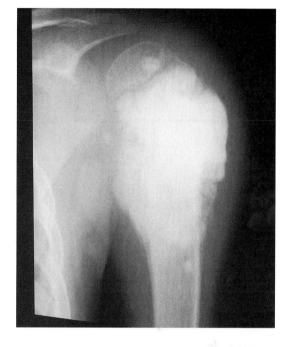

Fig. 5-25: A lateral projection of a boy, demonstrating an increase in bone density due to a sclerosing osteosarcoma. (Courtesy of Dr E.J. Becker.)

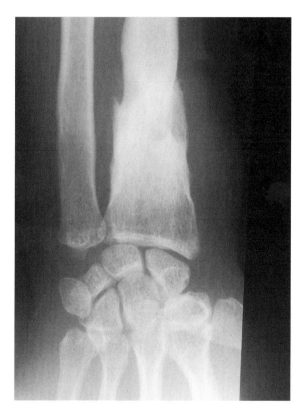

Fig. 5-24: An AP of the radius and ulna of a middle-aged man, demonstrating sclerosis of the distal radius secondary to chronic osteomyelitis.

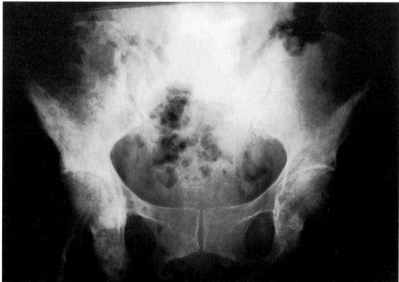

Fig. 5-26: An AP projection of the pelvis demonstrating multiple areas of sclerosis and radiolucency due to metastasis in an elderly woman.

A fibrous matrix results in the production of woven bone that radiographically has a ground-glass appearance [25]. In the initial stages of fibrous dysplasia the lesion is radiolucent [9, 13, 26], but as mineralization occurs during the later stages it takes on a ground-glass appearance (**Fig. 5-27** and **Fig. 5-28**).

Mineralization of a cartilage matrix results in a caricature of the provisional calcification followed by replacement by endochondral bone seen in endochondral ossification. Mineralization of the matrix itself results in a stippled or flocculent radiographic appearance [25], whereas replacement of areas of matrix by endochondral bone results in arc-shaped and ring-shaped radiodensities (**Figs. 5-29** to **5-31**).

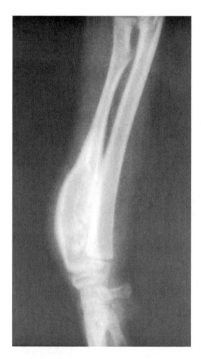

Fig. 5-27: A lateral projection of the distal ulna of a cat, demonstrating healing fibrous dysplasia. Centrally, the lesion has a ground-glass appearance.

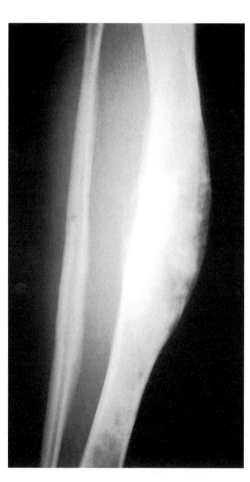

Fig. 5-28: A radiograph of a human tibia, demonstrating the ground-glass appearance of healing fibrous dysplasia. (Courtesy of Dr E.J. Becker.)

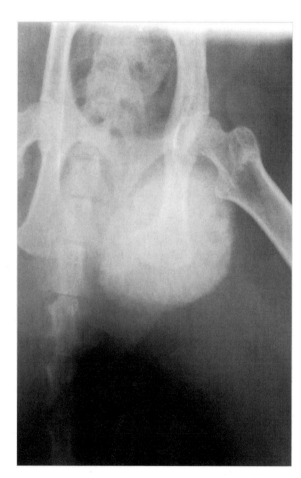

Fig. 5-29: A ventro-dorsal projection of the pelvis of a dog. The lesion is a chondrosarcoma. Compare with **Fig. 5-30**.

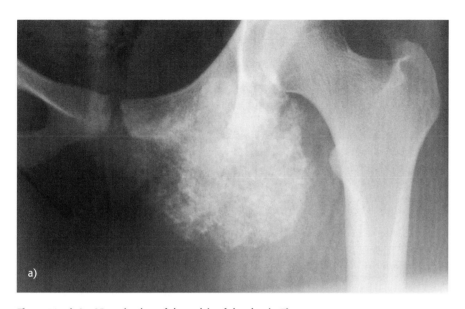

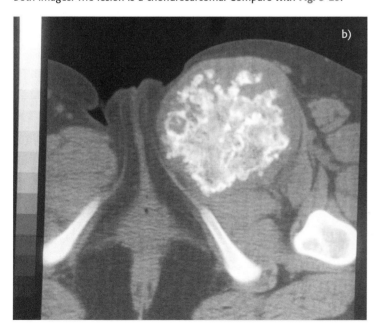

Fig. 5-30: a) An AP projection of the pelvis of the dog in Fig. 5-29, demonstrating a mineralizing mass.
b) A CT image of the lesion in (a). Note the arc-shaped radiopacities in both images. The lesion is a chondrosarcoma. Compare with Fig. 5-29.

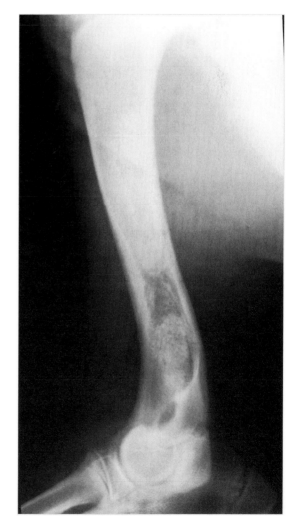

Fig. 5-31: A lateral projection of the distal humerus of a dog, demonstrating marked medullary sclerosis due to panosteitis.

Osteosclerosis

Osteosclerosis is a term used generally to describe a diffuse increase in bone density within the medullary cavity. The abnormality is relatively uncommon, particularly in animals. The more common causes include renal osteodystrophy, sickle cell disease, myelofibrosis, and osteopetrosis [27]. Focal osteosclerosis is more commonly associated with metastatic disease.

A condition specific to the growing dog, panosteitis, is characterized radiographically by focal increased medullary opacity [28] of the long bones (**Fig. 5-31**). Recently, canine distemper virus has been implicated in the etiology of this condition [29].

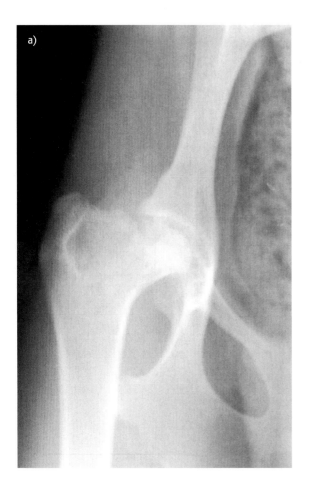

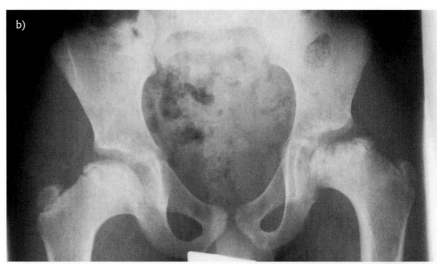

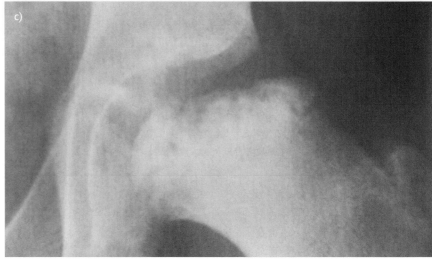

Fig. 5-32: Mottled lesions of the femoral head due to subchondral collapse and sclerosis due to Legg-Calvé-Perthes disease in (a) a 1-year-old poodle, (b) an 8-year-old boy and (c) a close up of (b).

In Legg-Calvé-Perthes disease, where multiple ischemic lesions coexist, areas of sclerosis and associated subchondral collapse give the femoral head a mottled appearance (**Fig. 5-32**).

The reparative stage of ischemic bone injury results in a focal increase in bone density. Since the necrotic tissue is by definition avascular, radiographically identifiable repair begins in the healthy peripheral bone with the development of a sclerotic border. In man and in the dog, following ischemic necrosis of the marrow cavity the radiographic appearance is characterized by the presence of serpentine radiodense tracts [30] within the cavity (**Fig. 5-33 and Fig. 5-34**). In people, a wide variety of causes of bone infarction are recognized, including occlusive vascular disease, sickle cell anemia, caisson disease, infiltrative disease, and infection [30]. In the dog, however, the

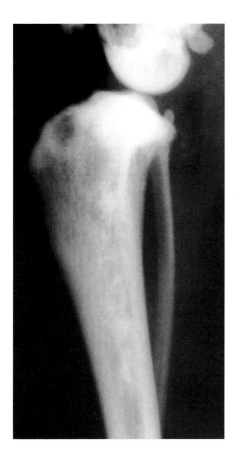

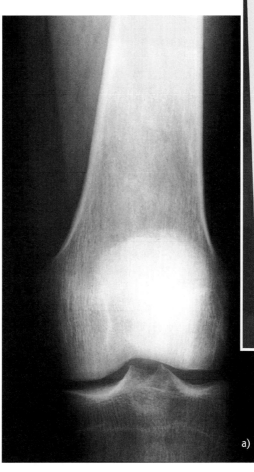

Fig. 5-33: A lateral projection of the tibia of a dog, demonstrating tortuous radio-densities located within the diaphyseal cavity. These abnormalities represent the reparative stage of ischemic necrosis.

Fig. 5-34: a) An AP projection of a human femur, demonstrating narrow cavity radiodensities typical of ischemic necrosis.
b) MRI of the same patient clearly demonstrates the presence of the lesion, indicating that the radiographic changes occur relatively late in the course of the disease. (Courtesy of Dr E.J. Becker.)

disease, in itself rare, is commonly associated with a primary malignant neoplasm [31]. It has been suggested that the infarction precedes the neoplastic change and that the two diseases are in some way related [32].

Within the center of a marrow infarct, dystrophic mineralization of necrotic fat may occur during the repair process, giving a patchy pattern of radiodensity. This radiographic abnormality, in conjunction with the marginal sclerosis, gives the lesion a "rising smoke" pattern of density [25].

Metaphyseal bands

The production of metaphyseal bands of increased radiopacity is an effect that occurs during bone growt, the results of which may remain visible well into adult life. This radiological abnormality is a feature of a number of specific and nonspecific diseases [9]. The primary abnormality is at the growth plate and is a dysfunction of the normally closely regulated interactions of chondroblastic, osteoblastic, and osteoclastic activities [33]. In most of these conditions the precise nature of the abnormality has not been identified.

In some instances, the normal invasion of the zone of provisional calcification by vascular tissue and its replacement with the primary spongiosa does not occur. Consequently, the zone of provisional calcification becomes wider and intensely mineralized. In vitamin C deficiency the widened zone of provisional calcification is seen in conjunction with a generalized osteoporosis and a ground-glass appearance, whereas it occurs as a single entity in congenital syphilis [9] (Fig. 5-35). On recovery, replacement of the zone of provisional calcification returns it to its normal width.

Hypertrophic osteodystrophy, or metaphyseal osteopathy, is an interesting condition, which appears to be unique to the dog and has historically been compared to vitamin C deficiency. The diseases have similarities in that a broad, heavily mineralized zone of provisional calcification exists. However, in hypertrophic osteodystrophy, subjacent to the zone of provisional calcification there exists a metaphyseal band of necrotic and infarcted bone, while further down the metaphysis an additional band of sclerosis exists [34], giving a series

of alternating radiodense and radiolucent bands (Fig. 5-36). The etiology of hypertrophic osteodystrophy remains unknown. However, infection with canine distemper virus has been implicated, and the virus transcripts have been histologically identified in metaphyseal osteoclasts in cases of the naturally occurring disease [35].

In lead poisoning, however, the replacement of the zone of provisional calcification is disorganized, and randomly oriented trabeculae are interspersed with intensely mineralized cartilage [33]. On recovery these so-called lead lines are not reabsorbed and move further down the metaphysis as normal growth proceeds. Previously, the increased radiographic density was ascribed to the incorporation of lead within the tissue. It is now recognized that although leadification does occur, it contributes

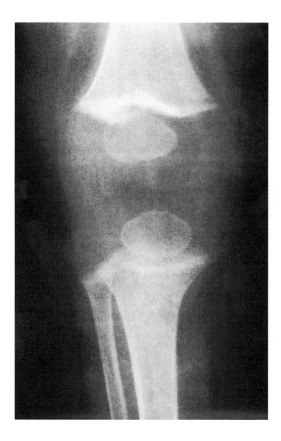

Fig. 5-35: An AP projection of the distal femur and proximal tibia of an African bush baby with scurvy. Note the increased density of the zone of provisional calcification and the general ground-glass appearance of the bones.

only 1/4 of the density of the band, the remainder being due to the abnormal calcification within the band [36].

Growth arrest lines have long been recognized as being subsequent to cessation of growth due to non-specific disease in people. They are not widely recognized in animals. They are also referred to as Harris or Park lines, as a tribute to the contributions of these two investigators [37, 38]. In the circumstances of non-specific growth arrest, cartilaginous growth stops while osteoblastic activity continues. Clearly, the continued formation of predominately longitudinal trabeculae, by replacement of cartilage, cannot continue, so the osteoblasts produce a transversely oriented band of trabeculae [33]. When normal growth resumes, this band will progress down into the metaphysis. Additional bone is also laid down on both surfaces of the band, increasing its width as it moves further down the metaphysis.

3.2.4 The periosteum

The periosteum consists of two layers of tissue which are not sharply defined. The outer layer consists of a network of fibrous tissue, extending into the cortex as Sharpey fibers. It contains a network of blood vessels. The inner layer is composed of loose connective tissue that contains osteoblasts or osteoblast precursors (**Fig. 5-37**). In response to injury, new bone production will occur, the pattern of which has diagnostic implications.

Periosteal reactions can either be classified as continuous and interrupted or they can be identified according to their spatial orientation (**Figs. 5-38** to **5-46**). Not uncommonly, several different periosteal reactions can be identified in a single lesion.

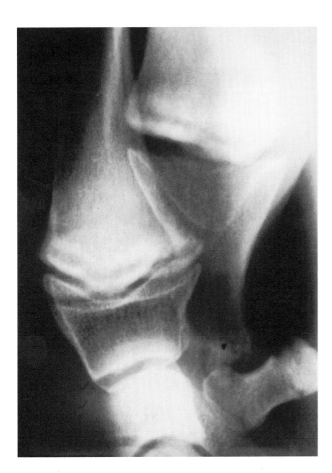

Fig. 5-36: A lateral projection of the distal radius and ulna of a dog with hypertrophic osteodystrophy. Note the alternating bands of radiolucency and radiodensity in the metaphysis immediately adjacent to the physis.

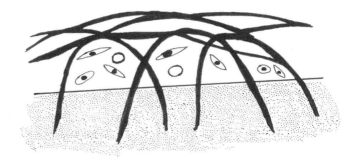

Fig. 5-37: An outline diagram of the histological structure of the periosteum. Note the outer fibrous layer and the inner cellular layer.

Lamellar periosteal reaction

A simple lamellar reaction occurs where the periosteum has been lifted from the surface of the cortex. New bone is produced which is seen radiographically as a linear radiodensity running parallel to the outer surface of the cortex (**Fig. 5-38** and **Fig. 5-47**). The radiolucent space can be occupied by inflammatory cells and exudate, hemorrhage, or occasionally neoplastic cells. Once the primary insult has been resolved, the radiolucent defect will be filled in with new bone, resulting in a solid periosteal reaction. Typically, this type of periosteal reaction is associated with a benign process.

Solid periosteal reaction

A solid periosteal reaction may be produced from a lamellar reaction as described above, or it may be produced by slow surface additions of new bone which become incorporated into the cortex. The characteristic feature of this type of reaction, which specifically indicates its benign nature, is its even, uniform, solid appearance, which is unchanged on sequential radiographs. Typical inciting causes include direct trauma, fracture repair, chronic osteomyelitis, and osteoid osteoma [39, 40] (**Fig. 5-39** and **Fig. 5-48**).

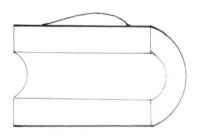

Fig. 5-38: An outline diagram of a lamellar periosteal reaction. Exudate, hemorrhage, or cellular tissue occupies the space between the periosteal new bone and the cortex.

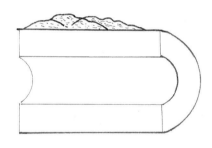

Fig. 5-41: An outline diagram of a solid cloaking periosteal reaction. This periosteal reaction is characterized by its uneven density and undulating margin.

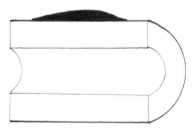

Fig. 5-39: An outline diagram of a solid periosteal reaction where a solid layer of new bone has been incorporated onto the cortical surface.

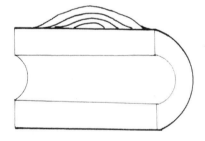

Fig. 5-42: An outline diagram of a lamellated periosteal reaction. It is recognized by concentric strata of new bone.

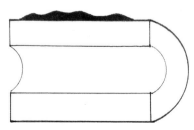

Fig. 5-40: An outline diagram of a dense undulating periosteal reaction.

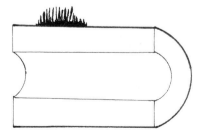

Fig. 5-43: An outline diagram of a perpendicular or "hair-on-end" periosteal reaction. This is produced by new bone being laid down midway between vessels running alongside Sharpey fibers.

Dense undulating periosteal reaction

A dense undulating periosteal reaction is commonly associated with venous stasis [39] (**Fig. 5-40**). Venous stasis results in a local lowering of oxygen tension, which induces osteoblastic activity [41].

Solid cloaking periosteal reaction

A solid cloaking periosteal reaction has been described in association with the glycogen storage diseases and chronic osteomyelitis [39]. This variation is characterized by an irregular density, analogous to the appearance of the folds of a cloak (**Fig. 5-41**).

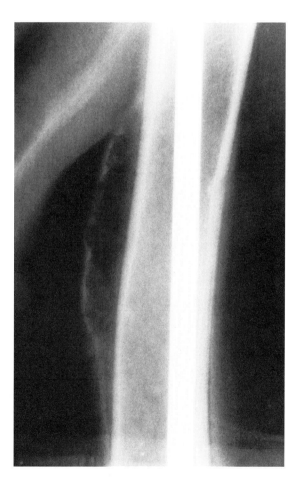

Fig. 5-47: A lateral projection of the femur of a dog that demonstrates a lamellar periosteal reaction due to elevation of the periosteum associated with a fracture. The fracture itself is not visible, but the intramedullary pin used in its repair can be identified.

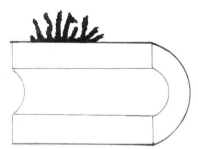

Fig. 5-44: An outline diagram of a sunburst periosteal reaction. It consists of a mixture of periosteal new bone that follows the distorted orientation of Sharpey fibers and tumor bone.

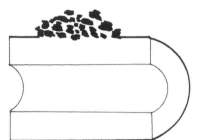

Fig. 5-45: An outline diagram of an amorphous periosteum where the periosteal new bone is frequently disorganized tumor bone. It is commonly associated with destruction of the adjacent cortex.

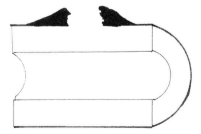

Fig. 5-46: An outline diagram of a Codman triangle. Periosteal new bone is being formed at the periphery of the lesion, resulting in the triangular-shaped collar. Centrally, periosteal new bone is being destroyed as fast as it can be formed.

Lamellated periosteal reactions

Lamellated or onion skin periosteal reactions occur where the pathological insult has a cyclical nature, such as in osteomyelitis, hypertrophic osteoarthropathy, or malignant neoplasms. Radiographically, it is identified by the presence of concentric strata of periosteal new bone (**Figs. 5-16**, **5-42**, and **5-49**). With time and resolution of the primary insult, the radiolucent layers will become less distinct.

In non-neoplastic lesions the lamellated appearance may, in fact, be the result of an active hyperemia which results in rapid cortical remodeling to increase the dimensions of cortical vascular canals [**42**].

The lamellated periosteal reaction has also been associated with periods of rapid growth in puppies [**43**]. The presence of a single periosteal lamella has been identified in normal children [**44, 45**]. Histologically, the lesions are identical in both species and are a manifestation of normal rapid growth [**43, 46**].

Perpendicular periosteal reactions

The interrupted periosteal reactions are also subdivided according to their radiographic characteristics. The perpendicular or "hair-on-end" pattern is characterized by new bone growing perpendicular to the surface of the parent bone (**Fig. 5-43**). Sections of the reaction made parallel to the bone

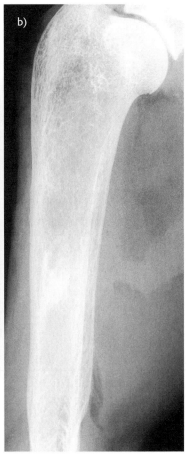

Fig. 5-48: A solid periosteal reaction on the femur of a dog (a) and the humerus of a man (b).

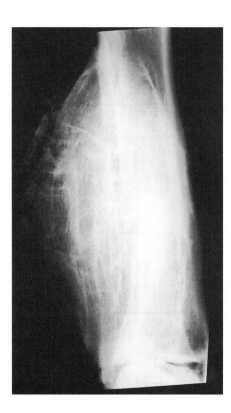

Fig. 5-49: A lateral projection of the metacarpus of a mature cow, demonstrating a lamellated periosteal reaction caused by chronic osteomyelitis.

surface demonstrate that it has, in fact, a honeycomb pattern. The "hairs" are due to the walls of the structure, lying parallel to the x-ray beam [42]. This configuration occurs because of the tendency of osteoblasts to become active midway between the vessels that lie alongside the radially oriented Sharpey fibers [42, 47]. Typically this reaction is associated with malignancy, classically Ewing Sarcoma. The new bone in this type of periosteal reaction is entirely of periosteal origin and not of tumor origin [9, 47].

Sunburst periosteal reaction

The new bone production of the sunburst [47] is of both periosteal and tumor origin (**Fig. 5-44** and **Fig. 5-50**). The periosteal new bone at the cortical surface becomes increasingly radiodense as mineralization progresses, and ultimately the sunburst appearance may disappear [42]. The presence of a sunburst periosteal reaction is highly suggestive of a diagnosis of osteosarcoma, but has been associated with other tumors, such as hemangioma [42]. Although this particular reaction is

well described in textbooks as the classical appearance of osteosarcoma, in clinical practice it is a relatively uncommon manifestation of this neoplasm.

Amorphous periosteal reaction

Although classified as a periosteal reaction, the amorphous form frequently represents tumor bone [39, 47]. These amorphous deposits, variable in both size and shape, usually denote malignancy (**Figs. 5-45**, **5-51**, and **5-52**).

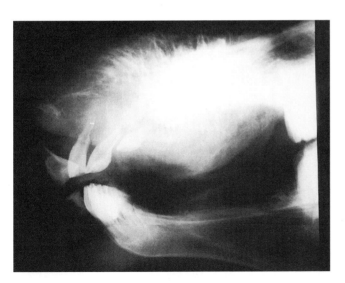

Fig. 5-50: A lateral projection of the maxilla of a foal, demonstrating a sunburst periosteal reaction caused by an osteosarcoma.

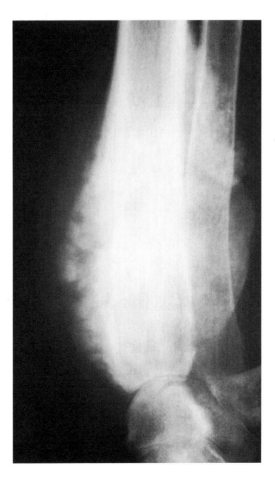

Fig. 5-51: A lateral projection of the distal radius of a dog with an osteosarcoma resulting in an amorphous periosteal reaction.

Codman triangle

The Codman triangle, or angle, is a radiographic feature that has acquired an air of mystique. It occurs when a pathological insult causes elevation of the periosteum. Centrally, destruction of periosteal new bone is occurring at a rate greater than osteogenic potential of the periosteum. At the periphery where the periosteum is simply lifted, mineralization will occur, forming a solid periosteal reaction (**Fig. 5-46**). Although this feature is associated with malignant neoplasms, it is also associated with benign and infectious processes (**Fig. 5-52**) [9, 42].

3.2.5 Cortical expansion

Cortical expansion is the term used to describe widening of the cortical outline. Unlike a balloon, the cortex cannot expand in response to internal pressure. Rather, it undergoes resorption from the endosteal surface with new bone being laid down on the periosteal surface. Localized thickening of the cortex may occur where the endosteal resorption is slower. Radiographically, these cortical ridges can give the false impression of trabeculation [42] within the lesion (**Fig. 5-53**).

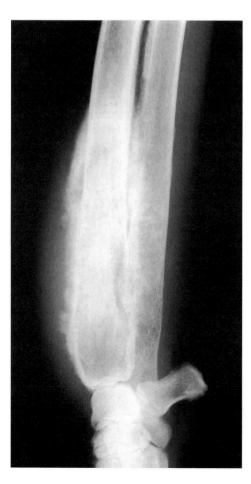

Fig. 5-52: A lateral projection of the distal radius of a dog. An osteosarcoma has resulted in an amorphous periosteal reaction distally. Proximally, a Codman triangle of solid periosteal new bone is present.

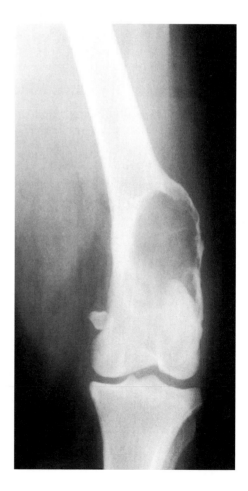

Fig. 5-53: A caudo-cranial projection of the distal femur of a dog demonstrating cortical expansion due to a fibrosarcoma.

4 Bibliography

Blue references indicate links to abstracts of articles available online:
http://www.aopublishing.org/BONE/5.htm

1. **Myer W** (1977) Radiographic review: Radiographic density. *J Am Vet Radiol Soc;* 18:138.
2. **Lavin M** (1993) Radiographic quality. *Radiography in Veterinary Technology.* 2nd ed. Philadelphia: WB Saunders Co., 43.
3. **Berbaum KS, el-Khoury GY, Franken EA, et al.** (1988) Impact of clinical history on fracture detection with radiography. *Radiology;* 168 (2): 507–511.
4. **Guibelalde E, Vano E, Llorca AL** (1990) Quality assurance of viewing boxes: proposal for establishing minimum requirements and results from a Spanish quality control programme. *Br J Radiol;* 63 (751):564–567.
5. **Keats TE, Smith TH** (1977) *An Atlas of Normal Developmental Roentgen Anatomy.* Chicago: Yearbook Medical Publishers.
6. **Schebitz H, Wilkens H** (1978) *Atlas of Radiographic Anatomy of the Horse.* 3rd ed. Toronto: WB Saunders Co.
7. **Keats TE** (1988) *Atlas of Normal Roentgen Variants That May Simulate Disease.* 4th ed. Chicago: Yearbook Medical Publishers.
8. **Goldschmidt MH, Thrall DE** (1985) Malignant bone tumors in the dog. In: Newton CD, Nunamaker DM, editors. *Textbook of Small Animal Orthopedics.* Philadelphia: JB Lippincott, 887.
9. **Greenfield GB** (1990) *Radiology of Bone Diseases.* 5th ed. Philadelphia: JB Lippincott.
10. **Jubb KVF, Kennedy PC, Palmer NC** (1985) *Pathology of Domestic Animals.* 4th ed. Toronto: Academic Press.

11. **Firth EC** (1983) Current concepts of infectious polyarthritis in foals. *Equine Vet J;* 15 (1):5–9.
12. **Rogers LF** (1993) Infections and inflammations of bones. In: Juhl PO, Crummy TB, editors. *Paul and Juhl's Essentials of Radiologic Imaging.* 6th ed. Philadelphia: J. B. Lippincott, 187.
13. **Jaffe HL** (1958) *Tumors and Tumorous Conditions of the Bones and Joints.* Philadelphia: Lea and Febiger.
14. **Madewell JE, Ragsdale BD, Sweet DE** (1981) Radiologic and pathologic analysis of solitary bone lesions. Part I: internal margins. *Radiol Clin North Am;* 19 (4):715–748.
15. **Handmaker H, Leonards R** (1976) The bone scan in inflammatory osseous disease. *Semin Nucl Med;* 6 (1):95–105.
16. **Sartoris DJ** (1989) Quantitative bone mineral analysis. In: Resnick D, editor. *Bone and Joint Imaging.* Toronto: WB Saunders Co., 202.
17. **Lodwick GS, Wilson AJ, Farrell C, et al.** (1980) Determining growth rates of focal lesions of bone from radiographs. *Radiology;* 134 (3):577–583.
18. **Resnick D** (1989) Tumours and tumour-like lesions of bone. In: Resnick D, editor. *Bone and Joint Imaging.* Toronto: WB Saunders Co., 1096.
19. **Miller WB, Murphy WA, Gilula LA** (1979) Brodie abscess: reappraisal. *Radiology;* 132 (1):15–23.
20. **Farrow CS** (1987) Primary benign bone tumour: Enchondroma. In: Farrow CS, editor. *Decision Making in Small Animal Radiology.* Toronto: BC Decker Inc., 38.
21. **Lodwick GS** (1964) Reactive response to local injury in bone. *Radiol Clin North Am;* 2:209.
22. **Helms CA, Munk PL** (1990) Pseudopermeative skeletal lesions. *Br J Radiol;* 63 (750):461–467.

23. **Morris JW** (1965) Skeletal fluorosis among Indians of the American Southwest. *Am J Roentgenol;* 94:608.
24. **Shupe JL, Olson AE** (1971) Clinical aspects of fluorosis in horses. *J Am Vet Med Assoc;* 158 (2):167–174.
25. **Sweet DE, Madewell JE, Ragsdale BD** (1981) Radiologic and pathologic analysis of solitary bone lesions. Part III: matrix patterns. *Radiol Clin North Am;* 19 (4):785–814.
26. **Gibson MJ, Middlemiss JH** (1971) Fibrous dysplasia of bone. *Br J Radiol;* 44 (517):1–13.
27. **Helms CA** (1994) Metabolic bone disease. In: Brant HC, Helms CA, editors. *Fundamentals of Diagnostic Radiology.* Baltimore: Williams & Wilkins, 958.
28. **Lenehan TM, VanSickle DC, Biery DN** (1985) Canine panosteitis. In: Newton CD, Nunamaker DM, editors. *Textbook of Small Animal Orthopedics.* Philadelphia: JB Lippincott, 591.
29. **Muir P, Dubielzig RR, Johnson KA** (1996) Panosteitis. *Comp Cont Educ Pract Vet;* 18:29.
30. **Bullough PG, Kambolis CP, Marcove RC, et al.** (1965) Bone infarctions not associated with caisson disease. *J Bone Joint Surg [Am];* 47:471.
31. **Riser WH, Brodey RS, Biery DN** (1972) Bone infarctions associated with malignant bone tumors in dogs. *J Am Vet Med Assoc;* 160 (4):414–421.
32. **Dubielzig RR, Biery DN, Brodey RS** (1981) Bone sarcomas associated with multifocal medullary bone infarction in dogs. *J Am Vet Med Assoc;* 179 (1):64–68.
33. **Follis RH, Park EA** (1952) Some observations on bone growth, with particular respect to zones and transverse lines of increased density in the metaphysis. *Am J Roentgenol;* 68:709.

34. **Woodard JC** (1982) Canine hypertrophic osteodystrophy, a study of the spontaneous disease in littermates. *Vet Pathol;* 19 (4):337–354.

35. **Muir P, Dubielzig RR, Johnson K** (1996) Hypertrophic osteodystrophy and calvarial hyperostosis. *Comp Cont Educ Pract Vet;* 18:143.

36. **Leone AJ** (1968) On lead lines. *Am J Roentgenol Radium Ther Nucl Med;* 103 (1):165–167.

37. **Harris HA** (1926) The growth of the long bones in childhood with special reference to certain bony striations of the metaphysis and to the role of vitamins. *Arch Intern Med;* 38:785.

38. **Ogden JA** (1984) Growth slowdown and arrest lines. *J Pediatr Orthop;* 4 (4):409–415.

39. **Edeiken J, Hodes PJ, Caplan LH** (1966) New bone production and periosteal reaction. *Am J Roentgenol Radium Ther Nucl Med;* 97 (3):708–718.

40. **Swee RG, McLeod RA, Beabout JW** (1979) Osteoid osteoma. Detection, diagnosis, and localization. *Radiology;* 130 (1):117–123.

41. **Bogumill GP, Schwam HA** (1984) *Orthopedic Pathology.* Toronto: WB Saunders Co.:161.

42. **Ragsdale BD, Madewell JE, Sweet DE** (1981) Radiologic and pathologic analysis of solitary bone lesions. Part II: periosteal reactions. *Radiol Clin North Am;* 19 (4):749–783.

43. **Volberg FM, Whalen JP, Krook L, et al.** (1977) Lamellated periosteal reactions: a radiologic and histologic investigation. *Am J Roentgenol;* 128 (1):85–87.

44. **Hancox NM, Hay JD, Holden WS, et al.** (1951) The radiologic "double contour" effect in the long bones of children. *Arch Dis Child;* 26:543.

45. **Shopfner CE** (1966) Periosteal bone growth in normal infants. A preliminary report. *Am J Roentgenol Radium Ther Nucl Med;* 97 (1):154–163.

46. **Hedhammar A, Wu FM, Krook L, et al.** (1974) Overnutrition and skeletal disease. An experimental study in growing Great Dane dogs. *Cornell Vet;* 64 (2):Suppl 5:5–160.

47. **Brunschwig A, Harmon PH** (1935) Studies in bone sarcoma. Part III: An experimental and pathological study of the role of the periosteum in the formation of bone in various primary bone tumors. *Surg Gynecol Obstet;* 60:30.

6 Bone infection

Joanne R. Cockshutt

1 Introduction

Osteomyelitis is defined as inflammation of cortical bone and the medullary cavity, including such soft-tissue elements as marrow, endosteum, periosteum, and the vascular channels of the bone. It occurs in both animals and humans, and the disease in the different species has many similarities. Despite advances in medical and surgical treatment, osteomyelitis can still be refractory to therapy and remains a serious clinical problem for physicians and veterinarians.

The disease appears in a variety of forms and has been variously classified by etiology, duration, and method of infection. This has resulted in confusing use of overlapping terms such as acute, chronic, hematogenous, posttraumatic, and postoperative in an attempt to describe the type of infection. Infection can reach the bone either directly or by hematogenous routes, and can be either acute or chronic in nature. Chronic osteomyelitis is frequently the result of inadequate treatment of acute osteomyelitis.

2 Route of infection

The lines of distinction between the routes of infection are often blurred, since micro-organisms can reach fractures via the blood stream and local soft-tissue infections can develop around, and then extend into, a surgically repaired fracture. However, the following are clinically recognized patterns of bone infection.

2.1 Hematogenous

The infective agent reaches the bone during a temporary bacteremia arising from a septic focus elsewhere in the body. Acute hematogenous bacterial osteomyelitis (AHOM) is a common and serious disease of prepuberal children and elderly humans [1, 2]. It is also common in foals and neonatal ruminants, but is rare in "companion animals", representing only about 6% of cases in dogs and cats [3, 4]. Vertebral osteomyelitis is a form of hematogenous osteomyelitis that is usually found in elderly human patients, but also occurs in children and animals [1, 5]. The infection may involve the intervertebral disk, vertebral bodies, or both (**Fig. 6-1**).

2.2 Local trauma

Posttraumatic or postoperative osteomyelitis occurs when a traumatic or surgical wound allows direct contamination of bone by exogenous organisms (**Fig. 6-2**). Typical traumatic injuries include open fractures and bite wounds. Osteomyelitis may also complicate open surgical repair of fractures and implantation of orthopedic prostheses: a leading cause of osteomyelitis in small animals and a major cause of morbidity in human and equine patients [2, 4, 6, 7].

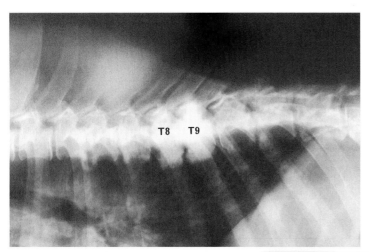

Fig. 6-1: Lateral spinal radiograph of a 2-year-old Rottweiler with discospondylitis. There is extensive new bone production involving the ventral borders of the eighth and ninth thoracic vertebrae. Also note the marked lysis, resulting in loss of the endplates of these vertebrae.

2.3 Extension

Infection can extend directly from an adjacent soft-tissue infection. Important causes [1] in both humans and animals are dental and sinus infections, and foot infections following a puncture wound (Fig. 6-3). In cattle and sheep [8], contiguous spread of infection to foot bones and joints commonly causes clinically and economically significant disease (Fig. 6-4). Osteomyelitis involving the foot is also a frequent development in people with diabetes and vascular insufficiency [1, 2].

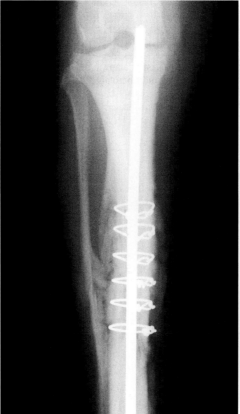
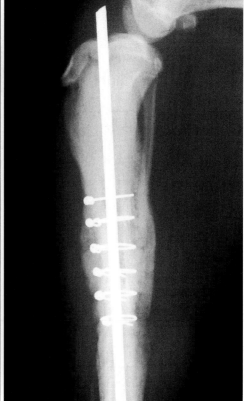

Fig. 6-2: Bacterial osteomyelitis of the tibia in an 8-month-old golden retriever 3 weeks after fracture repair. There is patchy periosteal new bone proliferation with areas of radiolucency.

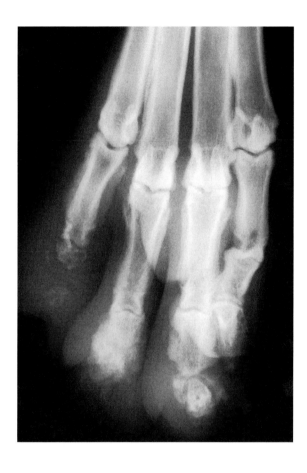

Fig. 6-3: Cellulitis and osteomyelitis involving the third, fourth, and fifth digits in a 4-year-old Labrador retriever. There is destruction of the third phalanx in each digit and periosteal new bone production involving the first and second phalanges.

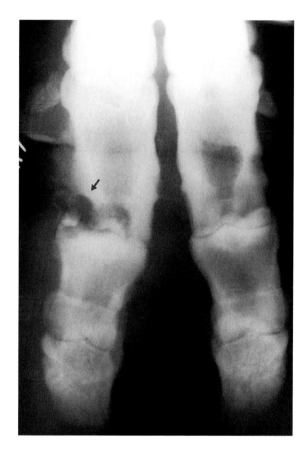

Fig. 6-4: Cellulitis and focal osteomyelitis of the 1st phalanx in a 3-year-old Charolais bull. There is severe bony lysis of P1 *(arrow)*. Lysis is also present in P2, and there is periosteal reaction involving both of these bones. (Courtesy of Donald Trout.)

3   Infecting organisms

Most cases of osteomyelitis involve bacterial agents, although other organisms and factors can contribute to the development of the disease. Infecting agents differ according to the age and species of the patient. Both monomicrobial and polymicrobial bacterial infections occur, and both aerobic and anaerobic bacteria may be isolated. Fungal osteomyelitis is common in cattle, but less so in other species [3]. Parasites and viruses rarely cause osteomyelitis. The condition may also result from corrosion of metallic surgical implants, or be promoted by other surgical materials that cause chronic tissue inflammation [5].

3.1   Human patients

Staphylococcus aureus is the most important cause of osteomyelitis in people of all ages [1, 2, 9, 10]. Less often, group A streptococci and *Haemophilus influenza* can cause acute hematogenous osteomyelitis in children [9]. Enteric Gram-negative bacilli, *Pseudomonas aeruginosa*, coagulase negative staphylococci and pneumococci are other common isolates. *Pasteurella multocida* infections may follow cat bites [1]. In vertebral infections, *Staphylococcus aureus* is the most frequent pathogen isolated, but the urinary tract is a common source of infection with Gram-negative enteric organisms [1]. Tuberculosis was formerly an important cause of vertebral osteomyelitis, but the incidence of the disease has decreased markedly in this century. This is attributable to the widespread practice of milk pasteurization, improved standards of living, and the development of effective antimicrobial agents. There has, however, been a resurgence of tuberculosis cases associated with HIV infections, and resistant tuberculosis strains have appeared.

Infections are polymicrobial in 35–50% of human cases [1, 2]. Anaerobic infections are common and are often associated with human bite wounds or osteomyelitis occurring after implantation of an orthopedic prosthesis. Anaerobic infections should also be suspected in osteomyelitis arising from dental, otolaryngeal, or intra-abdominal infections, decubitus or foot puncture wounds, or in any chronic mixed infection [1].

3.2 Veterinary patients

In dogs and cats, approximately 50% of infections are monomicrobial. As in humans, *Staphylococcus aureus* is the most commonly isolated aerobic bacteria, being present in almost half of pure infections [4, 5]. Other *Staphylococcus* spp, *E. coli*, beta hemolytic streptococci, *Proteus, Klebsiella,* and *Pseudomonas* spp are common aerobic agents. Polymicrobial infection with the above agents often occurs. Anaerobic bacteria are important causes of osteomyelitis, either alone or in combination with other bacteria, particularly when bite wounds are involved. Various anaerobes, including species of *Bacteriodes, Actinomyces, Clostridium, Peptostreptococcus,* and *Fusobacterium,* have been identified in at least 20% of infections and are likely present in the majority of bone infections in small animals [7, 11, 12].

Acute hematogenous osteomyelitis of foals and calves is usually polymicrobial and caused by Gram-negative enteric bacteria [6, 13, 14]. *E. coli, Salmonella* spp, *Klebsiella* spp, *Actinobacillus* spp and *Streptococcus* spp are frequent etiologies in neonatal foals, calves, and sheep. Infections in older foals may be caused by *Salmonella* spp or *Rhodococcus equi* [6, 13]. Gram-negative aerobic bacteria, singly or in combination, are regularly isolated in equine posttraumatic osteomyelitis, along with *Enterobacter, Streptococcus* and *Staphylococcus* spp and

Pseudomonas aeruginosa [3, 6, 14]. In cattle, *Actinomyces pyogenes* is the most common cause of digital osteomyelitis, while *Actinomyces bovis* is associated with infections of the jaw in this species [3, 13, 15].

Anaerobic organisms are also being recognized more frequently in large animal patients, as increased effort is being made to isolate them.

4 Pathology

AHOM occurs in immature individuals following either a systemic infection or a local infection such as omphalophlebitis, enteritis, or pneumonia. Bacteria spread hematogenously, typically to the metaphyseal or epiphyseal region of the long bones (Fig. 6-5). It is thought that the vascular architecture of the terminal branches of the metaphyseal arteries contributes to the preferential lodging of bacteria in the metaphyseal or epiphyseal areas, or in the vertebral endplates [4, 6, 16]. Small capillaries form tight loops as they empty into larger venous sinusoids. The resulting sluggish and turbulent blood flow may encourage local bacterial seeding. Additionally, the capillary endothelium is incomplete here, allowing extravasation of bacteria. A relative local paucity of phagocytic cells may also contribute to the establishment of infection [17]. Bacterial embolization results in venous stasis and retrograde progression of thrombosis. Local marrow necrosis produces a medium conducive to further growth of bacteria. In neonatal foals and ruminants, and in children under 1 year of age, vessels traverse the growth plate and enter the epiphysis. As a result, metaphyseal and physeal infections can spread to the joint [17]. Immature carnivores do not have well-developed transphyseal vessels, and septic arthritis rarely occurs in these species [4]. Septic arthritis is less common in growing children, since the growth plate forms a barrier to direct spread of infection from the metaphysis.

Bacteria can also reach bone from an external source, or by extension from an adjacent soft-tissue infection. However, healthy bone is very resistant to infection, and bacteria alone will not necessarily cause osteomyelitis. Other factors, such as vascular stasis, soft-tissue injury, an unstable fracture, or the presence of foreign material are important in the pathogenesis. Many of these contributing factors are present in surgical and trauma patients. Damaged soft tissue and necrotic bone are ideal media for bacterial growth. Ultimately, vascular obstruction is necessary for the development of osteomyelitis; this readily occurs as inflammatory exudate accumulates within the marrow cavity and vascular channels of the bone. The resulting increase in intramedullary pressure causes vascular thrombosis, bone necrosis, and abscess formation. Inflammatory byproducts, including cytokines, toxic O_2 radicals and prostaglandins contribute to tissue damage and vascular obstruction. Prostaglandins also promote osteoclastic activity, which increases cortical porosity and aids the spread of purulent exudate. Pus is forced into Volkmann and haversian canals and into endosteal and subperiosteal spaces, thus spreading the infection and further compromising cortical blood supply. In time, a segment of cortical bone can become isolated from its blood supply by this process; this avascular bone is called a sequestrum. Sequestra harbor bacteria and slow the healing process. Surrounded by purulent exudate, sequestra are protected from osteoclastic resorption and eventually become enveloped by granulation and fibrous tissue, and then by periosteal new bone. This shell of vascular new bone, surrounding the sequestrum, is known as an involucrum and can be apparent on radiographs as an indication of chronic osteomyelitis. Openings in the involucrum (cloacae) allow inflammatory exudate to exit through fistulous tracts to the skin: a classic sign of osteomyelitis.

External trauma also compromises the blood supply to bone and contributes to inflammation. If a fracture is present, the development of osteomyelitis is potentiated, particularly if the fracture repair is unstable. Instability, caused by inappropriate repair technique or by implant failure, allows ongoing interfragmentary motion, which impairs revascularization and promotes bone necrosis [5]. In a vicious cycle, osteomyelitis promotes bone necrosis and resorption of cortical bone at the fracture site, thus worsening the instability. This process must be interrupted if treatment of postoperative osteomyelitis is to be successful.

Other factors potentiate the development of osteomyelitis. Bacterial colonization is assisted by the presence of foreign materials such as metal plates and suture material. As well, certain pathogenic bacteria, particularly *S. aureus,* develop surface receptors (adhesins) for bone matrix, which aid bacterial adherence [2]. Bacterial persistence is also aided by the production of a mucoid polysaccharide biofilm (glycocalyx or "bioslime"). Glycocalyx binds bacteria to bone and metallic implants and protects them from host defenses such as phagocytes and antibodies [6, 7]. It also reduces the effectiveness of many antimicrobial drugs. Bacteria proliferating within glycocalyx express phenotypically enhanced growth, virulence, and resistance to antimicrobial treatment [2, 5, 16]. In addition to aiding bacterial survival, glycocalyx limits exfoliation of bacteria, thus interfering with diagnostic isolation efforts.

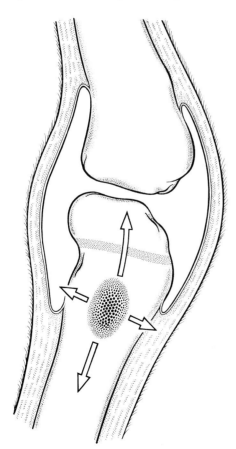

Fig. 6-5: Spread of infection in hematogenous osteomyelitis. Infection in the venous sinusoids of the metaphysis spreads to the periosteum sometimes with epiphysis and joint capsule involvement (drawn by Mr John Fuller).

5 Diagnosis

5.1 History and physical findings

The patient history and clinical signs are often sufficient to make a tentative diagnosis of osteomyelitis. There may be a history of trauma, fracture repair, or soft-tissue infection. A neonatal patient may have had an umbilical infection or systemic illness. The patient may have resided in, or traveled to, an area where pathogenic fungi are endemic.

Clinical signs of osteomyelitis are variable and depend upon the stage of the disease. In acute osteomyelitis, classic signs of inflammation (pain, heat, and swelling) develop in the affected area within 5–7 days of bone contamination and cause lameness. There is often evidence of systemic illness, including pyrexia and anorexia. In the postoperative patient, these findings help to distinguish between infection and inflammation secondary to surgical trauma.

Patients with chronic osteomyelitis usually have some degree of lameness associated with pain at the site of infection. There may be muscle atrophy or fibrosis depending upon the duration of the infection. A classic sign of chronic osteomyelitis is that of transcutaneous drainage from the infected region, and this is often the presenting complaint. If there is an underlying fracture or bone non-union, crepitation or bony malalignment may be detected. Systemic signs are not consistently present in chronic disease, although repeated and temporary episodes of anorexia and pyrexia will often occur. These signs probably coincide with episodes of septicemia occurring as exudate builds up within the bone [16]. Otherwise, although the inflammatory process can impinge on other structures, the clinical signs usually remain localized. Patients with discospondylitis may show neurological deficits caused by nerve or spinal cord compression. Such neurological disruptions may be the direct result of bony expansion, or be caused by pathological fracture of a vertebra.

5.2 Diagnostic imaging

Radiographic assessment of suspected osteomyelitis patients begins with survey radiographs. Soft-tissue swelling, the first sign of acute osteomyelitis, may be apparent within 48 hours of the appearance of signs in acute cases. However, bony changes will not be seen for 1 or 2 weeks, since conventional radiographs will not detect bone loss until at least 30% of bone matrix is destroyed [6, 18]. Areas of local bone resorption or lysine, with variable amounts of bone production, are seen in acute osteomyelitis, and are often more pronounced in young patients (**Fig. 6-6**). Occasionally, gas is visible in soft tissues or within the bone; while infrequent, this is a reliable sign of osteomyelitis. If there is a concurrent fracture, the radiographic changes associated with fracture repair and healing will make early diagnosis of osteomyelitis more difficult. However, areas of lucency around implants are strongly suggestive of infection, as are signs of fracture instability and implant loosening (**Fig. 6-7**).

The radiographic signs of chronic osteomyelitis include new bone production, lysis, and remodeling. Sequestra may be visible as radiodense fragments surrounded by a radiolucent area bordered by sclerotic bone. It generally takes several weeks or months for a sequestrum to become apparent on radiographs, but this is a virtually pathognomonic finding in chronic osteomyelitis.

Contrast radiographic techniques are sometimes helpful [7]. Fistulography can be used to outline transcutaneous fistulas, and to confirm their origin in the suspected bone lesion. Occasionally a fistulogram will outline a radiolucent foreign body. Unfortunately, fistulas may not fill completely with the contrast material, and false negative results are common.

While conventional radiography is appropriate for the initial evaluation, several other diagnostic imaging methods are used routinely in human patients. Cost and availability frequently excludes their use in animals. Ultrasound may be useful for detecting joint effusion or pockets of purulent exudate in AHOM but cannot distinguish between infected and non-infected fluid [9, 10]. Radionuclide bone imaging (scintigraphy) is highly sensitive for the early detection of acute osteomyelitis [2, 4, 19]. Bone-seeking radiopharmaceuticals (tracers) are given intravenously and gradually accumulate in bone, concentrating in areas of increased bone metabolic activity. Technetium 99m (^{99m}Tc) is the most widely used radioisotope; other scintigraphy techniques use gallium-67 or indium-111 labeled white blood cells [2, 6, 9]. Magnetic resonance imaging (MRI) and computed tomography (CT) are high-resolution techniques that reveal soft-tissue involvement [20], edema, and articular damage, as well as periosteal reaction and cortical destruction (**Fig. 6-8** and **Fig. 6-9**). Both techniques can detect osteomyelitis before scintigraphy or conventional radiography reveals positive findings. MRI is superior to CT for evaluating the extent of the infection, and can be used to plan surgical therapy by outlining fistulous tracts and abscesses [21].

CT, while less sensitive for evaluating soft tissues, is superior to MRI for detecting sequestra and cortical bone destruction [18, 21].

5.3 Laboratory evaluation

Hematological abnormalities in patients with acute osteomyelitis usually include a polymorphonuclear leukocytosis. The neutrophilia is usually more pronounced in younger patients; adult horses with osteomyelitis, for example, may have only a mildly elevated white blood count [6]. Hematology results are usually normal in patients with chronic infections.

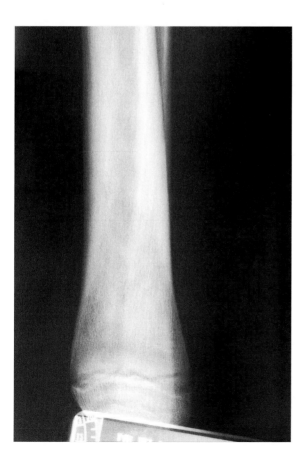

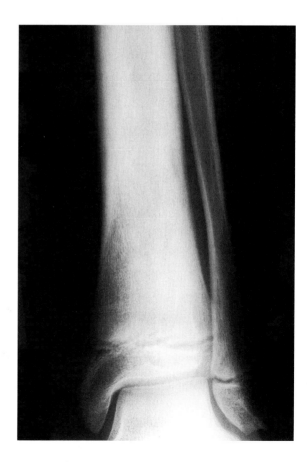

Fig. 6-6: Osteomyelitis in the tibia of a 13-year-old human patient. Areas of lucency in the metaphyseal region are typical of acute hematogenous osteomyelitis. (Courtesy of Lawrence Friedman.)

Cytological evaluation can aid early detection of acute osteomyelitis before radiographic changes are apparent. Inflammatory exudate, aspirated from the site by needle centesis, may contain toxic leukocytes and bacteria. Sterile deep-needle aspiration is also used to obtain samples for bacterial culture and antimicrobial susceptibility testing. Identification of the causative organism is helpful in confirming the diagnosis and essential to the selection of appropriate antimicrobial chemotherapy. In order to enhance the accuracy of culture results, antibiotic treatment should be discontinued for at least 24 hours prior to sample collection in acute cases, and up to 3 days in chronic infections. Samples should be cultured for both aerobic and anaerobic bacteria, with additional samples collected for immediate Gram staining. Samples for culture should not be obtained from transcutaneous sinuses. Skin bacteria often colonize fistulas, while the causative organism may be sequestered within glycocalyx. Sinus cultures are usually polymicrobial, and reflect the true pathogen in less than 50% of patients [7].

Where appropriate, tissues may be cultured, or biopsied, at the time of surgical wound débridement, and this may well provide the most accurate information. It remains the only precise method for distinguishing between infection and neoplasia, and special staining techniques can also identify

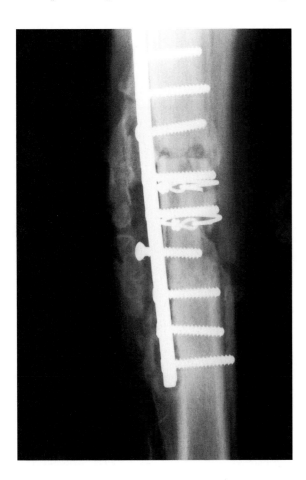

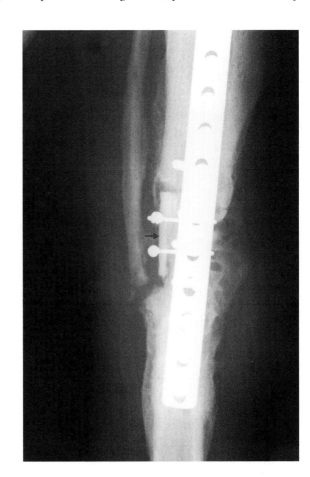

Fig. 6-7: Osteomyelitis of the tibia 8 weeks after fracture repair in a 2-year-old Doberman pinscher. There is considerable new bone production on all aspects of the tibia, and loosening of a plate screw. An isolated cortical bone segment (sequestrum) is present (*arrow*).

fungal elements. Also, when fungal infection is suspected, fungal cultures or titers may help to confirm the etiology.

Blood culture should be performed when systemic infection is suspected. In human patients with AHOM, about 50% of blood cultures are positive for Gram-positive organisms [9]. Since acute osteomyelitis is often associated with septic arthritis in the neonate, synovial fluid samples may be helpful in identifying the etiological agent.

In cases of suspected discospondylitis, blood and urine cultures should be taken. Positive cultures have been reported in 75% of blood samples and 25% of urine samples from affected dogs [4, 5].

6 Treatment

Treatment is aimed at eliminating the infection and usually requires a combination of medical and surgical therapy. Acute hematogenous osteomyelitis, and selected cases of postoperative osteomyelitis, may respond to conservative management with antimicrobial chemotherapy. In contrast, chronic infections rarely resolve without surgery.

In order to avoid the development of chronic osteomyelitis, early, aggressive treatment of acute osteomyelitis is essential. An empirically chosen antimicrobial is used initially, until the culture and antibiotic sensitivity tests are available. Intravenous

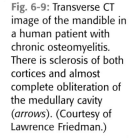

Fig. 6-8: Frontal MRI of a human patient with discitis. There is collapse of the intervertebral disk space and increased signal intensity in the vertebral endplate, which has undergone partial destruction (*arrow*). (Courtesy of Lawrence Friedman.)

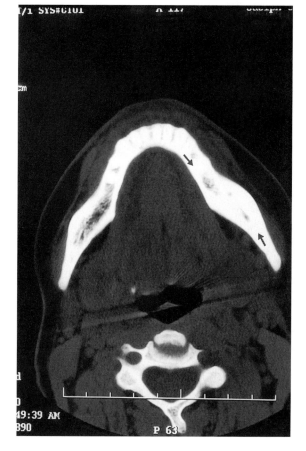

Fig. 6-9: Transverse CT image of the mandible in a human patient with chronic osteomyelitis. There is sclerosis of both cortices and almost complete obliteration of the medullary cavity (*arrows*). (Courtesy of Lawrence Friedman.)

administration of a broad-spectrum agent is recommended. Appropriate antibiotic treatment should then be continued for 1–3 months, depending upon the causative organism and the clinical response [1, 5, 14]. The choice of antibiotic should be based on minimizing toxicity and cost, while obtaining maximum specificity against the infecting agent. Some patients with acute infection require surgical drainage of the lesion. Subperiosteal abscesses should be debrided surgically and drained [9]. Surgical decompression of abscesses within the bone can be achieved by creating a window through the cortex into the medullary cavity.

Chronic osteomyelitis is a surgical disease, with complimentary antimicrobial treatment as an integral part of the therapy. Surgery consists of removal of all dead bone, sequestra, and devitalized soft tissue (saucerization), and drainage of abscesses. Débridement must be aggressive and continued until bleeding cortical bone is encountered. Chronic draining sinuses need not be excised entirely, but should be probed to ensure that all sequestra are found and removed. All foreign material should be removed, and tissue dead space eliminated. Postoperative drainage may be achieved by implanting irrigation-suction drainage systems, or by leaving the wound open. The latter technique is preferred by some surgeons since many drainage systems are inefficient and may promote ascending infections [5, 14, 16].

If saucerization results in large bone deficits, bone grafting is recommended [2, 5–7, 16]. Cancellous grafts fill the space left by débridement and promote revascularization. If heavy exudation is anticipated, a two-stage surgical approach is advised: débridement followed by autogenous cancellous bone grafting once the infection has been eliminated. Vascularized bone grafting is an alternative means of filling bone defects, as is the Ilizarov bone transport technique (see **Chapter 10**). Techniques that promote revascularization are the best method for preventing recurrent osteomyelitis. Local pedicle muscle flaps, free muscle flaps, and myocutaneous flaps are commonly used to cover bone and fill soft-tissue defects in people and wounds in animals that fail to close by second intention healing [7].

Appropriate antibiotic treatment is instituted following débridement, and continued for at least 4–6 weeks [2, 5, 7]. Antibiotics are usually given orally, but the use of either methylmethacrylate or biodegradable polymers to deliver gentamycin or other antibiotic to the infected area has become popular in both human and veterinary surgery [22, 23]. Chains of antimicrobial-impregnated acrylic beads are implanted in the surgical field and slowly elute antibiotic. The advantage of this technique is that high local antibiotic levels are achieved while at the same time maintaining low plasma concentrations and minimizing side effects [2, 6, 14, 23].

In cases of postoperative osteomyelitis, the surgical treatment goals must include the provision of fracture stability. A fracture will heal, albeit slowly, in the presence of infection, provided that adequate stabilization is achieved. Implants can be left in place if they, and the fracture, are stable. Otherwise, they should be removed immediately and replaced with a more stable fixation system. Successful fracture stabilization is the key to successful treatment of postoperative osteomyelitis; the specific fixation device chosen is of secondary importance. In both human and veterinary orthopedics, the favored stabilization methods in such cases are bone plating and external skeletal fixation (ESF). ESF has the advantage of providing good fracture stabilization while minimizing additional soft-tissue injury. Bone plates and screws may be preferred if there has not been extensive bone loss and soft tissues are healthy. Ultimately, to promote complete resolution of infection once the fracture has healed, all surgical implants that might harbor microorganisms should be removed [5, 14].

Amputation and joint arthrodesis are considered salvage procedures in most species. They are generally reserved for patients with unresponsive disease or non-reversible joint, nerve, or muscle dysfunction. However, they are common treatments for cattle and small animal patients with advanced digital infections [8, 15, 16]. Amputation may also be a consideration for a patient with extensive disease or severe underlying medical problems such as diabetes [1, 10].

7 Prevention

It is unlikely that preventive measures can reduce the post-surgical rate of infection to below 0.5% [2]. Most cases of postsurgical osteomyelitis are the result of errors in surgical and aseptic technique during fracture repair. Inadequate patient preparation, breaks in asepsis during surgery, and prolonged surgical times can all contribute to the development of infection. Adherence to Halsted's principles of surgery will minimize vascular injury and trauma to bone and soft tissues, and reduce susceptibility to invasion by micro-organisms. Perioperative administration of antibiotics is used in fracture repair surgery in order to provide inhibitory plasma levels from the time of the operation to 24 hours postoperatively [2, 14]. Complex fractures with extensive soft-tissue damage may require more prolonged treatment with antibiotics selected on the basis of known hospital pathogens.

8 Bibliography

Blue references indicate links to abstracts of articles available online:
http://www.aopublishing.org/BONE/6.htm

1. **Bamberger DM** (1993) Osteo-myelitis. A commonsense approach to antibiotic and surgical treatment. *Postgrad Med;* 94 (5):177–182, 184.

2. **Lew DP, Waldvogel FA** (1997) Osteomyelitis. *N Engl J Med;* 336 (14): 999–1007.

3. **Hogan PA, Honnas CM** (1996) Osteomyelitis. In: Smith BP, editor. *Large Animal Internal Medicine.* 2nd ed. St. Louis: Mosby Year Book, 1287.

4. **Radasch RM** (1993) Osteomyelitis. In: Harari J, editor. *Surgical Complications and Wound Healing in the Small Animal Practice.* Philadelphia: WB Saunders, 223.

5. **Johnson KA** (1995) Osteomyelitis. In: Olmstead ML, editor. *Small Animal Orthopedics.* St. Louis: Mosby Year Book, 261.

6. **Baxter GM** (1996) Instrumentation and techniques for treating orthopedic infections in horses. *Vet Clin North Am Equine Pract;* 12 (2):303–335.

7. **Fossum TW, Hulse DA** (1992) Osteomyelitis. *Semin Vet Med Surg (Small Anim);* 7 (1):85–97.

8. **Desrochers A, St Jean G** (1996) Surgical management of digit disorders in cattle. *Vet Clin North Am Food Anim Pract;* 12 (1):277–298.

9. **Dhar S** (1996) Septic arthritis and osteomyelitis in children. *Surgery;* 14:236.

10. **Nade S** (1997) Acute and chronic osteomyelitis. *Surgery;* 15:248.

11. **Johnson KA** (1994) Osteomyelitis in dogs and cats. *J Am Vet Med Assoc;* 204 (12):1882–1887.

12. **Muir P, Johnson KA** (1992) Anaerobic bacteria isolated from osteomyelitis in dogs and cats. *Vet Surg;* 21 (6):463–466.

13. **Trent AM, Plumb D** (1991) Treatment of infectious arthritis and osteomyelitis. *Vet Clin North Am Food Anim Pract;* 7 (3):747–778.

14. **Trotter GW** (1996) Osteomyelitis. In: Nixon AJ, editor. *Equine Fracture Repair.* Philadelphia: WB Saunders, 359.

15. **Trostle SS, Hendrickson DA, Stone WC, et al.** (1996) Use of antimicrobial-impregnated polymethyl methacrylate beads for treatment of chronic, refractory septic arthritis and osteomyelitis of the digit in a bull. *J Am Vet Med Assoc;* 208 (3): 404–407.

16. **Smith MM** (1993) Orthopedic infections. In: Slatter D, editor. *Textbook of Small Animal Surgery.* 2nd ed. Philadelphia: WB Saunders, 1685.

17. **Firth EC** (1992) Specific orthopedic infections. In: Auer JA, editor. *Equine Surgery.* Philadelphia: WB Saunders, 932.

18. **Jaramillo D, Treves ST, Kasser JR, et al.** (1995) Osteomyelitis and septic arthritis in children: appropriate use of imaging to guide treatment. *AJR Am J Roentgenol;* 165 (2):399–403.

19. **Ali SA, Cesani F, Nusynowitz ML, et al.** (1997) Skeletal scintigraphy with technetium-99m-tetraphenyl porphyrin sulfonate for the detection and determination of osteomyelitis in an animal model. *J Nucl Med;* 38 (12): 1999–2002.

20. **Erdman WA, Tamburro F, Jayson HT, et al.** (1991) Osteomyelitis: characteristics and pitfalls of diagnosis with MR imaging. *Radiology;* 180 (2): 533–539.

21. **Gold RH, Hawkins RA, Katz RD** (1991) Bacterial osteomyelitis: findings on plain radiography, CT, MR, and scintigraphy. *AJR Am J Roentgenol;* 157 (2):365–370.

22. **Calhoun JH, Mader JT** (1997) Treatment of osteomyelitis with a biodegradable antibiotic implant. *Clin Orthop;* (341):206–214.

23. **Evans RP, Nelson CL** (1993) Gentamicin-impregnated polymethylmethacrylate beads compared with systemic antibiotic therapy in the treatment of chronic osteo-myelitis. *Clin Orthop;* (295):37–42.

7 The adaptation of bone architecture to mechanical function

Matthew J. Pead & Lance E. Lanyon

1 Introduction

The art of orthopedics is primarily directed toward establishing or re-establishing optimal mechanical function within the musculoskeletal system. Knowledge of the dynamic relationship, which normally exists between structure and function in bone, is obviously of primary importance if this goal is consistently to be achieved.

The rigid form and apparent permanence of the skeleton, both during life and after death, often gives the impression of an inert structure better associated with buildings or bridges. This may be because, in common with tendon and ligament, the bone's cellular population contributes little if anything to the tissue's immediate mechanical performance. Bone can be removed from the body and be mechanically tested in similar ways to inanimate materials. However, it only takes superficial study to reveal that the impression of bone as an inert tissue is wrong. Bone is not only constantly renewing and adapting its structure, it is also metabolically important and actively contributes to the mineral homeostasis of the body. Indeed the metabolic function of bone has been studied in such depth that in much of the literature the skeleton's primarily supportive role is either forgotten or not recognized.

Unlike muscle, whose mechanical performance derives from the muscle cells, bone is the recipient of mechanical activity rather than the instigator. Loads are applied to bones either via their joint surfaces or through their fibrous insertions. The application of these loads deforms the parts of the skeleton just as the passing of every vehicle deforms the parts of a bridge. Only a totally incompetent engineer would build a bridge that collapsed under the load of its first vehicle. However, it takes more sophisticated design to ensure that no part of the structure is loaded to the extent where even the continual passing of vehicles will cause no damage. If the design is defective, then some parts of the structure may be repeatedly deformed to a degree that causes their failure. Although each individual deformation may not be large enough to cause damage, many such deformations will be above the finite "endurance" limit at which they can be repeated indefinitely without damage. Failure occurs in this situation because of accumulation and progression of the minor defects caused by each loading event. In such a situation the working life of the part concerned will depend upon the number of loading cycles imposed, and the amount of deformation that each one involves. An inanimate structure therefore relies for its longevity on a suitable design, and a sufficiently massive structure, to ensure that no part is repeatedly loaded in a way which allows minor damage to accumulate. Once built, such a structure can adjust neither its mass nor its shape to accommodate changes in load-bearing responsibilities. The best that can be expected is that, through regular maintenance activity, aging parts in which damage accumulates can be replaced.

The properties of bone material, and the construction of each whole bone, are almost certainly genetically programmed. If the bones of the skeleton relied for their shape, size, and structure on a design based solely on predetermined genetic information, then they would be in the same situation as the bridge. This is fortunately not the case as bones also have a capacity to adjust their mass, their internal organization, and in some circumstances their shape, according to the uses to which they are being put and before such use can inflict any damage. This appropriate match between structure and function is achieved by the cellular population of bone adapting, reinforcing, remodeling, and, if necessary, realigning the elements of the skeleton in response to various changes in their mechanical circumstances. The result of this adaptive capability is that structure may be matched to function without wasteful use of materials or potentially disastrous periods of incapacity for repair. Thus, although the bone's cells do not contribute to the immediate mechanical performance of the existing structure, it is only by their active agency that the mechanical competence of the structure is achieved and maintained.

How this adaptive response is controlled is still a matter for speculation and investigation. An attractive hypothesis is that the intermittent mechanical deformation (functional deformation), which results from musculoskeletal activity loading a bone (functional loading), is the stimulus, or engenders the stimulus, to which the cells responsible for controlling the adaptive process are sensitive. This would make good sense since the deformation or strain within the structure is the product of the applied load and the structure's shape, mass, and material properties. If load-induced strain does provide the controlling stimulus for adaptive change, then the repeated deformations to which bones are continually subjected are not entirely the destructive influences that they could be in an inanimate structure. Instead, they are a necessary functional input to the adaptive process responsible for the achievement and maintenance of the skeleton's structural competence.

The presence of an adaptive response sensitive to mechanical function is of particular importance in orthopedics since clinicians rely on the response to achieve their results. An empirical knowledge of the physiological changes that occur under various sets of mechanical circumstances is the basis of experience on which clinical judgements are made. Unfortunately, despite the importance of this structure/function relationship, it is not an easy one to study. Mechanical factors are not the only influences on the modeling and remodeling of the skeleton, as the cells responsible for these processes are also influenced by numerous metabolic factors. In addition, the relationships between mechanical, genetic, and metabolic factors may vary from one bone to another.

Viewing a bone in the same way as an inanimate mechanical structure such as a bridge is reasonable when considering the effect of an immediate mechanical demand. In clinical orthopedics it is the performance of the skeleton over time, such as a healing or training period, which is important. If performance over time is important, then the interaction of an adaptive response, genetic programming, and metabolic demands must be considered for a true perspective on the skeleton's mechanical performance.

2 The relationship between bone loading, function, and form

The architecture of a bone, its form, its shape, and the material properties of its matrix are critical to its ability to function as a mechanical element in the musculoskeletal system. A link between this form and the functional loading which the bone receives is important. If bone is clearly influenced by its mechanical circumstances, then the manner in which an adaptive response brings about such a link may be further investigated.

2.1 Effect of function on the development of bone form

There is abundant evidence that bone form and material properties are genetically determined. During growth and development of bone, the loads incurred by normal function also influence form. So the development of a normal bone requires an appropriate genetic inheritance and a loading history which falls within normal limits. Once growth has finished the genetic influence producing an appropriate bone form cannot be continually re-expressed, but functional demand could become the principal driving force toward an architecture optimized for mechanical function.

Most bones develop in, and eventually replace, cartilaginous precursors, which already conform roughly to the organ's final shape. Although some workers propose that the loading pattern of the fetal anlage has a significant effect on future development [1], it seems likely that there is a basic genetically driven pattern for each bone and that mechanical factors are unlikely to be the predominant influence on the early development of bone form [2]. The variation in the stage of skeletal maturity at birth in different species is an example of genetic programming. Those animals such as horses, cattle, and chickens, whose young have to be prepared to walk or run within a few hours of delivery, are considerably more advanced than those such as man, the cat, and the dog, whose offspring will be incapable of locomotion for weeks or months. However, movement and muscular effort undoubtedly occur in all these species in utero or in ova, providing an opportunity for preparturient conditioning [3]. In one series of experiments (Lanyon *et al.,* unpublished data), strain in the bones of fetal lambs was recorded. Surprisingly, but perhaps not to any mother, the strains caused by fetal movements in utero were as high as those engendered during locomotion after birth. Thus there is the opportunity from the start of growth for the skeleton to be influenced by the demands of function.

2.2   Response of bone to loading during development

The causal relationship between the development of bone form and loading history was admirably demonstrated by Uhthoff and Jaworski [4]. By immobilizing one forelimb in growing beagles they showed that the metacarpals in this limb did not develop their normal cross-sectional size or mass of bone tissue. When remobilized there was rapid new bone formation during which these functionally deprived bones caught up with their normally loaded controls. If one forelimb in adult dogs was immobilized, then bone was lost from the non-load-bearing metacarpals primarily by endosteal resorption. Again

restoration of load bearing resulted in restitution (at least in part) of the lost bone [5].

These overall changes in whole bones are quite striking and can be observed in radiographs of many clinical cases [6, 7]. The precise loading dependency of various features of bone architecture is not so obvious. One of the best-documented bony features known to develop in relation to normal use is the characteristic triangular form of the proximal tibia. In the human fetus and newborn the cross-section of the tibia is round. The triangular shape develops with the onset of function [8]. Normal function, however, involves at least two effects:

1. The loading and deforming of the bone tissue.
2. The intermittent pressure of active muscles directly onto the cells of the periosteum.

These two effects must not be confused.

Pressure on the periosteum will normally cause local bone resorption. Blood vessels pressing on the periosteum can form grooves for themselves, and teeth can be moved through the jaw by comparatively small pressures acting through the alveolar ligament [9]. In these situations there is pressure within the cell-rich periosteum, and the cells there, responsible for bone modeling and remodeling, may be directly influenced by it. It may be a similar mechanism that causes actively contracting muscles adjacent to the tibia to form a curved bed for themselves in the bone's cortex. Myotomy or paralysis in a growing animal affect the development of the normal triangular section of the tibia [8]. However, under these conditions both functional deformation and muscular pressure are both removed as functional deformation only exists in this and in other bones in the presence of an active musculature. Thus the separate effects of pressure proximity to the periosteum and functional deformation within the bone have not yet been satisfactorily delineated.

Although the cross-sectional shape of a bone is likely to be affected by the local presence of its adjacent muscles, its curvature may also develop in relation to function [10]. This development is less likely to be the result of muscle proximity since, in some bones at least, the curvature exists as much in the tendinous region as in the muscle belly. Also, although the characteristic curvature of several bones provides a curved concave bed for one group of muscles, this involves providing a convex surface for the muscle group adjacent to the opposite cortex. Insofar as long-bone curvatures are the result of function, it seems more likely that they are associated with the distribution of loads within the bone tissue than with the accommodation of adjacent musculature.

2.3 Functional loading as an influence on bone form

The mechanical relevance of the disposition of trabeculae, particularly those in the human vertebrae and femoral head (**Fig. 7-1**) aroused considerable interest in the nineteenth century [11–13]. The ideas put forward then culminated in a concept called the trajectorial theory. This theory, whose validity is still not entirely clear, relied on considering bones as homogeneous bone-shaped bodies and then calculating mathematically the distribution of stresses which would occur within them when subjected to loads presumed to be similar to those imposed during life. The initial controversy surrounding the trajectorial arrangement for trabeculae arose, unnecessarily, from an over-rigid statement of the trajectorial concept, and the idea that acceptance of this concept also involved accepting that trajectories themselves actually encourage bone formation. Trajectories in bone are no more real than isobars on weather maps; they merely represent theoretical lines of pure tension and compression stress within the structure. Koch [14] made a lengthy and careful analysis of the human femur using this principle. His calculations led him to conclude that "the trabeculae of the upper femur, as shown in frontal sections, are arranged in two general systems, compressive

Fig. 7-1: Trabecular organization. The trabeculae in the section of the human femoral head (a) can be clearly seen as organized tracts. Drawings of such arrangements (c) and their similarity with the mathematically calculated stress patterns in analogous objects such as Culman's crane (b) (reproduced from Wolff [13]), stimulated the idea that the trabecular structure might be mechanically orientated.

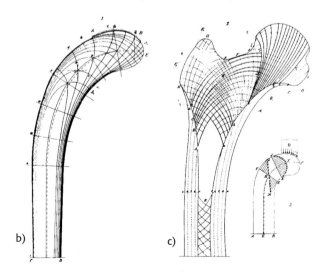

a)

b)

c)

and tensile, which correspond in position with the lines of maximum and minimum stress in the femur determined by the mathematical analysis of the femur as a mechanical structure".

2.3.1 Wolff's law of functional adaptation of bone

The principles of bone's mechanical suitability to its function and its capacity to adapt to changing functional demands are crucial to an understanding of skeletal development. These ideas have come to bear the name of one of their early proponents, Wolff. Unfortunately, with nineteenth century assurance, the recognition of the structure/function relationship was rather overstated and became known as Wolff's law [15]. This law is best considered as a general relationship embodying two concepts: Firstly, strategic placement of skeletal elements, and secondly adjustment of their mass.

The most specific statement of Wolff's law is the trajectorial theory mentioned in the previous section. Its implications are that by aligning themselves along the principal stress or strain directions, the plates and struts of cancellous bone avoid bending and provide the maximum structural support for the minimum osseous material. The advantages of such an arrangement and, more importantly, the adaptive capability of being able to achieve it, are obvious. There were a number of assumptions made in order to predict the trajectorial directions, notably that of considering bone as solid and homogeneous and presuming its manner of loading. These assumptions, together with the realization that much of the mathematical theory used in these early studies was incorrect [16], make the acceptance of Wolff's hypothesis as a "law" overoptimistic. However, the hypothesis generated by the work of Wolff and others, that the trabecular network is a structural system whose organization adapts to its loading environment, is important as a starting point for the link between form and function.

It was suggested that the deformation imposed upon the bones by mechanical function may be related to the stimulus which maintains their mechanical competence [17, 18], and thus provide part of the link between loading and the mechanical ability to resist that loading. If this is so, then functional deformation is indeed an important part of the jigsaw of influences acting on the skeleton. To determine the importance of functional deformation it must first be measured and then related to the capacity of the bone to adapt to its mechanical circumstances.

3 Functional loading and deformation

When a solid object has a load applied to it, it deforms. If the load is small then the deformation may be correspondingly insignificant. If the load is large, then the deformation may be sufficient either to break the object or to cause a permanent change in its shape. Bones must have a design that is competent to handle the loads normally imposed upon them, without deforming to the point of failure.

3.1 The relationship of load and deformation

If bone structure adapts according to its loading experience, then some physical consequence of loading must affect bone cells. The deformation, or strain, which is produced by loading, was suggested as a parameter suitable for this role [17]. The range of loading normally applied to bone imposes deformations within the elastic limit of the tissue. Thus, during the application of load deformation will be proportional to the load applied, and on unloading the original shape of the bone will be immediately restored. In fact this is a simplification, since bone is not an ideally elastic tissue, but it will suffice for our consideration here. The forces within the bone tissue, which resist the applied loads, are the stresses. The change in any of the bone's dimensions due to deformation of the bone, which gives rise to the stresses, may be expressed as strain. Each strain

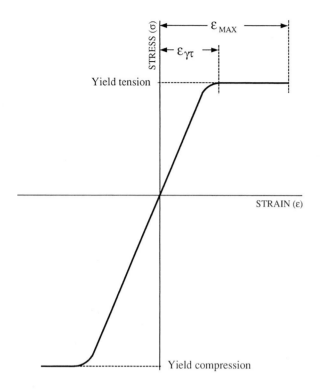

Fig. 7-2: Idealized plot of stress against strain for bone. The stress (σ - force per unit area) has a linear relationship to strain (ε - deformation) between the yield values in compression and tension. Over this linear part of the graph, bone acts as an elastic solid and stress is related to strain by the equation $E = \sigma/\varepsilon$ where E is the modulus of elasticity (Young's modulus). This relationship is the same for compression and tension. At the yield strain $\varepsilon_{\gamma\tau}$ the tissue becomes non-elastic and small increases in stress cause large deformations. ε_{MAX} is the ultimate strain for the material, and when this deformation is reached, the structure fragments. The yield strength for tension is about 7000 με, and the peak strains found in bone under normal functional loading in vivo are about 3000 με.

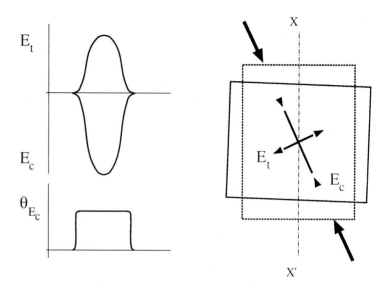

Fig. 7-3: Relationship of load to strain in a simple structure. A compressive load indicated by the large arrows deforms the block. E_c, the principal compressive strain, represents the decrease in the length of the block in the direction in which the force is applied; E_t, the principal tensile strain, represents the increase in the width of the block at right angles to E_c, and θ_{E_c}, the angle of the principal compressive strain to an axis (XX') through the block parallel with its sides. In the principal strain directions there is no shear, but when strain is measured in any other direction there will be a shear component.

is the ratio of change in that particular dimension to the original dimension (**Fig. 7-2** and **Fig. 7-3**).

Even if the external loading on an object is simple, as in **Fig. 7-3**, the pattern of stress and strain is more complicated. As the object is compressed in one direction, it is stretched in the other. At any point on its surface therefore, there are two directions of principal strain at right angles to one another, in one of which the strain is purely compressive and in the other purely tensile. In an isotropic material these principal strain directions are the same as the stress trajectories, the lines of maximum and minimum stress previously referred to. In any direction other than these principal directions there is a varying amount of shear strain that will be greatest at 45° to them.

3.1.1 Measurement of strain in vivo

The strain gauges most commonly used for measurements from bone consist of an electrical conductor arranged as a grid and mounted on a thin supporting base. The base is bonded to the structure being investigated so that it deforms as if it were part of the structure's surface (**Fig. 7-4**). The change in dimensions of the conductor alters its electrical resistance, and this alteration, which is proportional to strain, can be readily recorded. When such devices were first used on bone the bonding system was too cumbersome both to allow long-term

implantation and closure of the surgical wound over the implanted gauge [**19**]. With the advent of the rapidly poly-merizing cyanoacrylate bonding agents [**20, 21**], a number of strain gauges could be quickly bonded to the bone surface reliably in vivo and the incisions closed over them, allowing strain measurement without causing undue interference to the integrity of the system being investigated.

There are limitations on the potential of such a gauging system in bone. Strain on the bone surface is only one of the dimensional changes which occur during overall bone defor-mation, and gauges such as those described can only respond to changes in strain at the point to which they adhere and in the direction in which their grid is aligned (**Fig. 7-4**). If only one single-element gauge is attached to any point, it is not possible to infer the principal strain direction from its response or to discriminate between changes in the amount or direction of strain. Single-element gauges, therefore, are of limited practical use unless the loading direction is known. This is unusual in vivo; indeed, one of the objects of strain gauge instrumentation in vivo is to ascertain the changes in strain direction which occur during various activities. To do this, a multiple gauge consisting of three separate strain gauge elements is used. By recording the independent estimates of strain from these three gauges it is possible to calculate the size and changing directions of the principal surface strains throughout any deformation cycle [**22**]. In order to follow changes in the amount and direction of loading throughout a structure, three or more such 3-element rosette gauges must be placed around the structure's circumference.

Using the strain gauge technique in experimental animals, it has been possible to ascertain the strain patterns imposed on a number of bones during various activities [**20, 21, 23**], although there is still only one published report of in vivo, rosette strain-gauge data from a human during locomotion [**24**] (**Fig. 7-5**). A clearer picture of the way bones deform under load has emerged, allowing investigation of the relationship between the mechanical environment and bone architecture postulated in the 1890s [**15**].

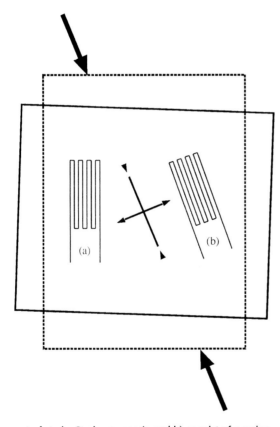

Fig. 7-4: Measurement of strain. Strain gauges (a and b) consist of a series of thin metal elements. These are bonded to the substrate which is to be measured, and when that substrate is deformed the gauges are also deformed. This changes their electrical resistance. Only a gauge arranged axially (b) to the principal strain direction would record that strain. A gauge at an angle to the principal strain direction will record only the proportion of the strain acting along the axis of the gauge.

3.2 Functional deformation and the orientation of cancellous bone

In the fetus and in those animals (or parts of animals) which, for some reason, do not develop normal activity, cancellous bone is arranged in a uniform, "uninfluenced" 3-D lattice. As functional loads are imposed upon this lattice, the trabecular tracts (**Fig. 7-1**) which are familiar in the adult appear. This trabecular system appears to have both mechanical suitability and an adaptive capability, making it an obvious target for investigation of the structure/function relationship in bone.

3.2.1 Experimental support for the trajectorial theory of bone architecture in cancellous bone

The principal problem in determining how structure and function are related in cancellous bone is the continuing difficulty of characterizing the behavior of individual trabeculae when the whole trabecular lattice is under load. With the use of recordings taken from strain gauges attached to bony surfaces in animals during their unimpeded activity, it became possible to measure the strain caused by functional loading in cortical bone. Since cortices enclose cancellous bone and this does not itself present an even surface to which a gauge could be attached, strain gauges cannot be applied to it directly but only to the overlying cortex.

In one series of experiments [25], the relationship between trabecular direction and strain direction was investigated by strain gauges attached to the lateral cortex of the sheep calcaneus (**Fig. 7-6**). Unlike the situation in the human, this bone has no contact with the ground but acts as a lever for the attachment of the Achilles tendon. Its shaft has no significant lateral attachments and so, during locomotion, it is deformed in the sagittal plane of the leg, parallel to its medial and lateral cortices. Beneath these cortices are two well-developed trabecular tracts arranged to cross each other, as in an arch. Because

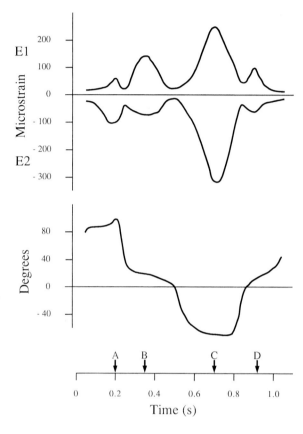

Fig. 7-5: Strain recording from a rosette strain gauge on the anteromedial aspect of the human tibia during a single walking stride [24]. The principal tension E_1, principal compression E_2, and the angle of the principal tension to the long axis of the tibia are shown. (A) is the impact of the heel on the ground, (B) weight bearing with the foot flat on the ground, (C) pushing forward with the heel up and the toes on the ground, and (D) the point at which the foot is lifted from the floor.

the bone is loaded in the sagittal plane it was thought acceptable to assume that the strain directions on the lateral surface reflected those in the same plane within its cancellous architecture.

During locomotion, the strain direction on the surface of the calcaneus changes little throughout each stride. The bone is deformed and then released at a constant angle. If trabecular architecture were to be related to functional strain direction,

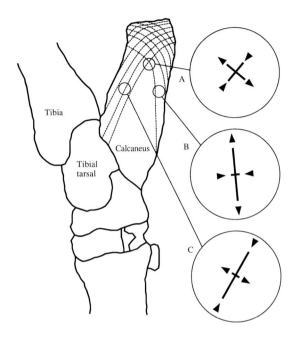

Fig. 7-6: Rosette strain-gauge analysis from the sheep calcaneus and its relationship to the trabecular tracts within the bone [25]. Strain-gauge measurement from site (C) shows a preponderance of principal compressive strain aligned with the dorsal trabecular tract. Strain gauge measurement from site (B) shows a preponderance of principal tensile strain aligned with the ventral trabecular tract. Measurement from site (A), where the dorsal and ventral trabecular tracts cross, shows similar values for the principal compressive and tensile strains, with the compressive strain still aligned with the dorsal tract and the tensile strain with the ventral tract. The tracts cross at right angles. This result supports the contention of the trajectorial theory that trabeculae are aligned with pure tensile or compressive forces, which means that they are not exposed to bending.

this was thought likely to be the direction concerned. Comparison between the direction of the larger principal strain on the bone's surface and the direction of the trabeculae beneath the cortex showed that they coincided well. On the plantar side of the bone the principal tensile strain seemed to be aligned with that of the plantar trabecular tract, and on the dorsal side the principal compressive strain was similarly aligned with the dorsal tract. In the bone's center the two tracts

crossed approximately at right angles, as do the principal strain directions (**Fig. 7-6**).

From this result it seems that, in one site at least, the most specific statement of Wolff's law, the trajectorial theory, survives the test of one of its major assumptions—that of the direction of functional loading. There is also support for the trajectorial theory from more recent mathematical analysis [26]. All this support, however, is only for coincidence in the direction of trabeculae and functional strain trajectories. It does not reinforce any hypothesis as to how such an arrangement is achieved.

3.2.2 The functional stimulus for the trajectorial arrangement mechanism in cancellous bone

In some parts of the skeleton, the agreement between the theoretically predicted and experimentally determined trajectories, and the trabecular orientation, is quite good. If trabeculae are arranged in the same direction as functional stress trajectories, then they will only be subjected to axial tension or axial compression, and will thus avoid bending. However, if trabeculae are arranged obliquely to these trajectories they will experience varying amounts of bending, which will produce an uneven strain distribution on their different surfaces. The assumption that trabeculae are aligned in relation to functional stress is underlain by the concept that this relationship is achieved by some feature of their loading environment. One hypothesis would be that pure tensile or compressive strain encourages bone formation. However, it seems more likely that the uneven strain pattern caused by bending stimulates deposition and removal of bone tissue until the trabeculae are so aligned that bending during functional loading is minimized or eliminated. When this situation has been achieved the trabeculae will have assumed a trajectorial arrangement [27].

For this explanation to be valid, it is necessary to accept that bone tissue can adjust its orientation in response to small changes in both the amount and distribution of intermittent deformation. If this is true, then trabecular architecture reflects an extremely important, mechanically related system of modeling/remodeling sensitivity. It is of course possible that the mechanism responsible for the adaptive response in bone is not just sensitive to changes in deformation but is also controlled by them.

The experimental evidence for the coincidence of trabeculae and functional stress trajectories has been augmented by intuitive [28] and strict mathematical analyses [29, 30]. It has been presumed in these studies that the mathematical variable that seems best satisfied must have also been the origin of the stimulus. However, this approach has not produced any explanation of the mechanism which has received any experimental support. Despite this, the coincidence between structure and function in the trabecular meshwork is enough for a causal relationship to be fairly certain. However, it is not only trabeculae of cancellous bone that assume a definite and characteristic shape with the onset of mechanical function; whole bones also only attain their "normal" size, section, and curvature in the presence of normal function. Whole bones do not enjoy the freedom to move their positions in the same way as the elements of the cancellous mesh. As a result they cannot avoid bending and torsion in addition to compression and tension. Thus, the explanations of the relationship of architecture and function in the trabeculae appear inadequate to explain long-bone form.

3.3 Functional deformation and the mass and orientation of whole bones

If solid trabeculae can align themselves in relation to the directions and amount of tension and compression, why should whole bones not be able to do the same? Frost [31] assumed that they could and that they do. He considered that bones have some appreciation of both the size and direction of functional deformation that occurs in their cortices, and that these cortices had a responsive mobility that allows them to arrange themselves so that during their predominant function they are subjected to overall compression. Frost's hypothesis, which he called the "flexure drift law", proposed that repeated intermittent, similarly aligned flexural strains induce cortical relocation until the flexural component of the overall loading is eliminated and axial compression is achieved. In other words, a trajectorial arrangement is achieved by the bone cortices similar to that which appears to occur in trabeculae. According to the flexure drift hypothesis the normal anatomical curvatures seen in adult bones represent an equilibrium position. In this position the bending effects of muscle groups on one side of the bone are countered by the bending effects within the bone due to end-on compression acting on a curved structure (**Fig. 7-7**). If such an arrangement did occur, it would have advantages, since bone, as a material, is much stronger in compression than in any other mode of loading, particularly bending. However, others have contested this view [27], believing that cortical position is more or less determined, and accepting that during loading some cortices are subject to compression and others to tension. In this model, bending did not represent an unstable situation likely to induce a change of shape, but could be a bone's normal circumstance under loading.

3.3.1 The "flexure drift law" and the limiting stress hypothesis

Although the responsive mobility of bone cortices to bending stresses was contested, most authors agreed on the response of bones to the magnitude of the loading imposed upon them. In cancellous bone, trabeculae are thought to become thicker and sturdier, move closer together, and develop more interconnections in regions that carry high loads. The opposite occurs if load bearing is reduced. Bone cortices also become thicker in areas where loading is increased and reduced in thickness when loading is diminished. This responsiveness of bone to the size of the mechanical loads placed upon it is the second principle of Wolff's law. It has become the generally accepted view that the amount of bone tissue present at any site is controlled by the amount of its mechanical loading in such a way that customary intermittent strains are adjusted to be within some tolerable, and presumably optimal, limit. It has been tempting to assume that the optimal limit is uniform regardless of location.

Pauwels [27] called this optimal stress range the "limiting stress", and Frost [32] used the term "minimum effective strain". Bassett [18] proposed that it is achieved and maintained as a result of a stimulatory pathway which controls the amount of bone present by means of a stress-sensitive or strain-sensitive feedback loop. If Pauwels [27] was correct in his hypothesis, some bones will be bent and some will not, but the customary stress within each cortex of every bone will be

constant, the "limiting stress". To achieve this uniform stress the amount of bone present and thus the thickness of each cortex will reflect its customary loading. If Frost [31] was correct, not only would the limiting stress be maintained, but also the cortices of bones would align themselves so that the stress would always be compressive.

An understanding of the curvature and deformation of long bones is not an abstruse or academic goal. The basis for much orthopedic management is an empirical understanding of bone's behavior under changing mechanical conditions, and the foundation for good surgical intervention rests on a sound appreciation of mechanical principles as they apply at any particular site (**Fig. 7-8a**). Naturally, if bone in different parts of the skeleton responds in a similar manner to certain generalized stimuli, knowledge of these and the response they engender would remove much of the guesswork from our intervention. Since the mechanical behavior of whole bones is to some extent reflected by the deformation on the surface of their cortices, it seems relevant to determine this in the only way possible at present and to measure them with strain gauges. This, of course, has to be done principally in experimental animals.

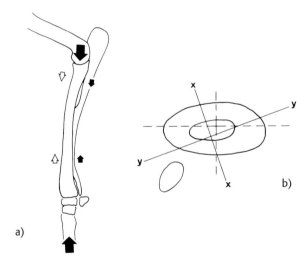

a) b)

Fig. 7-7: Strain in the sheep radius in vivo [46]. According to the flexure-drift hypothesis, the slight craniocaudal curvature of the radius should have been formed to achieve compression on each surface during functional loading *(lateral view: a)*. However, axial loading *(large solid arrows)*, causes bending, to which the flexor muscles *(small solid arrows)* which are active during loading, contribute and which is not counteracted by the relatively weak influence of the extensors *(open arrows)*. The result is that the convex anterior cortex is in tension (about 700 µe) and the caudal cortex is in compression (about –1200 µe). The cross-section *(b)* shows the axis of greatest resistance to bending y–y, and the least resistance x–x, which is the direction in which the bone is bent during loading in vivo. Thus, rather than cortical bone shape engendering the lowest possible uniform compressive strain, it appears to be orientated to engender uneven strain levels and relatively high strains.

3.3.2   Experiments on the curvature of long bones

If Frost's flexure-drift concept were true, then bone curvatures should be adjusted so that during repetitive functional loading the net strain on each cortex is compressive, when averaged over a period of time. Thus the curvature of a functional bone is likely to be different from one which develops in a non-load-bearing situation. This hypothesis has been tested by comparing the curvature of normal rat tibias with that in bones which developed in a non-loaded (paralyzed) situation [10]. This comparison confirmed that normal curvature developed only in response to normal function. However only in-vivo strain-gauge analysis could show whether this curvature resulted in uniform compression around the bone's circumference.

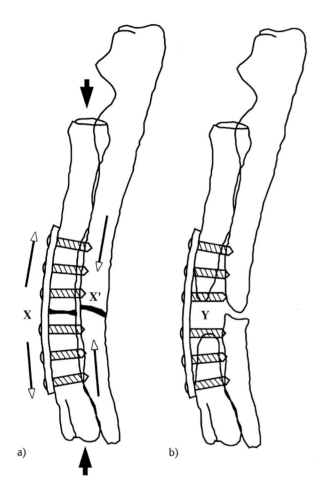

a)

b)

Fig. 7-8: Orthopedic considerations due to uneven strain distribution in bones. In the repair of the canine radial fracture XX' a well-contoured plate can be used on the anterior surface of the radius as a tension band (a). This surface of the radius is in tension under normal loading, and the plate is thus also loaded in tension, which is mechanically the most advantageous position as it is least vulnerable to fatigue. If dynamic compression is used in the placement of the plate, the cortex underneath the plate will be actively compressed, while loading of the limb will tend to compress the opposite cortex (X') resulting in compression across the whole fracture line. However, if the fixation is too rigid, the plate may take the entire load and the bone ends may not receive any strain stimulus for the adaptive mechanism. This can result in bone loss (Y) and malunion or non-union of the fracture due to "stress protection" (b).

Strain-gauge analysis of the radius of dogs, horses, and sheep confirms that the functional loading of this bone during locomotion subjects the convex cranial curvature to longitudinal tension and the concave caudal surface to longitudinal compression [33]. The tibiae of the same species have a cranially concave longitudinal curvature in the middle and distal thirds of their shaft. During functional loading, this part of the shaft is loaded by both bending and twisting forces. The result of the torsional force is that the larger principal strains on the cortices are not longitudinal but are aligned some degrees away from the bone's long axis. On the bone's cranial surface it is the principal tensile strain which is aligned nearer the axis; on the caudal surface it is the principal compressive strain. In contrast with the radius, the tension surface in the tibia is the concave cranial surface [34, 35]. The horse and sheep metacarpus are both relatively straight bones. During functional loading locomotion at a steady speed they are deformed so that each of their surfaces is subjected to longitudinal compression strain, although because of superimposed bending forces each cortex is not strained to an equal extent [36]. During acceleration and deceleration this bending is sufficient to place either the cranial or the caudal surface into longitudinal tension [37].

In these three separate bones there are three different relationships between curvature and customary loading direction. Plainly intermittent bending, to some bones at least, is a stable situation which does not induce adaptive change. Further, there appears to be no consistent relationship between the curvature of various bones and the functional bending imposed upon them.

3.3.3 Implications of the curvature of long bones

In the light of this variable relationship between loading and curvature it is reasonable to ask: What is the curvature there for? Frost's original idea that it was to eliminate strains due to bending [31] (**Fig. 7-7**) is clearly untenable, but does the curvature reduce bending? Again the answer is: apparently not.

Biewener [37] has calculated that in the radius some 85% of the locomotor strain is the direct consequence of end-to-end compression of a curved structure. In other words, without the curvature, functional strains would be reduced not increased. Examination of the cross-sectional shape of the radius shows that it is elliptical, but with the long axis being parallel to, rather than at right angles to, the axis of bending produced by the curvature. This means that both longitudinal curvature and cross-sectional geometry conspire to engender high functional strains rather than reduce them. The reason for this can only be speculated upon. However, the consequence is that the shape of the bone largely determines the strain distribution within it. Thus a comparatively wide range of loading situations results in a similar strain distribution. If functional strains are used as the controlling input for regulating adaptive changes in architecture, then having a large robust bone in which the strain input is high, and which increases steadily with increasing load, may be more useful than having a smaller bone in which strains are low and uniform during coordinated activity but high and unpredictable during buckling or off-axis loading [38].

The observations of mechanical function in normal bones have shown that uniform strains are not possible due to curvature and the bending under load which it dictates. A simple interpretation of the "limiting stress hypothesis", which considers the thickness of the cortices of bones to be controlled solely by the local customary load upon them, is not satisfactory. These studies do appear to show a link between the magnitude and distribution of functional deformation within a bone and its architectural properties. A clearer view of the influence of mechanical conditions on bone architecture was achieved by observation of altered functional deformation.

4   The adaptive response of bone to altered functional deformation

One classic method to determine the extent to which bones adapt to mechanical change is to alter their mechanical circumstances and to observe the result. A variety of such experiments have been performed [39, 40],which showed the osteogenic effect of increased loading. More specifically, in bending or compression, dynamic loading was osteogenic whereas static loading was not [41, 42], and dynamic loading could induce both intracortical [43] and periosteal modeling/remodeling [44]. However, prior to reliable in vivo strain gauging, the exact nature and extent of the changes in the stress/strain situation of the bone was impossible to determine. Once strain gauging became available, the strain situation of the bone could be related to the induced modeling/remodeling.

4.1   Experimental overload of limb bones in quadrupeds

In the antebrachium of most quadrupeds the radius and ulna both contribute to support during locomotion, although the proportion that each bone contributes varies between species. Removal of a section of one bone, usually the ulna, produces excessive strain in the other bone as part of the weight-bearing equipment of the leg is lost, although surprisingly the animals normally walk after the first week. Ulna osteotomy has been used as an experimental tool to study the adaptive response with in vivo strain gauging used to assess the relative overstrain

In a series of ulna osteotomies in young pigs [45], the mechanical result of removing the ulna was a compressive overstrain of some 2 to 2.5 times on the cranial cortex of the radius. After the osteotomy, the periosteum hypertrophied and the orderly circumferential deposition of laminar bone was converted to a rapid proliferation of bony fronds vertically from the bone's original periosteal surface. At the same time osteonal remodeling eroded much of the pre-existing cortex. This rapidly increased the area that the periosteum of the radius enclosed. Subsequently, widening of the medullary cavity, filling of the osteoporotic cortex, and endosteal remodeling greatly increased, and the cross-section of the radius changed from that of a "D" to a circle. Eventually the rate of new bone formation slowed, and that which was deposited had the original circumferential laminar appearance. At this stage the amount of strain imposed during locomotion on the cranial cortex of the hypertrophied bone was the same as that at the similar site on the normal bone of the contralateral limb [45]. This result supports a "limiting stress" hypothesis, or at least a constant target strain for that location.

In a similar experiment in adult sheep [46], removal of a section of the ulnar shaft only increased the locomotor strain on the bone's cranial surface (tension and convex aspect) by some 20–25%, and on the caudal surface (compression and concave aspect) by some 8%, due to the smaller contribution of the ulna to support in this species (**Fig. 7-9**). One of two things might have been expected to happen:

1. Both bone cortices could have drifted toward the induced concavity (caudally). The bone would then have become straighter, and the original amount of locomotor strain would have been restored. Such a sequence of events might have been expected from a consideration of the flexure drift hypothesis.
2. The cranial cortex could have hypertrophied to reduce its 20% overstrain to normal, and the caudal cortex could have behaved similarly to reduce its 8% overstrain. In this case the cranial cortex would have had to increase its thickness by far more than the caudal cortex.

In fact, there was periosteal new bone deposition on both the cranial and caudal cortices (**Fig. 7-9**). The thickness of new bone on the caudal cortex (8% overstrain) was some 10 times as much as that on the cranial cortex, in which the overstrain was 20%. This result was probably the most economical method of reducing the net overstrain on the whole segment of bone, but it represented neither a drifting response from mobile cortices nor a local hypertrophy response of two independent cortices whose spatial position was fixed.

The results of these experiments suggest that bone is exquisitely sensitive to the amount of customary intermittent strain to which it is subjected. The normal locomotor strain on the cranial cortex of the sheep radius is some 0.8 μm over a distance of 1 mm, and the initial and thus maximum overstrain induced by ulna osteotomy represents an additional 0.2 μm

in 1 mm. On the caudal cortex, the normal locomotor strain is 11 μm in 1 mm, and the initial overstrain in this case was only some 0.05 μm. Thus, repetitive increase or redistribution of strain, in quite minute proportions, will induce a coordinated and sustained osteogenic response which may be greatest in parts of the bone not necessarily themselves subjected to the greatest overstrain and, in some situations, perhaps not subjected to overstrain at all. The suspicion that the peak strain magnitude is only one of the variables affecting bone adaptation is confirmed in this same sheep experiment where the

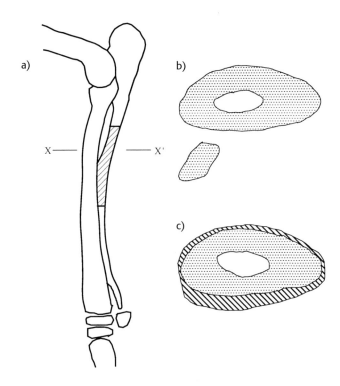

Fig. 7-9: Remodeling responds to overstrain [46]. a) shows the lateral view of an ovine radius and ulna, with the removed portion shaded. The transverse section (b) is the normal profile of the radius and ulna at level XX'. c) shows the section of the bone a year after removal of the ulna portion. Although the cranial *(uppermost)* surface experienced the greatest overstrain, new bone *(shaded area)* was predominantly deposited on the caudal surface.

peak strains on the cranial cortex after adaptation were actually smaller than normal. Presumably the strain environment of this cortex continues to provide a stimulus for cortical deposition of new bone, despite strains at this location already being below normal.

4.2 Significance of bone strain (in vivo)

Knowledge of the deformation or strain engendered in bone tissue during normal functional activity is important in understanding bone physiology because of the impact of strain on that physiology. Any material subject to repetitive cyclical strains may be susceptible to fatigue, that is, gradual mechanical failure at strains much lower than those required for a single instantaneous fracture (**Fig. 7-10**). Such failure results from microdamage to the material of the matrix, and bone may be affected by such microdamage even at the strain levels

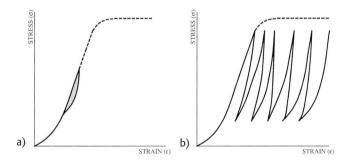

a)   STRAIN (ε)   b)   STRAIN (ε)

Fig. 7-10: Stress/strain curves (dotted line) and load/deformation curves (solid line) for two bone specimens undergoing cyclical loading. At the lower end of the stress/strain curve (a), repeated loading does not cause any damage and the loading curves are superimposed in a loop, indicating that there is no overall deformation building up over a period of time. At the higher end of the stress/strain curve, but still below the yield point, the bone sustains internal damage and some overall deformation at the end of each cycle.

induced by normal functional loading. If such damage is allowed to accumulate it will eventually result in failure and fracture, so it seems logical to assume that there is a physiological mechanism which repairs microdamage and prevents fatigue fracture. Additionally, the earlier part of this section shows the importance of strain as a stimulus for an adaptive response. Thus the principal effects of functional deformation on bone can be considered as twofold:

1. Functional strain is an influence in determining and maintaining skeletal structure; it may be the most important functional influence on the cellular behavior which ensures that bone structure becomes, and remains, suitable for its customary mechanical function. When the normal stimulus of intermittent deformation is altered, by even small amounts, the resulting osseous response is both marked and intuitively appropriate. Conversely, reduction of function by immobility or bed rest quickly leads to loss of bone. The "normal" skeleton therefore must be considered as only being maintained in its "normal" state because of its being constantly under the influence of a "normal" mechanical environment. This system of cellular reaction to mechanical stimulus can be called the adaptive response and may be particularly important in relation to orthopedic interference, especially that involving internal fixation or prosthetic replacement (**Fig. 7-11**).

2. Functional strains may cause skeletal damage, deterioration, and structural failure, even within the normal strain ranges found in vivo [47]. The accumulation of microdamage due to fatigue must be arrested in order to avoid the ultimate failure of the bone (**Fig. 7-10b**). Microdamage in bone is manifested as microcracks, and these appear to be associated with increased levels of remodeling [48]. It seems likely that areas of the matrix which contain microcracks can be specifically replaced by new matrix during remodeling; thus there must be a mechanism which recognizes the areas which need replacement and directs the remodeling processes toward them.

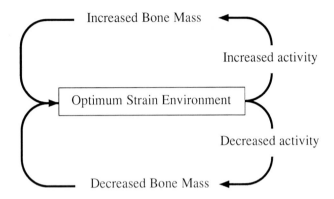

Fig. 7-11: Schema to show how a feedback influence on modeling/remodeling—from the strain caused by the loads imposed during activity—could control bone architecture in order to maintain an optimal strain environment.

Both adaptation of bone architecture to the prevailing loading environment and replacement of fatigued areas of bone involve the modeling/remodeling activity of the bone surface cells. It is thus possible that there is an interrelationship between these two effects of functional deformation, in the mechanism by which the response to them is coordinated.

If functional strains have this key role in bone physiology, it implies that the form of the bone, its curvatures and alignments, the thickness of its cortices, and the arrangement and density of its cancellous architecture are developed and maintained under the influence of an adaptive process sensitive to mechanical events. Some of these features remain capable of adaptive change and so will respond to alterations in their mechanical circumstances, although bone appears to become less responsive to functional stimuli with increasing age. Thus normal bone form needs not only a normal genetic inheritance and a metabolic environment which is biochemically appropriate, but also a loading history which falls within normal limits. In some conditions such as those occurring during disease, damage, or orthopedic interference, some elements of a bone may become abnormal, and the healthy balance between structure and function is lost. Understanding the mechanism which maintains the balance between structure and function is thus a key in understanding orthopedic disease.

5   A hypothesis for the mechanism of strain-related control which governs adaptive change in bone

We postulate that a group of cells are sensitive to strain in the matrix adjacent to them, and that they have the ability to communicate with one another in order to form an appreciation of the strain distribution throughout a volume of the bone tissue. We suggest that this information on strain distribution and waveform is the mechanical input to which bone modeling and remodeling is sensitive. The principal candidate for the strain-sensitive cell is the osteocyte/osteoblast population. These cells are spread over the surface and throughout the tissue and connect with each other via their cytoplasmic processes and gap junctions [49, 50]. We postulate that these cells compare the appreciation of the strain environment that they are experiencing with an innate, genetically programmed concept of the target strain environment for that location. On the basis of a mismatch between the current and target strain environment, the cell network can influence the surface cells and thus direct modeling/remodeling to eliminate the mismatch. The same network of cells would be suited to the transmission of a stimulus for remodeling from areas of microdamage to the surface sites where osteoclasts are recruited, and subsequently to convey the positional data necessary to target the secondary osteonal remodeling into the damaged area. Therefore, this hypothesis allows the possibility that both consequences of functional deformation, adaptive change and repair of fatigue microdamage, are mediated through the same mechanism.

The influence of the strain-sensitive cell population on the modeling/remodeling population must interact with other influences such as the systemic hormones that affect bone. In a normal adult bone, where resorption balances formation, there is likely to be an equilibrium between a potentially osteogenic stimulus from the strain-sensitive cells and the potentially resorptive influence of the systemic calcium-regulating hormones.

There are a number of phases in the adaptive mechanism:

1. A physical stimulus for the mechanism generated by the loading environment, or some part of the loading environment of the bone, and its transduction into cellular activity.
2. Integration of local strain-related activity throughout a volume of bone to form an appreciation of strain distribution.
3. Production of a strain-related stimulus, capable of influencing change in bone architecture through the agency of modeling and remodeling.
4. Interaction of that stimulus with other factors that affect remodeling. Thus a strain-related stimulus for modeling/remodeling might be opposed, enabled, or enhanced according to the local biochemical environment such as the hormonal milieu.
5. Adaptive modeling and remodeling. The coordinated activity of populations of osteoblasts and osteoclasts to adapt or modify bone architecture (**Fig. 7-12**).

6 Investigation of the mechanism of the adaptive response

It is evident from experiments such as those outlined earlier, and numerous observations of clinical and exercise situations in which the functional loading of bone is altered, that an adaptive response plays an important part in the control of bone architecture. Understanding the mechanism of this response must be a major goal in orthopedic research, as such an understanding may allow the manipulation of the response and intervention in any orthopedic disease where change of bone architecture is important. It appears that the adaptive response can recognize some physical consequence of loading and, under some circumstances, initiate and control a model-

Fig. 7-12: Schema to show the chain of events in the hypothesis for the mechanism of the adaptive response.

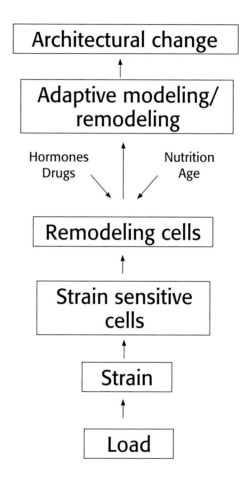

ing/remodeling reaction which results in a strategic change in bone architecture. As investigation of such a system attracts a wide range of approaches, from architectural mechanics to molecular biology, the constituent phases of the response have often been examined separately, and an overall picture is only now starting to emerge.

6.1 Physical parameters stimulating the adaptive response

Even a very simple strain regimen has a number of components, only some of which are likely to influence bone cells to produce adaptive change in bone architecture. A variety of mathematical techniques have been used to make theoretical predictions of the parameters that give rise to adaptive modeling/remodeling [51–54]. However, a series of assumptions have to be made in such predictions, and so in vivo experiments, where the adaptive response is observed in a bone undergoing a change in its customary loading pattern, have been important.

Lanyon and Rubin [42] tried to attribute the aspects of the strain waveform, which influenced bone modeling by using a surgically isolated, externally loadable turkey-ulna preparation.

If the isolated segment was not loaded, it became osteoporotic. However, interruption of disuse by extremely short periods of dynamic loading not only prevented resorption but also resulted in an increase in bone formation proportional to the peak strain magnitude [23] (Fig. 7-13). Only four consecutive 1 Hz loading cycles per day were needed to prevent resorption, and just 36 cycles per day saturated the osteogenic response at peak strains of about -2000 microstrain (μɛ) [55] (Fig. 7-14). Static load applied continuously produced no different effect from disuse [42]. Further experiments with compressive loading have suggested that the frequency of the strain wave-

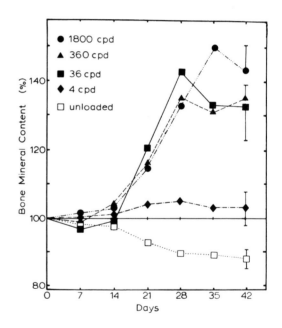

Fig. 7-14: Graph showing change in bone mineral content at the midshaft of the avian ulna preparation [55]. The results show different responses over a 6-week experimental period during which ulnae were loaded for different numbers of cycles per day (cpd) A lack resulted in a loss of bone, but only 4 cpd was enough to prevent this loss. 36, 360, and 1800 cpd. all resulted in an increase in bone mass and there were no differences in these effects. This indicates that the adaptive mechanism may be saturated by relatively low (36) numbers of cycles of a novel loading stimulus.

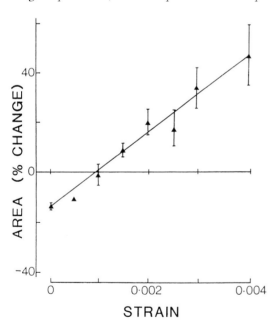

Fig. 7-13: Graph showing increase in bone cross-sectional area at the midshaft of the turkey ulna preparation [23]. The differing responses of ulnae loaded at different peak-strain magnitudes show a linear relationship between strain and adaptive response.

form and the rate of strain change are also important [56, 57], and Qin [58] has shown that resorption can be prevented at lower peak strain magnitudes (100 με) by employing more cycles per day (100,000).

The modeling response in these daily loading experiments initially consists of diffuse woven bone (**Fig. 7-15**), but if daily loading is maintained, this bone consolidates and undergoes haversian remodeling as it becomes a structurally integral part

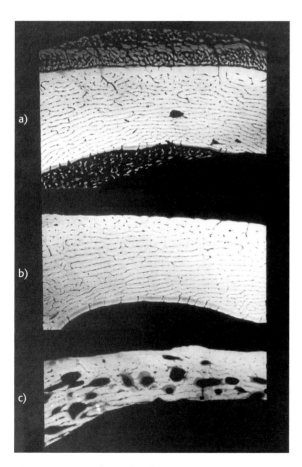

Fig. 7-15: Microradiographs of cortical segments of the avian ulna cortex. b) shows the normal cortex, a) and c) are from prepared ulnae, c) showing the osteopenia induced by the absence of loading and a) showing the increase in new bone induced by a 5-minute daily loading period over 8 weeks.

of the expanded cortex (Rubin personal communication). A single period of osteogenic loading, such as that used on a daily basis in the earlier avian ulna experiments, produces active formation of woven bone 6 days later [59]. Thus it appears that the formation observed in the long-term experiments is the result of the accumulation of a series of such packets of activation. The new bone formed in the long-term experiments did not occur at the site of the greatest strain [23, 46]. This indicates that the adaptive response may produce a strategic placement of new bone, rather than a simple response related to local peak strain magnitude. There is some confirmation of this in the finding that strain gradients may correlate with the deposition of new bone [60].

As new bone was formed at peak strain magnitudes less than those found in vivo, it was postulated that part of the stimulus for the adaptive response came from the difference between the strain distributions due the artificial loading and those due to normal activity. Apparently, appropriate placement of new bone also suggests the importance of strain distribution. Such a strategic response requires an appreciation of the mismatch between the actual and the desirable strain distribution for each location, rather than just the accumulation of all the differences in local peak strain magnitudes. A comparison of compressive and torsional loading in the turkey ulna showed that different loading modes, giving rise to different strain distribution patterns, produce different dose/response relationships between peak strain magnitude and change in bone cross-sectional area [61]. In addition, the nature of the architectural change was different between torsional and compressive loading. Bone loaded in torsion undergoes both formation and resorption resulting in a change in cross-sectional shape without an overall change in cross-sectional area [61].

The brief periods of stimulus by an unusual strain distribution, which are needed to saturate the adaptive response, suggest that bone architecture is controlled by avoiding error strains, rather than by highly repetitive normal strains. The finding that artificial application of normal strain distributions requires higher strains to initiate a response [62] tends to confirm this. Thus the adaptive mechanism appears to be error-driven [63]. When a novel strain environment is imposed on the bone, the mismatch between the normal and imposed strain distributions is high. This high-error strain stimulates a structurally appropriate architectural response, which if sustained will return the strain environment to normal [23, 46] (**Fig. 7-16**). Each period of loading initiates a packet of architectural change, the final response being the accumulation of all these packets. Each successive packet brings the bone architecture closer to the "target" required; thus each successive change will be smaller than the last. The large volume of woven bone initially produced, as seen in the single-loading experiments, might be considered as a way of quickly reaching a rough estimation of the new "target" shape which is then "fine-tuned" by the later changes. It is also possible that this

woven bone, which can be formed faster than other bone types, acts as a temporary "scaffold" until it can be remodeled as solid cortical bone.

Strain distribution, dynamic peak strain magnitude, and other components of the strain waveform related to functional loading appear to have a regulatory influence on bone architecture. Normal levels of bone mass will be maintained as long as intermittent loading occurs for a brief period at roughly daily intervals. Failure to maintain such exposure to functional loading results in disuse osteopenia. When a novel loading situation imposes an unusual or error strain environment on the bone, the adaptive mechanism can change the bone architecture to a more suitable configuration for the new load.

6.2 Possible mechanisms of strain transduction

Transduction must occur either directly from physical deformation to the cell, or via the intermediary of some strain-related phenomena. A number of strain-related phenomena including strain energy dissipation [30], hydrostatic pressure [64, 65], and local strain-generated changes in calcium solubility [51, 66], have been postulated as mechanisms for transduction. However, phenomena which can be generated in a strain-related fashion currently attract the most interest as potential transduction systems.

6.2.1 Strain-related electrical potentials in bone

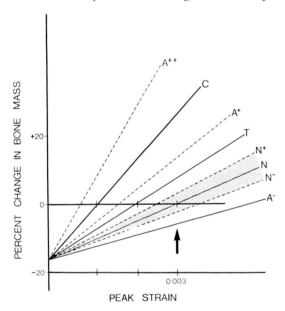

Fig. 7-16: A schema for the effect of strain distribution. Each line represents the response to increasing peak strain magnitude at a different strain distribution. The normal strain distribution (N) and a band of strain around it (shaded area) causes no increase in bone mass provided peak strains do not exceed 3000 microstrain. Other strain distributions may be more (A+) or less (A-) osteogenic. For example (c) a largely compressive strain distribution such as that imposed on the avian ulna preparation by axial loading is particularly osteogenic, provoking a large increase in bone mass at relatively low peak strains.

Deformation of bone tissue causes fluid flow through the microstructure of the bone which, as this fluid is charged, induces strain-generated potentials (SGPs) [67]. The size of the SGPs is dependent upon both the strain magnitude and the rate at which it changes (**Fig. 7-17**). The range of strain magnitude and rate over which the potentials are sensitive to change is similar to those magnitudes and rates found in bone in vivo.

Slow or causal locomotion only engenders small potentials, but vigorous activity engenders a pattern of electrical change reminiscent of the pattern of mechanical change which induced it [68] (**Fig. 7-17**). Changes in SGP magnitude and frequency have also been observed in association with different stages of healing in bone [69], indicating their potential for involvement in feedback during remodeling.

There is circumstantial evidence that potential changes may be important in controlling bone physiology from observations of the effects of pulsed electromagnetic fields (PEMFs) and capacitive coupling. The healing of certain types of fractures

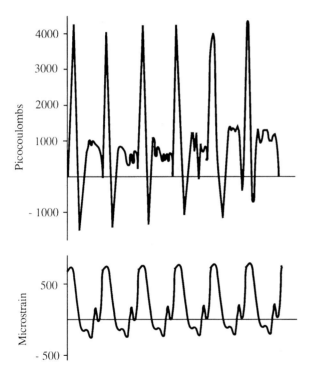

Fig. 7-17: Simultaneous potential and strain recording from the sheep radius [68]. The upper trace shows the SGP (silver chloride electrode) and the lower the strain in the longitudinal direction of the radius during fast walking. The increase in tension, which occurs as the animal places its leg on the ground, engenders a positive potential peak, which decays and eventually returns to zero as the leg is swung to the point of impact in the next stride. Each cycle takes approximately 0.5 seconds.

can be accelerated by application of such devices [70, 71], and their ability to affect the behavior of bone cells in vitro has also been demonstrated. Application of pulsed fields to the isolated avian ulna system induced an osteogenic reaction similar to that induced by loading, and varying in magnitude depending on the wavelength of the signal supplied to the field coils [72]. Application of a particular pulsed field to an isolated canine fibula preparation slowed resorptive activity at the periosteal surface, while a second field type not only slowed resorption but also induced new bone formation at the periosteal surface [73, 74].

Cells can be affected by changes in potential, and so the strain-related potential changes in bone might be important in a transduction mechanism. A mechanism dependant on potential fluctuation would fit well with the observation that dynamic and not static strains induce adaptation, and with high strain rates which induce strong potential differences, having an increased osteogenic effect [57]. The pattern of SGPs reflect the strain distribution [68] and they set up potential gradients across the bone tissue. An appreciation of these gradients might be a way in which the resident bone cells recognize strain distribution. There is therefore considerable circumstantial evidence for the importance of SGPs as an intermediary between strain and cellular activation, but until a definite link is established there is always the possibility that they are merely an irrelevant, albeit strain-related, phenomena.

6.2.2 Load-induced proteoglycan reorientation

The bone matrix proteoglycans have a high charge separation and might be affected by changes in electrical potential. Immediately after a single period of loading there is an increased orientation of the proteoglycan molecules within the cortical bone which, in the absence of further loading, persists for over 24 hours [75, 76]. Long-term disuse [77] and human clinical osteoporosis [78] are both associated with decreased proteoglycan orientation in bone tissue. Although it is possible that this phenomenon is an irrelevant byproduct of strain in bone, the bone cells could be stimulated by the reorientation of the proteoglycans around them. As this reorientation is a persistent phenomenon, it could provide a mechanism by which intermittent strain experienced in "real time" induces more persistent but recoverable strain-related changes in the bone matrix which could subsequently influence bone cell behavior. This could be interpreted as a "strain memory". Although there is as yet no positive evidence that strain-related proteoglycan orientation has any functional consequences, it is of interest that the degree of orientation of proteoglycans in the matrix appears to be deficient in bone specimens from human clinical osteoporosis patients [78].

6.2.3 Direct strain stimulation of bone cells

As a result of observations of osteoblasts in vitro, Jones and Bingmann [79] postulate that transduction can occur by the direct activation of phospholipase C (PLCγ-1). This activation is thought to be due to the deformation of the cells which occurs as a consequence of the deformation of the substrate to which they adhere. PLCγ-1 activation can lead to prostaglandin synthesis, and prostaglandin release has been demonstrated in the early part of the cascade of response to mechanical stimulus in bone and bone cells [80–82]. Another possibility for the direct activation of bone cells relies on a perturbation of their cytoskeleton. Osteocytes depend for their shape on a complex cytoskeleton [83], and there is a mechanism of mechanotransduction in osteoblasts which is dependent on the cytoskeleton [84].

6.3 Early strain-related changes in bone cells

If an assessment of strain distribution is important, then strain-derived information must be collated over a volume of bone. Osteocytes, with their wide distribution throughout the bone matrix, appear to be in a suitable position to receive strain-related stimulus from all parts of the bone. In the isolated avian ulna preparation, a single period of osteogenic loading capable of stimulating new bone formation [59] gave rise to a local strain magnitude-related increase in the number of osteocytes showing G6PD (glucose 6 phosphate dehydrogenase) activity, 5 minutes after loading. There was also an increase in the level of G6PD activity of periosteal cells [85]. G6PD activity is the rate-limiting step of the pentose monophosphate shunt, and an increase in G6PD activity is consistent with increased synthetic activity. Twenty-four hours after loading the number of osteocytes incorporating ^{3}H uridine increased by a factor of 6 [86]. This is consistent with increased synthetic activity in these cells. Whereas the G6PD activity 5 minutes after loading appears to occur in a local strain magnitude-dependent fashion, there is some evidence to suggest that the RNA response 24 hours after loading more closely parallels the disposition of subsequent new bone. The difference in these patterns of activity may represent the phase of "signal processing" which we suggest occurs within the osteocyte network to produce the appreciation of strain distribution, and perhaps the strain-related stimulus for adaptive modeling and remodeling. The means of communication are certainly present in osteocytes since they are interconnected by cytoplasmic processes which run through the canaliculi and posses gap junctions [50, 87]. Such connections are specifically designed for the passage of information from one cell to another. This system of connections also extends to the surface osteoblasts and so could allow "instructions" for modeling/remodeling activity from osteocyte to the effector cells.

6.4 Further cellular activity in the adaptive response

Once the strain sensitive cells are activated there must be a number of cellular interactions which can engender any modification of the bone architecture required. Although study of these cells in vivo ensures that all the potential influences on their normal function are present, it is often difficult to study the individual elements of any mechanism in such a complex system. In vitro studies allow more accurate investigation of individual interactions, although they may suffer from a lack of relevance due to their artificial nature. An important advance has been the use of in vitro systems in which biochemical changes are observed in association with mechanical loading which are similar to those observed in vivo.

6.4.1   Prostaglandin mediation

Since Yeh and Rodan [80] showed that prostaglandins are produced as a direct result of strain on bone cells in vitro, they and others [88] have suggested that prostaglandins might be the messenger that initiates the modeling/remodeling response. In addition, a number of authors have shown the importance of prostaglandins in the interactions of cells on the bone surface [89–92], further underlining the importance of prostaglandins in bone modeling/remodeling.

In vivo, a single dose of indomethacin at the time of osteogenic loading can reduce the activation of a quiescent periosteum [59, 93] and can be shown to affect load-induced remodeling when given either before or after osteogenic loading [94]. In vitro systems using cancellous cores and embryonic tibias have been used to further investigate this interference in the adaptive mechanism by suppression of prostaglandin synthesis. In these systems there is an increase in G6PD activity 5 minutes after loading and an increase in ^{3}H uridine uptake 6 hours after loading in resident bone cells, similar to that seen in vivo. The increase in G6PD activity in bone cores is inhibited by indomethacin. The loading-related uptake in ^{3}H uridine was reflected in an increase in the specific activity of ^{3}H uridine in the RNA extracted from the bone cores, and this too was substantially modified by indomethacin [95–97].

Such indirect evidence for the role of prostaglandins was augmented by the finding that within 5 minutes of the beginning of loading in bone cores there is a transient increase in prostacyclin (PGI$_2$) and prostaglandin E (PGE) in the perfusate (Fig. 7-18). There was also immunocytochemical evidence of the presence of PGE in surface cells, and PGI$_2$ in both surface cells and osteocytes [82]. PGI$_2$, but not PGE, added to the perfusate of bone cores produces within 6 hours an increase in

the specific activity of ^{3}H uridine in extracted RNA [98]. The finding that exogenous PGI$_2$, but not PGE, added to the medium in this preparation stimulates RNA production in the absence of loading indicates that PGI$_2$ may be released early in the mechanism to trigger a sequence of events leading to synthesis of control substances for remodeling. Early release of PGI$_2$ and increase in cellular G6PD activity has also been shown after loading bone cells in vitro [99]. In addition, ion channels appear to be involved in this early prostaglandin response [100], giving the possibility of a link between this mechanism and the potential effects discussed earlier.

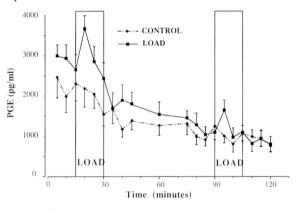

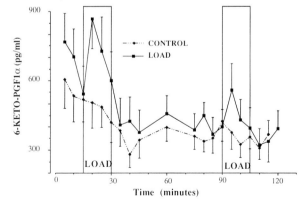

Fig. 7-18: Graphs showing the release of prostanoids from cancellous bone cores loaded in vitro [82]. The increased release of prostaglandin E (PGE) and prostacyclin (PGI) (as monitored by its metabolite 6-Keto-PGF$_{12}$), which is stimulated by a period of loading, is shown relative to unloaded controls.

6.4.2 Growth factors

As G6PD activity can reflect an increase in synthetic activity producing RNA, it is possible that these events are linked. The RNA could be coded for the production of a specific growth factor or cytokine, which might subsequently control remodeling by providing a link between osteocytes or between osteocytes and surface cells. Polypeptide growth factors such as in Insulin-like growth factor 1 and 2 (IGF-I and IGF-II) and transforming growth factor beta (TGF-β) can affect osteoblasts [101–105], and so could fulfil this messenger role. Prostaglandins released early in the adaptive mechanism might stimulate release of such factors. Expression of IGF-II does occur in conjunction with PGI_2 in loaded explants and bone cells in vitro [99].

6.5 Interaction of the adaptive response with other influences on bone

There is ample clinical evidence to show that the mechanically driven adaptive response interacts with systemic metabolic influences on bone. Female athletes, despite intensive exercise in training, suffer bone loss if they develop amenorrhea [106], and bone loss in postmenopausal women can be antagonized locally by exercise [107–109]. Experimentally, using the avian ulna preparation in egg-laying females, it has been shown that bone loss due to disuse is additional to that due to calcium insufficiency. However, this bone loss can be modulated by external loading [110] (**Fig. 7-19**).

There is no inflexion in the dose response curve between bone formation and strain magnitude (**Fig. 7-13**). This suggests that stimulation of new bone formation and inhibition of bone resorption may be dose-related aspects of the same adaptive response to strain. As disuse osteopenia occurs only in the presence of intact parathyroids [111], it appears that the stimulus for bone loss arises from the resorptive effect of the hormonal environment unopposed, at the site of interaction, by the conservation and potentially osteogenic effects of mechanical loading. The evidence from modulation of

calcium deficiency-induced bone loss by loading [110] (**Fig. 7-19**) shows the overwhelming effect that calcium-regulating hormones can have over mechanically derived, potentially osteogenic responses.

The systemic metabolic influences on bone mass must exert their control through the same osteoblast/osteoclast system

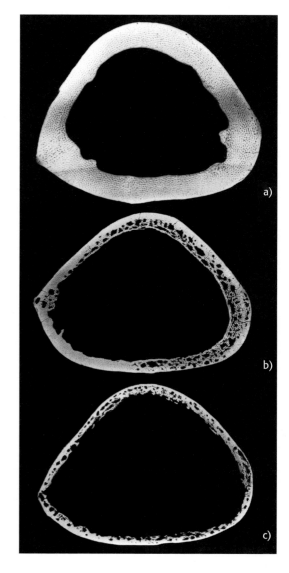

Fig. 7-19: Microradiograph sections from the avian ulna [110]. a) shows a normal avian ulna and (b) an intact ulna showing substantial remodeling due to calcium insufficiency. Section (c) is the contralateral, prepared isolated ulna which was not loaded. This shows the increased bone loss, which occurs when there is no loading to stimulate the adaptive response and protect the bone architecture.

used by the adaptive response, if they are to be able to modify bone architecture. It is likely that at some point in the adaptive mechanism these competing influences can interact. Osteoblasts have receptors for many messenger substances such as estrogens, prostaglandins, growth factors and parathyroid hormone [112], and such substances which have been shown to interact with the adaptive response [113]. These cells can synthesize a range of potential messenger substances [112, 114] and are the principal controlling cells in directing the actions of osteoclasts [115, 116]. Thus it seems likely that the osteoblast is the site of integration of the various influences on bone architecture, and there is experimental evidence to show the interaction of hormonal receptor pathways in the adaptive response at the osteoblast [117]. It is possible that direct systemic effects on osteoclasts, such as that of calcitonin, and on osteocyte, such as that postulated for estrogen [118], are integrated into the balance of systemic and adaptive effects.

6.6   Conclusions relating to the hypothesis for the adaptive mechanism

1. The physical stimulus for the adaptive response appears to depend on the mismatch or error of the strain distribution from normal, and the magnitude, frequency, and strain rate of the strain waveform.
2. There is evidence to support the idea that transduction of the physical stimulus into cellular activity occurs in the osteocyte/osteoblast network. The mechanism of this transduction is still not clear but a direct physical effect of strain on the cells or an effect related to strain-generated potentials appear to be strong possibilities.
3. There is some evidence for integration of osteocyte activity over a volume of bone via the interconnecting osteocyte network.
4. The adaptive mechanism can apparently produce a strain-related stimulus, capable of influencing change

in bone architecture through the agency of the surface remodeling cells. Prostaglandins are important in the chain of events which lead to this architectural change and cytokines may also be involved (**Fig. 7-20**).

5. Interaction of the strain-related stimulus with other factors that affect remodeling takes place, possibly at the level of the osteoblast. Thus a strain-related

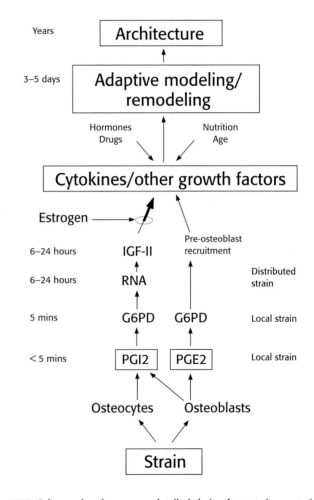

Fig. 7-20: Schema showing a more detailed chain of events in a putative mechanism for the adaptive response based on some of the in vivo and in vitro experimental work described in this chapter.

stimulus for modeling/remodeling might be opposed, enabled, or enhanced according to the local biochemical environment such as the hormonal milieu.

7 The function of the adaptive response in normal and abnormal bone

The normal adult skeleton has a stable architecture. This architecture can be viewed as the product of a bone correctly adapted to a normal loading environment, so that there is no requirement for adaptive change. Despite this apparent quiescence, the cellular processes of remodeling are still active, continually driving bone turnover for the replacement of damaged areas of matrix and allowing homeostatic control of systemic mineral ion levels. Although there is no adaptive change, there is still a role for the adaptive mechanism. It seems likely that processes of mineral ion release and repair of damaged matrix require some direction from a mechanically sensitive system. This would ensure that any remodeling involved in these processes does not adversely affect the bone architecture and its mechanical function. We propose that in an adult bone, the mechanically sensitive adaptive mechanism and general osteoprotective factors, such as estrogen and calcitonin, are in equilibrium with the resorptive drive of the calcium-regulating hormones such as PTH. Within this balanced system, remodeling occurs to allow repair or mineral turnover, but resorption is balanced by formation and the bone architecture remains unchanged. In the normal juvenile skeleton the situation is more complex because the genetic drive toward growth continually predisposes bone to formation. Any effect of the adaptive mechanism is therefore more difficult to distinguish [119].

If the equilibrium between osteogenic and resorptive factors is disturbed, the bone architecture will change until a new equilibrium position is reached. Such a disturbance might occur in normal bone undergoing a novel set of mechanical stimuli, such as that related to a new pattern of exercise. In this case,

the architecture at the new equilibrium position will be appropriate to the demands of the novel loading conditions. Some orthopedic problems and bone disease can also be interpreted as a disturbance of this equilibrium. Under these circumstances pathological factors may disturb the equilibrium, overriding the adaptive response, or an implant might disturb the normal strain distribution. The result is a new bone architecture, which may not be appropriate to the existing loading conditions. However, if the role of the adaptive response and the bone remodeling equilibrium is understood, it is possible to intervene with therapy designed to boost the adaptive response and restore a mechanically competent architecture.

7.1 The adaptive mechanism in normal bone turnover

Turnover occurs in bone to allow release of mineral ions or repair of damaged areas of the matrix. Bone removal is followed by equivalent formation, linked in the activation/resorption/formation (ARF) sequence [120]. At the surface of a bone osteoclasts resorb a hollow or pit, and in cortical bone this resorption can continue to form a tunnel. The hollow is subsequently filled in with a series of layers of bone, formed by osteoblasts. The filling of a tunnel results in the concentric laminae of a secondary osteone (haversian cylinder). As the adaptive mechanism can influence both osteoblasts and osteoclasts, it does not seem unreasonable to suppose that this mechanism could influence the remodeling activity of routine turnover.

The skeleton represents a large store of minerals which can be utilized systemically, especially when there is a particular requirement such as for calcium, during pregnancy, lactation, antler growth, egg-laying, or dietary insufficiency. The mineral is released by the physical destruction of bone tissue in the first phase of increased remodeling; this release is controlled hormonally [121]. In a mechanical and architectural sense, hormonally induced resorption will be indiscriminate in its effects on the skeleton, as there is no direct feedback to it from mechanical demand. However, local osteoprotective stimulus derived from the adaptive mechanism might delineate "preferred sites" at which the temporary loss of structural material would make the least impact on the load-bearing properties of the bone as a whole. An example of the apparent function of such a mechanism is the antler growth of deer. Here the bone loss during antler growth from the metacarpus, which is a bone with a primary mechanical role, is only a quarter of that from the ribs, although of course they must share a common hormonal environment [122].

Secondary osteonal bone is invariably weaker than the primary bone it replaces [123]. Thus, the only mechanical advantage of replacing primary cortical bone is as a method of repairing damaged tissue. It has been proposed that the existence of fatigue damage is a major stimulus for osteonal remodeling which replaces the damaged tissue [48, 124–126]. Such damage does occur in bone exposed to physiological strains [47], and it is not surprising that osteonal remodeling occurs most intensively in regions where either one would expect high strains, as around muscle insertions [127], or where high strains have actually been demonstrated, as in the caudal cortex of the sheep's radius [36].

Activation of osteoclastic cutting cones is increased as a result of disuse, microdamage caused by fatigue failure, and areas of devitalized bone [128]. The nature of the stimulus to activate and then target these cutting cones is not clear. Osteoclasts are activated by cells of the osteoblast lineage on the bone's surfaces [115]. As these cells can communicate with the osteocyte population, it is possible that a signal to activate, and perhaps subsequently guide, a cutting cone could come from osteocytes in the neighborhood of cracks. Alternatively, such a signal could be derived from the failure of osteocytes killed, or disabled by damage in their locality, to provide a continuing inhibitory signal to prevent osteoclast invasion. This latter interpretation fits better with devitalized bone also providing a stimulus for replacement. However, in areas of adaptation it is not uncommon for woven bone, established early in the adaptive process and containing recently deposited healthy osteocytes, to be selectively replaced by secondary osteons. It is possible therefore that osteonal targeting is achieved in response to a positive attracting signal or the absence of an inhibiting signal. Regardless of which process is involved, a communicating network of live cells would be required to transmit the need for remodeling to sites where osteoclasts may be recruited, and to convey the positional data necessary to target the cutting cone to the damaged area. Without some indication from the osteocyte network, either as a positive signal or absence of a negative one, it is difficult to see how osteoclasts, or the surface osteoblasts thought to control them, would have the relevant information for the targeting process.

While an attractive possibility, there is as yet no direct evidence that osteocytes influence the activation or subsequent targeting of osteoclastic cutting cones. Secondary osteonal remodeling in acellular teleost bone does not seem to require osteocytic direction [129]. However, it seems a reasonable hypothesis that the adaptive mechanism exerts an osteoprotective influence on remodeling activity occurring within bones which are not undergoing any overall change in architecture. Such an arrangement represents a feedback of information on physical parameters and might prevent unrestrained remodeling activity compromising the mechanical function of the bone.

7.2   Decreased strain/disuse osteoporosis

If a bone's customary level of strain is decreased, more bone is present than is warranted by the current mechanical demand and bone is lost from the skeleton. Bone loss occurs over a period during which the remodeling rate increases, and each remodeling episode replaces less bone than it removes. In cancellous bone this results in thinning of trabecular plates and loss of interconnections between them. In cortical bone, incomplete refilling of secondary osteones and endosteal resorption leads to a thinned porotic cortex. This swing toward resorption appears to be the result of hormonal stimulation no longer countered by the conservation effect of load-bearing [111]. The bone loss can occur at a local level, as in a patient with a cast limb, or at a general level such as in bed rest or space flight [130, 131]. In totally immobilized limbs a new equilibrium is reached after a few weeks and no further overall loss occurs, although the level of remodeling activity remains higher than in normal functional bone [6]. This base level may represent a minimum mass for a bone, representing the mass a bone attains without any functional stimulus. It is possible that this represents the basic genetically derived bone mass.

Experiments such as those of Jaworski and Uhthoff [5] have shown that remobilization can reverse disuse osteoporosis. Prolonged immobilization appears to make the restoration of normal bone cell activity a slow process [132], but if this activity is restored, there is a chance to reattain the original bone mass. The in vivo experiments described earlier [55] show that the onset of disuse osteoporosis can be antagonized by mechanical loading. The application of PEMFs to slow surface resorption (**Fig. 7-21**) [73, 74] or the use of capacitive coupling [133] also appear to be of some use in the control of bone loss. Thus it appears that there is the potential for stimulation via the adaptive response to re-establish the balance between resorption and formation, and this potential may become a useful basis for therapy in osteoporosis.

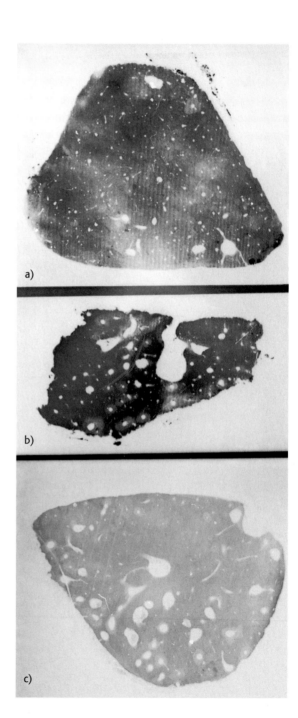

a)

b)

c)

Fig. 7-21: Disuse osteoporosis and the effect of PEMFs. a) is a microradiograph of the normal canine fibula and b) shows the remodeling and osteopenia induced in the contralateral fibula by 12 weeks isolation from functional loading. c) shows how the cross-sectional area of a fibula, similarly isolated from loading, was preserved by PEMF treatment for an hour every day over the 12-week period after isolation. Note that although the overall shape of the fibula cross-section was preserved, PEMF treatment did not arrest the increase in intracortical remodeling responsible for the increased cortical porosity.

7.3 Increased strains, cycle numbers, and change in strain distribution

There are numerous examples of increased loading, or unusual loading regimes, leading to adaptive bone modeling. Increase in bone mass has been noted in the humerus of the serving arm of tennis players [119, 134], the tibiae of weight lifters and ballet dancers [135], and in the wrists of subjects specifically exercising the area analyzed [136]. It is therefore possible that training regimes can be designed to increase bone mass in mechanically appropriate fashion. A general increase in physical activity is not always correlated with increased bone mass [137], but small amounts [138] or short bursts [139] of unusual or unaccustomed exercise do increase bone formation. These findings coincide with the experimental evidence that short periods of loading at unusual strain distributions are effective in activating and saturating the adaptive response. It is also clear that changing exercise patterns can change the material properties of bone and, therefore, its resistance to damage and fracture [140].

If bone is repeatedly deformed, even at a level well below its ultimate or yield strains (**Fig. 7-10**), microdamage may occur. The amount of this damage will depend on the number of loading cycles and the strain that each one involves. If the rate of accumulation of this damage exceeds the capacity of the bone physiology to repair it, a fatigue fracture will result. If the adaptive mechanism is primarily sensitive to low cycle numbers of error strains, there may be no mechanism to adjust bone architecture to the number of imposed cycles rather than their nature. Thus the only mechanism for protection against microdamage accumulation may be repair of the existing cortex.

7.3.1 Fatigue (stress) fracture

The fatigue fracture is a manifestation of microdamage accumulation and depends upon the location and nature of the mismatch between structure and function. Thus these fractures occur in the characteristic patterns which relate to the abnormal loading of a particular bone or a structural deficiency in a particular bone—in healthy, often young, individuals who embark upon an increased activity regimen such as a humans taking up a new sport, army recruits being introduced to training, and dogs and racehorses in athletic training [141, 142]. Under these conditions it is probable that the bone is strained to a higher level, in a different manner, and much more frequently than is usual. Such a change in activity may engender a new strain environment and adaptive modeling. The new "target" architecture may be suitable to withstand the increased cycle number as well as the new strain distribution for which we assume it is "designed". However, maintenance of the new activity at the initial high level will make the occurrence of any adaptive increase in cortical thickness impossible, before intracortical damage and increased remodeling lead toward progressive, radiologically apparent stress fracture.

Fatigue fractures are also common in athletes and ballet dancers at the height of their performance and during their most intensive training. Often the stress fracture is, however, precipitated by some change in training regimen [143], which, by loading the bone in a manner for which it was not prepared, causes substantial damage within the bone cortex. Such athletes undergo continuous training and their bone architecture is likely to be fully adapted to its strain environment, with cortical mass dependent on peak strain. However, under the extreme conditions of training, the number of strain cycles imposed on a bone is abnormally high. Fatigue failure is caused by a combination of the size and number of strain cycles; if the cortical thickness is determined by the peak strain and not the number of cycles, one would expect this level of activity to cause considerable damage which, in turn, would induce a high level of reparative remodeling. The combination of a high level of activity imposing high and frequent strains on a cortex containing resorption spaces is ideal for fatigue failure. Muscular fatigue reduces the efficiency with which the soft tissues can protect the hard tissues from high-impact loads. This effect in athletes pushing themselves to the limit would almost certainly increase the peak strains and further predispose to fatigue damage.

In the elderly, especially women, there is a progressive loss in the amount of bone tissue present in the skeleton [144]. The result of this is likely to be an increase in the amount of strain induced by each activity. Fatigue damage, including that in cancellous bone, can accumulate in areas such as the vertebrae and upper femur, leading to complete collapse of these structures under what would normally be the trivial loading of minor, everyday activities [50, 145].

The amount of strain for each activity is also likely to be increased when the structural or material strength of the bone is decreased by a pathological condition. The collapse of vertebrae or fatigue failure of femoral necks in postmenopausal osteoporosis and the buckling of thin-walled long bones in osteogenesis imperfecta are examples of this [146].

7.4 Sudden changes of strain distribution in trauma or implant surgery

The adaptive mechanism is unable to prevent fractures as it has no prior information of a fracturing overload to mount a strategic response to, and in a fatigue fracture situation it appears to be unable to stimulate enough modeling/remodeling to stop a failure. However, the normal bone conformation for which the adaptive mechanism is responsible has a considerable "safety margin" between the amount of strain normally imposed on the bone and the ultimate strain that the structure is capable of withstanding [147]. Fractures, the implants that are used to treat them, and other implants such as those used in arthroplasty surgery all cause an immediate disturbance in the normal strain environment of the bone. However, there is considerable evidence that the adaptive mechanism is involved early on in the reaction to such a disturbance.

7.4.1 Fracture, interfragmentary strain, and dynamization

When a fracture does occur, the normal strain environment of the bone is completely disrupted, and there will be little mechanical feedback to drive the adaptive response. Once a callus is established, the remodeling required to re-establish the normal cortical architecture presumably requires orchestration by the adaptive mechanism, as there is no other feedback system for mechanical information. Thus strain through the fracture is important to stimulate the adaptive response and complete fracture healing.

Although excessive motion at a fracture site can obviously lead to a failure of bone union, the natural process of fracture healing involving the formation of a stabilizing callus is stimulated by loading and motion [148, 149]. Motion and loading are thought to stimulate the inflammatory phase of fracture healing, especially revascularization [150]. These mechanical phenomena can affect the differentiation between primary and secondary bone union and lead to the correct differentiation of tissue in callus [151]. Not surprisingly, when motion and loading are removed by rigid internal fixation, healing can be adversely affected. The imposition of axial micromovement through a rigid fixation device can improve both the biological and mechanical healing of fractures, leading to faster and stronger repair [152]. Similarly, significantly increasing the stiffness of an external fixator frame can reduce the rate of fracture healing [153]; also, the reduction of frame stiffness, particularly after the first 4 weeks of repair, can increase the strength of that repair [154]. Such ideas underlie the gradual reduction of frame stiffness practiced in the process of dynamization [155]. Perhaps the most dramatic example of the effect of mechanical conditions on fracture repair is the process of distraction osteogenesis, where mechanical strain induced by lengthening under Ilizarov techniques induces osteoblast proliferation and matrix deposition in a process which is different from other methods of fracture repair [156].

7.4.2 "Stress protection" due to implants in fracture repair

It has become one of the objectives of modern fracture management to restore function to the affected parts as rapidly as possible and so avoid the disuse osteoporosis, muscle wasting, and joint stiffness which are common sequels to prolonged immobilization [157]. Rigid internal fixation of the fracture is one means of achieving this. The fracture is reduced and the fragments are held in place by wires, screws, or plates in such a manner that light functional loads may be transmitted through the bones almost immediately. There is a balance to be made between application of an implant which cannot carry the load normally withstood by the bone and which depends on load sharing with the repaired fragments, and implants which can resist all the applied loads, but which may protect the fracture from all mechanical influences. To understand this balance requires specific knowledge of the relationship between the shape and loading configuration of the bone in question (**Fig. 7-7a**).

Although correct application of implants may allow early mobilization of the whole limb, the presence of the implants inevitably affects the strain distribution in the treated bone. It has been shown that in sheep in which the radius was subjected to osteotomy and fixed with a compression plate, the intermittent surface strain during locomotion, once initial lameness was overcome, was reduced to 1/3 of normal directly beneath the plate, while being practically normal on the opposite cortex [**34, 158**]. This reduction in the normal functional stimulus of part of the bone is called stress protection or stress shielding (**Fig. 7-8**). It is often associated with, and presumed to be, the cause of a localized area of osteoporosis, which can become a point of weakness and potential fracture. This osteopenia does not increase indefinitely after application of an implant [**159**]. It is complicated by the fact that implants, such as plates which affect the bone surface directly, also cause a short-term local bone loss which is related to vascular disturbance [**160**]. Once the bone loss has reached a certain level it ceases, and this level presumably represents an equilibrium between the bone with its decreased functional demand and the implant with which it is now load sharing.

Stress protection is most commonly seen in conjunction with plate fixation [**149**]. Plates are often used as neutralization or buttress support for fractures and take a large proportion of any imposed load. External fixators used in a configuration which takes a large proportion of the bone load can also cause stress protection. Intramedullary nails, which act as a gliding implant, cause a significant proportion of applied load, especially axial compression, to be carried by the bone fragments; thus the loss of functional stimulus is avoided [**149**]. It may be possible to use a similar idea in plate fixation by devising plates with less bending stiffness, which will allow more load sharing with the bone [**161, 162**]. However, a loss of stiffness in bone plates to decrease osteopenia may conflict unfavorably with the use of plates for fracture reduction in which stiffness can be most useful. External fixators can be "dynamized" [**155**] to increase loading across the fracture site and thus reduce osteopenia once bridging has occurred. This process involves adjustment of the fixator frame, normally by removal of some of the fixation pins, which weakens the fixator and thus increases the proportion of the load which the bone carries.

The osteopenic area may be at most danger of fracture when its protective implant is removed [**163**], which has lead some authors to recommend a diminished number of plate removals [**164**] except with local complication related to the implant. However, providing there is no slowing of bone remodeling due to infection, avascularity, or old age, the porotic cortex should become rapidly and uneventfully filled in, as the adaptive response functions in relation to the restoration of normal activity. In practice, this means that the patient should have an initial regimen of splinting and reduced exercise, with a subsequent gradual return to normal function [**164**].

7.4.3 Change in strain environment due to permanent prostheses

Implants such as hip and knee prostheses distort the normal strain environment, as the load across the joint is transferred via the bone/implant interface rather than the normal trabecular bone network [165]. This change in the strain environment is more significant than that imposed during fracture healing as it is permanent. With such a change in the strain environment, an adaptive change in bone architecture might be expected, and this can cause problems both in loosening the current implant and in increasing the difficulty of placing a second implant during a revision procedure. Bone loss has been demonstrated in the proximal femur after hip arthroplasty using both cemented [165] and non-cemented [166] prostheses. This problem appears to be greatest in the non-cemented prostheses which are stiffer and consequently "stress protect" the proximal portion of the femur to a greater degree. Attempts to design prostheses which stimulate the adaptive mechanism and support bone formation have been made using finite element analysis to predict the biological response to different designs [167]. It is clear that some solutions to the bone/implant interface are much better than others in terms of load transfer. However, some of the best solutions have drawbacks in terms of implant loosening due to endosteal resorption. Stress shielding is not the only mechanism causing bone loss in the proximal femur, and factors such as wear debris and implant instability contribute to the problem [168]. The task of designing improved prostheses, especially non-cemented prostheses, is one in which the adaptive response and the correct conditions at the bone/implant interface must be brought together to provide a clinically improved implant.

7.5 The hormonal environment and bone architecture

The effects of systemic hormones on bone can frustrate or limit the effects of the adaptive response. Numerous systemic hormones can affect bone [121, 169], but most of these effects are on growth and are observed during bone development or seen during a hormonal imbalance due to systemic disease. Estrogens can induce new bone formation directly [170], but this appears to be independent of the adaptive response. There is however a hormonal effect which interacts with the adaptive response of major clinical importance, that is the loss of osteoprotective estrogens after the menopause which leads to bone loss in women.

7.5.1 Senile and postmenopausal osteoporosis

In senile and postmenopausal osteoporosis the main clinical problem is bone loss from the trabecular network of the vertebrae, long-bone epiphyses, and similar areas, which leads to an increased incidence of fracture. In the centers of the spinal vertebrae, loss of activity may result in loss of the off-axis loading of the tissue that generates error signals in the trabeculae. This may primarily affect the horizontal trabeculae that support the meshwork, rather than the vertical ones whose primary role is carrying the normal axial load. If the horizontal trabeculae "perceive" this as disuse, they will tend to be resorbed, especially if there is a hormonal environment such as loss of estrogen which facilitates resorption (Fig. 7-22). Age-related reduction and elimination of horizontal trabeculae [144], inability of axial loading exercise to increase spinal bone mass [171], and the ability of some exercise to increase spinal bone mass [172] are consistent with such a hypothesis. Without the horizontal trabeculae the vertebrae are much more vulnerable to crush fracture from occasional off-axis loading. Although the loading patterns of cortical bone are more complex—involving tension, compression, torsion, and bending—we believe that each bone recognizes a particular

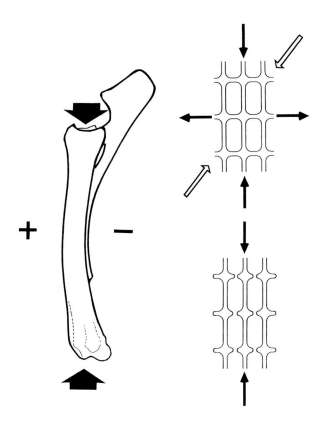

Fig. 7-22: Loading patterns in cancellous and cortical bone. The curvature of the long bone engenders bending and relatively high strains under axial loading *(large black arrows)*. Such high strains do not permit a "minimum structure" but the deformation of the bone is always in a predictable direction. The trabeculae of cancellous bone appear to be positioned to avoid bending. In many situations where trabecular bone is found, the vertical trabeculae are directly loaded and the horizontal trabeculae provide support to prevent buckling of the vertical tracts under high loads. Axial compressive loads *(solid arrows)* will only cause strain in the indirectly loaded horizontal trabeculae if they are high enough to engender buckling in the directly loaded vertical trabeculae. However, the horizontal trabeculae will be loaded by off-axis loads *(open arrows)*. In situations where axial strains are low, and abnormal loading resulting in off-axis strains *(open arrows)* is infrequent, the horizontal trabeculae may be lost through disuse. Such a pattern of activity is more likely in the older person. If the horizontal trabeculae are lost in this way, then the trabecular meshwork loses its ability to support loads that may buckle the vertical trabeculae and so is more vulnerable to failure.

strain environment as normal, and so a restricted range of normal (error-free) loading produces a minimal adaptive response. Thus, a decrease in the number of error cycles and their magnitude and strain rate will reduce the stimulus for formation and allow weakening of the bone by resorption.

During the process of aging the hormonal and nutritional climate moves toward bone resorption, particularly in post-menopausal women, due to the loss of osteoprotective estrogens. If this is accompanied by a loss in the vigor and variety of movement, then the stimulus for an appropriate bone architecture is also reduced and the influences leading to resorption are practically unopposed, allowing loss of bone to the point at which the skeleton becomes vulnerable to incidental fracture. Exercise can be used to maintain or increase bone mass in osteoporosis, particularly in postmenopausal women [107, 173–176]. In a review of a hundred exercise studies in humans [174], it was concluded that a combination of relatively vigorous aerobic and strength training was most effective, which is in accordance with a mechanism sensitive to error-strain stimulation. It appears that the osteogenic effect of the adaptive response to appropriate loading can be used to antagonize osteoporotic bone loss. Although such mechanical loading can provide a stimulus for an appropriate bone architecture, a sensible therapeutic strategy is to enhance the effects of this stimulus as much as possible. Thus calcium supplementation [177], and hormonal therapy where appropriate [178, 179], may enable and even enhance the effects of the mechanical stimulus [180].

Prevention of osteoporosis may involve treatment and exercise regimes throughout the period of potential bone loss. If the regulation of bone architecture is homeostatic, then the strategy of achieving high bone mass between 20 and 35 years of age may be redundant as the bone mass will be reduced to the target level as soon as the therapy is withdrawn, and there is evidence to support this as women with higher bone mass lose bone faster [181]. Individuals with a high bone mass may have a genetically more robust skeleton, or a more robust response to loading, and will lose bone more slowly. There is evidence for a hereditary component [182] in osteoporosis which has been related to specific gene expression [183], so the effect of individual characteristics such as a robust skeleton cannot be extrapolated to the whole population without an understanding of the individual's genetic makeup.

8 Conclusions

The concept of an adaptive response is central to the function of bone physiology, as it is the only system by which the elements of the skeleton can gain information concerning the mechanical demands upon them and thus adapt to meet these demands. The system appears to involve the osteocytes' sensitivity to the strain induced in the matrix by loading. These cells can interact to build a complex appreciation of the strain environment acting on a bone and can, if necessary, control a strategic change in the bone architecture to meet the demands of a novel strain environment. The adaptive response interacts with the genetic and systemic influences on bone to produce the best architectural solution to the imposed loads within the confines of systemic and genetic boundaries, which determine parameters such as size, weight, shape, and mineral availability.

The hypothesis for the mechanism of the adaptive response put forward here is the result of a large number of experiments, but also fits well with the way in which bone responds in a variety of clinical conditions. Understanding the adaptive mechanism is a primary goal in orthopedic treatment as it allows the clinical orthopedist to select treatments which enhance the ability of bone to adjust and readjust its architecture in a way appropriate to the demands placed upon it, rather than imposing a solution to the detriment of the normal physiology. By working with, rather than against, the complex physiology of bone we may hope to solve more of the problems of skeletal disease and induce fewer failures by intervening in the wrong place at the wrong time.

9   Bibliography

Blue references indicate links to abstracts of articles available online:
http://www.aopublishing.org/BONE/7.htm

1. **Carter DR, Blenman PR, Beaupre GS** (1988) Correlations between mechanical stress history and tissue differentiation in initial fracture healing.
   J Orthop Res; 6 (5):736–748.

2. **Currey JD** (1979) Mechanical properties of bone tissues with greatly differing functions.
   J Biomech; 12 (4):313–319.

3. **Hosseini A, Hogg DA** (1991) The effects of paralysis on skeletal development in the chick embryo. II. Effects on histogenesis of the tibia.
   J Anat; 177:169–178.

4. **Uhthoff HK, Jaworski ZF** (1978) Bone loss in response to long-term immobilisation.
   J Bone Joint Surg [Br]; 60 (3):420–429.

5. **Jaworski ZF, Uhthoff HK** (1986) Reversibility of nontraumatic disuse osteoporosis during its active phase.
   Bone; 7 (6):431–439.

6. **Garland DE, Stewart CA, Adkins RH, et al.** (1992) Osteoporosis after spinal cord injury.
   J Orthop Res; 10 (3):371–378.

7. **Vaananen HK** (1991) Pathogenesis of osteoporosis.
   Calcif Tissue Int; 49 (Suppl):S11–14.

8. **Ralis ZA, Ralis HM, Randall M, et al.** (1997) Changes in the shape, ossification and quality of bones from developing paralysed limbs. A clinico-pathological and experimental study.
   J Bone Joint Surg; 59:251.

9. **Roberts WE, Goodwin WC, Heiner SR** (1981) Cellular response to orthodontic force.
   Dent Clin North Am; 25 (1):3–17.

10. **Lanyon LE** (1980) The influence of function on the development of bone curvature. An experimental study on the rat tibia. *J Zool Lond;* 192:457.

11. **Roux W** (1885) Beiträge zur Morphologie der funktionellen Anpassung. 3. Beschreibung und Erläuterung einer knöchernen Kniegelenksankylose.
    Arch Anat Physiol.

12. **Culmann C** (1875) *Die Graphische Statik.* 2nd ed. Zürich: Meyer & Zeller.

13. **Wolff J** (1870) Ueber die innere Architecktur der Knochen und ihre Bedeutung fur die Frage vom Knochenwachstum.
    Virchow's Arch; 50:389.

14. **Koch JD** (1917) The laws of bone architecture. *Am J Anat;* 21:177.

15. **Wolff J** (1892) *Das Gestez der Transformation der Knochen.* Berlin: Verlag August Hirschwald.

16. **Roesler H** (1981) Some historical remarks on the theory of cancellous bone structure (Wolff's law). In: Cowin SC, editor. *Mechanical Properties of Bone.* New York: Am Soc Mech Engineering, 27.

17. **Frost HM** (1964) *The Laws of Bone Structure.* Springfield, Ill.: CC Thomas.

18. **Bassett CA** (1968) Biologic significance of piezoelectricity.
    Calcif Tissue Res; 1 (4):252–272.

19. **Evans FG** (1953) Method of studying biomechanical significance of bone form.
    Am J Phys Anthropol; 11:353.

20. **Lanyon LE, Smith RN** (1970) Bone strain in the tibia during normal quadrupedal locomotion.
    Acta Orthop Scand; 41 (3):238–248.

21. **Lanyon LE** (1976) The measurement of bone strain "in vivo".
    Acta Orthop Belg; 42 (Suppl 1):98–108.

22. **Dally JW, Riley WF** (1978) Analysis of strain-gage data. In: Dally JW, Riley WF, editors. *Experimental Stress Analysis.* New York: McGraw Hill.

23. **Rubin CT, Lanyon LE** (1984) Dynamic strain similarity in vertebrates; an alternative to allometric limb bone scaling.
    J Theor Biol; 107 (2):321–327.

24. **Lanyon LE, Hampson WG, Goodship AE, et al.** (1975) Bone deformation recorded in vivo from strain gauges attached to the human tibial shaft.
    Acta Orthop Scand; 46 (2):256–268.

25. **Lanyon LE** (1974) Experimental support for the trajectorial theory of bone structure.
    J Bone Joint Surg [Br]; 56 (1):160–166.

26. **Hayes WC, Snyder B** (1981) Toward a quantitative formulation of Wolff's Law in trabecular bone. In: Cowin SC, editor. *Mechanical Properties of Bone.* New York: Am Soc Mech Engineering, 43.

27. **Pauwels F** (1980) *Biomechanics of the Locomotor System.* Berlin Heidelberg New York: Springer-Verlag.

28. **Frost HM** (1990) Skeletal structural adaptations to mechanical usage (SATMU): 1. Redefining Wolff's law: the bone modeling problem.
    Anat Rec; 226 (4):403–413.

29. **Cowin SC** (1984) Mechanical modeling of the stress adaptation process in bone. *Calcif Tissue Int;* 36 (Suppl 1):S98–103.

30. **Carter DR, Fyhrie DP, Whalen RT** (1987) Trabecular bone density and loading history: regulation of connective tissue biology by mechanical energy.
    J Biomech; 20 (8):785–794.

31. **Frost HM** (1986) *Intermediary Organisation of the Skeleton.* Boca Raton: CRC Press.

32. **Frost HM** (1983) Pharmacology and the osteoporoses: a field in flux.
    Methods Find Exp Clin Pharmacol; 5 (1):5–16.

33. **Burr DB, Schaffler MB, Yang KH, et al.** (1989) The effects of altered strain environments on bone tissue kinetics. *Bone;* 10 (3):215–221.

34. **Lanyon LE, Bourn S** (1979) The influence of mechanical function on the development and remodeling of the tibia. An experimental study in sheep.
J Bone Joint Surg [Am]; 61 (2):263–273.

35. **Rubin CT, Lanyon LE** (1982) Limb mechanics as a function of speed and gait: a study of functional strains in the radius and tibia of horse and dog.
J Exp Biol; 101:187–211.

36. **Lanyon LE, Magee PT, Baggott DG** (1979) The relationship of functional stress and strain to the processes of bone remodelling. An experimental study on the sheep radius.
J Biomech; 12 (8):593–600.

37. **Biewener AA, Thomason J, Lanyon LE** (1983) Mechanics of locomotion and jumping in the forelimb of the horse (Equus): In vivo stress developed in the radius and metacarpus.
J Zool Lond; 201:67.

38. **Bertram JE, Biewener AA** (1988) Bone curvature: sacrificing strength for load predictability?
J Theor Biol; 131 (1):75–92.

39. **Sedillot CE** (1864) De l'influence des fonctions sur la structure et la forme des organes.
C R Acad Sci; 59:539.

40. **Hert J, Pribylova E, Liskova M** (1972) Reaction of bone to mechanical stimuli. 3. Microstructure of compact bone of rabbit tibia after intermittent loading.
Acta Anat; 82 (2):218–230.

41. **Hert J, Babicky A, Mertl F** (1972) Response of bone to mechanical stimuli changes in blood supply of compact bone during intermittent mechanical loading.
Physiol Bohemoslov; 21 (3):265–272.

42. **Lanyon LE, Rubin CT** (1984) Static vs dynamic loads as an influence on bone remodeling.
J Biomech; 17 (12):897–905.

43. **Hert J, Liskova M, Landa J** (1971) Reaction of bone to mechanical stimuli. 1. Continuous and intermittent loading of tibia in rabbit.
Folia Morphol (Praha); 19 (3):290–300.

44. **Liskova M, Hert J** (1971) Reaction of bone to mechanical stimuli. 2. Periosteal and endosteal reaction of tibial diaphysis in rabbit to intermittent loading.
Folia Morphol (Praha); 19 (3):301–317.

45. **Goodship AE, Lanyon LE, McFie H** (1979) Functional adaptation of bone to increased stress. An experimental study.
J Bone Joint Surg [Am]; 61 (4):539–546.

46. **Lanyon LE, Goodship AE, Pye CJ, et al.** (1982) Mechanically adaptive bone remodelling.
J Biomech; 15 (3):141–154.

47. **Schaffler MB, Radin EL, Burr DB** (1989) Mechanical and morphological effects of strain rate on fatigue of compact bone.
Bone; 10 (3):207–214.

48. **Burr DB, Martin RB, Schaffler MB, et al.** (1985) Bone remodeling in response to in vivo fatigue microdamage.
J Biomech; 18 (3):189–200.

49. **Doty SB** (1981) Morphological evidence of gap junctions between bone cells.
Calcif Tissue Int; 33 (5):509–512.

50. **Menton LJ, Riggs BL** (1986) Hip fracture: A disease and an accident. In: Uhthoff HK, editor. *Current Concepts of Bone Fragility.* Berlin Heidelberg New York: Springer-Verlag, 385.

51. **Carter DR** (1984) Mechanical loading histories and cortical bone remodeling.
Calcif Tissue Int; 36 (Suppl 1):19–24.

52. **Cowin SC, Van Buskirk WC** (1979) Surface bone remodeling induced by a medullary pin.
J Biomech; 12 (4):269–276.

53. **Cowin SC, Hart RT, Balser JR, et al.** (1985) Functional adaptation in long bones: establishing in vivo values for surface remodeling rate coefficients.
J Biomech; 18 (9):665–684.

54. **Brown TD, Pedersen DR, Gray ML, et al.** (1990) Toward an identification of mechanical parameters initiating periosteal remodeling: a combined experimental and analytic approach.
J Biomech; 23 (9):893–905.

55. **Rubin CT, Lanyon LE** (1984) Regulation of bone formation by applied dynamic loads. *J Bone Joint Surg [Am];* 66 (3):397–402.

56. **McLeod K, Rubin CT** (1990) Predictions of osteogenic mechanical loading paradigms from electrical response data.
Trans Biol Growth Repro Soc; 9:20.

57. **O'Connor JA, Lanyon LE, MacFie H** (1982) The influence of strain rate on adaptive bone remodelling.
J Biomech; 15 (10):767–781.

58. **Qin YX, Rubin CT, McLeod KJ** (1998) Nonlinear dependence of loading intensity and cycle number in the maintenance of bone mass and morphology.
J Orthop Res; 16 (4):482–489.

59. **Pead MJ, Skerry TM, Lanyon LE** (1988) Direct transformation from quiescence to bone formation in the adult periosteum following a single brief period of bone loading.
J Bone Miner Res; 3 (6):647–656.

60. **Judex S, Gross TS, Zernicke RF** (1997) Strain gradients correlate with sites of exercise-induced bone-forming surfaces in the adult skeleton.
J Bone Miner Res; 12 (10): 1737–1745.

61. Pead MJ, Lanyon LE (1990) Adaptive remodelling in bone: Torsion versus compression. *Orthop Trans;* 14:340.

62. Mosley JR, March BM, Lynch J, et al. (1997) Strain magnitude related changes in whole bone architecture in growing rats. *Bone;* 20 (3):191–198.

63. Lanyon LE (1987) Functional strain in bone tissue as an objective, and controlling stimulus for adaptive bone remodelling. *J Biomech;* 20 (11–12):1083–1093.

64. Jendrucko RJ, Hyman WA, Newell PH, et al. (1976) Theoretical evidence for the generation of high pressure in bone cells. *J Biomech;* 9 (2):87–91.

65. Bagi C, Burger EH (1989) Mechanical stimulation by intermittent compression stimulates sulfate incorporation and matrix mineralization in fetal mouse long-bone rudiments under serum-free conditions. *Calcif Tissue Int;* 45 (6): 342–347.

66. Justus R, Luft JH (1970) A mechanochemical hypothesis for bone remodeling induced by mechanical stress. *Calcif Tissue Res;* 5 (3):222–235.

67. Pollack SR, Korostoff E, Starkebaum W, et al. (1979) Microelectrode studies of stress generated potentials in bone. In: Brighton CT, Black J, Pollack SR, editors. *Electrical Properties of Bone and Cartilage.* New York: Grune & Stratton, 69.

68. Lanyon LE, Hartman W (1977) Strain related electrical potentials recorded in vitro and in vivo. *Calcif Tissue Res;* 22 (3):315–327.

69. MacGinitie LA, Wu DD, Cochran GV (1993) Streaming potentials in healing, remodeling, and intact cortical bone. *J Bone Miner Res;* 8 (11):1323–1335.

70. Brighton CT, Friedenberg ZB, Zemsky LM, et al. (1975) Direct-current stimulation of non-union and congenital pseudarthrosis. Exploration of its clinical application. *J Bone Joint Surg [Am];* 57 (3):368–377.

71. Bassett CA (1984) The development and application of pulsed electromagnetic fields (PEMFs) for ununited fractures and arthrodeses. *Orthop Clin North Am;* 15 (1):61–87.

72. Rubin CT, McLeod KJ, Lanyon LE (1989) Prevention of osteoporosis by pulsed electromagnetic fields. *J Bone Joint Surg [Am];* 71 (3):411–417.

73. Skerry TM, Pead MJ, Lanyon LE (1991) Modulation of bone loss during disuse by pulsed electromagnetic fields. *J Orthop Res;* 9 (4):600–608.

74. Pead MJ, Skerry TM, Rubin CT, et al. (1990) Treatment of disuse osteopaenia with pulsed electromagnetic fields. *Orthop Trans;* 14:435.

75. Skerry TM, Bitensky L, Chayen J, et al. (1988) Loading-related reorientation of bone proteoglycan in vivo. Strain memory in bone tissue? *J Orthop Res;* 6 (4):547–551.

76. Skerry TM, Suswillo R, el Haj AJ, et al. (1990) Load-induced proteoglycan orientation in bone tissue in vivo and in vitro. *Calcif Tissue Int;* 46 (5):318–326.

77. Dodds R, Skerry TM, Pead MJ, et al. (1990) Proteoglycan orientation in bone: Its relationship to loading, disuse and clinical osteoporosis. *Proc Ann Mtg Orthop Res Soc;* 36:572.

78. Ferris BD, Klenerman L, Dodds RA, et al. (1987) Altered organization of non-collagenous bone matrix in osteoporosis. *Bone;* 8 (5):285–288.

79. Jones DB, Bingmann D (1991) How do osteoblasts respond to mechanical stimulation? *Cells Matls;* 1:1.

80. Yeh CK, Rodan GA (1984) Tensile forces enhance prostaglandin E synthesis in osteoblastic cells grown on collagen ribbons. *Calcif Tissue Int;* 36 (Suppl 1):67–71.

81. Binderman I, Zor U, Kaye AM, et al. (1988) The transduction of mechanical force into biochemical events in bone cells may involve activation of phospholipase A2. *Calcif Tissue Int;* 42 (4):261–266.

82. Rawlinson SC, el-Haj AJ, Minter SL, et al. (1991) Loading-related increases in prostaglandin production in cores of adult canine cancellous bone in vitro: a role for prostacyclin in adaptive bone remodeling? *J Bone Miner Res;* 6 (12):1345–1351.

83. Tanaka-Kamioka K, Kamioka H, Ris H, et al. (1998) Osteocyte shape is dependent on actin filaments and osteocyte processes are unique actin-rich projections. *J Bone Miner Res;* 13 (10):1555–1568.

84. Toma CD, Ashkar S, Gray ML, et al. (1997) Signal transduction of mechanical stimuli is dependent on microfilament integrity: identification of osteopontin as a mechanically induced gene in osteoblasts. *J Bone Miner Res;* 12 (10):1626–1636.

85. Skerry TM, Bitensky L, Chayen J, et al. (1989) Early strain-related changes in enzyme activity in osteocytes following bone loading in vivo. *J Bone Miner Res;* 4 (5):783–788.

86. Pead MJ, Suswillo R, Skerry TM, et al. (1988) Increased 3H-uridine levels in osteocytes following a single short period of dynamic bone loading in vivo. *Calcif Tissue Int;* 43 (2):92–96.

87. Curtis TA, Ashrafi SH, Weber DF (1985) Canalicular communication in the cortices of human long bones. *Anat Rec;* 212 (4):336–344.

88. **Binderman I, Shimshoni Z, Somjen D** (1984) Biochemical pathways involved in the translation of physical stimulus into biological message. *Calcif Tissue Int;* 36 (Suppl 1):S82–85.

89. **Chambers TJ, Ali NN** (1983) Inhibition of osteoclastic motility by prostaglandins I2, E1, E2 and 6- oxo-E1. *J Pathol;* 139 (3):383–397.

90. **Ali NN, Melhuish PB, Boyde A, et al.** (1990) Parathyroid hormone, but not prostaglandin E2, changes the shape of osteoblasts maintained on bone in vitro. *J Bone Miner Res;* 5 (2):115–121.

91. **McSheehy PM, Chambers TJ** (1986) Osteoblast-like cells in the presence of parathyroid hormone release soluble factor that stimulates osteoclastic bone resorption. *Endocrinology;* 119 (4):1654–1659.

92. **Jee WS, Ueno K, Kimmel DB, et al.** (1987) The role of bone cells in increasing metaphyseal hard tissue in rapidly growing rats treated with prostaglandin E2. *Bone;* 8 (3):171–178.

93. **Pead MJ, Lanyon LE** (1989) Indomethacin modulation of load-related stimulation of new bone formation in vivo. *Calcif Tissue Int;* 45 (1):34–40.

94. **Chow JW, Chambers TJ** (1994) Indomethacin has distinct early and late actions on bone formation induced by mechanical stimulation. *Am J Physiol;* 267 (2 Pt 1):E287–292.

95. **el Haj A, et al.** (1988) Proteoglycans in bone tissue: Identification and possible function in strain related bone remodelling. *Orthop Trans;* 11:145.

96. **el Haj AJ, Minter SL, Rawlinson SC, et al.** (1990) Cellular responses to mechanical loading in vitro. *J Bone Miner Res;* 5 (9):923–932.

97. **Minter SL** (1991) *The use of in vitro techniques to investigate cellular responses to mechanical load in bone* [PhD]. Univ London.

98. **Rawlinson SC, Mohan S, Baylink DJ, et al.** (1993) Exogenous prosta-cyclin, but not prostaglandin E2, produces similar responses in both G6PD activity and RNA production as mechanical loading, and increases IGF-II release, in adult cancellous bone in culture. *Calcif Tissue Int;* 53 (5):324–329.

99. **Zaman G, Suswillo RF, Cheng MZ, et al.** (1997) Early responses to dynamic strain change and prosta-glandins in bone-derived cells in culture. *J Bone Miner Res;* 12 (5):769–777.

100. **Rawlinson SC, Pitsillides AA, Lanyon LE** (1996) Involvement of different ion channels in osteoblasts' and osteocytes' early responses to mechanical strain. *Bone;* 19 (6):609–614.

101. **Feyen JH, Di Bon A, van der Plas A, et al.** (1985) Effects of exo-genous prostanoids on the prolifera-tion of osteoblast-like cells in vitro. *Prostaglandins;* 30 (5):827–840.

102. **Finkelman RD, Mohan S, Jennings JC, et al.** (1990) Quantitation of growth factors IGF-I, SGF/IGF-II, and TGF-beta in human dentin. *J Bone Miner Res;* 5 (7):717–723.

103. **Wergedal JE, Mohan S, Lundy M, et al.** (1990) Skeletal growth factor and other growth factors known to be present in bone matrix stimulate proliferation and protein synthesis in human bone cells. *J Bone Miner Res;* 5 (2):179–186.

104. **Mohan S, Jennings JC, Linkhart TA, et al.** (1986) Isolation and purification of a low-molecular-weight skeletal growth factor from human bones. *Biochem Biophys Acta;* 884 (2):234–242.

105. **Pfeilschifter J, D'Souza SM, Mundy GR** (1987) Effects of transforming growth factor-beta on osteoblastic osteosarcoma cells. *Endocrinology;* 121 (1):212–218.

106. **Drinkwater BL, Nilson K, Chesnut CH, 3rd, et al.** (1984) Bone mineral content of amenor-rheic and eumenorrheic athletes. *N Engl J Med;* 311 (5):277–281.

107. **Simkin A, Ayalon J, Leichter I** (1987) Increased trabecular bone density due to bone-loading exercises in postmenopausal osteoporotic women. *Calcif Tissue Int;* 40 (2):59–63.

108. **Myburgh KH, Noakes TD, Roodt M, et al.** (1989) Effect of exercise on the development of osteoporosis in adult rats. *J Appl Physiol;* 66 (1):14–19.

109. **Smith EL, Reddan W, Smith PE** (1981) Physical activity and calcium modalities for bone mineral increase in aged women. *Med Sci Sports Exerc;* 13 (1):60–64.

110. **Lanyon LE, Rubin CT, Baust G** (1986) Modulation of bone loss during calcium insufficiency by controlled dynamic loading. *Calcif Tissue Int;* 38 (4):209–216.

111. **Burkhart JM, Jowsey J** (1967) Parathyroid and thyroid hormones in the development of immobili-zation osteoporosis. *Endocrinology;* 81 (5): 1053–1062.

112. **Rodan SB, Wesolowski G, Rodan GA** (1986) Clonal differ-ences in prostaglandin synthesis among osteosarcoma cell lines. *J Bone Miner Res;* 1 (2):213–220.

113. **Cheng MZ, Zaman G, Rawlinson SC, et al.** (1997) Enhancement by sex hormones of the osteoregulatory effects of mechanical loading and prosta-glandins in explants of rat ulnae. *J Bone Miner Res;* 12 (9):1424–1430.

114. **Russell RGG** (1990) Bone cell biology: The role of cytokines and other mediators. In: Smith EL, editor. *Osteoporosis*. London: RCP Publications, 135.

115. **Chambers TJ** (1985) The pathobiology of the osteoclast. *J Clin Pathol;* 38 (3):241–252.

116. **Rodan GA, Martin TJ** (1981) Role of osteoblasts in hormonal control of bone resorption—a hypothesis. *Calcif Tissue Int;* 33 (4):349–351.

117. **Damien E, Price JS, Lanyon LE** (1998) The estrogen receptor's involvement in osteoblasts' adaptive response to mechanical strain. *J Bone Miner Res;* 13 (8):1275–1282.

118. **Tomkinson A, Gevers EF, Wit JM, et al.** (1998) The role of estrogen in the control of rat osteocyte apoptosis. *J Bone Miner Res;* 13 (8):1243–1250.

119. **Haapasalo H, Kannus P, Sievanen H, et al.** (1998) Effect of long-term unilateral activity on bone mineral density of female junior tennis players. *J Bone Miner Res;* 13 (2):310–319.

120. **Parfitt AM** (1984) The cellular basis of bone remodeling: the quantum concept reexamined in light of recent advances in the cell biology of bone. *Calcif Tissue Int;* 36 (Suppl 1):37–45.

121. **Anderson DC** (1990) Hormones and the skeleton. In: Smith R, editor. *Osteoporosis*. London: RCP Publications, 135.

122. **Hillman JR, Davis RW, Abdelbaki YZ** (1973) Cyclic bone remodeling in deer. *Calcif Tissue Res;* 12 (4):323–330.

123. **Carter DR, Hayes WC, Schurman DJ** (1976) Fatigue life of compact bone—II. Effects of microstructure and density. *J Biomech;* 9 (4):211–218.

124. **Frost HM** (1966) *Bone Dynamics in Osteomalacia and Osteoporosis*. Springfield, IL.: CC Thomas.

125. **Carter DR, Caler WE, Spengler DM, et al.** (1981) Fatigue behavior of adult cortical bone: the influence of mean strain and strain range. *Acta Orthop Scand;* 52 (5):481–490.

126. **Carter DR, Caler WE, Spengler DM, et al.** (1981) Uniaxial fatigue of human cortical bone. The influence of tissue physical characteristics. *J Biomech;* 14 (7):461–470.

127. **Enlow DH** (1963) *Principles of Bone Remodelling*. Springfield, IL: CC Thomas.

128. **Jee WSS** (1964) The influence of reduced local vascularity on the rate of internal reconstruction in adult long bone cortex. In: Frost HM, editor. *Bone Biodynamics*. Boston: Henry Ford Hosp Intntl Symp, 42.

129. **Moss ML** (1965) Studies on the acellular bone of teleost fish. *Acta Anat;* 60:262.

130. **Krolner B, Toft B** (1963) Vertebral bone loss, an unheeded side effect of therapeutic bed rest. *Clin Sci;* 64:537.

131. **Tilton FE, Degioanni JJ, Schneider VS** (1980) Long-term follow-up of Skylab bone demineralization. *Aviat Space Environ Med;* 51 (11):1209–1213.

132. **Dickson RA** (1977) The effect of synovectomy on function and bone density in the rheumatoid hand. *J Bone Joint Surg [Br];* 59:378.

133. **Brighton CT, Tadduni GT, Goll SR, et al.** (1988) Treatment of denervation/disuse osteoporosis in the rat with a capacitively coupled electrical signal: effects on bone formation and bone resorption. *J Orthop Res;* 6 (5):676–684.

134. **Jones HH, Priest JD, Hayes WC, et al.** (1977) Humeral hypertrophy in response to exercise. *J Bone Joint Surg [Am];* 59 (2):204–208.

135. **Nilsson BE, Westlin NE** (1971) Bone density in athletes. *Clin Orthop;* 77:179–182.

136. **Beverly MC, Rider TA, Evans MJ, et al.** (1989) Local bone mineral response to brief exercise that stresses the skeleton. *Brit Med J;* 299 (6693): 233–235.

137. **Marcus R** (1996) Mechanisms of exercise effects on bone. In: Bilezikian JP, Raisz LG, Rodan GA, editors. *Principles of Bone Biology*. San Diego: Academic Press, 1135.

138. **Umemura Y, Ishiko T, Yamauchi T, et al.** (1997) Five jumps per day increase bone mass and breaking force in rats. *J Bone Miner Res;* 12 (9): 1480–1485.

139. **Eliakim A, Raisz LG, Brasel JA, et al.** (1997) Evidence for increased bone formation following a brief endurance-type training intervention in adolescent males. *J Bone Miner Res;* 12 (10):1708–1713.

140. **Reilly GC, Currey JD, Goodship AE** (1997) Exercise of young thoroughbred horses increases impact strength of the third metacarpal bone. *J Orthop Res;* 15 (6):862–868.

141. **Nunamaker DM, Butterweck DM, Provost MT** (1990) Fatigue fractures in thoroughbred racehorses: relationships with age, peak bone strain, and training. *J Orthop Res;* 8 (4):604–611.

142. **Brudvig TJ, Gudger TD, Obermeyer L** (1983) Stress fractures in 295 trainees: a one-year study of incidence as related to age, sex, and race. *Mil Med;* 148 (8):666–667.

143. **Orava S, Puranen J, Ala-Ketola L** (1978) Stress fractures caused by physical exercise. *Acta Orthop Scand;* 49 (1):19–27.

144. **Mosekilde L** (1989) Sex differences in age-related loss of vertebral trabecular bone mass and structure— biomechanical consequences. *Bone;* 10 (6):425–432.

145. **Parfitt AM** (1992) Implications of architecture for the pathogenesis and prevention of vertebral fracture. *Bone;* 13 (Suppl 2):41–47.

146. **Vetter U, Pontz B, Zauner E, et al.** (1992) Osteogenesis imperfecta: a clinical study of the first ten years of life. *Calcif Tissue Int;* 50 (1):36–41.

147. **Biewener AA** (1991) Musculoskeletal design in relation to body size. *J Biomech;* 24 (Suppl 1):19–29.

148. **Sarmiento A, Sobol PA, Sew Hoy AL, et al.** (1984) Prefabricated functional braces for the treatment of fractures of the tibial diaphysis. *J Bone Joint Surg [Am];* 66 (9):1328–1339.

149. **Cornell CN, Lane JM** (1992) Newest factors in fracture healing. *Clin Orthop;* (277):297–311.

150. **Wallace AL, Draper ER, Strachan RK, et al.** (1991) The effect of devascularisation upon early bone healing in dynamic external fixation. *J Bone Joint Surg [Br];* 73 (5):819–825.

151. **Cheal EJ, Mansmann KA, DiGioia AM, 3rd, et al.** (1991) Role of interfragmentary strain in fracture healing: ovine model of a healing osteotomy. *J Orthop Res;* 9 (1):131–142.

152. **Kenwright J, Richardson JB, Cunningham JL, et al.** (1991) Axial movement and tibial fractures. A controlled randomised trial of treatment. *J Bone Joint Surg [Br];* 73 (4):654–659.

153. **Goodship AE, Watkins PE, Rigby HS, et al.** (1993) The role of fixator frame stiffness in the control of fracture healing. An experimental study. *J Biomech;* 26 (9):1027–1035.

154. **Eggers EL, et al.** (1993) Canine osteotomy healing when stabilised with decreasingly rigid fixation compared to constantly rigid fixation. *Vet Comp Orthop Traumatol;* 6:182.

155. **Behrens F, Searls K** (1986) External fixation of the tibia. Basic concepts and prospective evaluation. *J Bone Joint Surg [Br];* 68 (2):246–254.

156. **Lammens J, Liu Z, Aerssens J, et al.** (1998) Distraction bone healing versus osteotomy healing: a com-parative biochemical analysis. *J Bone Miner Res;* 13 (2):279–286.

157. **Perren SM** (1989) The biomechanics and biology of internal fixation using plates and nails. *Orthopedics;* 12 (1): 21–34.

158. **Baggott DG, Lanyon LE** (1977) An independent 'post-mortem' calibration of electrical resistance strain gauges bonded to bone surfaces 'in vivo'. *J Biomech;* 10 (10):615–622.

159. **Terjensen T, Norby A, Arnulf V** (1985) Bone atrophy after plate fixation. *Acta Orthop Scand;* 56:416.

160. **Uhthoff HK, Foux A, Yeadon A, et al.** (1993) Two processes of bone remodeling in plated intact femora: an experimental study in dogs. *J Orthop Res;* 11 (1):78–91.

161. **Uhthoff HK, Finnegan M** (1983) The effects of metal plates on posttraumatic remodelling and bone mass. *J Bone Joint Surg [Br];* 65 (1): 66–71.

162. **Woo SL, Akeson WH, Coutts RD, et al.** (1976) A comparison of cortical bone atrophy secondary to fixation with plates with large differences in bending stiffness. *J Bone Joint Surg [Am];* 58 (2):190–195.

163. **Deluca PA, Lindsey RW, Ruwe PA** (1988) Refracture of bones of the forearm after the removal of compression plates. *J Bone Joint Surg [Am];* 70 (9):1372–1376.

164. **Richards RH, Palmer JD, Clarke NM** (1992) Observations on removal of metal implants. *Injury;* 23 (1):25–28.

165. **Lanyon LE, Paul IL, Rubin CT, et al.** (1981) In vivo strain measurements from bone and prosthesis following total hip replacement. An experimental study in sheep. *J Bone Joint Surg [Am];* 63 (6):989–1001.

166. **Engh CA, Bobyn JD, Glassman AH** (1987) Porous-coated hip replacement. The factors governing bone ingrowth, stress shielding, and clinical results. *J Bone Joint Surg [Br];* 69 (1):45–55.

167. **Weinans HH** (1991) *Mechanically induced bone adaptions around orthopaedic implants.* Univ Nijmegen, Netherlands.

168. **Joshi RP, Eftekhar NS, McMahon DJ, et al.** (1998) Osteolysis after Charnley primary low-friction arthroplasty. A comparison of two matched paired groups. *J Bone Joint Surg [Br];* 80 (4):585–590.

169. **Raisz LG** (1988) Hormonal regulation of bone growth and remodelling. 136. *Ciba-Foundation-Symp.;* Basel. Ciba-Geigy.

170. **Samuels A, Perry MJ, Tobias JH** (1999) High-dose estrogen induces de novo medullary bone formation in female mice. *J Bone Miner Res;* 14 (2): 178–186.

171. **Rockwell JC, Sorensen AM, Baker S, et al.** (1990) Weight training decreases vertebral bone density in premenopausal women: a prospective study. *J Clin Endocrinol Metab;* 71 (4):988–993.

172. **Snow-Harter C, Bouxsein ML, Lewis BT, et al.** (1992) Effects of resistance and endurance exercise on bone mineral status of young women: a randomized exercise intervention trial. *J Bone Miner Res;* 7 (7):761–769.

173. **Chow R, Harrison JE, Notarius C** (1987) Effect of two randomised exercise programmes on bone mass of healthy postmenopausal women. *Br Med J (Clin Res Ed);* 295 (6611): 1441–1444.

174. **Gutin B, Kasper MJ** (1992) Can vigorous exercise play a role in osteoporosis prevention? A review. *Osteoporos Int;* 2 (2):55–69.

175. **Pocock N, Eisman J, Gwinn T, et al.** (1989) Muscle strength, physical fitness, and weight but not age predict femoral neck bone mass. *J Bone Miner Res;* 4 (3):441–448.

176. **Smith EL, Gilligan C, McAdam M, et al.** (1989) Deterring bone loss by exercise intervention in premenopausal and postmenopausal women. *Calcif Tissue Int;* 44 (5):312–321.

177. **Kanders B, Dempster DW, Lindsay R** (1988) Interaction of calcium nutrition and physical activity on bone mass in young women. *J Bone Miner Res;* 3 (2): 145–149.

178. **Barlow DH** (1990) Hormone replacement therapy. In: Smith R, editor. *Osteoporosis.* London: RCP Publications, 135.

179. **Reeve J** (1990) Restoring trabecular bone mass in established osteoporosis. In: Smith EL, editor. *Osteoporosis.* London: RCP Publications, 143.

180. **Notelovitz M, Martin D, Tesar R, et al.** (1991) Estrogen therapy and variable-resistance weight training increase bone mineral in surgically menopausal women. *J Bone Miner Res;* 6 (6):583–590.

181. **Davis JW, Grove JS, Ross PD, et al.** (1992) Relationship between bone mass and rates of bone change at appendicular measurement sites. *J Bone Miner Res;* 7 (7):719–725.

182. **Soroko SB, Barrett-Connor E, Edelstein SL, et al.** (1994) Family history of osteoporosis and bone mineral density at the axial skeleton: the Rancho Bernardo Study. *J Bone Miner Res;* 9 (6):761–769.

183. **Grant SF, Reid DM, Blake G, et al.** (1996) Reduced bone density and osteoporosis associated with a polymorphic Sp1 binding site in the collagen type I alpha 1 gene. *Nat Genet;* 14 (2):203–205.

8 Biomechanics of fracture

Dennis R. Carter & Dan M. Spengler

1 Introduction

In any physical activity, a complex pattern of forces is imposed on the bones of the skeletal system. These forces are generally of three types:

- External forces acting on the body.
- Internal forces caused by muscle contraction or ligament tension.
- Internal reaction forces between bones.

The forces, also referred to as loads, cause small deformations of the bones on which they act. The mechanical response of a particular bone can be described by quantitatively assessing the relationships between the applied loads and the resulting deformations.

The relationships between forces and deformations reflect the structural behavior of the whole bone. In moderate loading situations, bone deformations are only present while the loads are being applied. When the loads are removed, the bone reassumes its original position and geometry. If the skeletal system is exposed to severe trauma, the loads imposed on a bone may become extremely high, resulting in large deformations and possibly in bone fracture. The major factors which determine the deformation characteristics and fracture resistance of a bone are the direction and magnitude of the applied forces, the size and geometry of the bone, and the material properties of the tissue which comprises the bone.

Large forces cause greater deformation, and the tendency toward fracture behavior of a long bone, when subjected to axial forces, is much different from when the bone is subjected to bending or torsional forces. The anatomical differences among the bones of the skeleton tend to reflect the types of forces which act on the individual bones. Large bones are much better suited to resist forces than small bones. Bones are specialized in their geometric configuration to resist forces in a particular direction.

The material properties of the tissue that comprises the bone are very important in determining the deformation and fracture properties of the bone. For example, an osteoporotic bone with the same geometry as a normal bone will experience greater deformation under loading and will fracture at lower force magnitudes.

This chapter will present some of the basic mechanical concepts related to bone fracture. However, before fracture biomechanics can be considered, it is necessary to understand some of the basic concepts that are used in examining structures exposed to mechanical forces. A more in-depth treatment of mechanics is provided by Timoshenko and Young [1] and Frankel and Burstein [2]. The material properties of bone tissue will be considered, the mechanical function of whole bones will be examined, and, finally, some fracture types observed clinically will be presented.

2 Basic mechanical concepts

2.1 Stress and strain

When forces are applied to any object, the object will be deformed from its original dimensions and internal forces will be produced within the object. The deformations created at any point in the object are referred to as the strains at that point. The internal force intensities are referred to as the stresses at that point.

Stresses = local force intensities
(dimensions = force per unit area, MN/m² or MPa).

Strains = local deformations
(dimensions = length per length).

The strains at any point in a bone subjected to forces are mathematically related to the stresses at that point. The quantitative relationships between stresses and strains are governed by the material properties of the bone tissue that comprises the whole bone. If the whole bone is loaded with very high forces, the stresses and strains at one region may exceed the ultimate stresses or strains that the bone tissue can tolerate. Mechanical failure will then occur at that point, and bone fracture will result. If a bone comprises tissue with poor material properties, such as osteomalacic bone, the tissue at the region of high stresses and strains will fracture at lower force levels than a bone consisting of normal tissue.

When a bone is subjected to forces, stresses and strains, which vary in a highly complex manner, are introduced throughout the bone structure. To characterize the stresses or strains at any one point completely, six stress values, which correspond to normal and shear strains on each of three independent planes passing through that point, must be specified. The concept of stresses and strains is simplified considerably if we restrict our consideration to stresses present on an imaginary plane through a point in the bone. **Fig. 8-1** demonstrates a human femur, which is subjected to a pattern of applied forces. Let us assume that we wish to examine the stresses at point O in this bone, which act on a plane passing through the diaphysis in a transverse direction. We can consider point O to consist of an infinitesimally small cube. The top face of this cube has an area that we will designate as A. Two types of internal forces may act on the top face of the cube. The first is a force (F) that is perpendicular to the face. This internal force results in a normal stress, which is equal to F/A. The other type of force which may act on this surface is shear force, which we will designate as S. This shear force results in a shear stress, which equals S/A. A normal stress can act either toward the face of the cube (compression) or away from the face of the cube (tension). The shear stress can likewise be oriented in any direction parallel to the top face of the cube, depending upon the loading condition imposed on the whole bone.

Normal stress = force per unit area acting perpendicular to a given plane (MPa).

Shear stress = force per unit area acting parallel to a given plane (MPa).

The two types of stresses illustrated in **Fig. 8-1** result in local deformations to the cube. A normal tensile stress will cause the front face of the cube to become longer and thinner. Normal compressive stresses cause the front face of the cube to become shorter and wider (**Fig. 8-2**). The normal strain in the cube can be defined as the ratio of the change in length (Δl) of the side of the cube to the original length of the side (l): normal strain $\varepsilon = \Delta l / l$.

The shear stresses imposed on the top face of the cube will cause the front face of the cube to be deformed from a square into a parallelepiped (**Fig. 8-3**). The shear strain is defined as the angular deviation of one side of the cube from its original right-angle position. This angle, expressed in radians, is approximately equal to $\Delta l / l$, as shown in **Fig. 8-3**. The amount of normal strain and shear strain experienced by the cube will be influenced by the magnitudes of the normal stress and shear stress on the top face of the cube, as well as by the inherent material properties of the bone tissue.

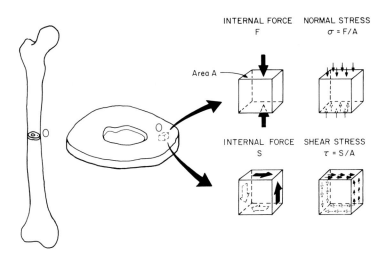

Fig. 8-1: Schematic representations of the stresses acting on a transverse plane through a point in the femoral diaphysis.

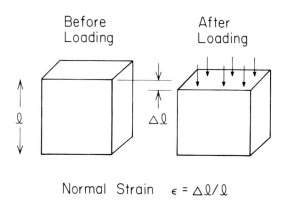

Fig. 8-2: Representation of the strain caused by compressive stresses. (From Carter DR, Spengler DM, 1978, Mechanical properties and composition of cortical bone, Clin Orthop [7].)

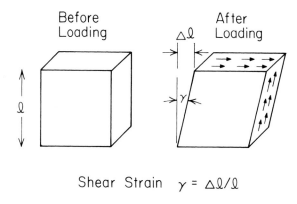

Fig. 8-3: Representation of the strain caused by shear stresses. (From Carter DR, Spengler DM, 1978, Mechanical properties and composition of cortical bone, Clin Orthop [7].)

In general, if the bone tissue is very well mineralized, the bone tissue itself will be very stiff and small strains will result from the application of stresses at that point. However, if the bone material is of poor quality, the same stresses will result in larger strains in the cube, since this bone material is softer and more compliant.

It should also be noted that we have thus far considered stresses at point *O* only on a transverse plane through the whole bone—that is, the top face of the cube. If we were to consider the stresses at point *O* acting on a plane which passes through the whole bone at an oblique angle, the stresses on that plane would differ from those on the transverse plane.

2.2   Tension and compression

Bones of the skeletal system are geometrically complex and are exposed to complex force patterns. These factors lead to very complex patterns of stresses and strains throughout the bone tissue. Simplified structures, which are loaded under well-defined conditions, can be used to demonstrate some basic mechanical concepts. **Fig. 8-4** demonstrates a bar of length (*L*) and a constant cross-sectional area (*A*) that is subjected to pure tensile loading (*F*). This loading condition results in a uniform, homogeneous pattern of stresses and strains throughout the structure at any cross-section. As load is applied to the bar, the bar begins to stretch.

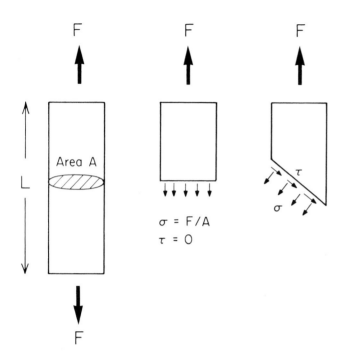

$\sigma = F/A$

$\tau = 0$

Fig. 8-4: Schematic representation of the stresses acting on a transverse and an oblique plane through a bar subjected to tensile forces.

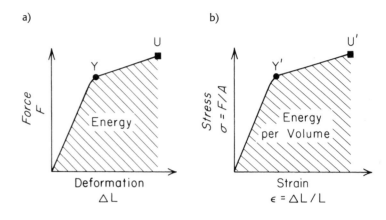

Fig. 8-5:
a) Force–deformation curve of a bar subjected to tensile loading.
b) The corresponding stress–strain curve of the material comprising the bar which is subjected to tensile forces.
(From Carter DR, Spengler DM, 1978, Mechanical properties and composition of cortical bone, Clin Orthop [7].)

The relationship between the applied force (F) and the increase in the length of the bar (ΔL) can be demonstrated on a force–deformation curve (**Fig. 8-5a**). The initial portion of the force–deformation curve is essentially linear. This linear portion of the curve represents the elastic behavior of the structure. If load is applied in the elastic region of the curve and is then released, the bar will return to its original length. If sufficient force is applied, however, internal damage will be created in the structure and the bar will begin to yield. Yield occurs at point Y on the force–deformation curve (**Fig. 8-5a**). Further loading beyond the yield point will result in marked deformation until total fracture occurs, point U (**Fig. 8-5a**). The total energy absorbed by the bar during the fracture process is represented by the area under the force–deformation curve.

The stresses and strains present on a transverse plane through the bar at any point may also be considered. Due to the simplicity of the loading situation, the stresses on this plane are identical over the entire cross-section. A stress–strain curve can be constructed for any point on a transverse plane through the bar (**Fig. 8-5b**). In this loading configuration the normal stress is equal to F/A and the normal strain is equal to $\Delta L/L$. No shear stresses or strains act on the transverse plane. The stress–strain curve is, in effect, a normalized curve, which reflects the mechanical behavior of the material that comprises the bar. If one were to double the cross-sectional area and triple the length of the bar, the force–deformation curve would be altered significantly.

Since the ultimate force, point U, is proportional to the cross-sectional area, the bar would be able to withstand twice as much force before it fractured. The bar would also deform three times as much before it fractured, since ultimate deformation is proportional to initial length. The stress–strain curve of this new bar, however, would be identical to that of the first bar. The yield strength and yield strain of the material, represented by point *Y*, as well as the ultimate strength and ultimate strain of the material, represented by point *U*, are independent of the size of the bar being loaded.

The force–deformation curve is therefore a representation of the mechanical behavior of the structure, while the stress–strain curve is a mechanical representation of the behavior of the material. In the elastic region, from *A* to *Y*, the "stiffness" of the material is measured by the slope of the stress–strain curve. This slope is called the elastic modulus, or Young's modulus of elasticity, and has dimensions of force per unit area. The elastic modulus of steel is approximately ten times greater than that of bone, and the ultimate tensile strength of steel is approximately five times greater than that of cortical bone.

It is important to realize that the stress in the bar (**Fig. 8-4**) is dependent upon the plane under consideration. If one considers a plane oriented at an oblique angle to applied load, shear stresses as well as normal stresses will be present on that plane. The maximum shear stresses acting in a bar under tensile or compressive loading are present on any plane, which is oriented 45° from the direction of loading. This fact becomes particularly important in considering the fracture behavior of cortical bone, since under tensile loading the bone tends to fracture on a transverse plane where the normal tensile stresses are greatest. However, in compression, the bone tends to fail along oblique angles; this pattern corresponds to failure along planes of high shear stresses.

2.3 Bending

A beam can be subjected to bending loads in two ways. These two types of bending are generally referred to as pure bending and three-point bending. **Fig. 8-6** demonstrates a simple beam that is subjected to pure bending loads. This loading situation can be thought of as if one were to grasp each end of the beam and twist it in such a manner as to produce a convex surface on one side of the beam and a concave surface on the other side. This action produces constant bending loading over the entire length of the beam.

The material on the concave side of the beam will be subjected to compressive strains, while the material on the convex side will be subjected to tensile strains. The strains produced at any cross-section of the beam will result in stresses at that cross-section. The concave side of the beam will be exposed to high compressive stresses, while the convex side will experience high tensile stresses.

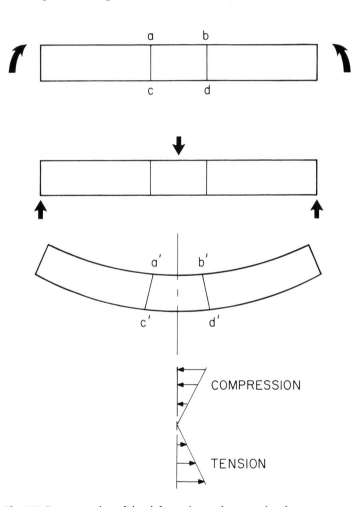

Fig. 8-6: Representation of the deformation and stresses in a beam subjected to bending forces. (From Carter DR, Spengler DM, 1978, Mechanical properties and composition of cortical bone, Clin Orthop [7].)

If the bar is loaded so that all the material is stressed only in the elastic region of the stress–strain curve, the distribution of stresses at any cross-section through the beam will be proportional to the distance from the center of the beam. Note that the material on the surface of the beam experiences the highest stresses. If the bending force is increased until the bar begins to fracture, fracture will be initiated at the surface of the beam, where the stresses are highest. Since pure bending is being applied, fracture may occur at any location along the length of the bar.

Pure bending as shown in **Fig. 8-6** rarely occurs in the skeletal system. Bending forces experienced by bones in vivo are better simulated by a single load applied to the beam which is supported at the ends, three-point bending. In such a loading situation the bending moment at a section through the beam is greatest at the point where the load is applied, and failure of the beam in bending will occur at that point. Three-point bending also introduces shear stresses on transverse planes through the beam, which would not be present in a pure bending situation. However, if the beam is much longer than it is thick, these shear forces will be negligible.

2.4 Combined bending and axial loading

Long bones in vivo are often subjected to combined compressive and bending loads. This loading situation can be illustrated by a bar subjected to a compressive force which is not directed through the center of the bar (**Fig. 8-7**). The resulting stresses on a transverse section through the bar can be found by merely summing the stresses caused by the independent actions of axial force and bending moment. High compressive stresses will be created on one side of the bar while the other side of the bar will experience either lower compressive stresses or tensile stresses, depending upon the relative magnitudes of the axial force and the bending load.

2.5 Torsion

A circular bar subjected to torsional loading will tend to be twisted about its axis. This twisting is evidence of shear strain on any transverse section through the bar (**Fig. 8-8**). The shear strains are associated with shear stresses in a transverse and axial direction. The magnitude of the shear stresses and strains varies linearly with the distance from the central axis of the bar such that the material on the surface of the bar experiences the greatest shear stresses. In considering the stresses on the surface of a circular bar in torsion, one generally thinks of the

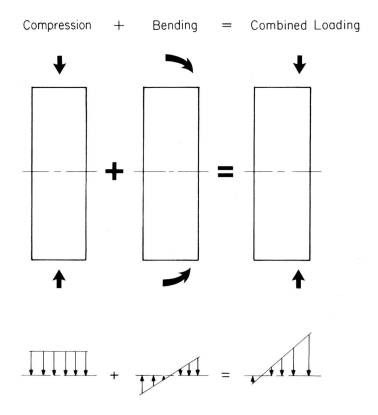

Compression + Bending = Combined Loading

Transverse Stress Distributions

Fig. 8-7: Stresses imposed on a transverse plane through a bar which is subjected to a combination of compressive and bending loading.

shear stresses in the transverse and longitudinal planes. However, it can be demonstrated that significant tensile and compressive stresses are present on oblique planes through the bar. If a bar is subjected to torsional loading and fractures along an oblique or spiral plane, then it can be assumed that failure occurred primarily because of high tensile stresses on this plane.

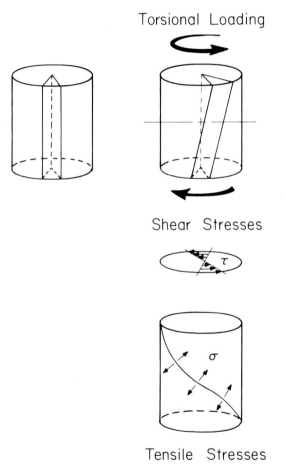

Fig. 8-8: Deformation and stress distributions in a cylindrical bar subjected to torsional loading. Sheer stresses are imposed on the longitudinal and transverse planes, while tensile and compressive forces are imposed on planes which make an oblique spiral through the bar.

3   Material properties of bone tissue

The fracture behavior of whole bones is strongly dependent upon the material behavior of the tissue that comprises the bone. To determine the material properties of bone tissue, small specimens can be extracted from the whole bone. Specimens can be loaded under well-defined conditions in the laboratory in such a manner as to produce uniform, known stresses throughout the specimen. Specimen deformation can be measured and strains calculated. The material properties of the tissues that comprise the bone specimen can thus be determined for the specific loading conditions imposed. This general approach to material testing has facilitated the documentation of bone material properties in tension, compression, bending, and torsion (shear).

Whole long bones are composed of bone tissue exhibiting two forms of structural organization. Cortical compact bone tissue forms the diaphyses of long bones and the thin shell of the bone ends. Cancellous (or trabecular) bone in the metaphyses and epiphyses is continuous with the inner surface of the cortical shell and exists as a three-dimensional network of bony plates and columns. The trabeculae divide the interior volume of bone into intercommunicating pores of different dimensions, producing a structure of variable porosity and apparent density. The classification of bone tissue as cortical or cancellous is based on bone porosity, which is the proportion of the volume occupied by non-mineralized tissue. Cortical bone has a porosity of approximately 5% to 30%; cancellous bone porosity may range from approximately 30% to more than 90%. However, the distinction between very porous cortical bone and very dense cancellous bone is somewhat arbitrary.

The chemical composition of cancellous bone is similar to that of cortical bone. The major difference in these two bone types is the high degree of porosity exhibited by cancellous bone. This porosity is reflected by measurements of bone-tissue apparent density, which is the mass of bone tissue divided by the bulk volume of tissue, including non-mineralized tissue spaces:

$$\textbf{Bone density} = \frac{\text{bone tissue mass}}{\text{bone bulk volume}}$$

3.1 Cortical bone

Laboratory testing has shown that the material properties of cortical bone are dependent upon the rate at which the bone tissue is loaded or deformed. A specimen of bone tissue, which is very rapidly subjected to forces, will have a greater elastic modulus and ultimate strength than bone tissue that is loaded more slowly (**Fig. 8-9**). In addition, bone tissue that is exposed to very rapid loading will absorb considerably more energy than bone tissue which is loaded more slowly. To quantify the rapidity of deformation, one can refer to the strain rate (dimensions: strain per unit time) to which the tissue is exposed during the loading process. In normal activities, bone is subjected to strain rates that are generally below 0.01/second. In traumatic bone fracture, however, strain rates may exceed 10.0/second. Materials such as bone whose stress–strain characteristics are dependent upon the applied strain rate are said to be viscoelastic materials. The elastic modulus and ultimate strength of bone are approximately proportional to the strain rate raised to the 0.06 power.

The stress–strain behavior of bone tissue is also strongly dependent upon the orientation of the bone microstructure with respect to the direction of loading. Several investigators have demonstrated that cortical bone is stronger and stiffer in the longitudinal direction, the direction of osteon orientation, than in the transverse direction. In addition, bone specimens loaded in a direction perpendicular to the osteons tend to fail in a more brittle manner, with little non-elastic deformation subsequent to yielding (**Fig. 8-10**). Long bones are therefore better able to resist stresses along the axis of the bone than across the bone axis. Materials such as bone whose elastic and strength properties are dependent upon the direction of applied loading are said to be anisotropic materials.

The viscoelastic anisotropic nature of cortical bone distinguishes it as a very complex material. Because of these characteristics one must specify the strain rate and the direction of applied loading when discussing bone material behavior.

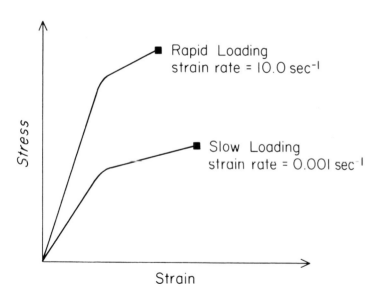

Fig. 8-9: The influence of strain rate on the stress–strain characteristics of bone tissue.

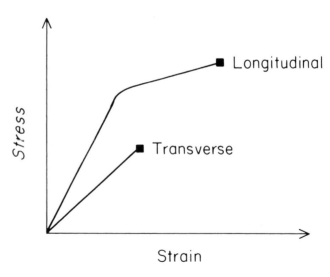

Fig. 8-10: The influence of the direction of the applied stress on the stress–strain characteristics of bone tissue.

3.1.1 Tension, compression, and shear

The most complete investigations of cortical bone elastic and strength characteristics were conducted by Reilly et al. [3] and Reilly and Burstein [4]. These studies also provided detailed information on the preparation and the testing of standardized bone specimens machined from whole long bones. Mechanical testing was conducted at strain rates between 0.02 and 0.05/second. The resulting stress–strain curve showed that cortical bone behaves in a manner similar to that of other engineering materials. Stress–strain curves in tension and compression consisted of an initial elastic region, which is nearly linear. This region was followed by yielding and considerable, non-elastic, "plastic" deformation before failure (**Fig. 8-10**). The non-elastic region of the stress–strain curve for the longitudinally oriented specimen reflected diffuse, irreversible microdamage created throughout the bone structure. Bone tissue that is loaded into this non-elastic region will not return to its original configuration after the load is removed. The mean value of the longitudinal elastic modulus was found to be approximately 50% greater than that of the transverse elastic modulus. The ultimate strength was greater in compression than in tension for specimens oriented in both the longitudinal and transverse directions. Specimens loaded in the transverse direction were significantly weaker in both tension and compression than the longitudinally oriented specimens. In addition, the transverse specimens tended to fail in a more brittle manner, with little non-elastic deformation subsequent to yielding.

To establish the shear properties of cortical bone, Reilly and Burstein [4] conducted torsional tests of square and cylindrical section specimens, which were oriented in the longitudinal direction. Estimates of the ultimate shear strength of the bone tissue from these torsional tests were complicated by the fact that the torque-displacement curves were non-linear. The ultimate shear strengths for the circular cross-sectional specimens were therefore calculated by applying the non-linear mathematical solution described by Nadai [5]. The results for the ultimate strength of adult, femoral cortical bone as determined by Reilly and Burstein [4] are summarized in **Tab. 8-1**. These results verify that the material strength of bone tissue is

Tab. 8-1: Ultimate strength of adult femoral cortical bone.*

Loading mode	Ultimate strength (MPa)
Longitudinal	
Tension	133
Compression	193
Shear (torsion test about longitudinal axis)	68
Transverse	
Tension	51
Compression	133

*Mean values from Reilly and Burstein [4]. Strain rate 0.02–0.05/second. Age span of population 19–80 years.

dependent upon the type of loading imposed, as well as the direction of the applied loading.

The various loading modes to which the bone specimens are subjected are associated with characteristic fracture patterns. **Fig. 8-11** demonstrates the fracture patterns for longitudinally oriented bone specimens that are subjected to tensile, compressive, torsional bending, and combined bending and compressive forces. Tensile specimens normally demonstrate a fracture pattern, which is approximately perpendicular to the direction of applied loading. The stresses imposed on the plane of fracture are tensile stresses. Tensile loading of longitudinally

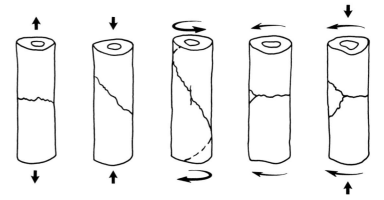

Fig. 8-11: Fracture patterns created in cortical bone due to tensile, compressive, torsional bending, and combined bending and compressive forces.

oriented bone specimens therefore results in fracture along planes of high tensile stresses. A bone specimen that is subjected to compressive forces will generally fracture along a plane, which is at an oblique angle to the direction of the applied loading. These oblique planes are subjected to significant shear stresses as the compressive forces are applied to the specimen. Compressive loading of the bone specimen therefore results in failure along planes of high shear stresses.

A bone specimen subjected to torsional loading demonstrates a more complex fracture pattern. Fracture is usually initiated at a small crack on the surface of the specimen that runs parallel to the specimen axis, on a plane of high shear stresses. After initiation of the fracture, the crack then runs in a spiral manner through the specimen, following planes of high tensile stresses. The final fracture surface appears as an oblique spiral, which is characteristic of torsional fracture of bone tissue.

A bone specimen subjected to bending forces will be exposed to high tensile stresses on one side of the specimen and high compressive stresses on the other side. The fracture pattern which results is consistent with that observed in tensile and compressive testing of longitudinally oriented specimens. A transverse fracture surface will be present on the tensile side of the specimen, while an oblique fracture surface may be created on the compressive side. The compressive side of the specimen may contain two oblique fracture patterns, creating a loose wedge of bone as the specimen is fractured. This fracture pattern is sometimes referred to as a "butterfly" fracture. The oblique fracture lines may be accentuated in situations wherein combined compressive and bending loads are imposed.

The fracture patterns shown for the bone specimens in **Fig. 8-11** are consistent with those observed in bone fractures clinically. Bone in vivo, however, is rarely subjected to idealized loading situations as illustrated in **Fig. 8-11**. Bone fractures seen clinically are usually caused by a complex loading situation, and the resulting fracture patterns are therefore numerous. It should also be noted that very high energy, rapid strain rate fractures result in significant comminution caused by the bifurcation and propagation of numerous fracture planes in the bone tissue.

3.1.2 Fatigue

The mechanical behavior of bones when exposed to a single application of high forces is of interest if one is concerned with the fracture behavior caused by a single traumatic episode. Bone tissue in vivo, however, is more commonly exposed to repetitive loading at stress levels less than those required to fracture the bone during a single traumatic episode. Repeated loading of bone in everyday activities or prolonged exercise, however, may lead to microscopic damage. If damage accumulates faster than biologic processes can repair it, fatigue fracture of bone may result. In a mechanical sense, fatigue is the progressive failure of the material under cyclic or fluctuating loads. Under cyclic loading, materials may fail at load levels less than those required to cause failure with a single applied loading. Fatigue fractures may occur during prolonged exercise such as marching or long-distance running, and are especially common in the metatarsals of young military recruits. Fatigue damage in bone due to repeated mechanical loading has also been implicated in the development of degenerative disorders, avascular necrosis, osteochondritis, senile femoral neck fractures, spondylolisthesis, pathologic fractures, and the failure of bone after orthopedic implant procedures.

Fatigue tests in the laboratory are often conducted by subjecting a number of identical specimens to constant amplitude cyclic stresses or cyclic strains of various magnitudes and noting the number of cycles to failure—that is, the fatigue life. The resulting plot of stress amplitude or strain amplitude versus cycles to failure serves to characterize the fatigue properties of the material under examination.

The yield strain of cortical bone at a strain rate of 0.01/second is approximately 0.006. Current studies in our laboratories are directed at examining the fatigue behavior of cortical bone at physiologic strain rates. Fatigue testing is being done at constant strain amplitudes, using a constant strain rate of 0.01/second. This procedure results in loading frequencies of less than one cycle/second for the test specimens.

The fatigue behavior of a representative human cortical bone specimen tested at a constant strain amplitude of 0.0035 is shown in **Fig. 8-12**. Fatigue loading initially caused a pro-

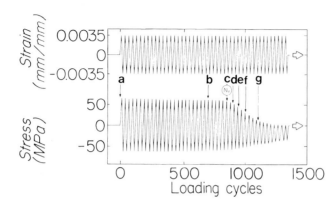 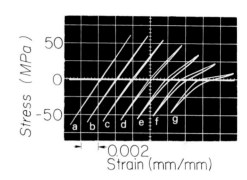

Fig. 8-12: Stress and strain characteristics of a human cortical bone specimen subjected to fully reversed axial loading at a constant strain amplitude of 0.0035. Strain rate 0.01/second. (From Carter and Spengler, 1978 [7].)

gressive, gradual decrease in the tensile stress amplitude. A smaller decrease in the compressive stress amplitude was observed. At approximately 850 loading cycles a dramatic decrease in tensile stress amplitude was observed; this was followed by a more gradual loss of compressive stress amplitude. The number of cycles to failure was selected to be 850, although complete specimen fracture did not occur. This convention for determining fatigue life is consistent with that established for fatigue testing of plastic materials. At approximately 1,300 cycles this specimen had essentially no tensile stiffness. The compressive stress amplitude was a little more than half the initial stress amplitude. The stress–strain curves corresponding to cycles a through g are shown in **Fig. 8-12**. The

loss of stress amplitude during constant strain-amplitude testing is indicative of progressive fatigue damage accumulation.

The monotonic single-loading tensile tests to failure result in widely varying yield strengths. However, the yield strains of all specimens have exhibited far less data scatter. This finding is consistent with the view of Currey [6], who suggested that bone failure is more strongly controlled by strain magnitude than by stress magnitude. The fatigue behavior of the bone specimens was also found to be much more dependent upon strain amplitude than upon stress amplitude. The plot of strain amplitude versus cycles to failure exhibits much less data scatter than the plot of initial stress amplitude versus cycles to failure (**Fig. 8-13**).

Fig. 8-13: The influence of strain amplitude and initial stress amplitude on the number of loading cycles to fatigue failure. Open and closed circles represent bovine and human bone, respectively. (From Carter and Spengler, 1978 [7].)

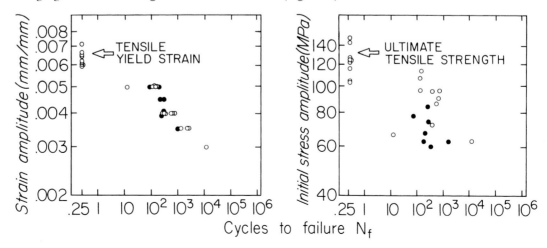

3.2 Cancellous bone

The major physical difference between cancellous bone and cortical bone is the high degree of porosity exhibited by cancellous bone. The apparent density (**Section 3**) reflects this porosity. **Fig. 8-14** demonstrates the influence of bone apparent density on the compressive stress–strain behavior of cortical and cancellous bone. The stress–strain characteristics of cancellous bone are markedly different from those of cortical bone and are similar to the compressive behavior of many porous engineering materials, which are used primarily to absorb energy upon impact. The stress–strain curve for cancellous bone exhibits an initial elastic behavior followed by yield, which occurs as the trabeculae begin to fracture. Yield is followed by a long plateau region that is created as progressively more and more trabeculae fracture. The fractured trabeculae begin to fill the marrow spaces and, at a strain of approximately 0.05, most of the marrow spaces have filled

with the debris of fractured trabeculae. Further loading of cancellous bone specimens after pore closure is associated with a marked increase in specimen stiffness.

The strength and elastic modulus of bone tissue are markedly influenced by the apparent density of the tissue. **Fig. 8-15** illustrates the influence of apparent density on the strength and elastic modulus of bone specimens tested in the laboratory. The data presented on these curves represent cortical bone with an apparent density of approximately 1.8 g/cm³, as well as numerous cancellous bone specimens with widely different apparent densities. These graphs indicate that the strength of all bone tissue in a skeleton is approximately proportional to

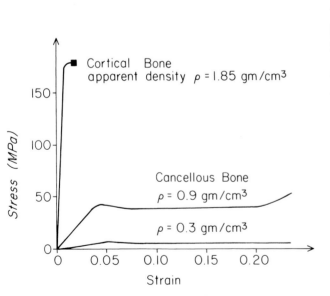

Fig. 8-14: The influence of bone apparent density on the compressive stress–strain behavior of cortical and cancellous bone.

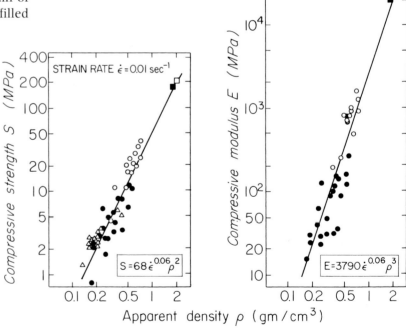

Fig. 8-15: The influence of apparent density on the compressive strength and modulus of cancellous and cortical bone. (From Carter and Spengler, 1978 [7].)

the square of the apparent density. The elastic modulus of bone tissue is approximately proportional to the cube of the apparent density. Although these relationships were initially derived from compressive tests, recent tensile tests of cancellous bone in our laboratories indicate that the strength of cancellous bone in tension is approximately the same as that in compression. In addition, the elastic modulus of cancellous bone is approximately the same in tensile loading as in compressive loading.

Fig. 8-16 is a force–displacement curve, which was generated during tensile testing of a cancellous bone specimen. The stress–strain behavior of cancellous bone in tension is markedly different from that in compression. Yielding is followed by progressive fracture of trabeculae, which causes the tensile load to diminish rapidly at fairly low levels of strain. At the point of total fracture, the two ends of the cancellous bone specimens separate, and the specimen can neither sustain additional loading nor absorb additional energy. Although the tensile strength and modulus of cancellous bone are similar to the compressive strength and modulus, the energy-absorbing capacity of cancellous bone in tensile loading is markedly less.

Fig. 8-17 demonstrates the energy absorbed by cortical and cancellous bone (apparent density 0.4 g/cm³) when the speci-

mens are loaded to strain levels of 0.036 and 0.50, respectively. At a strain of 0.036 the cortical bone, both in tension and compression, is fractured and therefore can absorb no more energy with increasing deformation. The cancellous bone is also totally fractured in tension and can absorb no further energy with increasing deformation. The cancellous bone in compression, however, has failed but will continue to absorb considerable energy with increasing bone deformation. This increasing energy absorption of cancellous bone in compression is demonstrated by the bar graphs for energy absorbed at 50% strain. It can be seen that the energy absorption capability of cancellous bone in compression is considerable and may even exceed the energy absorption capacity of cortical bone.

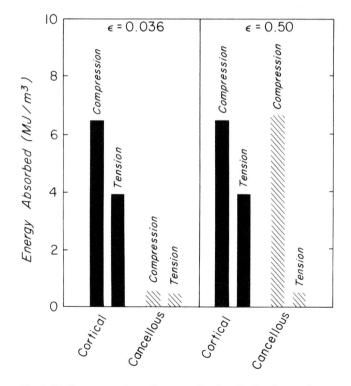

Fig. 8-17: The energy absorption capacity of cortical and cancellous bone in tension and compression. Apparent density of cancellous bone equals 0.4 g/cm³.

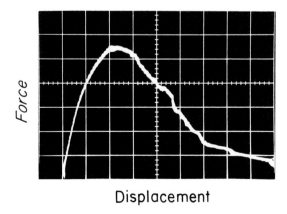

Fig. 8-16: Force–displacement curve of cancellous bone loaded in tension.

3.3 Influence of composition and microstructure

Bone composition and structure may vary significantly. These variations can be characterized by assessing differences in bone-tissue microstructure, porosity, mineralization, and bone matrix. Many investigations of the material behavior of bone have been based explicitly or implicitly on an examination of the influence of one or more of these parameters. However, it should be noted that in vivo these parameters seldom vary independently and are usually observed to vary simultaneously. It is much easier to demonstrate a correlation between a particular characteristic of bone tissue and its mechanical behavior than to positively identify a direct cause and effect relationship between a single parameter and the material properties of the bone tissue. In this section the effect of bone composition and microstructure on material properties will be examined briefly. Carter and Spengler provide a more in-depth treatment [7].

3.3.1 Age

Bone mineral content is low in children but increases rapidly and is high throughout the middle adult years. After the age of 40 years, bone mass declines [8]. Rarefaction is especially marked in postmenopausal females, since the osteogenic effect of estrogens is no longer present. The loss of bone in the elderly is common and is referred to as physiologic osteoporosis. If mineral loss is severe, the condition is called pathologic osteoporosis, although the distinction between physiologic and pathologic osteoporosis may be somewhat arbitrary.

The loss of bone mass in the elderly results in a reduction of the cortical thickness of the long bones and a decrease in the apparent density of cancellous bone. The most obvious changes seen clinically in osteoporotic patients are in the spine, where multiple chronic fatigue fractures may occur. The vertebral bodies are composed primarily of cancellous bone. As discussed earlier, the strength of cancellous bone is approximately proportional to the square of the apparent bone density. Small changes in the apparent density of vertebral bodies therefore cause significant losses of vertebral strength and fatigue resistance. What follows is progressive collapse and shortening of the vertebral bodies. In the lumbar spine this condition may lead to multiple collapse fractures, while in the dorsal spine vertebral wedge fractures are created. There is an overall reduction in the height of the patient and a characteristic dorsal kyphosis ("Dowager's hump"). Chronic back pain is a common finding.

There is also a marked increase in the frequency of fractures in the peripheral skeleton of an osteoporotic patient. These fractures often occur in the hip and may lead to serious complications. The incidence of cervical or trochanteric fracture increases dramatically with age, whereas the severity of the precipitating violence generally diminishes [9].

Changes in the material properties of cancellous bone are affected primarily by an increase in bone porosity and a decrease in apparent bone density. Changes in the material properties of cortical bone tissue are caused by gradual changes in bone composition and bone microstructure and a reduction in cortical thickness. A continuous process of cortical bone remodeling occurs throughout life and serves to change the internal microstructure of the bone tissue. This process is initiated by the osteoclastic resorption of bone and results in anastomosing tubular cavities, which are longitudinally oriented. Osteoblasts on the surface of these cavities then deposit successive layers of new bone with an orderly collagen fiber orientation. The caliber of each activity is thereby gradually reduced until only a small single vascular canal remains.

The newly formed cylinders of bone are called secondary haversian systems or secondary osteones. Secondary osteones consist of concentric sheets of laminated bone. These osteons are always bounded by a thin amorphous cementing substance, which is formed where osteoclastic activity ceases and osteoblastic bone formation resumes. The irregular area of bone between secondary osteones is called interstitial bone and consists of remnants of the bone that previously occupied the area.

Due to the remodeling phenomenon in cortical bone, aging is associated with an increase in the number of osteons and osteon fragments in a given area of bone. This results in a greater number of cement lines for a given area of bone. Numerous researchers have shown that cement lines are sites of mechanical weakness in cortical bone. It therefore appears that the extensive remodeling of bone with age results in a microstructural pattern which is less effective for resisting mechanical stresses. Remodeling of bone during aging also produces variations in bone porosity through the cortical thickness. In the aged individual, bone near the endosteal surface is more porous than the more recently formed, less extensively remodeled periosteal bone [10]. Variations of porosity through the cortical thickness result in a coincidental distribution of mechanical properties: the bone near the periosteal surface is stronger and stiffer than the more endosteal bone tissue.

Aging also causes significant changes in collagen cross-linking and mineralization in cortical bone. There is a gradual increase in the degree of collagen cross-linking and bone mineralization. These age-dependent changes tend to make the bone tissue stiffer and stronger than bone tissue of younger individuals. However, the amount of strain to failure generally decreases. The decrease in ultimate strain is associated with the decrease in the energy-absorbing capacity of the bone tissue. The tissue is therefore slightly more brittle than the bone of younger individuals.

The microstructural and compositional changes in cortical bone tissue associated with aging result in an overall reduction in the material properties of the bone tissue. The mechanical strength of cortical bone is greatest in the age range from 20–39 years. Further aging is associated with the loss of strength and stiffness as well as energy-absorbing capacity. The loss of strength and stiffness is not due to a decline of the strength and stiffness of the mineralized bone, but rather to a slight increase in bone porosity. The loss of energy-absorbing capacity is partly due to the increased brittleness of the mineralized tissue caused by increasing collagen cross-linking and mineralization.

3.3.2 Disease

Disease processes can alter the mechanical response of bones by altering either bone geometry or the bone-tissue material properties. Disease processes alter the material properties of bone tissue by changing the chemical composition of the bone matrix and/or the bone mineral. Bone tissue can be considered a two-phase composite material consisting of mineral and collagen. Increases in collagen cross-linked density are generally associated with an increase in mineral content. The resulting bone tissue is made much stronger and stiffer, not only by the increased mineral content but also by the stiffening of collagen matrix. Disease processes that tend to inhibit collagen cross-linking are often associated with a decrease in mineralization and a weakening of the bone tissue. In some disease processes the primary deficiency leads to a direct decrease in the amount of bone mineralization, which causes significant weakening of the bone. This situation may occur in diseases such as vitamin-D-deficiency rickets.

Defects in collagen metabolism may be responsible for changes in the mechanical properties of pathologic bone. For example, Russell et al. [11] reported a decrease in rat bone collagen cross-linking in the uremic state and suggested that this defect may explain the osteodystrophy observed in chronic uremia. Mechanic et al. [12] reported defective collagen cross-linking in the vitamin-D-deficient state. A defect in collagen cross-linking has also been reported in patients with osteogenesis imperfecta. In these patients, changes in collagen type have also been reported.

The influence of fluorosis on the mechanical properties of bone has received considerable attention. In certain experimental systems, sodium fluoride increases bone formation and would appear to be a reasonable substance to influence favorably osteopenic bone disease. However, considerable controversy exists concerning the mechanical properties of fluorotic bone. Results to date suggest that severe fluorosis causes a decrease in the strength of cortical bone and an increase in the strength of cancellous bone. The increase in cancellous bone strength is a result of the increase in apparent density of cancellous fluorotic bone. The actual strength of the trabeculae present, however, is probably reduced in a manner consistent with the reduction in bone strength seen in cortical fluorotic bone.

4 Whole bone fracture

4.1 Influence of bone size and shape

When the skeletal system is exposed to severe trauma, the bones are subjected to very high forces. Fracture occurs when the stresses in one region of the bone exceed the ultimate strength of the bone material. Bone fracture can therefore be thought of as an event which is initiated at the level of the material. The size and shape of the bone under loading determine the distribution of stresses throughout the bone. A large bone is more resistant to fracture simply because it distributes the internal forces over a larger volume of bone material. The stresses at any one location are therefore less than those in a smaller bone loaded under similar conditions.

A notable physical characteristic of long bones is that their diaphyses are tubular in shape. A tubular structure can better distribute the stresses imposed by bending and torsional loading than a solid cylindrical structure.

A given structural member (bar) can better resist torsional and bending loads if the material which comprises that member is distributed at a distance from the central axis.

The distribution of mass about the center of a structural member can be quantitatively described by the moment of inertia.

Tubular structures have a larger moment of inertia both in bending and torsion than cylindrical structures with the same amount of mass. **Fig. 8-18** illustrates three bars composed of the same material. Bar A is cylindrical and has a cross-sectional area of one square unit. Bar B has the same mass and cross-sectional area as bar A. However, bar B has a hollow interior and therefore a greater moment of inertia. Bar C has twice the mass and therefore twice the cross-sectional area of bars A and B. Since the additional mass of bar C is at the perimeter of the bar, far from the center, this will result in a much greater moment of inertia.

The tensile and compressive strength of the three bars illustrated in **Fig. 8-18** is directly proportional to the cross-sectional area. Therefore, when exposed to tensile or compressive loading, bars A and B will have the same strength and bar C will be twice as strong as A and B. In torsional or bending loading, however, the favorable distribution of mass in bars B and C makes these bars much stronger than bar A. In these loading modes, bars B and C will be 210% and 459% stronger than bar A, respectively.

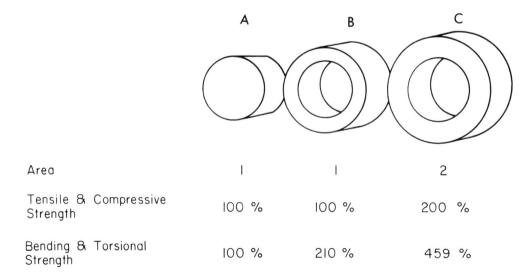

	A	B	C
Area	I	I	2
Tensile & Compressive Strength	100 %	100 %	200 %
Bending & Torsional Strength	100 %	210 %	459 %

Fig. 8-18: The influence of cross-sectional geometry on the structural strength of circular bars.

The influence of the moment of inertia on the structural strength of long bones is particularly relevant when the bone shape during fracture healing is considered. During the healing process, a fracture callus consisting of newly mineralizing bone tissue is formed at the fracture site. This callus bridges the gap between fractured bone ends and tends to produce a cuff of bone with a significantly greater diameter than that of the normal bone (**Fig. 8-19**). During healing the fracture callus is not as well mineralized as the normal bone, and therefore has inferior material properties. The high moment of inertia offered by the fracture callus, however, tends to compensate for this lack of material integrity and is an important factor in establishing stability at the fracture site. As the fracture heals, the fracture callus becomes progressively more mineralized and gradually increases in material strength. The excessive bone material around the perimeter of the callus is then progressively resorbed. With time, the healing bone reassumes its normal material properties and geometry.

4.2 Bone defects

Certain surgical procedures, as well as naturally occurring pathologic bone lesions, may create defects in the normal bone geometry, which significantly affect the fracture resistance of whole bones. Specific examples of these defects include screw holes, surgically excised bone slots, and bone cysts. Such defects reduce the strength of the bone by removing bone mass, causing the internal forces to be distributed over a smaller volume of bone tissue. Additionally, and often more importantly, bone defects tend to produce a pattern of poorly distributed stresses within the bone so that very high stresses are created near the defect. In such cases, the defect is said to produce stress concentrations in the bone when forces are applied and the bone tissue material strength near the defect is exceeded under relatively low forces.

Burstein et al. [13] studied the effects of screws and screw holes on the torsional material properties of rabbit bones. Drilling a hole in the bone diaphysis and inserting a screw created a 70% decrease in energy storage capacity. This decrease in energy absorption capacity was caused by the stress concentration effect produced by the surgical procedure. Eight weeks after the insertion of the screw the stress concentration caused by the hole and the screw had been alleviated by significant bone remodeling around the screw. However, when the screw was removed, the screw hole in the cortex again served as a stress concentrator and the strength of the bone was again significantly reduced. With time, such screw holes are filled in with mineralized tissue and the normal bone material properties, geometry, and strength are restored.

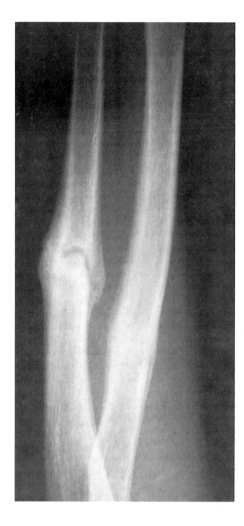

Fig. 8-19: Fracture callus in a healing bone. The greatly increased moment of inertia helps to stabilize the fracture site.

Fig. 8-20 illustrates a fractured femur that was treated by open reduction and internal fixation with a metal plate. After the initial fracture had healed, the metal plate and screws were removed, leaving the bone in a healed but significantly weakened condition. Refracture of the bone then occurred, with relatively minor trauma. The fracture line can be seen to have begun at one of the screw holes, which served as a stress concentrator.

Fig. 8-21 illustrates a torsional fracture through the tibia, which also occurred with minor trauma. The open section defect created by the excision of a cortical window produced a structure that had a drastically different and inferior stress distribution near the defect [2]. The very poor distribution of stresses in torsional loading resulted in bone fracture with very little applied force.

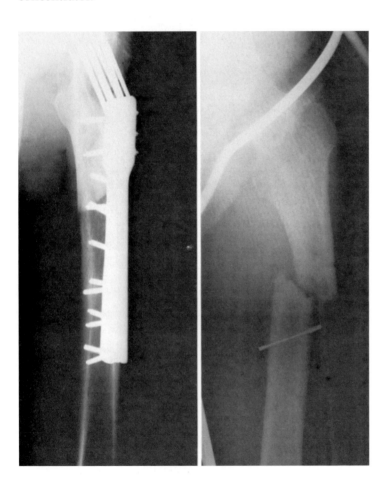

Fig. 8-20: Refracture of the femur caused by the stress concentration due to the presence of a screw hole after the removal of the bone plate.

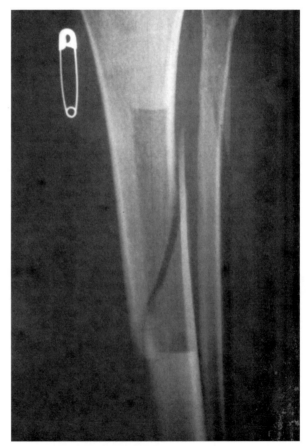

Fig. 8-21: Torsional fracture through an open section defect which was surgically created in the tibia.

4.3 Fracture patterns

In clinical practice, it is common to evaluate patients who have sustained bone fractures but cannot recall the specific injury mechanism. Knowledge of the events that caused injury, however, is important in assessing the patient and suggesting appropriate fracture management.

Some insight into the mechanism of injury can be gained from careful evaluation of the patient's radiographs, which can yield two important kinds of biochemical information. First, the orientation of the fracture lines can provide information on the type of loading which caused the fracture, such as tension, compression, torsion, bending, or combined loading. Second, the degree of fracture comminution allows a reasonable estimate of the energy absorption to failure. For example, a highly comminuted fracture with multiple fragments indicates a large amount of energy dissipation and quite likely a very rapid loading rate, such as is seen in high-speed vehicular accidents (**Fig. 8-22**). In such fractures, a great deal of soft-tissue injury generally accompanies the bone fracture. This section examines some common fracture patterns and relates these patterns to the mechanical events that caused the fracture.

4.3.1 Tension and compression

Tensile stresses are always present in bone subjected to torsional and bending loading. Bone fracture caused by tensile loading along the bone axis, however, is extremely uncommon in the long bone diaphyses. Directly applied tensile forces are associated with avulsion fractures in cancellous bone. Avulsion fractures in metaphyseal areas are encountered at sites of major ligamentous and tendinous attachment, such as the medial malleolus and the peroneus brevis insertion on the fifth metatarsal. An example of pure tensile failure of a patella is demonstrated in **Fig. 8-23**. This fracture, which was produced by forceful contraction of the quadriceps muscle rather than by externally imposed trauma, resulted in a transverse fracture on a plane of high tensile stresses.

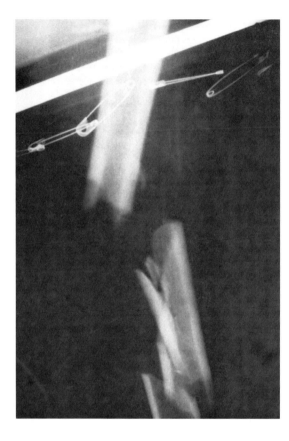

Fig. 8-22: Severe fracture comminution indicating high-energy bone fracture.

A common site of compression fracture in cancellous bone is the vertebral body. **Fig. 8-24** illustrates a severe compression fracture resulting in significant shortening of a lumbar vertebra. As suggested in **Fig. 8-17**, this compression fracture of a vertebral body resulted in a much greater absorption of energy than the tensile fracture through the cancellous bone shown in **Fig. 8-23**.

Cortical bone fracture caused by compressive loading along the long bone axis is sometimes observed in the diaphyses of long bones. Axial compression results in high shear stresses on planes, which are oblique to the long bone axis. Bone fracture due to axial compression occurs along these shear

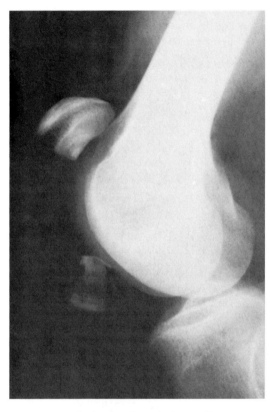

Fig. 8-23: Tensile fracture through the patella.

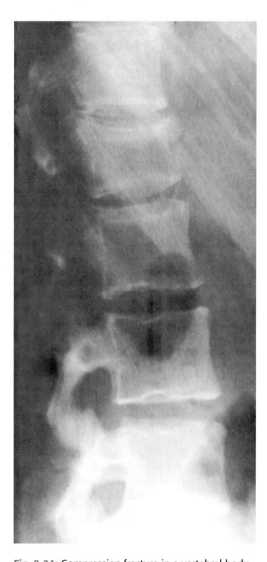

Fig. 8-24: Compression fracture in a vertebral body.

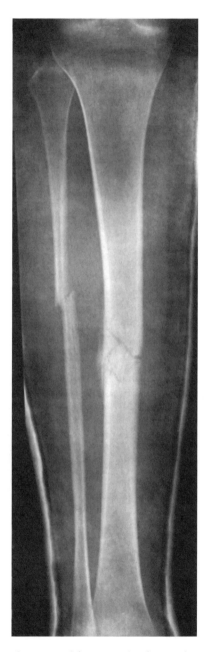

Fig. 8-25: Axial compression fracture in the tibia and fibula.

planes, producing an oblique fracture pattern in the diaphyses. **Fig. 8-25** illustrates a compression fracture in the tibia and fibula under axial loading conditions. Numerous oblique fracture lines are present.

4.3.2 Torsional, bending, and combined loading

Torsion is a commonly encountered loading situation which results in diaphyseal bone fracture with a spiral oblique appearance. Compare the radiograph of a human tibia (**Fig. 8-21**) and a human femur (**Fig. 8-26**) to the photograph of an experimentally produced in vitro torsional fracture in a dog femur (**Fig. 8-27**). In each of these cases a spiral fracture pattern was created; however, the degree of comminution is different in each fracture. The degree of comminution reflects the relative degree of trauma and force imposed on each of the bones. The fracture illustrated in **Fig. 8-21** was produced with relatively minor trauma and was primarily a result of the weakening of the bone caused by the open section defect. **Fig. 8-26** shows slightly greater comminution, which suggests that the fracture was caused by significantly higher forces and greater energy. The in vitro fracture illustrated in **Fig. 8-27** was produced at a very rapid loading rate, which led to more comminution and higher energy absorption. As stated previously, the spiral oblique pattern produced in torsional fractures is caused by bone failure along planes of high tensile stresses (**Fig. 8-11**).

High bending forces that create tensile stresses on one aspect of the cortex and compressive stresses on the opposite side often cause fracture in long bones. **Fig. 8-28** illustrates a fracture in the mid-diaphysis of the femur. A primarily transverse fracture is seen through one cortex, and a large "butterfly" fragment is seen on the opposite cortex. The butterfly fragment was formed by the propagation of two cracks on oblique fracture planes. The size of the butterfly fragment suggests that, in this case, significant axial compressive forces may have been acting in addition to bending forces.

Most fractures seen clinically are not produced by the simple loading mechanisms described, but are produced by a more complex loading situation. **Fig. 8-29** illustrates a fracture

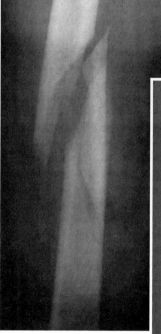

Fig. 8-26: Torsional fracture in the diaphysis of the femur.

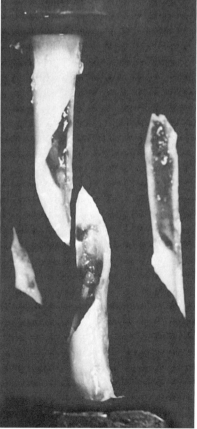

Fig. 8-27: Torsional fracture created in a canine long bone under rapid loading conditions.

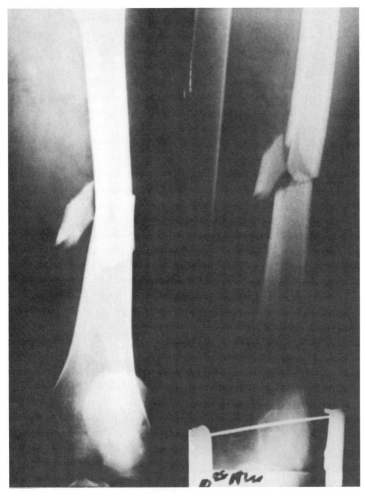

Fig. 8-28: Diaphyseal fracture caused by bending forces. A "butterfly" fragment was provided on the side of the bone subjected to compressive stresses.

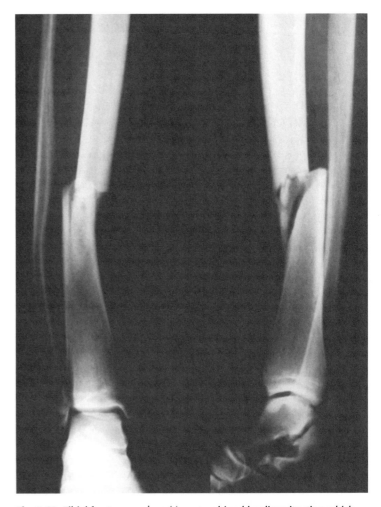

Fig. 8-29: Tibial fracture produced by a combined loading situation which probably included torsion, axial compression, and bending. Note the residual deformation of the fibula caused by yielding.

in the tibial diaphysis, which consists of a spiral fracture surface through one cortex and a transverse fracture through the opposite cortex. Also present are several small oblique lesions in the proximal bone fragment. This fracture was probably caused by a combination of torsional, bending, and compressive forces. The transverse fracture through one cortex was probably caused by tensile stresses produced by bending forces.

Torsional loading was probably responsible for the spiral oblique fracture surface. Fracture of the tibia and the subsequent tibial shortening resulted in significant residual deformity of the fibula. This residual bending in the fibula suggests that the bone material of the fibula was loaded beyond its yield point, but not sufficiently to produce complete fibular fracture.

4.3.3 Fatigue fracture

Fatigue (or stress) fractures are commonly observed in clinical practice. Patients with these fractures generally present with complaints of pain and localized bony tenderness. Initial radiographs may be normal, although a bone scan often reveals locally increased metabolic activity which reflects a localized increase in bone turnover. Fatigue failure of bone in vivo occurs when the accumulation of bone microdamage caused by mechanical stress surpasses the bone's ability to repair that damage. Fatigue fractures have commonly been reported in military recruits who were presumably in marginal physical condition, yet performed rigorous tasks such as carrying another individual rapidly over a long distance. When fatigue fracture is initiated in the hip area, significant morbidity may result. Early recognition and treatment are essential to prevent complications. In most situations prompt treatment consisting of elimination of weight bearing or immobilization results in healing.

The fracture patterns created in fatigue fractures are consistent with those previously described for the fracture of bone in severe trauma. **Fig. 8-30** illustrates a fatigue fracture consisting of a transverse lesion in the midtibial diaphysis. Biomechanical studies have shown that during running this area in the tibia is subjected primarily to tensile stresses along the bone axis. The production of a transverse lesion is consistent with the predicted fracture pattern caused by longitudinal tensile stresses. In other locations of the skeleton, such as the medial aspect of the femoral diaphysis, longitudinal compressive stresses are present during rigorous activity. In these locations fatigue fractures generally present as oblique lesions which form on planes of high shear stresses [14].

4.3.4 Pathologic fractures

The presence of underlying tissue abnormalities can significantly alter the mechanical response of bones. Pathologic changes can affect the mechanical behavior by causing a decrease in bone mass (osteoporosis, osteogenesis imperfecta), an altered bone quality (osteomalacia, osteogenesis imper-

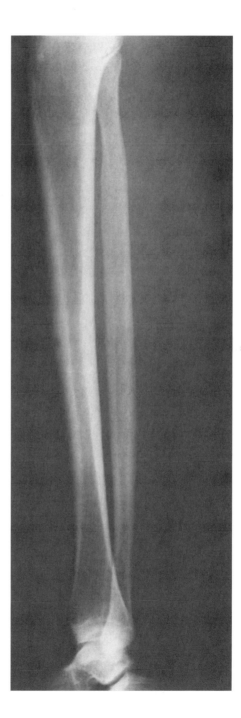

Fig. 8-30: Fatigue fracture in the anterior tibial diaphysis.

fecta), or changes in the distribution of bone mass (acromegaly). Pathologic fractures generally have little comminution, since the pre-existing abnormalities markedly impair the ability of the bone to absorb energy.

Fig. 8-31 illustrates a bone fracture through an area of metastatic carcinoma. Note the extensive bony destruction and minimal comminution. The presence of distal cortical destruction involving the lateral cortical wall suggests the necessity of using an internal fixation device that will safely reinforce the entire area.

Fig. 8-32 illustrates multiple fractures in various stages of healing in a patient with osteogenesis imperfecta. Note the

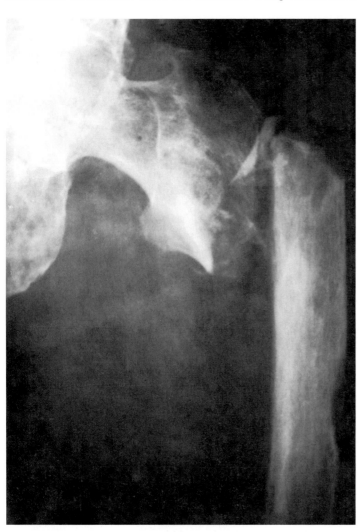

Fig. 8-31: Pathologic fracture through a region of bone significantly weakened by metastatic carcinoma.

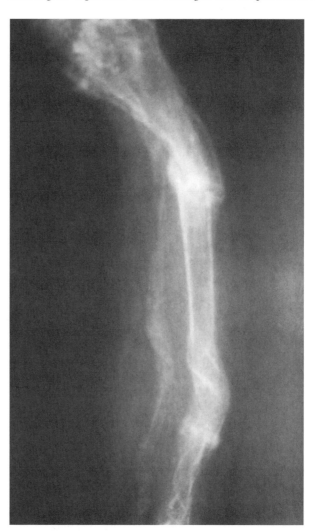

Fig. 8-32: Multiple fractures in various stages of healing in a patient with osteogenesis imperfecta.

extreme loss of apparent bone density, the gross bone deformity, and the paucity of soft tissue. Osteogenesis imperfecta is a systemic disease, which markedly impairs bone strength by altering bone composition and bone geometry.

Senile osteoporosis is a commonly encountered condition that impairs bone strength by increasing the bone porosity and decreasing the cortical thickness, even though no alterations in bone mineralization appear to occur. The loss of total bone mass is associated with an increase in the intramedullary area and periosteal diameter of long-bone diaphyses. The redistribution of bone mass further from the bone axis tends to maintain a high moment of inertia, which partially offsets the decline in bone strength caused by the loss of bone mass.

5 Bibliography

Blue references indicate links to abstracts of articles available online:
http://www.aopublishing.org/BONE/8.htm

1. **Timoshenko S, Young DH** (1968) *Elements of Strength of Materials.* New York: Van Nostrand.
2. **Frankel VH, Burstein AH** (1970) *Orthopaedic Biomechanics.* Philadelphia: Lea and Febiger.
3. **Reilly DT, Burstein AH, Frankel VH** (1974) The elastic modulus for bone. *J Biomech;* 7 (3):271–275.
4. **Reilly DT, Burstein AH** (1975) The elastic and ultimate properties of compact bone tissue. *J Biomech;* 8 (6): 393–405.
5. **Nadai A** (1950) *Theory of Flow and Fracture of Solids.* New York: McGraw-Hill.
6. **Currey JD** (1970) The mechanical properties of bone. *Clin Orthop;* 73:209–231.
7. **Carter DR, Spengler DM** (1978) Mechanical properties and composition of cortical bone. *Clin Orthop;* (135):192–217.

8. **Rose GA** (1970) Irreversibility of Osteoporosis. In: Barzel US, editor. *Osteoporosis.* New York: Grune & Stratton, 37.
9. **Alffram PA** (1964) An epidemiological study of cervical and trochanteric fractures of the femur in an urban population. *Acta Orthop Scand (Suppl);* 65:1.
10. **Smith JW, Walmsley R** (1959) Factors affecting the elasticity of bone. *J Anat;* 93:503.
11. **Russell JE, Avioli LV, Mechanic G** (1975) The nature of the collagen cross-links in bone in the chronic uraemic state. *Biochem J;* 145 (1):119–120.
12. **Mechanic GL, Toverud SU, Ramp WK** (1972) Quantitative changes of bone collagen crosslinks and precursors in vitamin D deficiency. *Biochem Biophys Res Commun;* 47 (4): 760–765.
13. **Burstein AH, Currey J, Frankel VH, et al.** (1972) Bone strength. The effect of screw holes. *J Bone Joint Surg [Am];* 54 (6):1143–1156.
14. **Carter DR, Hayes WC** (1977) Compact bone fatigue damage: a microscopic examination. *Clin Orthop;* 127:265–274.

9 Bone healing: histological and physiological concepts

Berton A. Rahn

1 Postfracture situation

A fracture means that the continuity of a bone is disrupted. Force transmission through the bone is no longer possible in any direction. Tension, bending, or torque will lead to displacement of the fragment ends, although compression perpendicular to the fracture plane is still possible.

The displacement of the fragment ends is determined by the initial trauma, the site of the fracture, external forces, and the pull of the muscles and other soft tissues which are attached to each single fracture fragment. In shafts of long bones external forces, as well as muscle pull, act with long lever arms to displace the fragments. Shortening and angular and rotational deviations therefore occur frequently. In metaphyseal

fractures impaction of the cancellous bone is more often seen. This impaction of cancellous bone mechanically results in a situation which allows only a little interfragmentary motion. In long bones external forces continuously produce interfragmentary motion. Initial immobilization of a fracture is induced by pain: the more painful a fracture, the more careful the individual is in not moving the injured limb. Shortening of a fractured long bone also helps in immobilization. Overlap of the fragment ends provides a more favorable lever arm situation for acting against dislocation (**Fig. 9-1**).

In most cases the disruption of the bone's integrity is not the only damage which occurs during a fracture. Concomitant

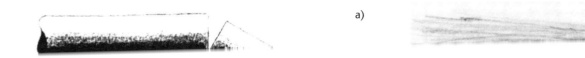

a)

b)

Fig. 9-1: Stability in spontaneous healing. The insufficient early stability (a) is improved by overlap of the fragment ends (b), which provides a more favorable lever-arm situation to minimize dislocation. Muscle contraction assists stabilization.

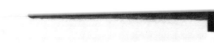
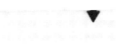

Fulcrum

injuries may markedly influence the further course of healing. Lesions of nerves can, for example, lead to a change in the mechanical loading situation, and it is known that the absence of function results in a porosis of bone. Severe trauma to the skin and soft-tissue cover of a bone may produce circulatory disturbances and may also favor infection. The extent of the vascular damage depends upon the level at which the circulation is interrupted. Disruption of large vessels leads to a hemorrhage into the soft tissues, resulting in a more or less extended hematoma. Because of its local swelling, a hematoma adds somewhat to the stability of the fracture. On the other hand the circulation on the low-pressure side is also impeded, which could retard the healing process. The coagulated blood makes a good growth medium for bacteria and, in the presence of infection, is not desirable.

In later stages the hematoma is replaced by scar tissue, and mechanical disturbances may then occur. Not only may the interruption of circulation in a larger vessel impede regional bone nutrition, but the microcirculation within the bone is also influenced by the trauma. The vessels of the haversian and Volkmann canals are occluded over a distance of a few millimeters from the fragment ends within the first few hours following injury (**Fig. 9-2**).

2 Reasons for fracture treatment

Bone does not necessarily need to be treated to unite, but function may be impaired owing to the deformity. The main point of all fracture treatment is to obtain final function as close to the prefracture situation as possible. The optimum would be obtained by an identical anatomical situation. This would mean that realignment has to be perfect and that, ideally, the immobilization must not allow any motion. Different means of treatment exist which result in different degrees of immobilization. The choice of method must adapt to the requirements of the local situation and to prognostic criteria. In a fracture of a long bone in a young individual, for example, a slight angular deformity still may be tolerated, since compensatory bone remodeling can lead to a normal anatomical structure. No lack

of congruity may be tolerated in an articular fracture. Even a small step in a joint will not allow normal joint function and, in later stages, this will result in degenerative articular changes

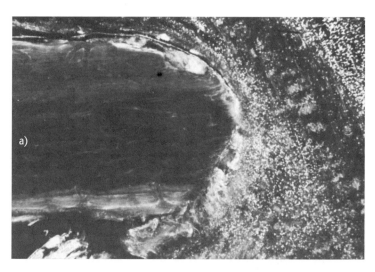

Fig. 9-2: Disruption of circulation in the fragment ends. Approximately 1 hour after fracture, the vital stain, which was injected intravenously, is not seen in the vessels of the fragment ends (a). At a distance of a few millimeters from the fragment ends, the vascular elements and the osteocytes are stained (b), demonstrating intact nutritional pathways.

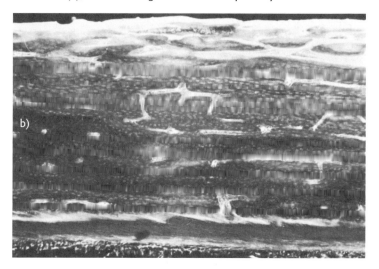

(**Fig. 9-3**). Another example that does not tolerate dislocation is a fracture of the mandible. Here only perfect occlusion of the teeth permits normal mastication and helps to avoid disturbances in the temporomandibular joint.

Not only does the reduction of motion in a fracture area result in better healing of the bone, but soft-tissue healing is also improved when there is no major mechanical irritation. The relief of pain is another reason for the immobilization of a fracture.

3   Tissues in bone healing

During the course of healing, different types of tissues can be seen in a fracture area, whereby one substitutes the other. This leads to a gradually increasing stiffness and strength and to gradually decreasing tolerance to deformation of the healing fracture area.

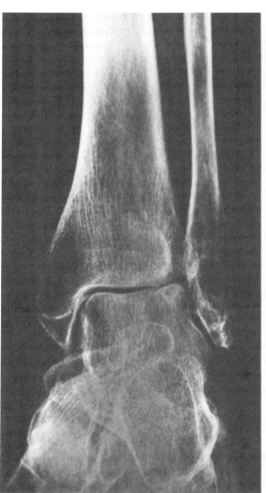
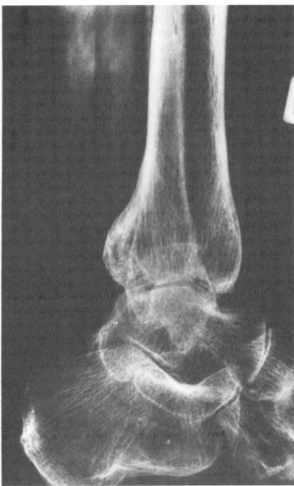

Fig. 9-3: Sequel to articular incongruency resulting in joint degeneration. After an articular fracture the joint surface was not adequately reconstructed. This later led to arthritic complications. (Courtesy of T. Rüedi.)

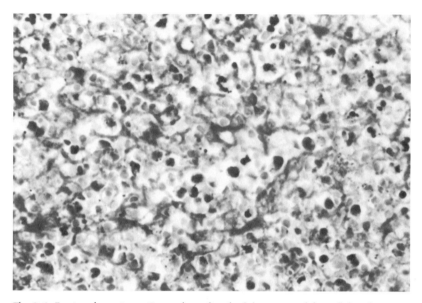

Fig. 9-4: Fracture hematoma. Some days after the injury most of the cellular elements of the blood clot have disintegrated, since they are no longer supplied by oxygen. Erythrocytes and leukocytes can still be distinguished.

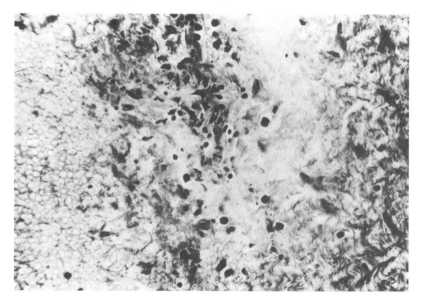

Fig. 9-5: Organization of the hematoma. The hematoma (*left*) is replaced by granulation tissue, which progressively matures to connective tissue (*right*).

3.1 Hematoma

Initially, a hematoma (**Fig. 9-4**) is found between the fragment ends. The blood coagulum as a "tissue" has mechanical properties which are negligible in respect to fracture mechanics. The function of the hematoma in the future of fracture healing is still controversial. There is some evidence that the leukocytes within the blood may transform into fibroblasts and other cells of the supporting tissue system [1], but the hematoma might well act as a guiding structure which, as a spacer, determines the size and shape of the callus. The occurrence of fibroblasts within a hematoma is a fact, whether they immigrate or are locally differentiated. The idea that circulating blood cells may form a mobile reserve of cells, which can help locally in tissue repair, is intriguing.

3.2 Granulation tissue

During the first few days the hematoma changes to become granulation tissue (**Fig. 9-5**). Present are capillary sprouts, mononuclear cells, fibroblasts, and fibrocytes. Not much is yet known about the mechanical properties of granulation tissue. Perren and Boitzy [2], in their theoretical analysis of fracture-healing mechanics, substituted the mechanical parameters of parenchyma as published by Yamada [3]. Granulation tissue is assumed to tolerate an elongation to about double its length and to withstand a maximum force of 0.1 Nm per mm^2 of cross-section until it fails in tension. Its resistance to a change in shape (stiffness) is small (modulus of elasticity $E = 0.05$ Nm/mm^2).

3.3   Connective tissue

During the process of healing, a maturation of this granulation tissue is observed and it is transformed into connective tissue with its collagen fibers (**Fig. 9-6**). This maturation results in an increase in stiffness. The modulus of elasticity (E) for connective tissue reaches values between 16.7 (perichondrium) and 1000 Nm/mm² (tendon), the ultimate tensile strength varies between 2 and 60 Nm/mm², and the elongation to rupture is found to be between 5 and 17%. Fibrous tissue is found in areas where tensile forces act while, according to Pauwels [4], cartilage is formed in zones of hydrostatic pressure.

3.4   Fibrocartilage

The fibrocartilage (**Fig. 9-7**) found in a fracture callus is a multipurpose tissue, which resists compression as well as some tension. The ultimate tensile strength (4–19 Nm/mm²), the modulus of elasticity (20–800 Nm/mm²), and the elongation at rupture (10–12.8%) are in the same order as for connective tissue.

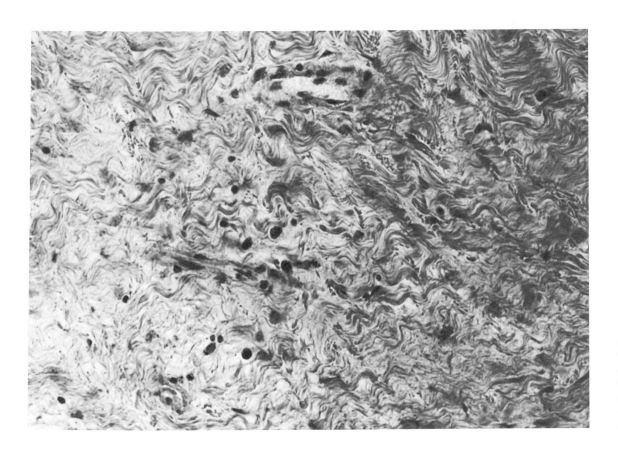

Fig. 9-6: Connective tissue. The connective tissue that developed at the site of the former hematoma shows curled collagen fibers with oval or spindle-shaped cells and small blood vessels.

3.5 Mineralization

During the progress of healing in both fibrous tissue and fibrocartilage, mineralization occurs (**Fig. 9-8** and **Fig. 9-9**). In fibrocartilage the mineralization progresses from the fragment ends toward the center of the fracture gap. The mineralization of the ground substance is followed by local resorption of the

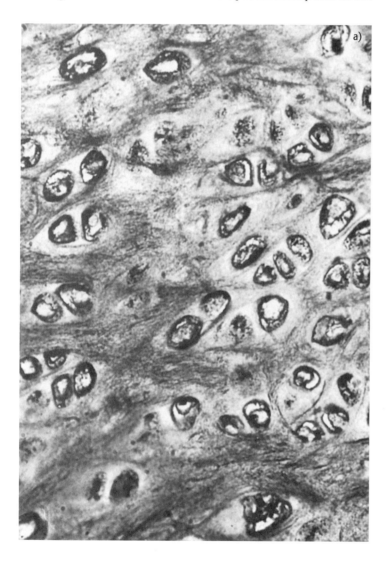
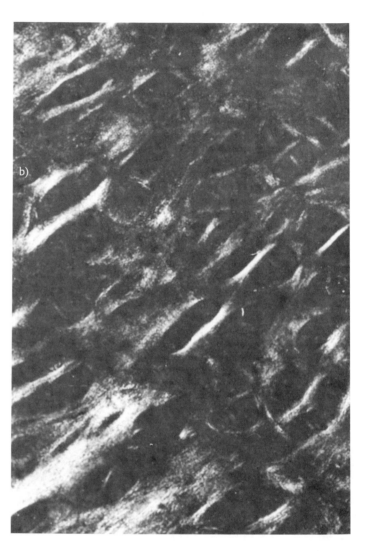

a)

b)

Fig. 9-7: Fibrocartilage. The cartilage found between the fragment ends is rich in fibers that are arranged between the chondrocytes (a). The polarized microscopic picture of the same site demonstrates the pattern of these fibers (b).

mineralized cartilage, whereby new vessels (**Fig. 9-10**) enter the fracture area (see **Chapter 11** on non-union). The walls of the resorption spaces are then covered with lamellar bone, thus forming new bone trabeculae. A further bone deposition combined with local resorption leads to a reshaping of those trabeculae. This mechanism and the resulting structure strongly resemble the bone formation in the zone of growth.

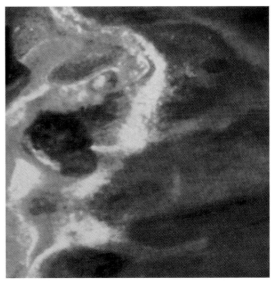

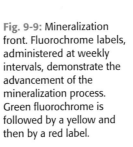

Fig. 9-9: Mineralization front. Fluorochrome labels, administered at weekly intervals, demonstrate the advancement of the mineralization process. Green fluorochrome is followed by a yellow and then by a red label.

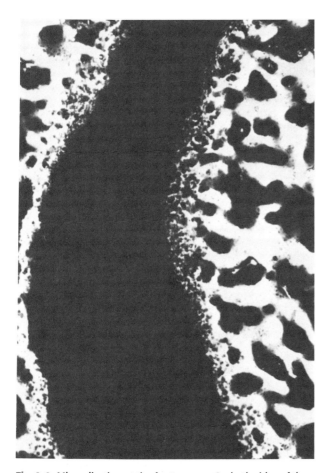

Fig. 9-8: Mineralization at the fracture gap. On both sides of the gap the mineral salts are deposited within the fibrocartilage. Later this mineralized fibrocartilage is remodeled into bone.

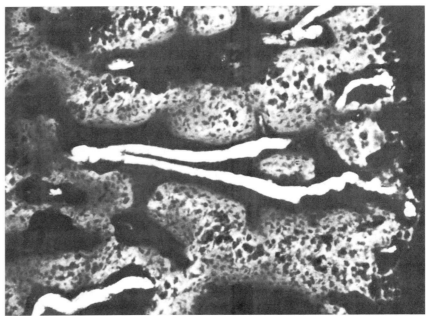

Fig. 9-10: Blood supply to the mineralization front. The vessels shown, filled with barium sulfate to produce radiographic contrast, penetrate the newly formed bone and the mineralized cartilage to transport new supplies for further mineralization.

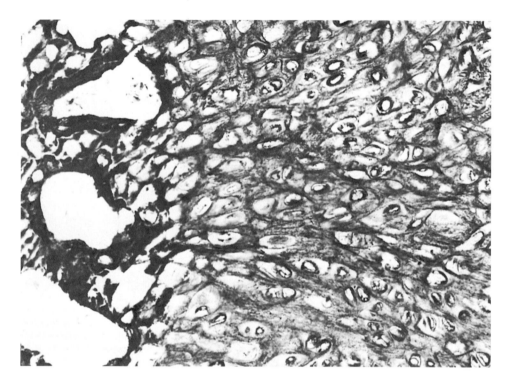

In fibrous tissue the mineralization takes place between the fibers (**Fig. 9-11**). During calcification the fibrous structure (**Fig. 9-12**) is still visible. The increased mineral content leads to an increase in stiffness of the tissue.

However, exact mechanical data in regard to this calcified connective or fibrous tissue are not available.

Fig. 9-11: Mineralization within the fibrous callus. Calcification follows the arrangement of the connective-tissue fibers. The mineralized tissue is soon remodeled to a cancellous structure.

Fig. 9-12: Formation of fibrous bone. As a first step, mineral is incorporated between the connective-tissue fibers. A network of fibrous bone results. By this mechanism, a relatively large area can be mineralized simultaneously. The entire area, labeled in yellow, was formed 10 weeks before the specimen was harvested, while the orange area on the left is 2 weeks old.

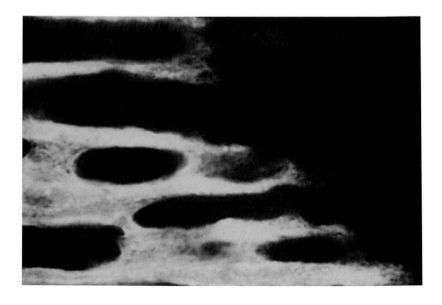

3.6 Cancellous and compact bone

Mineralization of both fibrous tissue and fibrocartilage result in the formation of cancellous bone structures. These structures are not permanent ones; in their spaces the deposition of lamellar bone occurs, which leads to a strengthening of the whole structure and finally to the formation of compact bone (**Fig. 9-13**). Thus a gradual increase in strength and stiffness occurs, along with a reduction of the ability to elongate. The ultimate tensile strength of compact bone is found to be in the order of 130 Nm/mm², the modulus of elasticity in tension at 10,000 Nm/mm², and an elongation of only 2% is possible before it ruptures.

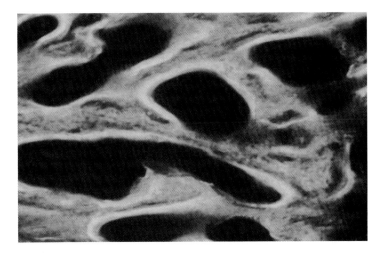

Fig. 9-13: Reinforcement of the initial bony callus. The fibrous bone network (*orange*) is reinforced by the deposition of lamellar bone (*yellow*) on its internal surfaces. This filling of the meshes may continue until the callus consists entirely of compact bone.

4 The role of strain in fracture healing

It seems evident that a tissue cannot exist under conditions which exceed its limits of elongation at rupture. Every movement in the fracture area would lead to an immediate destruction of this tissue. It is, therefore, a fair assumption that a tissue will not form under conditions which would not allow its existence. Perren and Cordey [5, 6] and Perren and Boitzy [2] started from these theoretical considerations to analyze the gradual changes in the mechanical properties of reparative tissues and the replacement with "stronger" tissues during fracture healing.

In long-bone fractures, forces acting with long lever arms tend to dislocate the fracture. The lever arm provided by the cross-section of the fractured bone provides little resistance to displacing forces—for example, bending (**Fig. 9-14**). To keep the fracture fragments in place and to immobilize them completely a strong and rigid material is used. Among all the tissues present during fracture healing, only compact bone fulfills these requirements. Bone tissue, however, cannot be formed initially because of the sizable elongation properties required. In fracture healing, nature uses several "tricks" to overcome these difficulties.

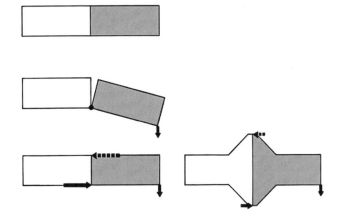

Fig. 9-14: The lever-arm situation during fracture healing. After a fracture of a long bone even a small external force can, by means of the long lever arm, displace fracture fragments. Transmission of compression across the fracture plane is still possible. To counteract the dislocating force, a high tensile force (*interrupted arrow*) is necessary to maintain the fragments in place. No tissue found initially in fracture healing would be able to resist such forces; the fragments would be torn apart immediately after their formation. The increased lever arm, provided by the increased cross-section of the external callus, permits the smaller forces to still reduce the relative motion between the fragments.

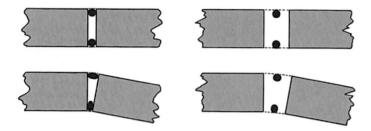

Fig. 9-15: The effect of interfragmentary strain. On bending of a healing fracture, the cellular elements in a fracture gap are deformed; on one side they undergo compression, on the other side distraction. At a given angle of bending, in a wide gap the cellular elements undergo less deformation than in a small gap, since the ratio between change of distance to total distance is smaller.

4.1   Fragment-end resorption

As a first trick, nature transforms the initial situation between the fragment ends to a more suitable one. A good example is a gap area between the fragment ends, which holds cellular elements (**Fig. 9-15**). When an angulation occurs, the cellular elements in the gap are compressed on the concave side and distracted on the convex side. The amount of deformation depends upon the initial gap width. In a small gap the ratio between the change of width to the total width (strain) is high—that is, the cellular element undergoes high deformation. For exactly the same angular deformation in an initially wider gap the deformation of the cellular elements is much smaller, since the change in width is distributed over a larger distance and the single elements have to take over only part of the total change. During spontaneous fracture healing, a widening of the interfragmentary gap by resorption of the fragment ends is a common finding when there is interfragmentary motion (**Fig. 9-16**). This mechanism of fragment-end resorption makes sense, since the tissue in the gap (**Fig. 9-17**) is less deformed and therefore less strained.

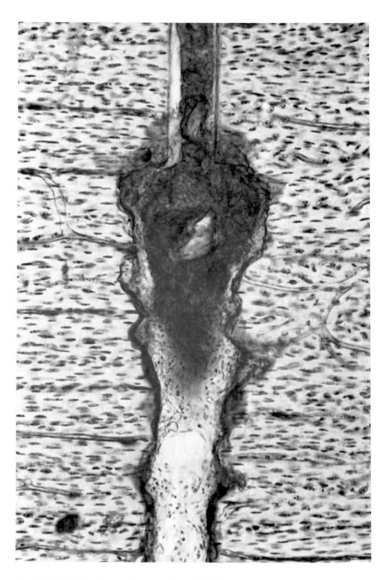

Fig. 9-16: Motion-induced resorption. With interfragmentary motion, resorption of the fragment ends is a common finding. This results in a wider gap between the fragment ends, which means less tissue deformation within the gap.

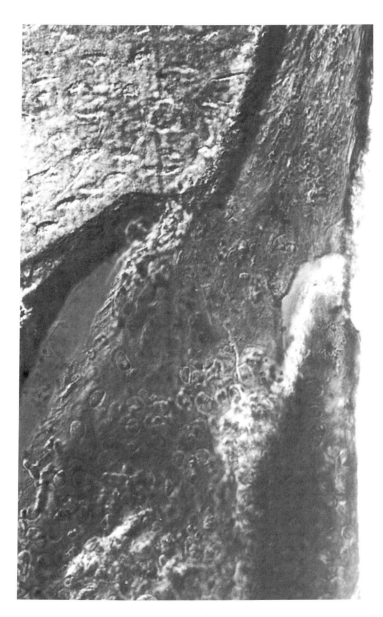

4.2 Formation of tissues suitable for mechanical conditions

As a second trick, nature only builds tissues which can exist under the given mechanical conditions. The comparison of a healing fracture to the construction of a bridge is correct for more or less static conditions (**Fig. 9-18**). As long as there is still motion left between the two parts of the bridge, it is not

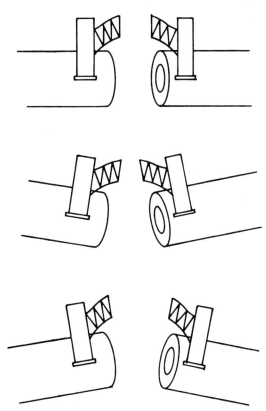

Fig. 9-17: The effect of strain on tissue differentiation. An interfragmentary gap has been partially widened. The tissue found in the narrow part, where the strain is high, is fibrous. In the widened part the strain has decreased. Here the cells are rounded, and the intercellular substance shows signs of mineralization. This is a more mature stage in bone healing.

Fig. 9-18: Bridging under adverse conditions. In spontaneous bone healing the foundations of the forming bridge are under continuous motion. Bridging of the gap may start on both sides, but the union becomes difficult because the distance between the two ends of the arch is continuously changing. Provisional fixation between the two ends (connective tissue and fibrocartilage) facilitates creation of the definitive structure. (After a fracture model by Urist and Johnson, 1943.)

possible to unite the two ends by means of the definitive material. The connection by a material which tolerates elongation and, at the same time, reduces the motion to a certain extent is still possible. This connection is then gradually exchanged and replaced by a tissue, which can exist under the new conditions. The gradual exchange continues until the elongation of the fracture gap is smaller than 2%, which finally allows the formation of lamellar bone. The example of a bone of 30-mm diameter should illustrate this situation. Granulation tissue would still allow an angulation of approximately 40°, fibrocartilage about 5°, and bone would tolerate an angle of only 0.7°.

4.3 External callus formation

Nature's third trick consists of the elaboration of external callus (**Fig. 9-14**). This increases the diameter and therefore increases the ability of the lever arm to resist bending. Perren [**5**] has shown the gain of stability, which is provided by placing the repair tissue away from the axis of the fractured bone: the strength efficiency increases by the third power of the distance of the center of rotation or bending, and the rigidity efficiency increases by the fourth power. By means of this elongated lever arm, even weak tissues can contribute efficiently to immobilization.

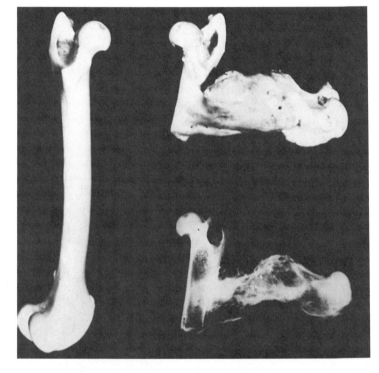

Fig. 9-19: Spontaneous healing in extreme angulation. Bony union usually occurs, even without treatment. The function, however, may be severely altered by malunion, as seen in this chamois, a type of mountain goat. (Courtesy of U. Geret.)

5 Healing patterns

5.1 Healing under unrestricted motion

Under spontaneous healing conditions bony union is usually not a major problem, but the dislocated fragment ends can assume and maintain extreme positions (**Fig. 9-19**).

In many cases fragment motion reaches a high degree. This situation influences the healing pattern in the original fragment ends, in the interfragmentary space, and in the periosteal and endosteal surroundings. During the whole course of

healing, two different stages can be observed. In the first phase the main effort consists of obtaining, in spite of interfragmentary motion, a bony bridge. This allows the return of limb function. The second phase, partially overlapping the first, consists of remodeling of the united bone to result in an anatomically optimal structure.

5.1.1 Formation of a bony bridge

In the first phase, the blood supply of the fragment ends slowly recovers (**Fig. 9-20**). The recovery is based in part upon a recanalization of existing but thrombosed vascular canals in the bone (see **Fig. 9-44**). In larger occluded areas, vascular recovery is linked to intracortical remodeling activities. This remodeling leads to a permanent or temporary loss of bone substance and there fore the fragment ends lose radiological density (**Fig. 9-21**).

The extremities of the fragments often do not regain a connection to the vascular network. Radiologically it may be observed that during the first weeks the fragment ends are rounded and shortened and the fracture gap increases in width. This shortening of the fragment ends, observed in radiological pictures, is due to osteoclastic activity. The resorption starts from the sides, whereby the osteoclasts undermine the fragment ends (**Fig. 9-22**). There is evidence that this "sequestration" takes place in the border zone between areas with and areas without a blood supply.

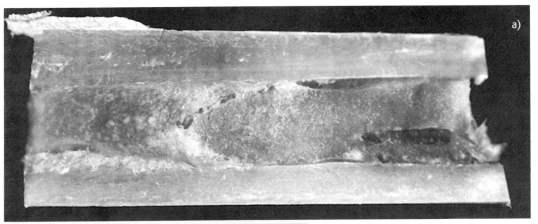

a)

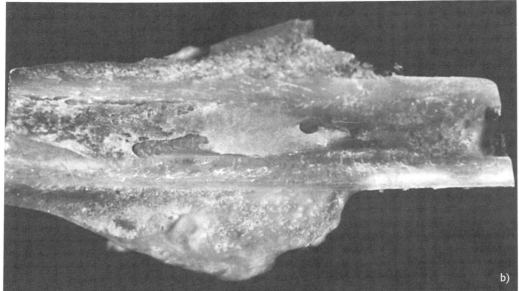

b)

Fig. 9-20: Disturbance and recovery of the blood supply of the fragment ends after osteotomy. Vital staining with disulphine blue shows that the fragment end (*right*) is without circulation for the first few days after the trauma (a). The recovery goes on slowly during the following weeks. Even after 3 weeks (b), extensive areas of the fragment ends still lack a blood supply. (Courtesy of M. Gunst.)

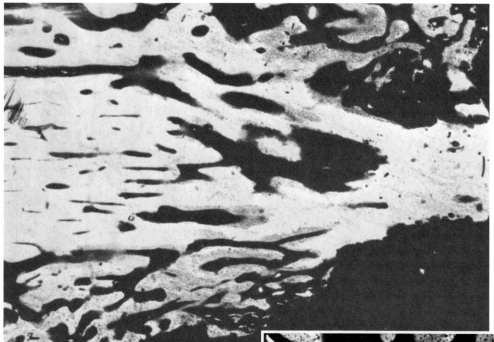

In the interfragmentary space the full spectrum of tissues (**Section 3**) may be observed. From the surrounding soft tissues, vessels sprout into this space, and granulation tissue replaces the hematoma. Granulation tissue matures to fibrous tissue and fibrocartilage. In the interfragmentary fibrocartilage, mineral is incorporated into the ground substance. This increases the stiffness of the tissue and decreases the interfragmentary motion. A resorption of the mineralized cartilage takes place locally, and small canals are formed. Capillaries follow the resorbing cells. Into these resorption canals new bone is deposited on the surface of the remaining trabeculae, and the small trabeculae become large. In the area of

Fig. 9-21: Changes in radiological density of the fragment ends. The border zone of intact circulation shows much increased remodeling activity, whereby a localized osteoporosis temporarily occurs. This microradiograph of a non-decalcified section shows this osteoporosis as well as resorption of the extreme fragment end.

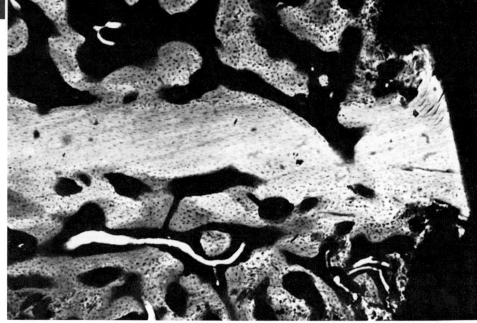

Fig. 9-22: Undermining of the fragment end. Remodeling activity at the fragment ends may become very intense, resulting in undermining or, in extreme cases, sequestration of the fragment ends.

the future cortex the spaces become completely filled to form compact bone, while in the area of the future medullary cavity more resorption activity takes place.

The medullary vessels are interrupted. The interfragmentary fibrocartilage layer forms a barrier to the circulation within the medullary cavity. During fracture healing new vessels enter the cartilage after it has mineralized and been resorbed. The first bridging of vessels occurs on a capillary level, and the reconstruction of a new medullary artery takes some time since the callus tissue in the medullary cavity has first to be resorbed.

The interfragmentary fibrous tissue is arranged in a more or less diagonal pattern (Fig. 9-23). This arrangement allows a higher elongation than the material proper ties of

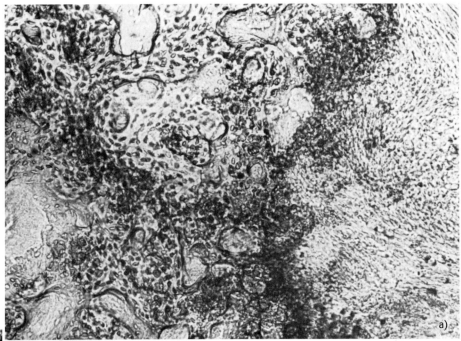

a)

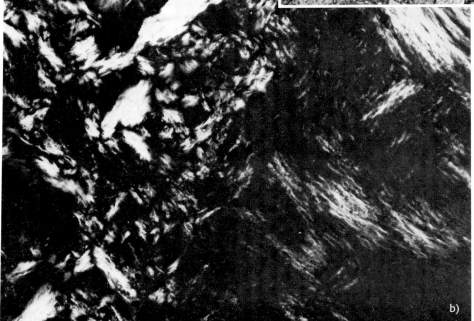

b)

Fig. 9-23: Transformation of fibrous tissue into fibrous bone. The interfragmentary fibrous tissue is arranged in a more-or-less diagonal pattern, and the mineralization follows this arrangement. The border between fibrous tissue and fibrous bone becomes clear in the bright-field micrograph (a). Under polarized light the connective-tissue fibers become apparent (b).

fibrous tissue would permit. The formation of fibrous bone (**Fig. 9-24**) by incorporation of apatite crystals follows this arrangement. Thus, more deformation is tolerated than compact bone would permit. The lower mineral content of fibrous bone will probably contribute as well to the higher deformability.

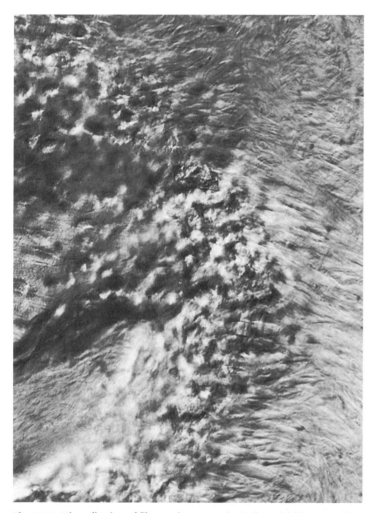

Fig. 9-24: Mineralization of fibrous tissue. Apatite is deposited between the fibers, and the fibrous tissue is thereby transformed into bone.

On the periosteal side callus starts to build up far from the fracture (**Fig. 9-25**). At first a network of fibrous tissue is formed. The fibrous tissue incorporates mineral to become fibrous bone. The parts which have been formed first are the most dense, since lamellar bone is incorporated into the network of fibrous bone. This callus continues to become denser and approaches the fragment ends. It forms a cuff (**Fig. 9-26**) outside of the original bone shaft. Radiographically this callus appears as an arch. The two segments of the arch build up from both sides until they bridge the fracture gap in the middle.

The fracture line in the radiograph loses its sharp outline. This is, on the one hand, due to the overlay effect of the callus, and on the other hand is an effect of bone loss within the original cortices and of the incorporation of mineral in the fibrocartilage and fibrous tissue.

5.1.2 Remodeling of the united bone

After bridging by fibrous bone from one fragment end to the other, stability is obtained and some function is allowed. The mechanical situation now permits bone to be formed wherever it is necessary, and definitive ones can replace provisional structures.

The callus still continues to become denser and, during the following months and years, a continuous change may be observed. Haversian remodeling starts to reconstruct the lamellar direction of the bone, parallel to the long axis of the limb. The callus is resorbed in places where it will not be needed in the future. Therefore, Howship lacunae may be found on the surface of the callus as well as in the region of the future medullary cavity. The diameter of the callus is reduced. In the area of the medullary cavity the bone becomes less dense; while in the area of the original cortices the callus becomes denser (**Fig. 9-27** and **Fig. 9-28**). This finally leads to a reconstruction of the tubular shape of the bone.

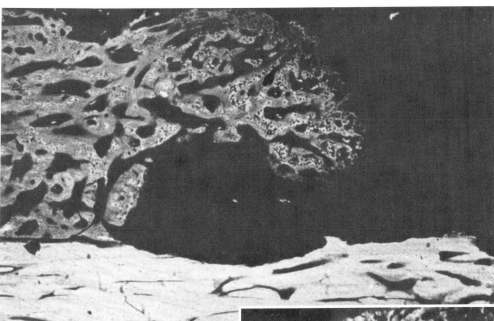

Fig. 9-25: Periosteal callus formation. Formation of periosteal callus usually starts at a distance from the fragment end and grows in the shape of an arch toward the other fragment end.

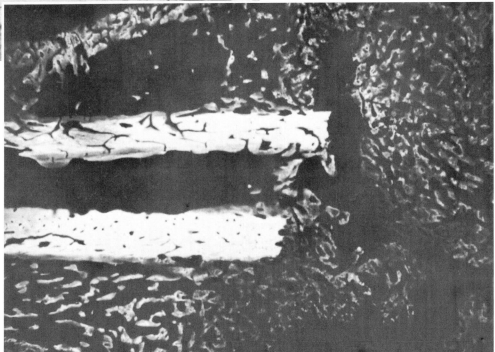

Fig. 9-26: Callus after bridging. The callus forms a cuff around the original bone shaft. The interfragmentary space is not yet completely mineralized.

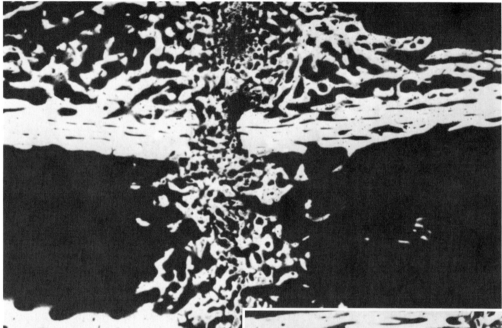

Fig. 9-27: Maturation of the callus. After bony bridging in the interfragmentary space, the callus gets denser in the area of the cortices, and becomes less dense on periosteal and endosteal aspects.

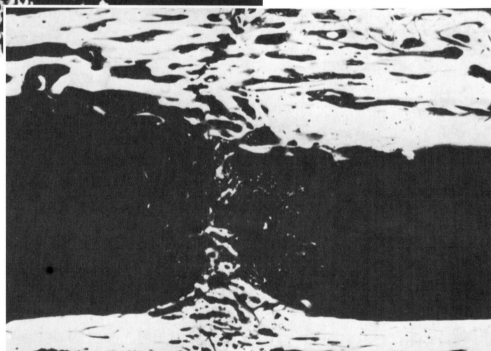

Fig. 9-28: Resorption of the callus after solid union. Intraosseous remodeling leads to reconstruction of axially arranged bone structures in the cortex area. Endosteal, as well as periosteal, callus undergoes resorption.

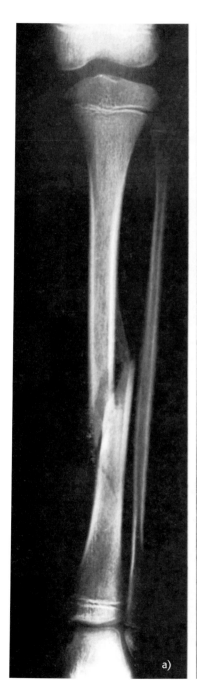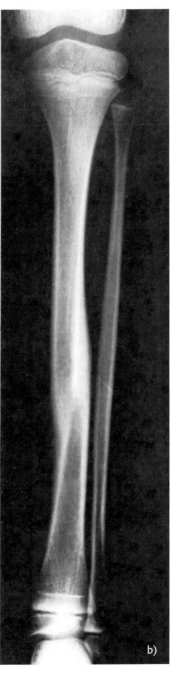

After spontaneous healing in adult individuals malalignment may have to be accepted. In children angular deformations are corrected spontaneously by bone resorption on convex sites and bone deposition on concave sites (**Fig. 9-29**). Shortening can be compensated by epiphyseal overgrowth in children younger than 12 years, while in older children the compensatory growth is not sufficient [7]. In no case will rotation be corrected spontaneously.

5.2   Healing under limited motion

Any fracture treatment aims toward healing in a good position with minimal displacement of the fragments. Some situations tolerate motion more, and some less, to guarantee a clinically acceptable result. The indication for one or the other method of treatment has to consider factors such as the age of the patient, localization and type of the fracture, personal experience of the surgeon, environment, and facilities for the special form of treatment, the risk of complications, etc. Between the two extremes of full motion and absolutely no motion, all intermediates are possible. The healing pattern found in these situations is somewhere between the callus-free healing after absolute stabilization and the type which is representative for spontaneous healing. Any intermediate pattern is possible, depending upon the stability offered by the method of treatment. The pattern of healing in a plaster cast is very similar to the aspect found in spontaneous healing, except that the dislocation is kept to a minimum. The medullary nail, typically, still allows some motion. Healing in this case takes place via a callus, and a resorption of the fragment ends may be seen. In addition, reaming of the medullary canal and the introduction of an intramedullary nail interferes with the circulation of the inner part of the cortex [8]. This zone will then present an intense remodeling (**Fig. 9-30**).

Fig. 9-29: Spontaneous disappearance of angular deformity of a fracture in a child. The angle in the tibia still present 4 weeks after a spiral fracture (a) has almost completely disappeared after 40 weeks (b). Bone deposition on the concave side and bone resorption on the convex side produced this result. (Courtesy of P. Matter.)

Fig. 9-30: a) Remodeling pattern after medullary nailing. At the border zone of disturbed circulation, as revealed by vital staining, remodeling starts with great intensity and enters the non-supplied zone. This shows especially well in the plexiform bone of the sheep tibia. (Courtesy of U. Pfister.) b) The progress of remodeling is well visible in the higher magnification of the microradiograph. At the bottom, resorption canals enter the zone where there is no circulation present. In the middle of the figure, these canals are partially refilled, and on top they are completely refilled. (Courtesy of U. Pfister.)

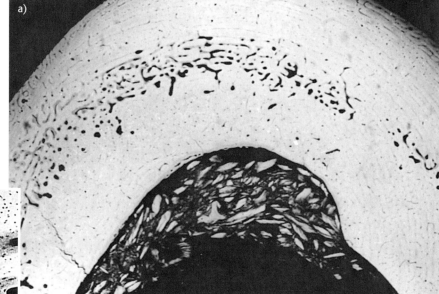

Healing with callus formation after plate fixation may be observed when a plate is placed in an unsuitable position, or when the rigidity of the plate is too low for a given situation. This was experimentally demonstrated by Hutzschenreuter et al. [9], who employed flexible plates on the "non-tension side" of the bone in the sheep. In consequence, resorption of the fragment ends and callus formation could be seen. A stiff plate on the same "non-tension side", however, presented only small amounts of callus (Fig. 9-31).

A plate may provide absolute stability in certain areas but, owing to the elastic deformability of bone, certain areas may be present where relative motion (see Fig. 9-34) or slight instability are present. Here, resorption commences by entering along the fracture plane. Simultaneously callus builds up, as is seen in spontaneous healing. The resorption stops as soon as the callus has bridged the fracture. The gap that is produced by the resorption may then be filled again (Fig. 9-32). A slight initial instability of a screw in the bone will also lead to relative motion between bone and implant (Perren et al., 1975)[10].

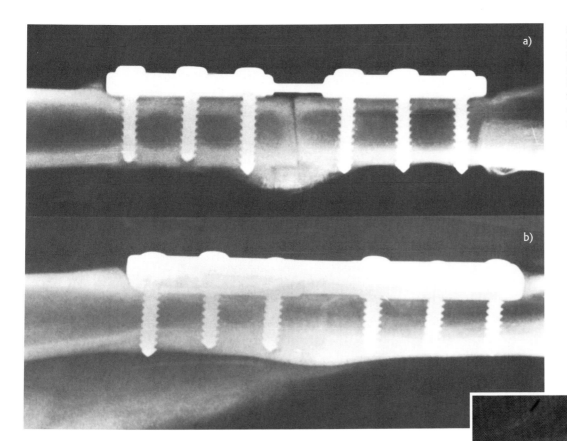

Fig. 9-31: Plate rigidity and healing type. Fixed with a less rigid plate (a), a fracture is still visible after 7 weeks. The fragment ends are resorbed, and periosteal callus has formed. Using a more rigid plate (b), the fracture has disappeared and little callus was formed. (From Hutzschenreuter et al., 1969.)

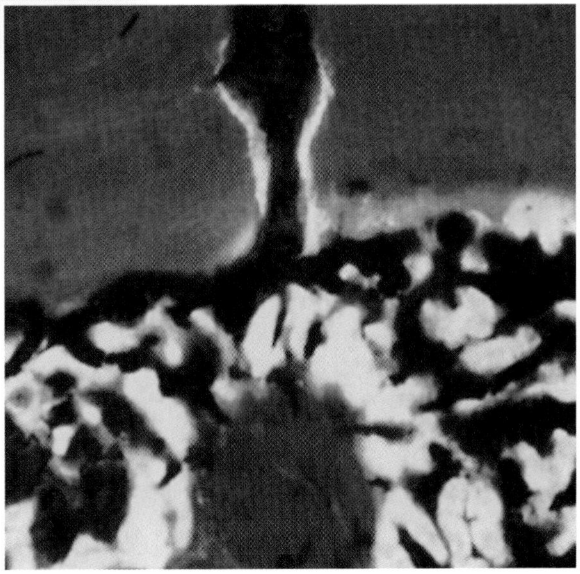

Fig. 9-32: Resorption and callus bridging. Fragment-end resorption can be observed as long as relative motion between the fragments is present. Meanwhile the formation of periosteal callus starts. Motion-induced resorption stops as soon as the periosteal callus has united the fracture. Here, new bone is labeled yellow by tetracyclines. It demonstrates that bone formation in the gap started the moment the callus had bridged the fracture.

Resorption of the original cortex will result (**Fig. 9-33a–c**), and callus around the screw can be observed in the medullary canal. Almost no resorption will result in places that correspond to the center of rotation of that screw (**Fig. 9-33d**).

Cerclage wires or wire sutures, except in situations where they act exclusively as tension bands, do not provide absolute stability. They serve for adaptation and reduction of motion. The callus thus is smaller but otherwise the aspect is similar to that of spontaneous healing.

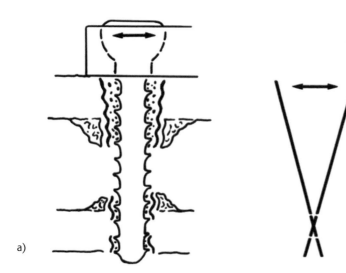

a)

Fig. 9-33a–c: Effect of implant motion on bone. An initial instability leads to relative motion between bone and implant. At the site of the largest excursion a maximum of resorption takes place (a). In addition to the resorption of the cortex, formation of callus in the medullary cavity can be observed (b). The special plate design serves to monitor the stability. Histologically, resorption of the bony interface may be seen, and the bone is replaced by soft tissue (c). (From Perren et al., 1975 [10]).

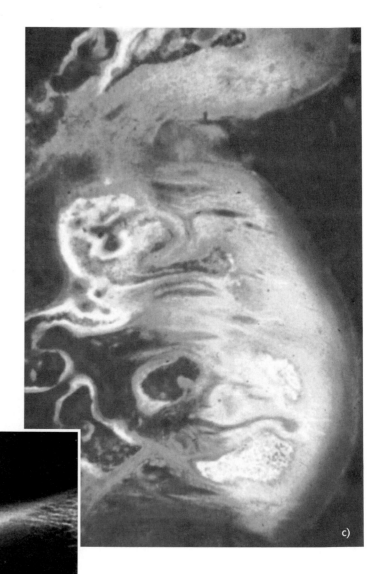

c)

b)

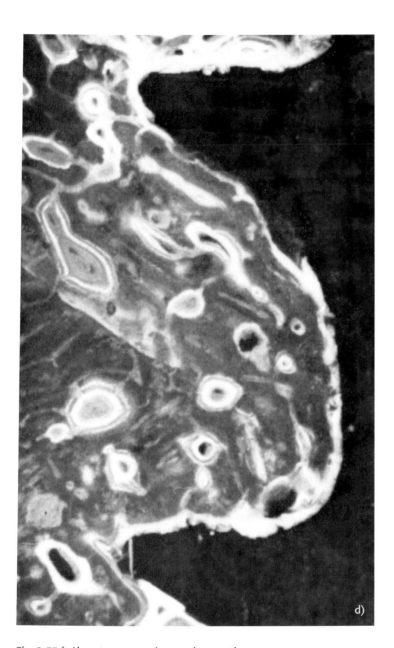

Fig. 9-33d: Almost no resorption results near the assumed center of rotation of the screw (d).

5.3   Healing under absolute stability

Healing under absolute stability is an extreme case in the whole spectrum of fracture healing, and is bound to special technical considerations. Bony contact between the fragments is necessary to maintain stability. Transmission of compression across the fracture is still possible while the implant takes over the tensional forces. Interfragmentary compression leads to the production of friction, which helps to resist lateral shear and torsional forces.

Contact areas and gap zones of different widths (**Fig. 9-34**) characterize the morphologic situation between the fragment ends. Between the compressed fragment ends in the contact area, no motion is allowed as long as the effect of the preload is higher than the effect of the external force. In the neighboring non-loaded areas (gap > 0) a minimal amount of

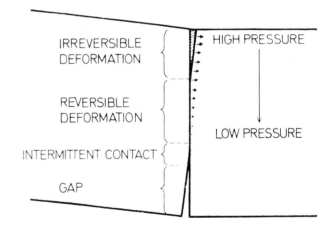

Fig. 9-34: Schematic representation of the mechanical situation at the fracture site following axial compression. This schematic drawing is based on the assumption of a straight plate compressing a transversely cut straight bone. The greatest pressure is found immediately beneath the plate. In some cases the ultimate compressive strength of bone may be exceeded and irreversible bone deformation may result locally. In the remaining contact area bone undergoes reversible deformation. As long as the preload is higher than the superimposed functional load, no relative motion between the fragment ends will result. The elastic deformability of the contact areas will permit slight relative motion in the low-pressure contact areas and in the gap zones.

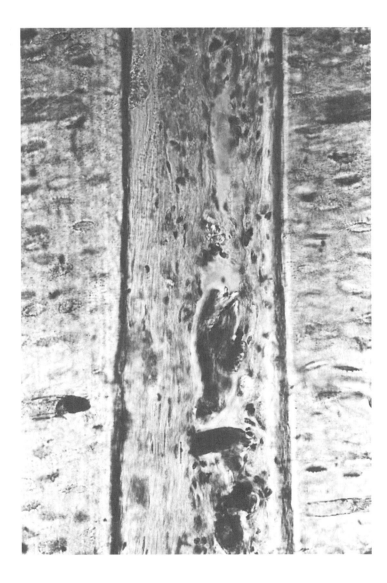

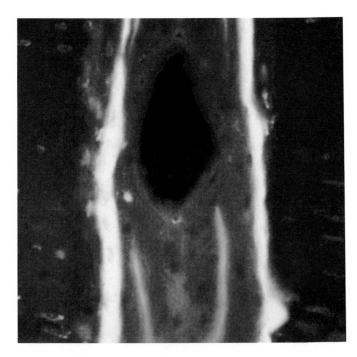

Fig. 9-35: Initial filling of a gap by loose connective tissue. During the first 2 weeks, gap areas, which are stabilized by neighboring contact areas, are entered by blood vessels, and loose connective tissue is formed. The dark areas in the gap are the remainders of the bone debris produced by the osteotomy.

Fig. 9-36: Primary bone formation in a stabilized narrow gap. Lamellar bone formation starts during the second week at the walls of the gap and continues to fill the gap at a speed of 1–2 μm per day. Blood vessels (*black area*) persist in the center of the filled gap.

motion is possible, but it is limited to the elastic deformability of the neighboring contact zones.

As long as there is no destruction of bone in the contact areas, the motion in the gap is small enough to keep interfragmentary strain smaller than 2%. This allows the existence of bone and therefore permits the formation of bone as well.

Within the gap a granulation tissue appears first, bringing in new blood supply. While loose connective tissue (**Fig. 9-35**) can be observed in the center of the gap, the deposition of lamellar bone starts early on the surface of the fragment ends. This lamellar bone deposition continues until the whole gap is filled (**Fig. 9-36**).

The formation of a more mature form of bone in a stabilized gap is usually called gap healing, which is one form of so-called primary bone healing. In larger gaps a network of fibrous bone (**Fig. 9-37**) is first observed. This may be due to the influence of the surrounding soft tissues, which transfer some motion into the gap. In a secondary stage the fibrous bone meshes are filled by lamellar bone (**Fig. 9-38**). The arrangement of the bone in the gap is gap-oriented, not in the long axis of the bone. Although this bone is primarily formed bone (i.e., not formed via fibrocartilage), the fracture is only united by bone tissue the bone is not yet healed at all. The apposition of bone lamellae onto the fragment ends is mechanically still an inferior type of union. Intracortical (haversian) remodeling through the bone-filled gap will later on lead to reconstruction of the original integrity.

Fig. 9-38: Filling of a wide gap. Phase II: The meshes of fibrous bone are filled by lamellar bone in a second stage.

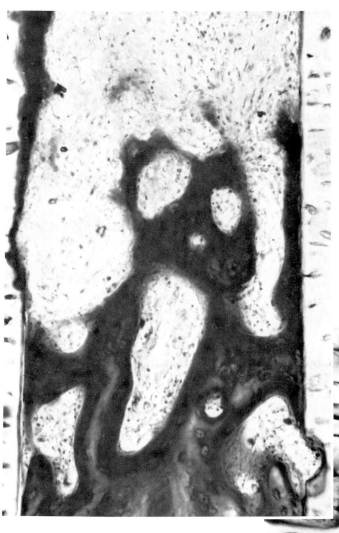

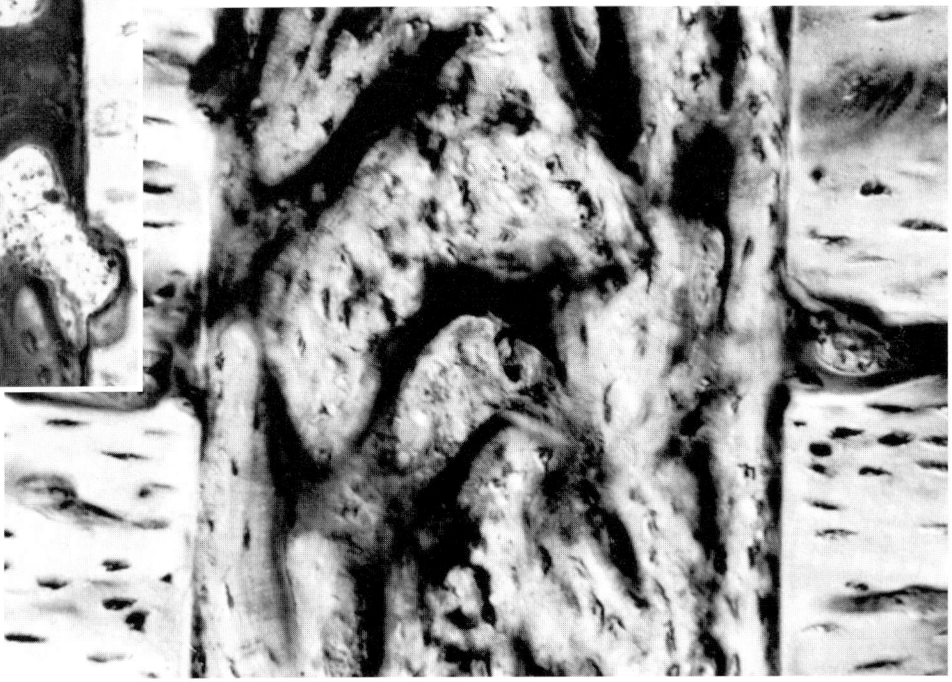

Fig. 9-37: Filling of a wide gap. Phase I: Fibrous bone formation. In a stabilized wide gap a network of fibrous bone is formed, which subdivides the whole space into smaller compartments. The holes in this network are approximately the size of osteons.

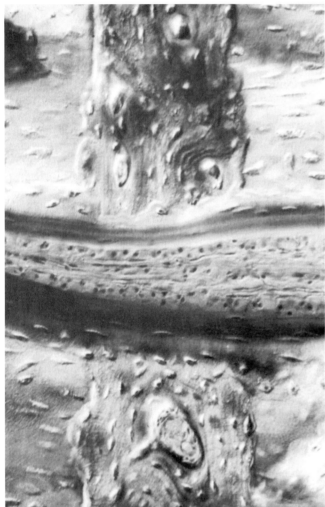

Two types of connecting osteons can be observed: the new osteon originates in one fragment end, crosses the bone-filled gap, and enters the other fragment end (**Fig. 9-39**); or an osteon originates in the filled gap and enters one of the fragments (**Fig. 9-40**). The mineralization during the gap filling starts in the first week, while the remodeling of the filled gap does not usually occur before the third week. The high remodeling activity of the old cortices is limited to a distance of a few millimeters from the fragment ends (**Fig. 9-41**). This area corresponds to the zone of initially disturbed blood supply. In these areas near newly formed osteons, many osteocyte lacunae appear. The lacunae are dark in transmitted light, and bright in dark-field illumination. They are assumed to represent dead osteocytes.

Fig. 9-40: Filling of a gap. Phase IIIb: New osteons originating in the gap. New bone structures can enter the fragments from the gap side, where the blood supply is recovering earlier than in the fragment ends. These plugs help to unite the fragment ends.

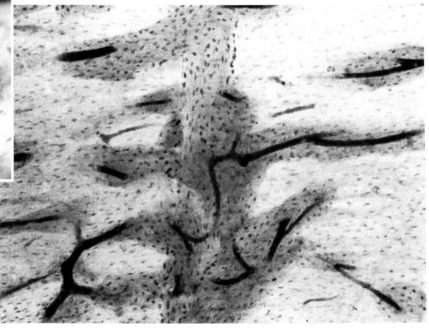

Fig. 9-39: Filling of a gap. Phase IIIa: Remodeling of a filled gap. Part of the new osteons originate in one of the fragments, cross the filled gap, and enter the other fragment. Thus, the fragments are united by lamellar bone structures, which are arranged in the long axis of the bone.

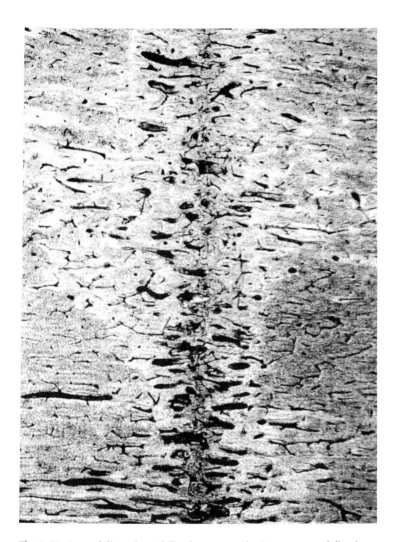

In contact zones the haversian remodeling proceeds through the fracture plane. This leads to a direct bony bridging by a structure, which is already mature bone and is oriented in the normal axial direction (**Fig. 9-42**). The process is called contact healing, the other finding in primary bone healing [**11, 12**]. Here as well, the high intensity of intracortical remodeling is limited to only a few millimeters on either side of the fracture. Although there is no resorption of the fragment ends, as in spontaneous healing, the zone around the fracture loses radiological density while the fracture line slowly disappears. In its first stage, the haversian remodeling removes bone by resorption; later on new bone is deposited in the resorption cavities. This new bone is still less dense during the first few months; therefore the fracture area remains visible radio-logically. No periosteal callus appears during the whole process of bone union, an effect that Danis [**13**] called "soudure autogene"—autogenous welding. The complete remodeling of the fracture area takes from a few months up to a few years, depending upon the species (**Fig. 9-43**).

The stability provided by internal fixation permits a rapid recovery of the medullary circulation. Ganz and Brennwald [**14**] have shown that in transversely cut rabbit tibiae the medullary artery may be reconstructed within 2 weeks. Such a repair is possible only if there is no interfragmentary motion.

Fig. 9-41: Remodeling of a stabilized gap area. The intense remodeling is restricted to a narrow zone in the vicinity of the now bone-filled gap. The area involved in the remodeling process corresponds to the area where the blood supply has been interrupted. This zone is a lighter shade of grey since the osteocytes are likely dead and unable to accept the fuchsin stain.

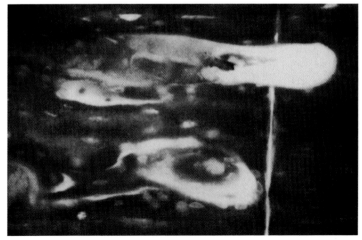

Fig. 9-42: Contact healing. In contact zones, immobilized even at the microscopic level, direct crossing of osteons from one fragment to the other is possible. This results in primary reconstruction of the fractured bone by axially oriented, mature lamellar bone elements.

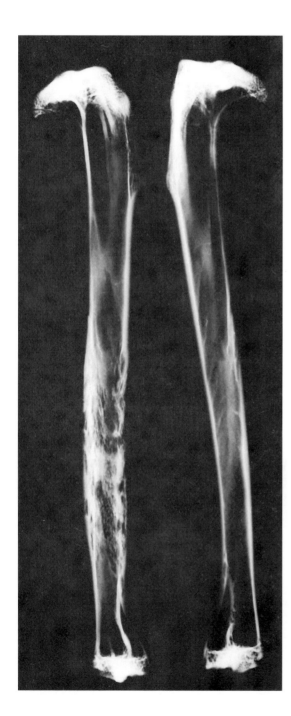

Fig. 9-43: Remodeling of united bone. After the union of a fracture is obtained, the bone has not yet regained its original internal structure. A long phase of intracortical, periosteal, and endosteal remodeling activity is necessary to transform the bone back to its original strength and structure.

Complete immobilization of the fracture is also a prerequisite for the direct crossing of capillaries, from one fragment end into the other, during intracortical remodeling. Plates and screws also produce large areas where circulation is damaged. In all those areas and in the fragment ends the existing vascular canals are closed to circulation. Recanalization seems to take place when the area recovers. Prior to bone remodeling, in part of the canals, resorption around the vessels may be observed which does not include the full size of the surrounding osteon [15–17]. The small new canal is later refilled with bone. This is comparable with internal renovation of existing osteons (Fig. 9-44).

In addition to this intracanalicular renovation mechanism of the haversian and Volkmann systems, the resorption of normal osteon-sized canals is also observed. This remodeling leads to temporary porosis of zones where the circulation has been damaged, and starts in the third week after the trauma. All the resorption cavities are refilled after approximately 1 year, or even more, depending upon the species.

At a later stage another reduction of bone mass under the plate is observed. This may be due to mechanical factors [18]. It is seen especially when heavy implants are used—for example, in double plating—and is a form of "stress protection". It might be the reason why the bone is rarefied. After plate removal in those areas a so-called refracture can occur, even with an otherwise inadequate amount of trauma. This refracture is usually not really a fracture through the old fracture plane, but a fracture in the area where repair processes have been taking place (Fig. 9-45a/b). The total bone mass in the region of the refracture is usually reduced. In addition, the bone structure is not homogeneous. The juxtaposition of fibrous and lamellar bone, new osteons, and porosity might lead to stress concentration (Fig. 9-45c/d).

When internal fixation is used the following aspects have to be considered.

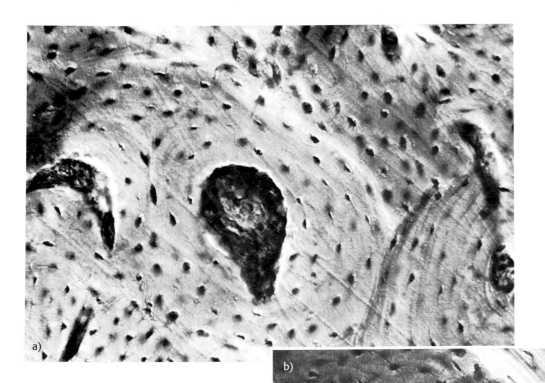

Fig. 9-44: "Renovation" of existing haversian systems. The central canal, in an existing osteon, is widened by bone resorption (a). This enlarged canal is then refilled by new bone lamellae (b). This type of intracortical remodeling is frequently observed in areas with a disturbed blood supply.

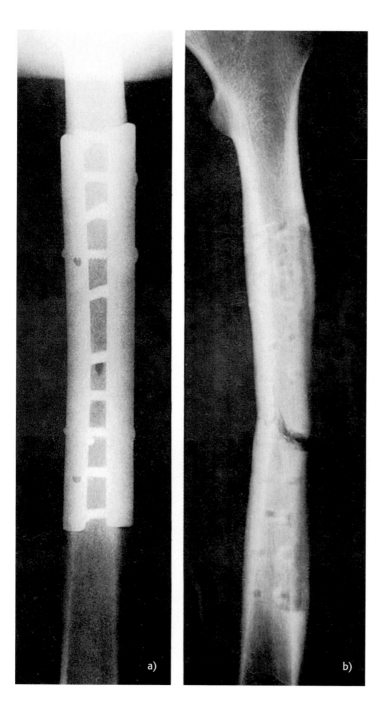

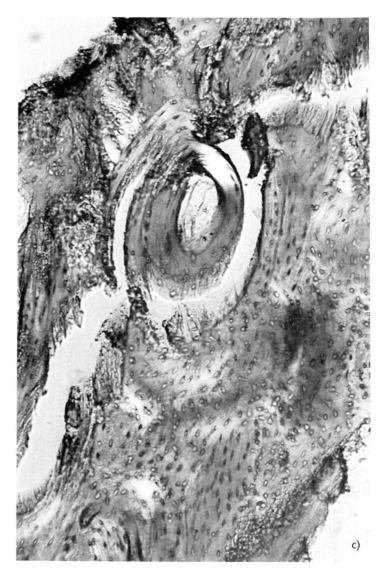

a)

b)

c)

Fig. 9-45: a) "Stress protection" as a cause of refracture. After the use of two plates in the repair of a femoral fracture, the bone under the plates was rarified. b) After the removal of the plates, a small amount of trauma was sufficient to produce a refracture. The rarefaction of the cortex may be explained as being caused by the absence of functional load in the bone. It seems that the two plates, positioned at a right angle, took over a large amount of the load. This case stems from an era when these problems

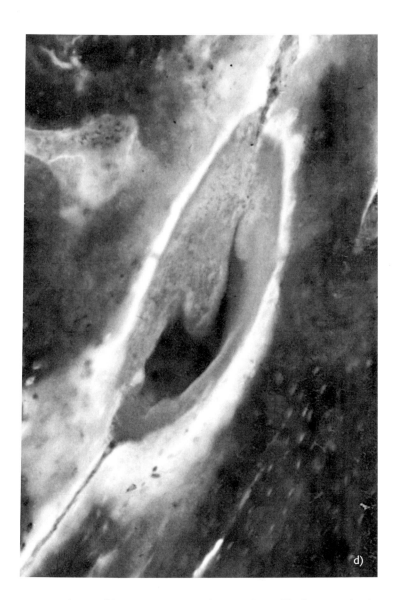

d)

were not then well known. The term "refracture" is used in the sense that it describes a fracture in an area where repair processes have been taking place, and it is not limited to fractures through the original fracture plane. c/d) During the remodeling process new osteons (c) or porosity (d), as well as former screw holes, disturb the homogeneity of the bone structure. When bony failure occurs, the site of the fracture plane will be determined by this lack of homogeneity.

5.3.1   Positive aspects of internal fixation

- The medullary circulation is re-established sooner.
- The anatomical reduction is maintained (joint fractures, jaw fractures).
- Early mobilization of the limb is possible (no fracture disease, Sudeck atrophy).
- Polytrauma is more properly manageable.
- No exuberant callus is formed (nerves).

5.3.2   Negative aspects of internal fixation

- The growth in the juvenile is affected. In spontaneous healing the overgrowth usually makes sense to compensate for shortening. After anatomical reduction the limb usually grows too long.
- Nerve damage (humerus, maxillofacial region) might occur during operation.
- Additional vascular damage is produced by drilling and by positioning plates.
- The strength of the bone cross-section in the fracture area takes longer to reach normal values than by callus formation.
- Osteoporosis may occur as a result of possible stress protection.
- Open treatment always bears the risk of infection.
- In special cases the implantation of foreign materials may not be tolerated, whether due to local toxicity or to allergic reaction.

Which situations allow the occurrence of so-called primary bone healing? It has been observed after plate fixation [11, 13, 19], and after the use of compressing medullary nails [20]. Both are procedures which, by pre-loading the fractured area, guarantee stability. Primary healing is usually linked to operative treatment, but is also possible under other special conditions, which provide sufficient stability. A special situation would be, for instance, the healing of bone fissures or fractures in the rabbit forearm, where the radius and ulna are almost rigidly linked by the interosseous membrane. If one of the two bones is fractured experimentally, there will be almost no dislocation (**Fig. 9-46**). The healing may then proceed with the minimum amount of callus (**Fig. 9-47**), and lamellar bone formation can be observed in the fracture gap (**Fig. 9-48**).

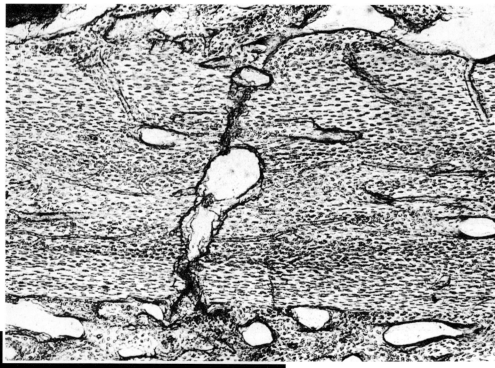

Fig. 9-46: Spontaneous healing with and without callus. Following a fracture of both forearm bones in rabbits, a large amount of callus is seen after 5 weeks (*bottom*). Spontaneous healing without any treatment of the isolated fracture of the radius may be observed to proceed with almost no callus formation (*top*).

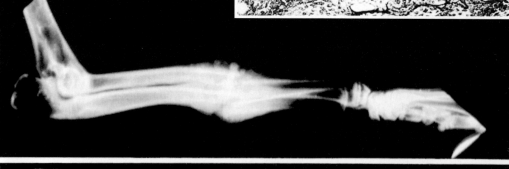

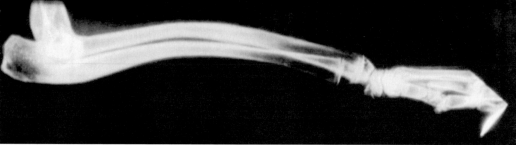

Fig. 9-47: Spontaneous healing without displacement. Under special conditions, such as in an isolated fracture of the radius in the rabbit, the intact ulna and a strong interosseous membrane may maintain the alignment. The early formation of periosteal callus preserves this alignment during the entire healing process.

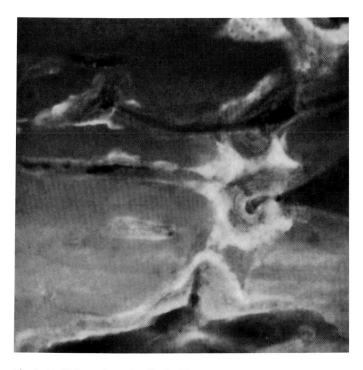

Fig. 9-48: "Primary bone healing" without treatment. Under conditions where naturally sufficient stability is offered, a healing pattern is observed that strongly resembles the one found after operative stabilization. The natural occurrence of so-called "primary bone healing" indicates that the mechanical situation at a fracture site, and not the operative treatment alone, is responsible for this healing pattern.

6 The role of bone resorption in bone healing

When considering bone healing one automatically thinks of bone formation, forgetting that both modeling and remodeling processes are involved in the reconstruction of the original anatomical situation. In both extreme patterns of bone healing, resorption has its special role. In the callus-free type, without interfragmentary motion, only filling of the gap is possible without resorptive activities. The essential part of the healing process, the remodeling across the fracture, is based upon groups of osteoclasts which first "drill" holes into the cortex. These canals are later filled by lamellar bone (**Fig. 9-49**). Without resorption, healing would not take place.

In spontaneous healing after bony bridging of the fracture, a callus of fibrous bone reinforced by lamellar bone is present. This bone is not entirely axially directed, and it will be restruc-

Fig. 9-49: "Cutter head" responsible for intracortical remodeling. A group of osteoclasts resorbs a canal into the compact bone. A "front" of osteoblasts that are arranged in a conical shape enters this canal to refill it with lamellar bone. Intracortical remodeling cannot take place without previous resorption.

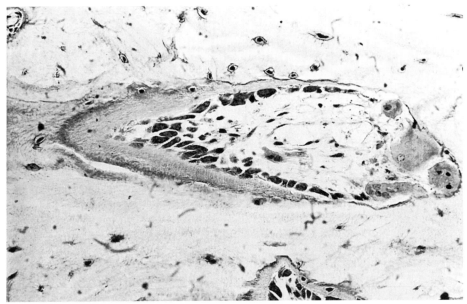

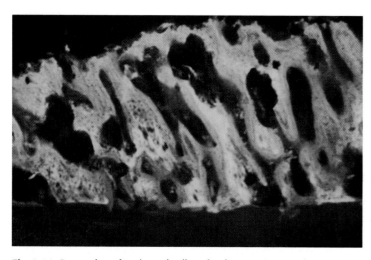

Fig. 9-50: Resorption of periosteal callus after bone union. On the outside, as well as within this periosteal callus, strongly indented surfaces are visible. These lacunae indicate osteoclastic activity, reducing the callus and restoring more normal contours. (Courtesy of M. Chapman.)

tured by the mechanism of haversian remodeling. Without resorptive activities the primitive callus structures would be maintained. The replacement of the fibrocartilage between the fragment ends is made possible only by the local resorption of the mineralized cartilage. While the bone of the callus becomes denser and stronger, especially by the incorporation of longitudinally directed haversian systems, the geometric advantages of the larger diameter are no longer needed. In consequence, a resorption on the periosteal side of the callus can be observed (Fig. 9-50). The reopening of the medullary cavity and the establishment of a normal medullary circulation is possible only after removal of the medullary callus.

In both types of healing, the removal of dead bone would not be possible without resorption. Although dead bone is mechanically not so different from living bone, replacement is important, since, with time, fatigue fractures may occur. In living bone a permanent reconstruction by intracortical remodeling takes place; while in dead bone, microfractures could aggregate and result in a real fatigue fracture.

7 Healing of bone defects

In minor defects occurring in connection with a fracture, a normal fracture healing will take place. In large shaft defects, it is possible that they will not be bridged, and non-union may result. In an articular fracture the cancellous bone in the epiphyseal and metaphyseal areas will be compressed. Bony healing in the cancellous bone is not usually a major problem, and it heals relatively quickly. A defect will be maintained within the joint space, which will lead to serious problems. Therefore, an anatomical reconstruction of the joint is necessary and is useful to support the reconstruction by grafting of cancellous bone.

Some defects may have an iatrogenic origin. Drill holes weaken the bone mechanically. After implant removal, the drill holes sometimes remain visible radiologically for months or even years. Johner [21] and Schenk [22] investigated the healing of small fresh drill holes. They found that holes of a diameter up to 300 µm are filled over the whole thickness of the cortex. In these holes, lamellar bone is deposited concentrically and, in a cross-section through the holes, they conform to the configuration of an osteon. Larger holes, up to a diameter of 1 mm, show subdivisions by fibrous bone trabeculae. In these smaller units the deposition of lamellar bone takes place. Thus larger holes are filled in almost the same time as the smaller ones, and almost the full thickness of the cortex is filled. These two mechanisms are comparable with gap healing under a stable situation.

In larger holes (>1 mm) fibrous bone is formed on the surface of the wall. Lamellar inserts are deposited into the fibrous net work. The center of the hole is usually not filled over the full thickness of the cortex. The radiologic visibility of such holes is due to the fact that there is less material, and the filling material consists of young bone which is less mineralized and therefore less dense.

An incomplete recovery from iatrogenic defects may also be seen after removal of large pieces of bone from the iliac crest for transplantation purposes [23]. Here, the healing process leads to only a rounding and smoothing of the edges, and takes place by the apposition of fibrous bone on the edges of the defect. This bone is reinforced by the incorporation of lamellar bone and is then remodeled to produce the new contours.

Another iatrogenic defect is produced purposely when a limb has to be lengthened to equalize its contralateral partner. After an initial fracture or osteotomy, the fracture gap is gradually enlarged by means of external devices. This enlargement should not take place too quickly because the soft tissues (tendons, nerves, vessels) would then suffer. At the same time it should not be too slow, or else bony bridging may occur before the desired length is obtained. The filling of such a gap is comparable with spontaneous fracture healing (hematoma, granulation tissue, fibrous tissue, fibrous bone trabeculae, lamellar bone). The whole finally undergoes haversian remodeling, as in callus healing. When the distraction device provides good stability, almost no periosteal callus is visible. New bone formation may be observed at the fragment ends, similar to a periosteal callus, and also in the region of the medullary cavity. In the medullary cavity area bone formation starts about 2 weeks after the beginning of the lengthening procedure. Fibrous bone originates in the medullary cavity from a depth of about 0.5 mm from the fragment ends and enters the defect in a cone shape. Further healing progress depends then upon the stability of the fixation. Every aspect, from total absence of external callus to the classical callus healing and even to a non-union, may be observed.

8   Complications in bone healing

8.1   Mechanical overload

Bone as a material has a given strength. In operative treatment, high mechanical loads are used for stabilization. Under certain conditions, it may be possible for the limits of strength to be passed. Especially in porotic bone, a stripping of the screws can occur during tightening. The judgment of the holding power on the basis of the radiograph under standardized laboratory conditions provides reproducible results [24] but is difficult to perform in clinical situations. Since in osteoporosis the bone is rarefied mainly on the endosteal side of the cortex, surface

hardness determinations will not present any correlation to the holding power for screws. The thickness of the cortex is a good parameter only when the cortex is homogeneous, but not in osteoporosis. In addition to the radiologic criteria, an experienced surgeon can "feel" when the bone deformation passes the yielding point from elastic to plastic deformation, and can then adapt the torque to the given bone [6].

Another type of overload of bone, even employing a careful technique, is not always avoidable. Perfect adaptation of a fracture at the microscopic level may still leave incongruities. When compression is applied to stabilize the fracture, the force concentrates on small areas. In these small areas the pressure passes the ultimate compressive strength of the bone and the bone collapses locally or undergoes irreversible deformation. Thus, a larger area comes into contact, the pressure (force per unit area) becomes smaller, and the stability can be maintained. If the stability is assured, the deformed zone will be included into the haversian remodeling (**Fig. 9-51**) [25]. Under unstable conditions the deformed fragment ends will undergo resorption, as do other fragment ends under unstable conditions.

8.2   Operative fracture treatment and infection

Every opening of the skin in a case of a fracture bears the risk that the fracture area will be contaminated. This is true for fractures that are initially open (compound) as well as for those that are opened surgically. The greatest risk of infection occurs in situations in which the soft tissues are also traumatized. The implantation of a foreign body favors the beginning of, or at least aids in maintaining, infection. Experimental investigations [26, 27] have shown that the stability offered by an implant is beneficial for fracture healing in spite of the fact that the infection stops only when the foreign body is removed. It was demonstrated that bony union could be obtained under rigid fixation in the presence of infection. It was even shown that the sequestra at the fragment ends were smaller than those formed under spontaneous healing conditions of an infected fracture.

In our own experience with infected mandibular fractures in sheep, we have also seen the importance of absolute

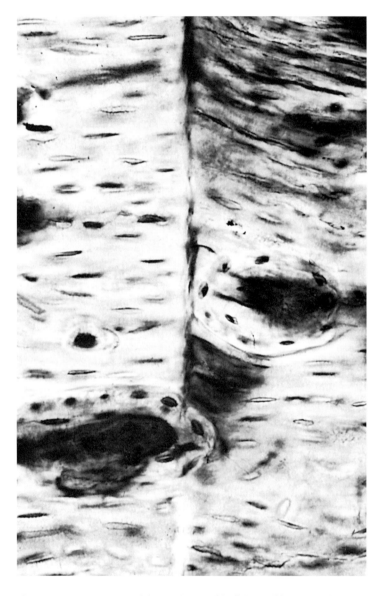

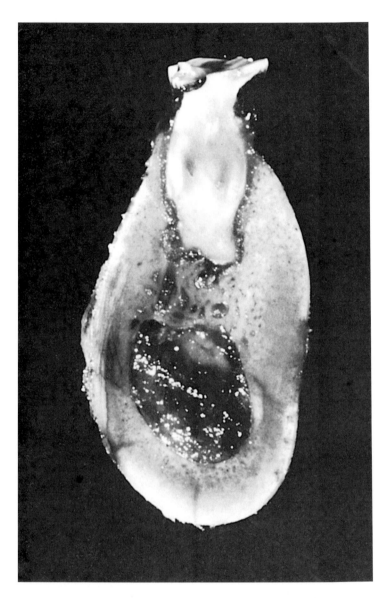

Fig. 9-51: Haversian remodeling in irreversibly deformed bone. Local overload has led to a triangular zone (*top right to bottom center*) of irreversible bone deformation. The contact area, remaining intact, has insured the stability of the fixation, and the deformed zone was included in the normal haversian remodeling.

Fig. 9-52: Disturbed circulation within a plated bone. The vital staining, with disulphine blue, could not enter the region below the plate, since the vessels in this area were not open at the time of dye administration. The dark area at center is due to erythrocytes that accumulated.

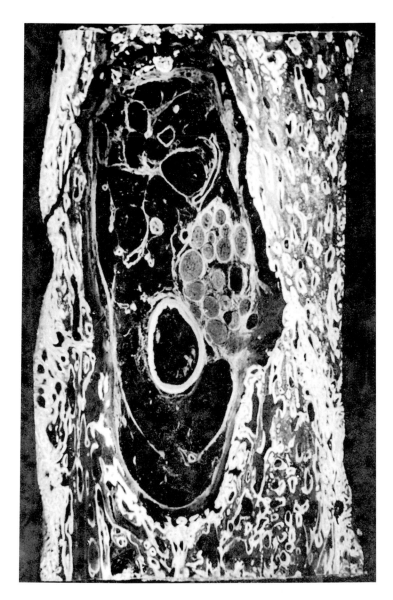

Fig. 9-53: Direct bony union in spite of infection. The buccal cortex of this infected sheep mandible was sequestered in the area under the plate where the circulation was interrupted. In spite of the sequestration of the cortex under the plate, the lingual cortex shows primary union. At a few sites, even direct crossing of new osteons from fragment to fragment may be observed.

stability. The use of a heavy plate, the type usually used in human femurs, permitted normal function from the beginning. In the area where the blood circulation was disturbed, that is, in the area under the plate (**Fig. 9-52**), a large sequestrum developed, and in all the cases the wound was draining. The lingual cortex, where circulation was normal, showed good healing progress (**Fig. 9-53**) and the plate could be removed after 9 weeks. There were loose sequestra and impacted food remains under the plate, but the lingual cortex was stable enough to allow normal function. After removal of the plate and the sequestra the wound was left open. The stability offered by the healed cortex provided optimal conditions for the healing of the infection. The defect filled with granulation tissue and, afterwards, the regeneration of the bone began by formation of fibrous bone trabeculae (**Fig. 9-54a**) which were the basis of a future cortex. The newly formed bone assumed an absolutely normal shape (**Fig. 9-54b**).

In addition to these complications, there is also the possibility of non-union occurring. This topic is given more detailed consideration in **Chapter 11**.

9   Summary

The pattern of fracture healing depends upon the mechanical situation at the fracture site. No tissue can be formed which could not exist under the given mechanical condition. This means, for instance, that the formation of lamellar bone cannot begin until the tissue elongation within the fracture gap is smaller than 2%. The healing passes through different tissue stages with decreasing deformability and increasing stiffness and strength. If there is no initial stability provided by treatment, the process of healing has to undergo all stages of tissue differentiation. In addition, external callus forms, which provides a longer lever arm for the early repair of tissues. If the method of treatment provides some stability, the callus formation is only minor and the healing stages may be abbreviated. Under absolute stability, bone, as the least deformable tissue, can be formed right from the beginning. If, for any reason (vascular, mechanical), the process of immobilization does not occur, a delayed non-union will result.

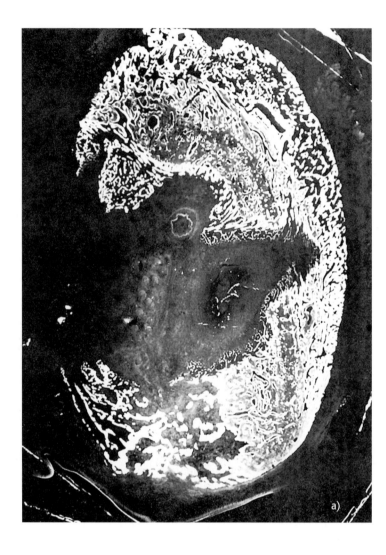

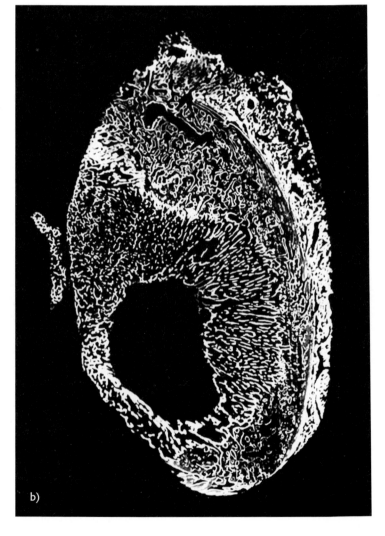

Fig. 9-54
a) Regeneration of sequestrated cortex. After the bony union of the lingual cortex, the plate and the sequestra were removed and the wound was left open. Under the protection of the united lingual cortex, the bone regeneration started at the borders of the surviving bone.
b) Bone formation continued to reconstruct a normal cross-section around the mandibular canal.

10 Bibliography

Blue references indicate links to abstracts of articles available online:
http://www.aopublishing.org/BONE/9.htm

1. **Allgöwer M** (1956) *The Cellular Basis of Wound Repair.* Springfield, IL: Charles C. Thomas.

2. **Perren SM, Boitzy A** (1978) Cellular differentiation and bone biomechanics during the consolidation of a fracture. *Anatom Clin;* 1:13.

3. **Yamada H** (1970) *Strength of Biological Materials.* Baltimore: Williams & Wilkins.

4. **Pauwels F** (1965) *Gesammelte Abhandlungen zur funktionellen Anatomie des Bewegungsapparates.* Berlin Heidelberg New York: Springer-Verlag.

5. **Perren SM** (1979) Physical and biological aspects of fracture healing with special reference to internal fixation. *Clin Orthop;* (138):175–196.

6. **Cordey J, Rahn B, Perren SM** (1980) Human torque control in the use of bone screws. In: Uhthoff HK, editor. *Current Concepts of Internal Fixation of Fractures.* Berlin Heidelberg New York: Springer-Verlag, 235.

7. **Osterwalder A, Beeler C, Huggler A, et al.** (1978) [Lengthwise growth of the lower extremities after shaft fractures in children]. *Helv Chir Acta;* 45 (1–2):23–26.

8. **Pfister U, Rahn BA, Perren SM, et al.** (1979) Vaskularität und Knochenumbau nach Marknagelung langer Röhrenknochen. *Aktuel Traumatol;* 9:191.

9. **Hutzschenreuter P, Perren SM, Steinemann S** (1980) Some effects of rigidity of internal fixation on the healing pattern of osteotomies. *Injury;* 1:77.

10. **Perren SM, Ganz R, Reuter A** (1975) Oberflächliche Knochenresorption um Implantate. *Med Orthop Tech;* 95:6.

11. **Schenk RK, Willenegger H** (1963) Zum histologischen Bild der sogenannten Primärheilung der Knochenkompakta nach experimentellen Osteotomien am Hund. *Experientia;* 20:593.

12. **Rahn BA, Gallinaro P, Baltensperger A, et al.** (1971) Primary bone healing. An experimental study in the rabbit. *J Bone Joint Surg [Am];* 53 (4):783–786.

13. **Danis R** (1949). *Theorie et Pratique de l'Osteosynthese.* Paris: Masson.

14. **Ganz R, Brennwald J** (1972) L'osteosynthese du tibia du lapin. In: Boitzy A, editor. *Osteogenese et Compression.* Bern: Hans Huber.

15. **Piret N** (1976) L'os compact du vieux chien. Etude histologique et microradiographique: 1. Exploration morphologique et fonctionelle du sequelette. In: CEMO, editor. *CEMO Symposium.* Geneva: CEMO, 1.

16. **Gunst MA, Suter C, Rahn BA** (1979) [Bone perfusion after plate osteosynthesis. A study of the intact rabbit tibia with disulfin blue vital staining]. *Helv Chir Acta;* 46 (1–2): 171–175.

17. **Eitel F, Schenk RK, Schweiberer L** (1980) [Cortical revascularization after medullary nailing in dog tibiae (author's transl)]. *Unfallheilkunde;* 83 (5):202–207.

18. **Uhthoff HK, Dubuc FL** (1971) Bone structure changes in the dog under rigid internal fixation. *Clin Orthop;* 81:165–170.

19. **Lane WA** (1914) *The Operative Treatment of Fractures.* London: Medical Publishing Co.

20. **Olerud S, Danckwardt-Lilliestrom G** (1971) Fracture healing in compression osteosynthesis. An experimental study in dogs with an avascular, diaphyseal, intermediate fragment. *Acta Orthop Scand Suppl;* 137:1–44.

21. **Johner R** (1972) [Dependence of bone healing on defect size]. *Helv Chir Acta;* 39 (1):409–411.

22. **Schenk RK** (1973) Fracture repair-overview. In: Czitober A, Eschberger J, editors. *9th Symp Calcif Tiss.* Wien: Baden, 1.

23. **Habel G, Rahn BA, Perren SM** (1980) Zur spontanen Knochenneubildung im Defektbereich nach Beckenspanentnahme. *Dtsch Z Mund-Kiefer Gesichtschir;* 4:139.

24. **Rahn BA, Matter P, Mikuschka-Galgoczy E, et al.** (1978) Relationship between radiological density, hardness, holding power of screws, and microscopic structure in human cortical bone. In: Asmussen F, Joergensen K, editors. *Biomechanics.* Baltimore: University Park Press.

25. **Rahn BA, Gallinaro P, Schenk RK, et al.** (1972) Compression interfragmentaire et surcharge locale de l'os. In: Boitzy A, editor. *Osteogenese et Compression.* Bern: Hans Huber.

26. **Rittmann WW, Perren SM** (1974) *Corticale Knochenheilung nach Osteosynthese und Infektion.* Berlin Heidelberg New York: Springer-Verlag.

27. **Friedrich B** (1979) [Biomechanical aspects in infected fractures]. *Hefte Unfallheilkd;* 138:156–159.

10 Concepts of fracture stabilization

Joseph Schatzker (1982)
Updated by John E.F. Houlton (1999)

1 Introduction

The mechanical function of bone is to transmit load. This may be applied as pure compression, as a bending force—which places one side of the bone under compression and the other under tension—or as a twisting force or torque. Bone is also subjected to avulsion or tensile forces, particularly at the site of ligamentous and tendinous attachments.

Bone failure is the result of mechanical overload. The resultant fracture configuration is influenced by the material properties of the bone, the type and magnitude of the force, and the rate of loading.

1.1 Material properties of bone

The skeleton acts as a rigid framework for the protection of soft organs and allows for locomotion. To achieve this, bones must have both strength and stiffness. Bone is approximately 10% as strong as steel. It is a complex tissue composed largely of organized collagen fibers and a hydroxyapatite mineral matrix. Its compressive strength is derived largely from this apatite structure, while its tensile strength comes largely from the somewhat weaker collagen fibers.

The strength of a bone will be influenced by its shape and by the distribution of its cancellous component. The strength of cancellous bone is very variable, but is usually less than 10% of cortical bone [1]. Thus, the tibia is 20% weaker in tension than in compression; in contrast, the radius is stronger in tension [2].

A significant biomechanical quality of bone is its brittleness. In this respect, bone behaves similar to glass, since it will only elongate around 2% before it breaks.

Bone is a viscoelastic material. Thus its failure depends not only upon the force but also upon the rate of force application. The faster and greater bone is loaded, the stronger and stiffer it becomes. If the force is applied slowly, over a long period of time, a much lower force is required to fracture a bone than if the force is applied rapidly. This force is stored and when the bone finally breaks it is dissipated in an explosive fashion. Such high velocity fractures are usually multiple and whatever force is not dissipated in fracturing the bone is absorbed by the soft-tissue envelope.

When a material is not homogeneous, its mechanical behavior is influenced by the direction of loading forces relative to its orientation. Such materials are called anisotropic. The anisotropy of bone, i.e., its different mechanical properties along different axes, does not play a major role in the fixation of fractures and will not be discussed further.

1.2 Bone fracture

Bone is strongest in compression, and fractures as a result of pure compression are rare. They occur only in cancellous bone with a thin cortical shell, such as the metaphyses or vertebral bodies.

Transverse, oblique, and spiral fractures are the common fracture types seen in tubular bone. Transverse and short oblique fractures are the result of a bending force, while oblique or spiral fractures are the result of torque. All three types may be associated with small triangular fragments, the so-called "wedge" fragment, or there may be many fragments. The degree of comminution depends upon the energy stored in the bone prior to the mechanical overload and the rate of loading. Fractures are frequently the result of a mixture of forces, and, therefore, often have a mixed pattern.

Bone is able to withstand the rapid application of force because it stores the energy within itself. However, when a bone fractures, its structural integrity is destroyed within fractions of a millisecond and the stored energy is dissipated in an explosive fashion. The degree of energy release influences not only the degree of bone fragmentation but also the associated soft-tissue damage. The latter is caused by a phenomenon called implosion, resulting in cavitation similar to that seen in gunshot wounds.

Direct forces, such as those generated in motor vehicular injuries, kicks, falls, etc., generally result in significant soft-tissue damage. Indirect fractures, where the bone fractures as a result of an internally generated force, are usually associated with much less soft-tissue damage. Since fractures due to direct trauma are frequently the result of a mixture of force application, their configuration is far more variable than the reasonably predictable injuries caused by indirect trauma.

1.3   Effects of a fracture

A fracture results in loss of the structural continuity of bone, and a loss of its weight-bearing capacity. Essentially, a fractured bone, particularly one of the lower limb, becomes mechanically functionless.

Immediately after the fracture, a number of protective and vascular disturbances occur; of these, local inflammation, pain, and reflex guarding of the limb are the most important.

Local inflammation is associated with an outpouring of fibrinous and proteinaceous fluid which fills the potential spaces between tissue planes. If the limb is not mobilized, this fluid will become organized and obliterate the fascial planes, resulting in intermuscular adhesions and a further loss of function. Muscle atrophy as a consequence of disuse will aggravate the problem; together, these processes may also encourage adhesions between soft tissues and bone. The end result is a potentially crippling joint stiffness.

Pain causes a reflex guarding of the limb and contributes to initial limb immobility. However, when joints are immobilized for long periods of time the articular cartilage atrophies, the joint capsule thickens, and the joint space becomes obliterated. The end result is a fibrotic joint with a reduced range of joint movement and loss of limb mobility.

It can therefore be seen that long-term limb dysfunction is more a reflection of the consequences of damage to the soft tissues than of the damage to the bone itself. A clinical syndrome of stiff joints, atrophic and/or fibrotic muscles, and osteoporosis of disuse has been described as "fracture disease" [3]. This can only be prevented by early function.

The most serious complication of a fracture is infection. This may prevent or, at best, delay healing of the bone. Prolongation of fracture healing will increase the likelihood of fracture disease. Moreover, the effects of the infection on the soft tissues will be to encourage fibrosis and further scarring.

2   Fracture treatment

The aim of any fracture treatment should be to restore full function to the affected region. Thus, the basic goal is to return the bone to its proper anatomical shape by a strong osseous union. With respect to diaphyseal fractures, proper anatomical shape may mean its exact previous form, or it may mean the restoration of the correct overall length of the bone and the re-establishment of the proper alignment of its associated joints. When dealing with intra-articular fractures, precise reconstruction of the articular surfaces and interfragmentary compression is always the goal.

It should be re-emphasized that whatever the fracture, the goal of treatment remains the same—solid bone union and, equally important, early and full recovery of function. This dictates that any preoperative fracture plan includes the management of the soft-tissue injuries as well as of the bone.

2.1 Early return of function

Full, active, pain-free limb movement is required to achieve a rapid return of normal blood supply, both to the bone and the soft tissues. It also enhances articular cartilage nutrition and decreases posttraumatic osteoporosis by restoring equilibrium between bone resorption and bone formation. It is therefore imperative to choose a fixation technique that permits early mobilization of the fractured area. The technique must restore the function of the soft-tissue envelope around the fracture, permit early weight-bearing forces to be transmitted through or across the fracture site, and encourage joint movement.

External fixation may, in some instances, permit early return to function. This can be achieved by the application of a cast or cast brace, or by the application of an external skeletal fixator. Casts and cast braces act by splinting the bone in a rigid "soft tissue–bone" complex, i.e., the cast provides an exoskeleton to immobilize the fracture. In contrast, external skeletal fixators immobilize the bone with the aim of having a minimal effect on the soft tissues.

There are clearly many limitations to the use of the "soft tissue–bone" concept, not the least in those fractures where the bones are surrounded by large amounts of muscle. It is impossible to immobilize such fractures due to distance between the cast and the bone. A further limitation of the exoskeleton principle is that casts are poor at controlling rotational and shortening forces. They are, therefore, really only suitable for fractures of the lower limb, where bending forces need to be controlled. These forces are most significant at the level of the joints since these are the areas where the limb tends to flex.

Casts may be strengthened in a number of ways. The overall thickness of the cast may be increased, or it may be strengthened in those areas that are subjected to the greatest forces. The latter technique has the advantage of increasing the area moment of inertia without adding too much weight.

The amount of padding under the cast will also influence the splinting effect of the cast, just as in the soft tissue–bone complex above. The greater the stiffness of this padding, the more support the cast provides. High stiffness is achieved by using little or no padding. However, this advantage must be weighed against the increased possibility of pressure sores.

Internal fixation of fractures to permit full, active, pain-free mobilization of muscles and joints has been a prime objective of the AO group for the last four decades. Anatomical reduction of the fracture fragments, particularly in joint fractures, and stable internal fixation designed to fulfill the local biomechanical requirements remain the first two principles of this group.

Anatomical reduction is important in a number of respects. In all joint fractures it is imperative to achieve perfect articular congruency and primary bone union, if osteoarthrosis is to be avoided. Anatomical reduction is also important when restoring the correct length and alignment of metaphyseal and diaphyseal fractures. It is particularly important when fixing such fractures with lag screws, with or without a neutralization (protection) plate to protect the repair. To achieve optimal mechanical strength, the cortical circumference must be fully reconstructed and placed under interfragmentary and axial compression.

Early return to function may also be achieved by internal splintage, using constructs where the implant(s) take most, if not all, of the weight-bearing forces. Such constructs must, of necessity, be stronger than where there is load sharing between the bone and the implants.

2.2 Implant materials and design

There is continuing interest in discovering new materials for implants, although stainless steel and titanium remain the conventional metals. The application of the latter is still somewhat limited in veterinary medicine, but its use in man is well accepted and there is no doubt that it is the superior material of the two. It is half the weight of steel, has a higher elasticity, improved corrosion resistance, and does not produce any known associated allergies.

According to the ISO standard 5832-2 unalloyed titanium, containing 99% titanium, is available in five grades. The grades are distinguished by the different amount of light elements that they contain, such as nitrogen, hydrogen, and oxygen. These light elements influence the mechanical properties of the material.

Implant stiffness, and its association with stress protection, continues to be the subject of much interest. Stress protection is the term used to describe the histological events that occur in a bone that has been rigidly immobilized. Such bone undergoes a loss of mass without a reduction in size. This is the result of an intense haversian proliferation so that each cross-sectional area of the compact lamellar bone is seen to contain many more haversian canals than normal. Thus, the basic assumption is that bone, deprived of necessary functional stimulation by reduced mechanical load, loses strength (Wolff's law) and becomes osteoporotic.

Stress protection should not be confused with stress shielding. The latter describes the problem from a purely mechanical aspect, unlike stress-induced osteoporosis which appears to be multifactorial. Surgical trauma, the placement of screws and rigid internal implants, the vascular impairment of the plate/bone contact area, and pressure distribution all make significant contributions to its pathogenesis.

The problem of implant stiffness was initially addressed by Gautier et al. [4] who substituted standard metal plates with softer plastic versions that fitted more closely to the surface of the bone. Rather than reducing plate-induced cortical osteoporosis, these authors demonstrated an actual increase in plate-induced osteoporosis after "flexible" plating. Reduced periosteal vascular supply under the plate, due to the greater contact between the softer plastic plate, was thought to be the reason. This provided the stimulus to conduct further research in implant design and to seek methods of improving the vascular supply under bone plates.

The problem of plate-induced osteoporosis has been approached by the development of the limited contact dynamic compression plate (LC-DCP). Contact between the plate and the bone is reduced by the presence of grooves on the underside of the plate, thereby improving the vascular supply. These grooves also encourage the development of a small bone bridge beneath the plate and a circumferential shell of callus around the fracture site. This reduces the existence of stress risers at implant removal.

The LC-DCP is constructed of titanium for improved tissue tolerance and is the culmination of recent research in biological plating by the AO group. Further development of this concept has resulted in the production of the PC-Fix (point contact fixator), which is essentially a plate acting as an internal fixator. The implant is held from the surface of the bone by mono-cortical screws that lock into the plate, thereby minimizing any vascular disturbance. The matter of plate contact areas and vascular supply is still being debated (see **Chapter 15**).

2.3 Bone healing

Bone will heal spontaneously by callus formation, but in the absence of adequate treatment a malunion is the likely outcome. However, any attempt to restore the original anatomy of the bone must respect the biological environment of the fracture and understand the mechanical forces that need to be counteracted.

The mechanical environment will influence the type of fracture healing. Under conditions of instability, spontaneous indirect healing occurs by the formation of callus. Initially, granulation tissue forms around and between the bone fragments. The fracture gap then widens due to resorption of the bone ends. Finally, bone forms through a series of steps from granulation tissue through to fibrocartilage, unmineralized callus, mineralized callus, and eventually cortical bone. The greater the instability at the fracture site, the greater the amount of callus that is produced before healing occurs.

Direct (or primary) bone healing occurs under the stable conditions provided by interfragmentary compression. Such conditions are produced by lag screw fixation, with or without a neutralization plate or an axially loaded dynamic compression plate.

Danis [5] was the first to demonstrate that diaphyseal fragments, if stabilized by a plate that exerted axial compression, were immobilized to such a degree that union occurred without any radiologically visible callus. He referred to this type of union as primary bone healing. Schenk and Willenegger [6] subsequently demonstrated that such conditions could be reproduced experimentally if a diaphyseal osteotomy is fixed with a plate that exerts axial compression. Healing of these experimental osteotomies occurs without the formation of a significant periosteal or endosteal callus. The healing is the result of a proliferation of new osteons which grow parallel to the long axis of the bone through the necrotic bone ends and then across the fracture. In this way bony continuity is once again re-established. There is no net resorption in this type of union. For every bit of necrotic bone removed, new bone is laid down. Under these circumstances, internal fixation does not lead to a relative distraction of the fragments because absolute resorption does not occur. Indeed this type of union is so similar to bone remodeling that it was previously questioned whether primary bone union could be regarded as union, or whether it represented only an accelerated bone remodeling. Such rigid internal fixation maintains the fragments in a state of absolute stability, and it is by the mechanism that it enhances union.

Healing occurs by internal remodeling in contact zones (contact healing) and by the filling of stable gaps with lamellar bone which subsequently remodels (gap healing). The amount of contact healing is limited to a small percentage of the total cross-section of the fracture plane and is directly related to the amount of compression applied [7].

The internal remodeling of the haversian system uniting the fragment ends is the only process in direct healing that results in solid union. Therefore, direct healing does not lead to faster union, but it is characterized radiologically by the virtual absence of callus formation.

The biological environment will also influence fracture healing. Live pluripotential mesenchymal cells in the region of the fracture and an adequate local vascular supply are both required for a successful outcome. Thus, there is a balance to be struck between accurate anatomical reduction and preservation of the vascular supply to the bone fragments. This is particularly relevant in the repair of multi-fragment fractures where the surgical time and intraoperative trauma required to reduce and immobilize all of the fragments must be balanced against the devascularization of the bone fragments. This has

lead to the idea of "biological fixation" or "bridging osteosynthesis". The latter term is perhaps the better, since all fracture healing depends upon the biological environment of the fracture.

All methods of fracture fixation must provide adequate stability in order to maintain length and correct joint alignment. Whatever the type of internal fixation, the implants must be sufficiently strong to withstand the early functional forces, and not fail due to mechanical overload. The repair must also be resilient enough to last until osseous union is achieved.

2.4 Compression of fractures

Key [8] and Charnley [9] were the first to introduce compression as an aid to stable internal fixation. Cancellous surfaces, such as those of an arthrodesis, united rapidly when compressed. Compression was first looked upon as providing an osteogenic stimulus to bone. However, early attempts to secure similar union in the cortex failed. It was thought that the resorption around the pins of the external fixator employed to compress the diaphyseal fragments represented bone necrosis secondary to pressure. There was general acceptance of the thesis that cancellous and cortical bone behaved differently and that they probably united by different mechanisms.

Since then it has become recognized that under stable conditions both cancellous and cortical bone heal by primary bone union. The external fixator applied to bone close to the broad flat surfaces of an arthrodesis was able to achieve absolute stability, which led to rapid primary bone union. The external fixator, applied to diaphyseal bone, resulted in a system of relative instability with micromotion. The resorption around the pins and at the fracture was due to motion and not to pressure necrosis.

Compression does not have any osteogenic properties. It merely exerts its beneficial effect on bone union by creating an environment of absolute stability where relative micromotion does not exist between the bone fragments. Interfragmental compression, because it results in impaction of the fragments and in a marked increase in their frictional resistance to relative motion, is the most important method for restoring functional continuity to bone. Such a method of internal fixation, which restores the functional continuity of bone, also decreases the forces borne by an internal fixation device. The load transfer occurs directly from fragment of bone to fragment of bone; the load is no longer borne by the implant. The function of the implant is to hold the bone fragments under compression, which restores the functional continuity to bone and enables it to function mechanically as if the fracture were not there. Stable internal fixation imparts stability and enhances the native stability of the bone.

2.5   Biologic fixation of fractures

Biological internal fixation or biological plating of fractures was first described by Mast et al. [10]. It is a somewhat poor term since all fractures require a suitable biological environment if they are to heal. However, the terms emphasize the biological environment of the fracture as opposed to the mechanical environment that is so important in the accurate recon-struction of multi-fragment fractures.

Clearly, in any internal fixation, there is a fine balance between the degree of stabilization and the surgical trauma associated with the repair. Biological fixation favors the pre-servation of the soft-tissue envelope surrounding the fracture site and therefore minimizes the surgical insult to the vascular supply of the area. The technique is particularly suited to the repair of very multiple fractures. Sufficient stability must be provided for the fragments to heal while the length of the bone and the correct orientations of the articular surfaces are maintained. Early callus formation is encouraged to reduce implant failure that may otherwise occur with early weight bearing.

3   Methods of interfragmentary compression—Internal skeletal fixation

3.1   The lag screw

The simplest way of compressing two fragments of bone together is to lag them together with a lag screw. Thus, the lag screw is the simplest and most widely used form of inter-fragmentary compression. Indeed it is the building block of any stable internal fixation. It is used in every instance where two fragments of bone are to be compressed, even if the overall fixation, because of the required strength, would demand other means such as a neutralization plate or buttress plate.

The best example of a lag screw is the wood screw, which in bone surgery finds its counterpart in the cancellous bone screw. This type of screw may have a smooth shank near its head and a threaded portion near its tip. When used as a lag screw, the smooth shank passes through one fragment and the threaded portion gains purchase in the other. Thus, when the screw is tightened, the two fragments are compressed and interfragmentary compression is generated. The cancellous bone screw, as its name implies, is used in cancellous bone. It finds its main application in epiphyses and metaphyses because the trabeculae of cancellous bone are thin. In order to increase the surface area of contact between the screw and bone and thus increase its holding power, the ratio between the outer diameter and the core is greater than that found in a cortex screw. Thus, the large cancellous bone screw developed by the AO group has an outer diameter of 6.5 mm and a core of 3.0 mm.

In other instances a screw with a fully threaded shaft may be employed if the cis-cortex is over-drilled to permit passage of the thread (**Fig. 10-1**).

The insertion of a screw into bone results in local damage, which the bone promptly repairs. Histologically this is seen as formation of new bone, which closely followed the profile of the screw. After the insertion of the screw, as healing occurs, there is a gradual rise of the holding power; this peaks between the sixth and eighth week. The holding power then gradually declines to a level well above the holding power at zero time [11]. This occurs because, as bone matures and becomes organized, much of the early woven bone laid down about the screw is resorbed.

The cortex in the epiphyseal and metaphyseal areas of bone is thin. Consequently, at the time of screw removal the cancellous thread is able to reverse cut its way into the cancellous bone and the thin cortex without difficulty.

The cancellous bone screw could be used as a lag screw in cortical bone. A difficulty would arise, however, at the time of screw removal. Although able to cut its way out of cancellous bone and the overlying thin cortex, the cancellous bone screw cannot back out through compact lamellar bone because it is unable to cut itself a thread in lamellar bone. The torque, which is generated when screw removal is attempted, invariably rises above the strength of the screw and the screw breaks. In order to overcome this difficulty in cortical bone, fully threaded cortex screws are used as lag screws. To fulfill the role of a lag screw, the thread must gain purchase only in one fragment. Because the cortical screws are fully threaded, the hole in the fragment next to the screw head has to be over-drilled to such a size that the screw thread will not gain any purchase in it. Such a hole is called a gliding hole. If the near cortex were not over-drilled then, the screw would maintain the gap between the fragments, no matter how much one attempted to tighten the screw, and compression would not be generated. The screw thread is made to gain purchase only in the far cortex. This hole is then referred to as the thread hole. As the screw is tightened, it turns freely in the gliding hole. It gains purchase in the thread hole, and interfragmentary compression is generated just as with a cancellous bone screw. At the time of screw removal, because the formation of new bone closely follows the profile of the whole screw, there is no obstruction in the gliding hole and it is removed without difficulty.

Cortex screws are smaller in their outer diameter than the corresponding cancellous bone screws and have a lower ratio between their outer diameter and the core. Thus, the large cortex screw, developed by the AO group, is 5.5 mm in its outer diameter and its core is 4.0 mm. By comparison, the large 6.5 mm cancellous bone screw has a core diameter of 3 mm. Because the holding power of screws is governed by the relationship of the screw diameter to the overall diameter of the bone and to cortical thickness, the screws come in different sizes for different areas and different bones of the skeleton.

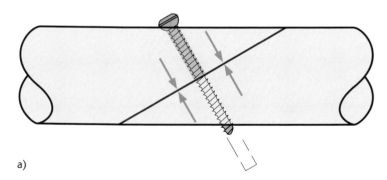

a)

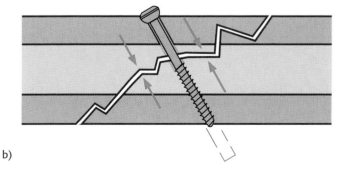

b)

Fig. 10-1: Lag screw effect using fully threaded screws.
a) By overdrilling the bone thread in the near fragment to the size of the outer diameter of the screw thread, the threaded part of the bone screw is enabled to glide in relation to the bone. When this technique is used for an inclined screw whose head rests on a surface parallel to the long axis of the bone (e.g., in DCP or LC-DCP), then one component of the axial screw force acts along the long axis of the bone. It tends to shift the screw head toward the fracture. The screw thread within the gliding hole may then engage, and compression is lost to a varying degree. This has led to the development of a cortex screw with a shaft corresponding to the outer diameter of the thread—the shaft screw (b).
(From Rüedi et al., 2000 [12].)

Screws may be either self-tapping or non-self-tapping. It was formerly thought that self-tapping screws provided a poorer hold in bone than non-self-tapping screws. It was felt that they created more damage and often became embedded in fibrous tissue rather than in bone [13]. This has been shown to be incorrect. Size for size, the buttress thread of a non-self-tapping screw has the same holding power as the V thread of a self-tapping screw [11]. The advantage of the non-self-tapping screw does not lie in its increased holding power but in the far greater precision with which it can be inserted into bone. This leads to better placement of the screw and often results in far better holding power and stability.

Lag screws must be inserted into the center of fragments. If they are inserted obliquely, instead of generating pure compression they can also produce shear (**Fig. 10-2**). This not only leads to a decrease in compression but also to a decrease in stability and may, at times, even lead to a loss of reduction because of displacement of the fragments due to shear. To exert the most effective interfragmentary compression, in addition to being inserted into the center, the lag screw must also be inserted at right angles to the fracture plane. Under axial load, however, displacement can still occur. Therefore, whenever axial stability is required some of the compression must be sacrificed, and the lag screw must be inserted at right angles to the long axis of the bone (**Fig. 10-3**).

A single lag screw is never enough to achieve a sufficiently stable and strong fixation of diaphyseal tubular bone. A minimum of two, and preferably three, lag screws is required. This means, therefore, that only long oblique and spiral fractures can be stabilized with lag screws alone and only if these

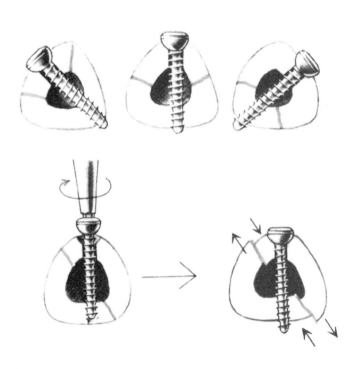

Fig. 10-2: Lag screws must be inserted in the center of fragments. (From Müller et al., 1979 [14].)

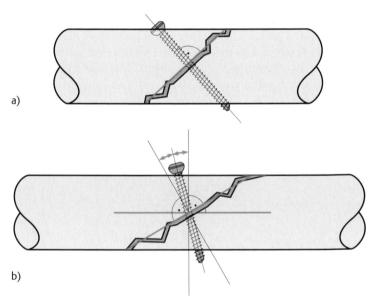

a)

b)

Fig. 10-3: Optimal inclination of the screw in relation to a simple fracture plane.
a) Shows a lag screw oriented perpendicular to the fracture plane. This is an ideal inclination in the absence of forces along the bone axis.
b) Shows an inclination half way between the perpendiculars to the fracture plane and to the long axis of the bone. This is an inclination which is better suited to resisting compressive functional load along the bone long axis.
(From Rüedi et al., 2000 [12].)

involve short tubular bones. If lag screws alone are used for the fixation of bones such as the humerus or femur, they almost always end in early failure because of mechanical overload. Only spiral fractures of bones such as the phalanges, metacarpals, metatarsals, or malleoli lend themselves to fixation with lag screws alone. The most common use of lag screws is in the fixation of shaft fractures but they are used in combination with neutralization plates, which protect the lag screws from overload.

3.2 Neutralization plates

A neutralization plate, as its name suggests, conducts all of the forces from one main fragment to the other and, in this way, protects the fracture from the forces of bending, shear, and torque. As outlined in **Section 3.1**, any two fragments should be first stabilized by means of a lag screw or screws. If the fixation is deemed mechanically insufficient, because of comminution or because of the bone involved, then the primary internal fixation with lag screws has to be protected with a protection or neutralization plate.

The term "neutralization" or the terms to be introduced subsequently, "buttress plate" and "tension band", do not refer to any specific plate but to the function of the plate. Thus, a straight plate or an angled plate can be a neutralization plate, a buttress plate, or a tension band plate. In some instances, a plate can even combine functions and be a neutralization and a tension band plate at the same time.

3.3 Compression and tension band plates

A short oblique or transverse fracture does not lend itself to lag screw fixation. Such a fracture can be stabilized by means of compression, but the compression has to be in the long axis of bone. Such compression can only be generated by a plate. The fracture is reduced, and the plate is fixed to one of the two fragments. A tension device is then fixed to the other fragment and is hooked up to the plate. As the tension device is tightened, it exerts a pull on the plate and places it under tension. This results in the two fragments being compressed. Such compression is static.

Axial compression may also be generated by means of a tension device or by the insertion of a load screw in a self-compressing plate (dynamic compression plate or semitubular plate). When such devices are used, the bone is brought under axial compression. Initially both cortices of the bone are equally compressed but, as tension increases, the bone bends slightly toward the plate.

Compression in the cortex opposite the plate decreases correspondingly, and, at maximum compression, a slight gap often appears in the cortex opposite the plate. To overcome this effect when a straight compression plate is applied to a straight bone, the plate must be contoured to a slight convexity at the fracture. When first applied to bone, a plate so contoured forces the opposite cortices to come into contact and the ones immediately next to the plate to gap slightly. As axial compression is generated, the cortices opposite the plate remain in contact and the ones next to the plate are gradually brought under compression. At peak axial compression, the opposite cortex remains compressed, rather than gapping, and the axial load is exerted not only on the cortex next to the plate but also equally on the whole fracture interface.

Pauwels [15] made the observation that certain long bones are eccentrically loaded. He postulated that, despite the interplay of muscles and gravity, the net loading of such bones would result in the side closest to the load being under compression and the other side being under tension. Thus, in these bones, the load generates not only compression because of its weight, but also internal compressive and tensile stresses because of the bending. If such a bone breaks, it assumes a characteristic position of deformity because of a fairly constant interplay of forces.

Pauwels [15] borrowed an engineering principle, which is applied to the reduction of the internal stresses of structures as a result of bending. This principle is called tension band, and internal fixation of bone which makes use of this principle is referred to as tension band fixation. Pauwels showed schematically, with the aid of a simple I-shaped column, how the neutralization of the internal stresses occurs

Fig. 10-4: To illustrate the effectiveness of the tension band principle, Pauwels used photo-elastic models. Eccentric loading produces a stress-strain differential within the material. These differentials can be equalized by a tension band applied to the tension side. It acts as a counterweight to eccentrically applied compression.
a) Eccentric force (K) is applied at a distance from the neutral axis (0), producing a tensile force of 79 kp/cm² (Z) and a compression force of 94 kp/cm² (D).
b) A weak tension band (G) is applied to the tension side (left column), producing a resultant force (R) more closely aligned with the neutral axis of the material. The tensile force Z is reduced to 47 kp/cm² while the compression force D is decreased to 79 kp/cm².
c–f) The application of a progressively stronger tension band (G) produces and intensifies the shift of forces toward the neutral axis. The resultant force (R) is shifted toward neutral force 0 until the tension-optical lines become collinear as seen in (f). There is now an equally acting compressive force of 30 kp/cm².
(From Pauwels, 1980 [16].)

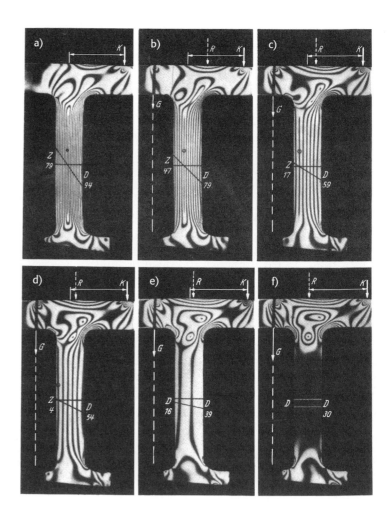

(**Fig. 10-4**). Pauwels' postulates relating to the tension and compression side of bone have, with the aid of strain gauges affixed to bone, been confirmed in vivo [17].

Transverse fractures fixed with a compression plate applied to the tension side of bone show an increase in the axial compression on weight bearing. This means that this mode of fixation makes use of eccentric forces and converts the forces of displacement into forces of stability.

Axial compression increases with loading. Thus, this type of fixation is referred to as dynamic compression. Because a compressive force applied on the side opposite to the compressive load functions as a tension band, the compression plate applied to the tension side of bone is called a tension band plate.

Certain bones such as the radius, ulna, humerus, and femur are eccentrically loaded. The strain on the cortices of these bones is not in equilibrium [17]. The medial cortex is loaded in compression and the lateral cortex in tension. During the stance phase of the gait cycle, the maximum deformation (i.e., the maximum compressive strain) is greater in the medial cortex than the maximum tensile strain in the lateral cortex. To exert axial compression in an eccentrically loaded bone, the pre-stressed plate must be applied to the cortex loaded in tension as explained above (**Fig. 10-5**). In this position it acts as a tension band; under dynamic load it converts the tensile forces into axial compressive forces, to such a degree that at peak load the compressive strain in the cortex deep to the plate can exceed the compressive strain in the medial cortex normally loaded in compression [17].

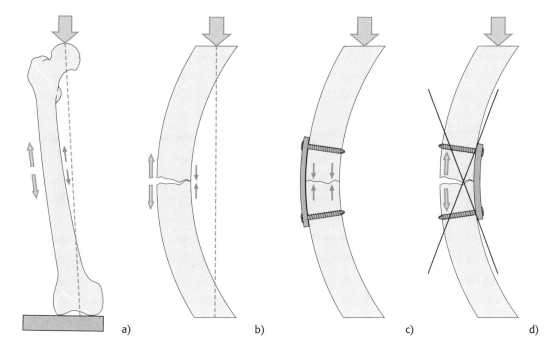

a)   b)   c)   d)

Fig. 10-5:
Tension band principle at the femur.
The intact femur (a) is an eccentrically
loaded bone with distraction or tensile
forces laterally and compression on the
medial side. In case of a fracture (b) the
lateral fracture gap will open, whereas the
medial will be compressed. If a plate is
place alongside the linea aspera of the
femur (c), it will be under tension when
loaded, thereby compressing the fracture
gap, provided there is bony contact
medially. If the plate is placed to the
compression side (d), it is not able to
prevent opening of the lateral gap
(instability). If the medial cortex is not
intact (e), the tension band principle
cannot work because of lack of buttress.
(From Rüedi et al., 2000 [18].)

3.4   Tension band wire

The principle of tension band fixation can be applied to
avulsion fractures such as the transverse fracture of a patella
or olecranon, or to the avulsion fracture of the greater trochanter, or the lateral or medial malleolus.

A tension band wire, like the tension band plate, must be
pre-stressed and inserted on the tension side of bone. Under
functional load, like a muscular contraction, it will convert a
tensile distracting force into dynamic forces and result in axial
interfragmentary compression. It is a secure and stable form of
internal fixation that permits early use of the involved part
without fear of displacement. The tension wire applies a purely
axial compressive force; it does not have any torsional stability.
To provide rotational stability, the tension band wire is frequently combined with two parallel Kirschner wires, which
function as internal splints.

4   Non-compressive stabilization

4.1   Internal splintage

4.1.1   Intramedullary nails

Intramedullary nailing, the introduction of Kirschner wires into
metaphyseal areas of bone in children, and the insertion of
angled devices into the proximal femur in order to stabilize
subcapital or intertrochanteric fractures are forms of internal
fixation referred to as splintage.

Such fixation merely splints the reduction and the stability
obtained by impaction. It is sufficiently stable to permit early
function but never provides the stability, which can be obtained by compression. The biological expression of stable

internal fixation is primary bone healing, which is clinically seen as the gradual disappearance of the fracture line without the appearance of radiologically discernible periosteal or endosteal callus.

The instability associated with the intramedullary splintage is reflected by the amount of callus produced. A large intramedullary nail that is tightly wedged into the medullary canal may result in sufficient stability to effect primary bone healing. Most often a variable amount of periosteal callus is seen. The stability that an intramedullary device bestows relies on the principle of a tube within a tube. Therefore, it is dependent upon the length of contact for its resistance to bending, and upon friction and the interdigitation of the fracture fragments for rotational stability. Thus, in human patients it is common practice to employ intramedullary reaming. This enlarges the medullary canal to a size large enough to permit the insertion of sufficiently large intramedullary nails, which not only provide sufficient stability but are also sufficiently strong to take over the function of the bone which they are replacing. Small nails adapted to the size of the isthmus, which in young patients is often narrow, are rarely strong enough, and are usually too flexible. They do not give the required stability and their use leads to complications such as nail migration, nail bending, nail fracture, delayed union, and non-union.

Intramedullary nailing provides distinct advantages in a weight-bearing extremity. Because it is a load-sharing device, it enables a much earlier return to function than is possible to achieve with other means of internal fixation. Because of its design and mode of application, an intramedullary nail is much stronger than a plate and consequently will withstand loading for a much longer period of time before failure. Therefore, it is possible to await union for a longer period of time than with a plate without fear of the implant going on to fatigue failure.

Because of its mode of application and immobilization of the fracture, an intramedullary nail is suitable only for fractures which occur in the middle third of long bones. The proximal and distal portion of long tubular bones broadens into cancellous bone. In these areas, the reamed nailing provides neither angular nor rotational stability. In the middle third, the nail is the most suitable means of immobilization of transverse or short oblique fractures. As long as there is contact between the main fragments, even comminuted fractures can be nailed, particularly if the comminuted fragments are secured with lag screws or cerclage wires. Some of the disadvantages of the "reamed nailing" have been overcome by employing interlocking nails (see **Section 4.2.4**).

Segmental defects of the femur can, under exceptional circumstances, be stabilized with intramedullary nails, but this technique requires the combination of the intramedullary nail with a plate to maintain length and rotational stability. By segmental defects we mean fractures with extensive multiple segments and only rarely with true bone loss. The techniques described for fractures, other than simple transverse and oblique, can be used only in nailing of the femur. In the middle third of the tibia, fracture patterns, other than transverse or oblique, should be stabilized by a combination of lag screws with a neutralization plate. In the femur, where the displacing forces are overwhelming, the nail is a preferable means of fixation because it is stronger mechanically and will not fatigue and fail as early as a plate. Non-unions of the middle third of the femur and tibia, if not associated with angular or rotational deformities, are ideally suited for intramedullary nailing. When angular or rotational deformities are present, these must be corrected before nailing.

The splinting of fractures by means of Kirschner wires in children always, and in animals sometimes, requires the additional support of external coaptation. These fractures often unite rapidly, particularly if they are in metaphyseal areas. This allows for removal of the wires within 2–3 weeks. The stability gained from angled devices inserted as splints into the proximal femur is insufficient to provide adequate stability if the fragments are merely lined up and not impacted.

The stability of these fractures must be achieved by impaction. This restores bone continuity and allows the bone to function as a structural unit. The plate functions as an internal splint and is used to maintain the fragments in their stable position, but not to provide stability to the fracture. If called upon to provide stability, such plates frequently fail with the resultant complication of malunion or non-union.

4.2 Bridging osteosynthesis

Internal splinting using the principle of bridging osteosynthesis has become widely accepted in recent years. The fundamental principle is to leave the fracture fragments undisturbed. The technique relies upon the soft-tissue envelope to reconstruct an approximate cylinder of bone fragments, while the major proximal and distal fragments are distracted and pulled out to length. No attempt is made to realign or immobilize any fracture fragments, thereby leaving their tenuous soft-tissue attachments undisturbed.

Bridging osteosynthesis can be achieved by a number of techniques. A conventional plate can bridge the complex fracture zone with only three or four screws anchored proximally and distally in the intact parts of the fractured bone. Alternatively, splinting can be achieved by plate/rod fixation, the use of an interlocking nail (**Section 4.2.4**), or by the application of an external fixator (**Section 4.3**).

4.2.1 Bridging plates

The concept of the bridge plate was first described by Brunner and Weber [19]. These authors noted two advantages of the technique. Firstly, as the plate spans a long fracture zone, the load on the underside of the plate not fixed to the bone is distributed over an extended distance. This reduces stress risers and avoids sites of excessive deformation prone to fatigue failure. Secondly, since the plate is applied at a distance to the bone, it permits better vascular access to the repair tissue and benefits more from the mechanical support provided by the repair tissue due to better leverage (**Fig. 10-6**).

Fig. 10-6: Bridging plate.
a) Bridging callus is evident 20 weeks after repair of this femoral fracture using a 4.5 narrow lengthening plate (NLP).
b) A comminuted diaphyseal fracture of the tibia/fibula.
c) The fracture has been repaired using a 4.5 narrow lenthening plate and three lags screws. An autogenous cancellous bone graft was used in conjunction with the fracture repair.
d) The plate and two lag screws were removed 6 months after surgery. The fracture is clinically and radiographically united. (From Miller et al., 1989 [20].)

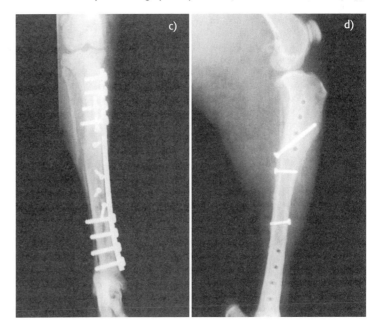

4.2.2 Buttress plates

Reconstruction of comminuted fractures with lag screws and neutralization plates carries a number of inherent risks—both from a mechanical and biological perspective. If fracture reduction is incomplete and a small gap exists in the transcortex, that is, the cortex opposite the plate, high local strains will occur as forces are concentrated in this small gap. Paradoxically, if the area of comminution is not reduced, the forces are distributed over a much greater area, thereby lowering interfragmentary strain. However, if the bony column is not reconstructed, the bone plate must transmit all the weight-bearing forces until callus formation occurs. Such a plate is termed a buttress plate.

If a standard bone plate is used as a buttress plate, empty screw holes over the area of multiple fractures will act as stress concentrators and encourage plate failure. This risk can be reduced by using lengthening plates that have round holes at their ends and a solid central portion devoid of screw holes.

In metaphyseal areas of bone where the cortex is very thin, fractures require protection. Axial overload could result in deformity because the thin cortex, which itself is often comminuted, would crumble. Plates used in these areas for this purpose are also referred to as buttress plates.

Metaphyseal areas of different bones, unlike the diaphysis, which is tubular, differ in configuration. This has resulted in the development of different buttress plates designed for different metaphyses. Thus, there is a special T-plate for the proximal humerus, a special "spoon" and "cloverleaf" plate for the distal tibia, a special T-plate and L-plate for the proximal tibia, and a special buttress plate for the distal femur.

When a buttress plate is applied to bone, it must be very carefully adapted to the shape of the bone because the plate is functionally designed to distract and support, and not to compress. If it were to compress, it would result in the deformity it is designed to prevent. Additionally, since the reduction of many small fragments may destroy their vascular supply, thereby increasing the possibility of implant failure, it is recommended buttress plates be applied using the biological plating principles. The soft-tissue envelope must remain undisturbed while limb alignment is restored. Large fragments may be "lassoed" with absorbable, synthetic suture material to pull them into reasonable alignment provided soft-tissue dissection is kept to a minimum (**Fig. 10-7**).

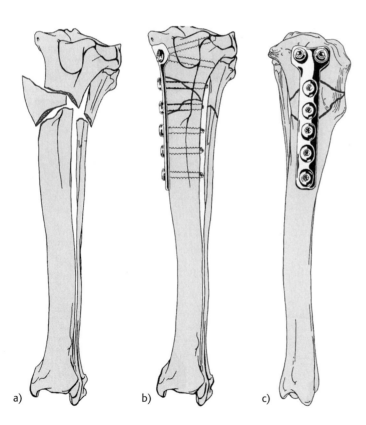

a)

b)

c)

Fig. 10-7: Buttress plate
a) A multiple fracture of the proximal end of the tibia with a wedge segment.
b/c) Repair was accomplished using a T-plate, which was employed so as to restore length of the bone and the support to the tibial plateau incorrect alignment. Medial view of the proximal tibia, showing the T-plate.
(From Brinker et al., 1998 [**21**].)

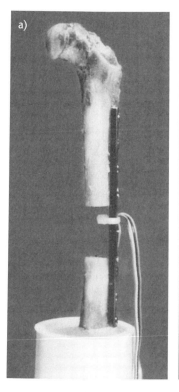

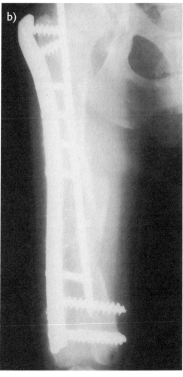

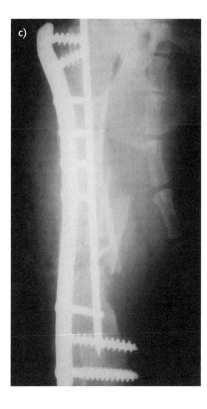

Fig. 10-8: Plate rod
a) Photograph of a plate/rod construct as it would be prepared for mounting into the materials testing machine. Note the strain gauges placed on the surface of the bone plate; one gauge is positioned in the solid section of the bone plate and a second gauge positioned adjacent to an empty plate hole. (From Hulse et al., 2000 [22].)
b) Multiple fracture of a canine femur treated by a combined plate/rod system. Immediate postoperative radiograph.
c) The same fracture 12 weeks following the operation. The fracture is consolidated and dynamic loading of the site may now be commenced by removing the intramedullary pin. (Figs b and c, Courtesy of A. Johnson.)

4.2.3 Plate rod fixation

In order to reduce the risk of a plate failing in the buttress mode, a plate/rod construct has been suggested [22].This construct is particularly suited to those fractures where biological assessment indicates that fracture healing will be slow, while mechanical assessment dictates that the implants must withstand maximum stress (Fig. 10-8).

The size of the intramedullary pin has a significant influence on the strength of the construct. A pin that occupies 50% of the diameter of the medullary cavity will reduce the stress on the plate by 50% or more. Moreover, it will extend the fatigue life of the plate by at least ten-fold. However, an intramedullary pin that only occupies 25% of the medullary cavity will only reduce the stress on the plate by 10%. Generally, pins which occupy 30–40% of the medullary cavity are employed. The

spatial alignment of the pin will also influence its protecting role on the plate. The greater the distance between the plate and the pin, the greater mechanical advantage the pin will have. Thus, pins should be inserted in a normograde or retrograde fashion with this in mind.

4.2.4 Interlocking nails

The interlocking nail has its origins in the Küntscher nail, popularized in the 1940s by Dr Gerhard Küntscher [23] who was the first to describe fixation of diaphyseal fractures of the femur with a solid interlocking nail.

There are several systems of interlocking nails and instrumentation, but they all have a common design. The nails are solid, 6 mm or 8 mm in diameter, and made from stainless steel. They are available in a variety of lengths. One end has a trocar point and the other keying flanges with an internal thread for attachment to an aiming device. Alternatively, nails may not have an external guiding system and the screws are introduced under fluoroscopic guidance.

At each end of the nail there are two holes though the nail to allow for the insertion of transversely orientated locking screws. If these screws engage the nail/bone only on one side of the fracture, the locking nail acts in a dynamic mode. When screws are present on both sides of the fracture, the pin will function in a static mode of fixation. By locking the main proximal and distal fragments to the nail with screws, axial collapse and rotation are resisted. Moreover, since the intramedullary pin is in the central axis of the bone, it is better positioned to resist bending forces in all directions (**Fig. 10-9**).

The interlocking nail has supplanted plate fixation for many fractures in man, and closed nailing of femoral and tibial fractures is now considered the treatment of choice. More recent nailing systems are anatomically designed, but this clearly increases the problem of attached guidance systems. In animals, the range of sizes and shapes of the various long bones will make such customized systems prohibitively expensive, unless fluoroscopic units and radiolucent drill extensions become widely available.

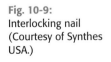

Fig. 10-9:
Interlocking nail
(Courtesy of Synthes
USA.)

4.3 External skeletal fixation

There has been a considerable resurgence in the use of external skeletal fixators in recent years. The fixators consist of a series of percutaneous, trans-osseous, transfixing pins that penetrate both cortices of the bone in which they are drilled. They may, or may not, penetrate the skin on both sides of the limb. The pins may be smooth, or they may be threaded centrally or at one end. Classically, they are connected to an external connecting bar(s) by clamps—the entire apparatus being called a construct or montage (**Fig. 10-10**).

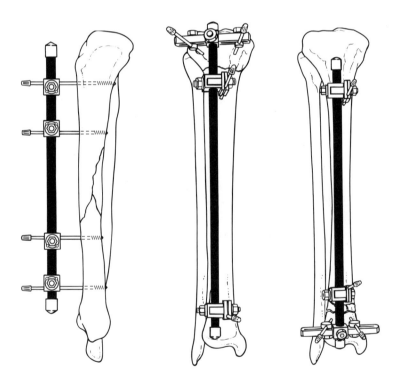

Fig. 10-10: External Fixator (Courtesy of Synthes USA.)

Clamps may be single or double, open or closed. Alternatively, the pins may be joined to connecting bars composed of acrylic resin (methylmethacrylate, dental acrylic, etc.). This has the advantage that the pins do not need to be in a single plane. Hence, acrylic frames have a greater versatility where multiplanar pin fixation is required.

Acrylic frames have been the subject of considerable research with regard to their strength compared to stainless steel [24]. In the fracture model explored, a 1.91-cm diameter acrylic connecting bar was stronger than the standard medium-size Kirschner apparatus using 4.8-mm standard connecting bars.

Ring fixators, of which the Ilizarov is perhaps the best known, provide an alternative approach to external skeletal fixation. These fixators use a number of very small pins that are inserted through the limb and are connected to encircling or hemi-circumferential connecting bars. The pins are tensioned before tightening the clamps on the rings, thus markedly increasing their strength. Although these frames are generally used to correct growth deformities and to lengthen limbs by distraction osteogenesis, they are very versatile in fracture management [25, 26]. Their main disadvantage relates to the greater difficulty in constructing the frame and their bulk (**Fig. 10-11**).

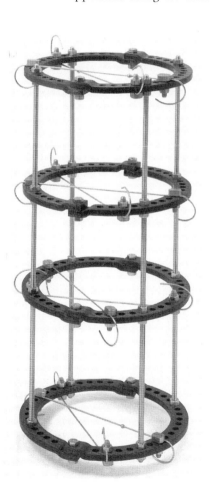

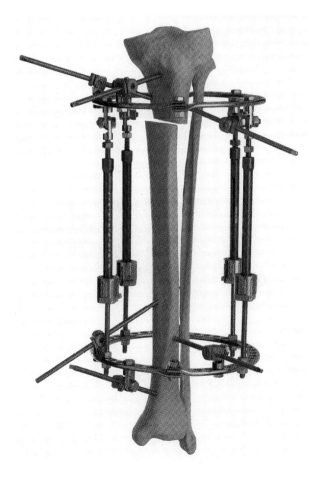

Fig. 10-11: Ilizarov fixation device (Courtesy of Smith & Nephew Richards, Inc.)

Axial compression can be applied by means of external skeletal fixators, which force the pins together. Indeed, this was the first clinical application of compression [6, 7]. This type of fixation is stable only over short lengths of bone and only when broad flat cancellous surfaces are being compressed, such as the surfaces of arthrodeses or metaphyseal osteotomies. When applied to tubular cortical bone, such fixation does not result in absolute stability. Although not absolutely stable, the external skeletal fixator is extremely useful under certain clinical circumstances, such as in the treatment of open fractures which may not be suitable for internal fixation. The external fixator provides sufficient stability to permit functional use of the extremity while it maintains bones in their reduced position. The stability is sufficient to render the fracture painless and to encourage soft-tissue rehabilitation.

External skeletal fixation is also useful in circumstances where comminution is too severe to permit internal fixation and where better stability is required than that obtainable by cast fixation or traction. Common examples of such clinical situations are the badly fragmented Colles fractures (fracture of the lower end of the radius), certain femoral or tibial fractures, and certain pelvic fractures. Because external skeletal fixation, when applied to cortical bone, does not result in absolute stability, such fixation has to be supplemented by bone grafting to ensure union, or it has to be converted to a stable type of internal fixation as soon as the clinical situation permits.

5   Implant failure and bone grafting

Metal plates or other devices, no matter how rigid and thick, will undergo fatigue failure and break if subjected to cyclical loading. In a stable internal fixation, bone continuity is re-established and maintained by compression. In this way, bone resumes its function as a load-bearing structure, minimizing the load borne by the internal fixation. Metal is best able to withstand tension, whereas bone is able to best withstand compression. Thus, in an ideal internal fixation, the biomechanical design must be such that bone is loaded in compression and the internal fixation in tension.

If a defect occurs in a bone, and if it occurs in the cortex opposite the plate, then, as loading occurs, the fulcrum moves closer and closer to the plate. The larger the defect, the closer the fulcrum moves to the plate, until eventually the fulcrum falls within the plate. Consequently, with repetitive loading, even if only due to muscular contraction and not to weight bearing, the implant is repeatedly cycled (**Fig. 10-12**).

Thus, an internal fixation can be viewed as a race between bone union and implant failure. If a defect is accepted, bone union will be delayed. This is related to the size of the defect, the degree of fragmentation, and the degree of devascularization of the fragments. In the presence of a defect the implant is cycled and goes on to the inevitable fatigue failure, with loss of fixation.

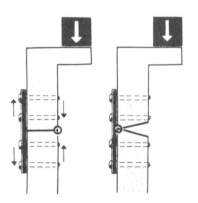 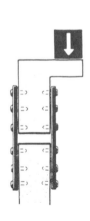 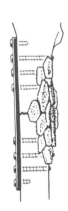

Fig. 10-12: Mechanism of plate failure and its prevention by bone grafting.
A defect in the cortex opposite the plate results, under load, in a bending with the fulcrum falling within the plate. This cyclic bending can be prevented by the application of a plate to the defective cortex or by bone grafting. Once the bone graft is incorporated and becomes a bony bridge it acts like a second plate. (From Müller et al., 1970 [13].) Alternatively, the lateral element may be temporarily spanned with an external fixator to "protect" the plate. In such cases the medial plate is not applied, but the medial defect is packed with bone graft material.

In order to prevent this predictable sequence of events whenever a defect occurs, there is comminution or devitalization of fragments, or enormous forces have to be overcome, such as in the femur, one should use autogenous cancellous bone grafting at the time of the internal fixation. Such a bone graft, once it becomes incorporated into an osteoid bridge opposite the plate, rapidly hypertrophies and matures because it becomes subjected to compressive forces. As it re-establishes the continuity of bone opposite the plate, it acts mechanically as a second plate and prevents the cycling and inevitable fatigue failure of the implant. In this way the internal fixation is maintained until union proceeds to completion, with ultimate revascularization and remodeling of all fragments until the bone architecture returns to normal.

6 Implant removal

Primary bone healing is different from healing by callus, but not better. It is a biological expression of stability. Early on, following fracture, bone that has undergone primary bone healing is weaker than that united by callus. A callus, because of its spatial disposition, is further away from the central axis of the bone and is at a mechanically more advantageous position to resist force. Primary bone healing, which consists of the growth of new osteons across the fracture, can be likened to intracortical dowels joining the cortical fragments together. These are closer to the central axis of the bone and are mechanically in a less advantageous position. Once the internal architecture of the cortex returns to normal, in mature diaphyseal bone usually by 18 months following fracture, it becomes mechanically as strong as the bone which is healed by callus.

Bone healing under conditions of stable fixation is not only weaker by virtue of the disposition of the new osteons, but also by virtue of the fact that such bone is subject to tremendous remodeling, manifested by the proliferation of the haversian canals. Thus, such bone, although unchanged in its cross-sectional diameter, contains less bone per cross-sectional area because of the great proliferation of the haversian canals. This continues until the accelerated remodeling ceases and the architecture gradually returns to normal. This usually occurs some 12 months from the time of fracture. Factors which prolong the remodeling phase are the patient's age, degree of fragmentation, degree of devitalization, size of the gaps, accuracy of the reduction, stability of the fixation, and whether or not bone grafting has been carried out.

Furthermore, it is important to note whether there were any signs of instability during the time of healing or whether the fracture progressed uneventfully to union.

All of these facts must be borne in mind when considering the removal of an implant. If the implant is removed prematurely, the bone will inevitably fail and a re-fracture will occur. Following removal of an implant, bone must be protected from an overload. The screw holes function as points of stress concentration. Thus, if suddenly loaded, the bone may fail. Similarly, the ridges that frequently develop on each side of the plate should not be removed. Any excessive callus may be used for "on site" grafting of the empty screw holes. Clinical experience suggests that long bones should be protected by restricting the amount of loading for 6 weeks following removal of an implant. Implant removal is advised in younger patients, even if the implant is completely non-irritating. This is also true of implants used in non-weight-bearing extremities. Such implants clearly change the physical properties of the bone and expose the individual to dangers of fractures at the point where the plates end and normal bone begins.

7 Bibliography

Blue references indicate links to abstracts of articles available online:
http://www.aopublishing.org/BONE/10.htm

1. **Yamada H, Evans FG** (1970) *Strength of biological materials.* Baltimore: Williams & Wilkins.

2. **Knets IV, Pfafrod GO, Saulgozis JZ** (1980) *Deformation of Biological Hard Tissue (in Russian).* Riga: Zinatne.

3. **Lucas-Championiere J** (1907) Les dangers de l'immobilisation des membres – fragilite des os – alteration de la nutrition du membre – conclusions pratiques. *Rev Med Chir Pratique;* 78:81.

4. **Gautier E, Rahn BA, Perren SM** (1986) Effect of steel versus composite plastic plates on internal and external remodelling of intact long bones. *Orthop Trans;* 10:391.

5. **Danis R** (1947) The operative treatment of bone fractures. *J Int Chir;* 7:318.

6. **Schenk R, Willenegger H** (1963) Zum histologischen Bild der sogenannten Primärheilung der Knochenkompakta nach experimentellen Osteotomen am Hund. *Experientia;* 19:593.

7. **Ashhurst DE** (1986) The influence of mechanical conditions on the healing of experimental fractures in the rabbit: a microscopical study. *Philos Trans R Soc Lond B Biol Sci;* 313 (1161): 271–302.

8. **Key JA** (1932) Positive pressure in arthrodesis for tuberculosis of the knee joint. *South Med J;* 23:909.

9. **Charnley J** (1953) *Compression Arthrodesis.* Edinburgh: E & S Livingstone.

10. **Mast J, Jacob R, Ganz R** (1989) *Planning and reduction techniques in fracture surgery.* Berlin Heidelberg New York: Springer-Verlag.

11. **Schatzker J, Sanderson R, Murnaghan JP** (1975) The holding power of orthopedic screws in vivo. *Clin Orthop;* (108):115–126.

12. **Perren SM, Frigg R, Hehli M** (2000) Lag screw. In: Rüedi TP, Murphy WM, editors. *AO Principles of Fracture Management.* Stuttgart–New York: Thieme, pp160, 163.

13. **Müller ME, Allgöwer M, Willenegger H** (1970) *Manual of Internal Fixation.* Berlin Heidelberg New York: Springer-Verlag.

14. **Müller ME, Allgöwer M, Schneider R** (1979) *Manual of Internal Fixation 2nd ed.* Berlin Heidelberg New York: Springer-Verlag.

15. **Pauwels F** (1958) *Über die therapeutische Anwendung neuer Erkenntnisse auf dem Gebiet der funktionellen Anatomie bei Erkrankungen des Stütz- und Bewegungsapparates (Aschoff Vorlesung).* Freiburg i Breisgau.

16. **Pauwels F** (1980) *Biomechanics of the Locomotor Apparatus.* Berlin Heidelberg New York: Springer-Verlag.

17. **Schatzker J, Sumner-Smith G, Clark R, et al.** (1978) Strain gauge analysis of bone response to internal fixation. *Clin Orthop;* (132):244–251.

18. **Wittner B, Holz U** (2000) Plates. In: Rüedi TP, Murphy WM, editors. *AO Principles of Fracture Management.* Stuttgart–New York: Thieme, p183.

19. **Brunner CF, Weber BG** (1981) *Besondere Osteosynthesetechniken.* Berlin Heidelberg New York: Springer-Verlag.

20. **Miller CW, Kuzma AB, Sumner-Smith G** (1989) The Narro Lengthening Plate for Treatment of Comminuted Diaphyseal Fractures in Dogs. *V.C.O.T.;* 3:108–112.

21. **Brinker WO, Olmstead ML, Sumner-Smith G** (1998) *Manual of Internal Fixation in Small Animals. 2nd ed.* Berlin Heidelberg New York: Springer-Verlag.

22. **Hulse D, Ferry K, Fawcett A** (2000) Effect of intramedullary pin size on reducing bone plate strain. *V.C.O.T.;* 13:185–190.

23. **Huckstep RL** (1972) Rigid intramedullary fixation of femoral shaft fractures with compression. *J Bone Joint Surg [Br];* 54:204.

24. **Willer RL, Egger EL, Histand MB** (1991) Comparison of stainless steel versus acrylic for the connecting bar of external skeletal fixators. *J Am An Hosp Ass;* 27:541.

25. **Ilizarov GA** (1976) *Results of Clinical Tests and Experience Obtained from the Clinical Use of the Ilizarov Compression-Distraction System.* Moscow: Med Export Moscow.

26. **Latte Y** (1994) Application of the Ilizarov method in veterinary orthopaedic surgery. *Prat Med Chir Anim Comp;* 29:545.

11   Non-union of fractures

Section A

Geoff Sumner-Smith

 1   Introduction to pathogenesis and treatment of non-union

Despite the advent of modern techniques, individual fractures occasionally refuse to heal and a non-union or pseudarthrosis occurs. The problem is not new; the oldest known case was reported by Moodie [1]. The pseudarthrosis was seen in the radius of a small primitive Paleocene ungulate of the Eocene epoch, known as Ectocanus. The same author also reported the occurrence of a case of non-union in the fossilized skull of an ancient pig-like animal, Arthaeotherium, from the later Oligocene epoch. This fossil was discovered in the South Dakota Badlands.

When the first Egyptian expedition opened some of the tombs belonging to the dynasties of 2500 to 3000 BC, they found evidence of non-union in bones of skeletons therein. The condition was certainly recognized by Hippocrates, who mentioned it in his classic report on fractures some 400 years BC. In the year 1756, the English surgeon Sir Percivall Pott wrote one of his many monographs. He had, himself, suffered a fracture of the midshaft of the tibia. His writings of that date were concerned with the management of fractures, and in particular with the fracture which has since borne his name. Pott had already recognized that this was a common site at which the fragments frequently failed to unite, and where malunion and also pseudarthrosis might be a sequel. Strangely enough, it appears that the more modern and sophisticated treatments have become, the greater the incidence of non-union. Bonnin [2], speaking of tibial fractures, asked: "What has caused the delay in consolidation in 6 weeks and consolidation in 11 weeks between 1840 and 1940?"

2   Fracture union–osteosynthesis

At this point, it must be clearly understood that what appears to be firm clinical union, with a lack of spring in the fracture and disappearance of tenderness, as mentioned by Tippett [3], does not correspond with uniform mineralization of the callus. Mineralization is not complete until many weeks later. In 1912 Robert Jones wrote: "we must realize that the academic period of consolidation, authoritatively asserted, is not accurate; and that bones which appear firm to the hand will yield, after many weeks, to incidence of body weight" (quoted by Tippett) [3].

Braschear [4] stated that "a state of non-union exists when repair has stopped completely and that surgery is required to bring about union". The statement implies a clear-cut end point but, in reality, this point is impossible to define since it is a combination of radiographic and clinical findings; "delayed union" implies a longer healing time than is usual for "that particular fracture".

3 Nomenclature and identification of conditions

The healing process may be classified into four separate entities: union, malunion, non-union, and pseudarthrosis.

The nomenclature accorded to healing of bone and the absence of healing continues to cause problems in interpretation, particularly when a language barrier is encountered. The student should appreciate that, when reading some European literature, a difference between non-union and pseudarthrosis may not be mentioned; these conditions are described as "Pseudarthrose" in the European literature. This term is meant to cover both non-union and the formation of a "false joint", whereas in the English literature it is usual to differentiate between the two conditions.

The term "Pseudarthrose" (German) is not synonymous with non-union as described in English. "Pseudo" is taken from the Greek and means "false".

3.1 Terms

Hence the correct terms are, more properly:
- Union: a healing fracture.
- Malunion: a healed fracture, but anatomically incorrectly aligned.
- Delayed union: a healing fracture, although healing very slowly.
- Non-union: failure to unite.
- Pseudarthrosis: "false joint" formation.

The synonyms found in German texts are, therefore:
- "Heilung" (union).
- "Verzögerte Heilung" (delayed union).
- "Pseudarthrose" (non-union).
- "Falsches Gelenk" or "Neoarthrose" (pseudarthrosis).

"Pseudarthrose" as used in German is incorrect, and should be reserved for the condition where a true "false joint" is formed.

The decision to classify a fracture as undergoing delayed union, a case of non-union, or pseudarthrosis has been described by Cave [5] and Wray [6]. Cave [5] described delayed union as being determined almost entirely by radiography and by certain bones showing evidence of healing in a more or less prescribed period of time. The best evidence of healing is callus formation, as shown in the radiograph.

Identifying the conditions in detail, they may be described as follows:

3.1.1 Union

This term is used to describe a fracture that has united. It is usually reserved for the state in which fracture ends have completely united; in other words, the fracture is "properly healed" (see **Chapter 10**).

3.1.2 Malunion

The fracture has united but the union is incorrectly aligned. The parts are not, therefore, in their proper anatomical position. For instance, a shaft fracture has healed on an angle instead of being straight, or a suprachondral fracture has healed without proper contiguity of the joint surfaces.

3.1.3 Non-union

This occurs when the apposed ends of the fracture have failed to unite and to ossify. The amount of healing that has occurred may vary from a cartilaginous bridge, which has failed to ossify, to fibrous-connective tissue, or to an absolute lack of bridging whatsoever. Each type will be examined later in the text.

3.1.4 Pseudarthrosis

This is a term that indicates a true false-joint formation when bone ends are joined by a fibrous joint-capsule-like structure, which contains synovial-like fluid originating from local serum production.

3.2 Classification of fracture non-union

Classifying fractures as either biological failures or technical failures, Frost [7] deplored the fact that there has been an increase in the number of technical failures since the early part of the century, and rather ruefully stated that "after all, a major upgrading in the orthopedic knowledge, education and practice has taken place in the last 40 years. As a result, the group termed biological failures now forms approximately 50% of those patients referred to most large medical centers for fracture non-unions".

There is a natural human failing for surgeons to classify their own failures as being due to biological factors rather more frequently than they would accord that reasoning to a fracture handled by another surgeon! Weber and Čech [8], in an admirable treatise, have classified non-unions according to their biological reactions. This system is particularly suitable for the clinician since it has a bearing on the treatment of the problem; consequently, it will be followed in this dissertation.

Although the basic principle of treatment of non-union is that of stable fixation, the ability of the bone to respond to a biological reaction is very relevant. With this in mind, Weber and Čech [8] have classified fractures that are undergoing a "disturbance in union" into two major groups:

- Capable of biological reaction—i.e., non-viable.
- Incapable of biological reaction—i.e., non-viable.

The ability to judge into which major group a fracture falls is relevant to the type of treatment that should be instituted.

3.2.1 Viable non-union

The Weber-Čech classification [8] lists three types (**Fig. 11-1**):

- The hypertrophic type of non-union possesses an abundant callus with a profusion of blood vessels and is known as an "elephant foot" non-union. It results either from insufficient stabilization or premature weight bearing (**Fig. 11-1a**, **Fig. 11-2**, **Fig. 11-3**).
- The second type, slightly hypertrophic, is described as a milder form of "elephant foot" callus and hence is given the name "horse hoof" callus. It is usually the

result of resorption underneath a plate, and often the plate breaks since the initial immobilization was insufficiently stable (**Fig. 11-1b**).

- The oligotrophic (no callus) type of non-union is not an atrophic non-union. It may be the result of major displacement followed by too much extension or incomplete reduction of a fracture. Healing is impaired, although the ends may be joined by fibrous tissue containing blood vessels. After 2–3 months the ends of the fracture cortex round off, resorb, and later decalcify. Scintimetry of such fractures reveals that they are indeed viable and capable of biological activity, although radiographically they appear inactive and without any callus formation (**Fig. 11-1c**, **Fig. 11-4**, **Fig. 11-5**, **Fig. 11-6**).

All of these types of viable non-union may follow conservative or operative treatment. The lack of union generally results from instability or lack of reduction at the fracture site.

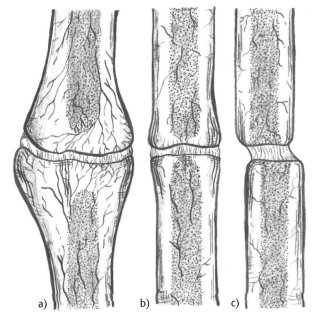

Fig. 11-1: Weber and Čech classification of viable non-union. a) Elephant's foot. b) Horse hoof. c) Oligotrophic. (Courtesy Weber and Čech [10].)

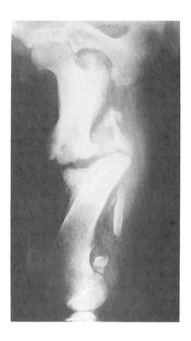

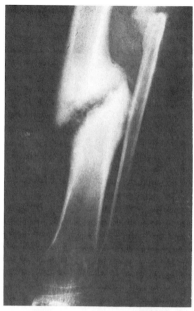

Fig. 11-2:
Hypertrophic non-union of a 4-month-old fracture in the femur of a Collie dog. Hypertrophy of the periosteal callus is visible, and a wedge fragment is positioned caudal to the fracture. The fracture gap is extensive. At surgery a sigmoid-like structure was exposed (pseudarthrosis) and excised, the medulla was opened, and the fracture was reduced and stabilized under compression with a plate. Healing ensued.

Fig. 11-3:
Hypertrophic non-union of a fracture of human tibia 2 years after the original fracture, which had been treated in a walking long-leg cast. (Courtesy J. Schatzker.)

Fig. 11-4:
a) Oligotrophic non-union fracture of the radius and ulna in a 4-year-old poodle 12 weeks after the accident. The fracture was originally stabilized by the local practitioner by means of a portion of a K-wire which broke. Disuse atrophy of the carpal and metacarpal bones is visible.
b) Lateral view displaying disuse atrophy of the carpal bones.
c) The same fracture following reduction stabilization with a 5-hole plate and 2-mm screws.
d) The healed fracture 22 months after the original trauma and 19 months after plating. The radiograph was taken immediately after removal of the plate. The portion of the original broken pin is visible.

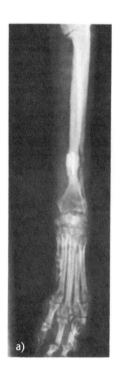

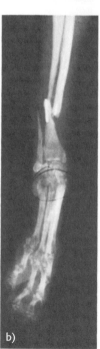

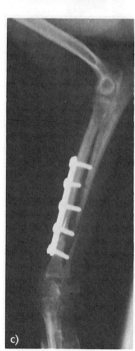

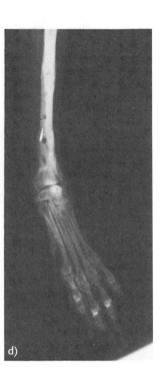

a)   b)   c)   d)

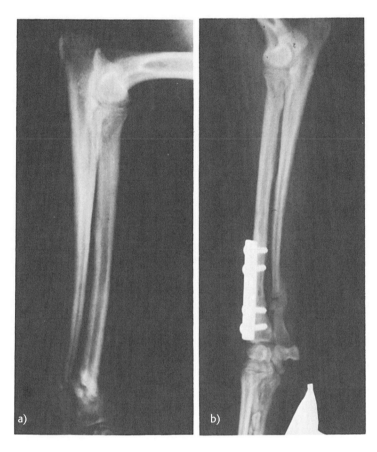

Fig. 11-5:
a) Oligotrophic non-union of a fracture of a radius and ulna of a 4-year-old terrier 10 weeks following the initial break.
b) The same fracture 6 weeks later following reduction and stabilization with a plate. There is minimal callus formation on the radius. The gap between the ulna segments has been united by a periosteal callus. The screw hole used for the tension device in the radius proximal to the plate has still not been completely filled by mineralized bone.

3.2.2 Non-viable non-union

The Weber-Čech classification divides these into four types (**Fig. 11-6**):

- In dystrophic cases an intermediate fragment exists which has, owing to interference in its blood supply, healed to only one major fragment, with the consequence that its blood supply is received from only one side. Hence, the poorly vascularized portion of the fragment is incapable of sufficient osteogenesis to bridge the gap with the second major fragment. Instability at this particular fracture line may be followed by implant failure if such has been used. Torsional forces will occur if external fixation has been employed (**Fig. 11-6a**).
- The necrotic type of non-union is generally the result of multiple fragmentation, with the consequence of major deficiencies in blood supply to some of the fragments. Even though such fragments may be stabilized, they do not form a callus. A gap between the fragments may not be visible on a radiograph, but at the same time a callus is not present. The particular piece or pieces of bone become more radiopaque than the surrounding bone and die with the possible consequence of implant failure or, in the case of external fixation, sequestration (**Fig. 11-6b**).
- The defect type of non-union occurs when a small, or major, section of bone is lost, either at the time of the original trauma owing to sequestration or following surgical excision of neoplasms. The resulting gap between the remaining viable bone ends is too great to be bridged without specific remedial surgical intervention (**Fig. 11-6c**).
- The atrophic type of non-union usually results from one of the three previous types classified as non-viable. The inactivity at the site results in osteoporosis of the bone and a loss of vascular supply, with a consequent loss of all osteogenic activity (**Fig. 11-6d**, **Fig. 11-7**, **Fig. 11-8**).

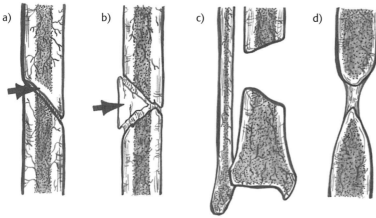

Fig. 11-6: Weber and Čech classification of non-viable non-union.
a) Dystrophic
b) Necrotic
c) Defect
d) Atrophic
(Courtesy of Weber and Čech.)

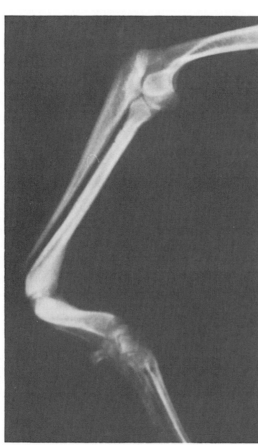

Fig. 11-7:
Atrophic non-union of a 5-year-old poodle radius and ulna. Despite re-plating and repeated bone grafting, the fracture did not heal, although treated for more than 2 years.

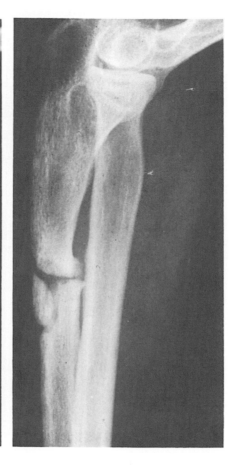

Fig. 11-8:
Monteggia fracture involving the ulna of a man 1 1/2 years following the original accident. The fracture had been treated by placing the limb in a long arm cast. (Courtesy J. Schatzker.)

4 Predisposing causes of non-union

No problem in orthopedics has evoked such profuse discussion as that of non-union, and the causes of non-union that have been listed, discussed, and suggested are legion. These may be divided into two main groups: physical causes at the fracture site and systemic conditions of the patient.

4.1 Physical factors at the fracture site

These include: comminution, infection, ill-advised open surgery, hyperemia, too much hardware, ischemia, reaction to implants, distraction of fragments, improper application of metal, imperfect reduction, too early ambulation, excessive compression, too early weight bearing, avascular necrosis, injury to soft tissue, periosteal stripping, functional disuse, loss of bone, osteoporosis, plugged medulla, senile changes, insecure immobilization, ambulatory effect of synovial fluid, interposition of soft tissues, radiation, and burns.

These suggestions have been discussed by McMurray [9], McMurray [10], Hobson [11], Anderson and Burgess [12], Watson-Jones and Coltart [13], Wray [6], Wong [14], Cameron [15], Hickman [16], Piermattei [17], and Whittick [18]. It appears to be generally agreed that no one single factor is necessarily the cause of pseudarthrosis, and that a common combination of factors is involved. These physical factors may be summarized:

- Failure to reduce the fracture,
- Failure of adequate uninterrupted immobilization,
- The surgeon.

Although fracture healing is essentially a local process, many other factors have been investigated as contributing to pseudarthrosis.

The present divided opinion of the place of movement in fracture healing has been admirably summarized by Hicks [19], who stated that "one of the greatest points of contention between the conservative and radical schools concerns the effect of movement on the process of union. The conservative school believes that movement favors union; the radical school believes that movement stimulates callus formation, which is not the same thing, and sometimes provides non-union."

4.2 Systemic factors

The influence of calcium and phosphorus metabolism has been reported by Tisdall and Harris [20], Watt [21], Harris [22], and Ham et al. [23]. Primary hyperparathyroidism (adenoma) occasionally predisposes to non-union [7] and, in such cases, blood calcium levels may vary cyclically from normal to abnormal. The suggestion that defects in mineral deposition are important causes of non-union was refuted by Wray [6]. Other items that have been studied included diet and general metabolic deficiency [24], cortisone and ovarian secretion [25, 26], and vitamin deficiency [27, 28]. The influence of local and plasma phosphatase has also been studied [29].

The biochemistry of a healing callus is similar to that of the growth plate cartilage, and the hormonal effects in the morphology of bone healing follow a similar pattern. Defects in the hormonal influence on fracture healing may thus result in non-union [30]. It has also been suggested that alkaline phosphatase activity at the site, normally at a peak 5 days following a fracture, may be considerably reduced at the site and in the circulatory system in individual cases that subsequently progress to a non-union [31].

Frost [7] discussed some patients with biological failures of healing and noted that they present a special problem for bone grafting. Results are 50% less successful than grafted non-unions in patients classified as having technical failures. This is not dependent upon the type of graft employed, allograft or homograft. Lacroix and Urist (quoted by Frost) [7] suggested that there is a special, yet unidentified agent which they term osteogenin or bone induction factor (see Chapter 14)

Frost [7] reported six cases of patients who "simply did not make any new osteoblasts or chrondoblasts, at least not anywhere near adequate numbers". This information was obtained by "labeling" and biopsying the eleventh rib of these individuals. Frost suggested that there is some fundamental disturbance in the mesenchymal stem cells of such individuals. One patient displayed this phenomenon in four successive fractures.

For an up-to-date study of the role of enzymes and hormones in fracture healing, the reader is referred to the current texts on these subjects.

5   Etiology

Pauwels [32, 33] has stated that the ossification of the fracture site occurs only when tension and compression forces act upon the scaffolding of the site and when contrary forces are absent. The disturbance of ossification and callus production at the site of the fracture undergoing torsional forces is understood. It would appear that a fracture can withstand a considerable amount of bending at the site, compression, and some tension, but torsional wrenching forces delay and impair healing. Severe torsional forces tear across the uniting capillary and fibroblastic network.

This phenomenon has been demonstrated both clinically and experimentally. In man, if a fracture of the distal tibia occurs and the fibula remains intact, shearing forces occur at the fracture site in the tibia. Experimentally, the same situation has been demonstrated in the radius of the dog by Schenk et al. [34]. The distal ulna of dogs was sectioned and the radius left intact, thereby producing shearing force in the site of the osteotomy of the ulna. Similar experiments have been carried out by the author of this chapter who sectioned the radius and ulna of dogs, the radius alone, and the radius with associated stripping of the periosteum. Following osteotomy some of the limbs were restrained in plaster-of-Paris casts and some were left free and allowed to bear weight. The shearing force occurred in the plaster-of-Paris cast cases because of rotation within the cast of the upper segment, while the lower forelimb was held firm. Experimentally, the animals whose fractures had not been immobilized externally united more rapidly than those in casts did. Bending moments occurred at the fracture

site of these animals, but there were minimal shearing forces in the form of torsion. When the radius alone was sectioned, there appeared to be little in the way of torsional forces, since the site chosen was at the junction of the middle and lower thirds and the interosseous muscle acted to stabilize the situation at this site [35]. In clinical cases in dogs, it is known that when fractures of the radius and ulna are immobilized externally by casts, the carpus must be placed into slight varus and the elbow included in the cast in order to minimize rotation at the fracture site.

When compression forces also exist, as in the case of the fracture in man of the distal tibia with intact fibula, these forces prevent the proper invasion of the callus by blood vessels, the microcapillaries being persistently occluded and severed by the movements of squeezing and compression. This type of situation leads to occlusion of the medullary cavity at the site by a layer of fibrocartilage and sometimes fibrous bone.

A classic description of the periosteal callus of pseudarthrosis was made by Martin [36] and quoted by Weber and Čech [8]: "It comes to the gap and climbs on it like a wall that it cannot penetrate". In this situation, the actual vascular activity may be demonstrated by scintigramography [37]. Clinically, it is appreciated that if all forms of shearing at the fracture site and preferably all instability is eliminated, then the fibrocartilaginous non-union will go on to ossify and will totally unite.

6   Sites of non-union

The most common sites of pseudarthrosis are readily agreed upon by all the authorities in the field of human orthopedics, as quoted by Cave [38], Blumfield [39], and Henderson [40]. These are in the following order: (1) lower tibia, (2) femoral neck, (3) radius and ulna, and (4) radius.

Results of investigations into the clinical incidence in the veterinary field by Vaughan [41] and Sumner-Smith [42] agree that in the dog the incidence, in descending order, is: radius and ulna 60%, tibia 25%, femoral shaft 15%. According to

Cave [5], there appears to be a distinct age incidence of pseudarthrosis in man, highest in the 20–30-year age group, although pseudarthrosis of the femoral neck is most common in the elderly. The limited number of cases in dogs, as reported by Vaughan [41], do not really show any age incidence, although 70% were adult animals.

7 Incidence

An accurate figure as to the overall incidence of non-union, in any species, is impossible because not all fractures are reported, and only those that go on to non-union are treated at referral centers. This provides an inaccurate impression of the total incidence if measured against all fractures treated at the center.

Frost [7] has suggested that in human patients non-union is most commonly seen in the 40–60-year age group, and that such fractures have usually received adequate technical treatment but failed to heal normally.

8 Diagnosis of non-union

The following factors should be taken into account when considering classification of a fracture as undergoing non-union.

8.1 Lack of rigidity

Consideration should be given to the duration of existence of a fracture and, on handling, the amount of rigidity anticipated at that time should be determined. Unfortunately, the amount of rigidity at the site has to be determined rather empirically, but the clinician is usually able to ascertain whether natural or excessive movement is occurring at a site that should, by that time, have become quite stable.

8.2 Profuse or absent callus formation

The different types of fracture callus that may occur have already been described; therefore, on clinical examination, it follows that the site may display a very profuse and palpable callus or none whatsoever.

8.3 Blood supply

The role of the blood supply is also mentioned by Frost [7], who noted that cases due to biological failure bleed quite briskly and display osteoporosis radiographically. Examples of non-union due to poor blood supply also exist. The shearing type of situation with severing of the macrocirculation and formation of cartilaginous callus is a good example.

8.4 Pain at site

On manipulation pain will invariably be present in early cases of non-union and yet, as the situation progresses and particularly in cases of pseudarthrosis, the amount of pain is minimal.

8.5 Weight bearing

If the non-union fracture affects a weight-bearing long bone, the bone will be unable to receive a load without suffering mechanical failure.

8.6 Deformity

It follows that if a fracture is incorrectly aligned, or is still undergoing movement, the gross appearance of the area will be anatomically unnatural.

8.7   Muscle atrophy

In that the area involved in a non-union fracture will not be carrying out its proper function, disuse muscle atrophy will have occurred and will continue to be in evidence until the area regains its normal function and is able to rebuild the surrounding muscle bulk.

9   Radiographic features of non-union

9.1   Plain films

Some or all of the following features will be evident on radiographic examination of a non-union fracture; which of the features do appear will depend upon the site and the character of the non-union.

- Despite the production or absence of callus, if non-union has occurred, then radiographic evidence of a fracture gap will remain. It must be remembered that fibrous tissue will not ordinarily be evident on a radiograph of fracture healing.
- Sclerosis of the fracture ends often occurs as a result of osteoblastic inactivity, and is visible on the radiograph.
- The marrow cavity adjacent to the fracture site becomes obliterated and this obliteration is visible on the radiograph. This is particularly true in a hypertrophic non-union (see **Fig. 11-2** and **Fig. 11-3**).
- Osteomalacia of the neighboring bone may occur, owing to the surrounding inactivity of the neighboring muscle.
- If a callus is present it will be of the non-bridging variety, showing productive periosteal callus formation with failure to unite across the gap.
- Many non-union fractures are displaced, and consequently the radiograph will demonstrate a lack of apposition of the fracture ends.

- In advanced cases of non-union the early formation of a pseudarthrosis is visible on the radiograph, which may well display a faint picture of inflammatory soft tissue that will form the so-called false joint.

The diagnosis of metaphyseal non-union may, on occasion, be very difficult as overlapping hardware may obscure the site. In such cases, stressed views and examination under fluoroscopy are more reliable [43].

9.2   Osteomedullography

The technique of intraosseous phlebography, known as osteomedullography, is another method for assessing bone healing and consequently the diagnosis of non-union. In such cases the contrast medium does not flow between the fragment ends. The technique is recommended as a reliable method of determining callus activity in fractures, in which primary osteosynthesis and bone grafting are followed by difficulties in estimating the progress of fracture reunion [44]. Determination of the rate of healing by this method may make it possible to avoid the development of non-union by instituting remedial action.

In normally healing fractures, an interosseous flow of contrast medium develops within 10 weeks of the fracture occurring. It is recommended that if contrast material is not crossing the gap by 12 weeks, grafting of the site should be performed.

The picture of the osteomedullogram will not return to normal for 9–18 weeks, since the medullary canal remains plugged with endosteal new bone. However, as previously stated, in normal healing abundant venous flow should be present across the site of a normally healing fracture, even if displacement is present. These observations confirm those of Wilson (**Chapter 2**) concerning the importance of the intramedullary vascular connection for the healing of fractures.

9.3 X-ray absorptiometry

In a canine ostectomy model the atrophic non-union has been shown to be predictable by means of dual energy x-ray absorptiometry by Markel et al. [45].

10 Treatment

The disadvantages of open reduction of a fracture have been summarized as possibly leading to postoperative infection, delayed union or non-union, and failure of fixation [46]. The disadvantages of closed reduction are the increased possibility of malunion and loss of function. Sarmiento [46], an exponent of the stabilization of fractures by a snugly functional braced cast, has noted that such casts produce stability of the fracture fragments and permit them to heal while at the same time the extremity continues to function in a normal physiological environment. This is conducive to uninterrupted osteogenesis. Firm compression of the soft tissues plays a major role in stabilizing fractures by this technique and has a hydraulic effect on the blood supply to the site.

Watson-Jones [13] has stated that "because of the high risk of infection following surgery consideration should be given to closed reduction splintage before open surgery is performed" and also that non-union is "a failure of the surgeon rather than a failure of osteogenesis". At the same time he indicated that continuous traction of a conservatively treated fracture, such as a tibial shaft, results in a poor blood supply to the distal fragment and distraction of the fracture, even with consequent slow union and a likely absence of non-union.

The purpose of any form of treatment of a fracture that has not united must be the return, as near as possible, to full function and anatomical alignment of the skeletal part involved. In the first place, it is necessary to determine if the site really is in a state of non-union and is not one of delayed union which, with adjunctive conservative therapy, will go on to unite. Although the majority of cases of non-union will, in fact, require open surgery, some may be successfully treated by an alteration of the conservative external fixation. Patients may not have obeyed the clinician's instructions and, in the case of animals, may well have interfered with restraint support.

In such cases, it is necessary for the clinician to decide whether or not a non-union, which has become a painless pseudarthrosis, should in fact be left alone. The decision will depend upon the functional activity of the pseudarthrosis. In other words, because a fracture has failed to unite it is not always imperative that it receives attention to bring about that union. Functional pseudarthrosis of such fractures as unilateral fracture of the mandible or femoral neck may, although unstable, have become acceptable to the patient. As with all cases of elective orthopedic surgery, the general state of health and age of the patient will have a distinct bearing on a decision concerned with treatment of a fracture non-union.

Much has been written concerning the optimum time that a fracture should be stabilized operatively, and it has often been propounded that this should preferably occur within 4–8 hours of the fracture occurring. However, statistical evidence has been produced to indicate that this may not be the proper time to "interfere". In 1959 Smith [47] produced probably the first report indicating that delay of surgery reduces the incidence of non-union. This report was quickly followed by similar studies supporting the concept of delaying the operation [48, 49]. Wilber and Evans [50] reported the results of a survey of 89 fractures of the femoral shaft. They found that of their patients treated by early operative management, 18% suffered delayed union and a further 18% suffered non-union, whereas of those treated by delayed operative management, only 3% suffered delayed union and not one suffered non-union.

Wilber and Evans [50] also reported that "all 10 non-unions, 10 of the 11 delayed unions, and 5 of the 6 infections occurred in the early operative group". The incidence of delayed union was twice as high in open fractures as in closed fractures, and the incidence of non-union was four times as high in open fractures as in closed.

The one instance of delayed union in a patient treated by delayed stabilization occurred in a fracture that had received a bone graft.

While the recommended amount of time that stabilization of a fracture should be delayed varies from 2 to 14 days, the probable optimum time is not more than 5 days. It is to be appreciated that increased difficulty in reduction of a fracture may occur following a delay of more than 5 days, owing to the presence of abundant connective and fibrous tissue.

For the sake of convenience, the treatment of non-union fractures will be divided into separate groups, two concerned with uninfected fractures, two with infected fractures, and cases involving the metaphysis. These are non-displaced, displaced, infected (without drainage), infected (drainage present), and metaphyseal.

10.1 Non-displaced fractures

- Stabilize the fracture under compression using the tension-band principle. The compression device may be employed, if indicated (**Fig. 11-9** and **Chapter 10**).
- Leave the fibrous union intact, even if the site has formed a pseudarthrosis. The stabilizing implant, an internal tension-band plate, or the external compression clamps of a half-pin device, is applied on top of or through the callus, as appropriate.
- Cancellous bone grafts should be "seeded" around the non-union site in order to stimulate healing.

10.2 Displaced fractures

- The site of fracture should be opened in order to permit reduction.
- Any excessive amount of callus pad that impairs reduction should be excised. The rest of the callus should be left alone.
- The medullary cavity will probably be occluded by fracture callus. This should be reamed open to permit the invasion of fresh blood vessels across the fracture site (**Fig. 11-10**).

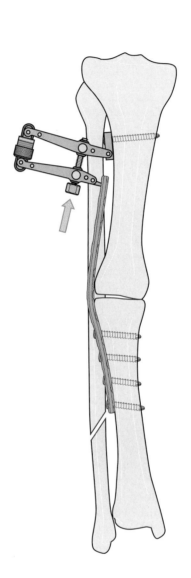

Fig. 11-9:
Compression device (from Rüedi and Murphy 2000 [51]).

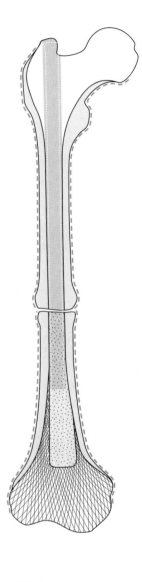

Fig. 11-10:
Opening the medullary cavity to permit the invasion of fresh blood vessels (from Rüedi and Murphy 2000 [51]).

- The ends of the fragments, when reduced, should be examined carefully and fashioned in order to combat shear forces.
- Fix the fracture with either a neutralizing plate or an intramedullary nail and screw. Cerclage wire fixation must be used with a neutralizing plate.
- Wedge fragments should be fixed by stable internal fixation and preferably lagged to the adjacent bone.
- If the fracture site is atrophic, then cancellous bone should be grafted to stimulate healing [52].

Where there has been considerable bone loss, Watson showed that carefully staged reconstruction leads to successful outcomes [53].

10.3 Infected non-union without drainage

Essentially the treatment of an infected fracture that is not draining is similar to the two previous types, with the addition of the requirement that dead bone must be removed. Therefore, plan to:
- Excise dead bone.
- Treat and stabilize with the same basic principles mentioned above.
- "Seed" with a cancellous bone graft and also, provided the rest of the bone is of sufficient size, perform decortication of the cortex.

In the 1930s, a technique was developed, in Russia, by Ilizarov [54], which combines both mechanical and biological factors for the treatment of fractures. The method is also used in the treatment of non-unions. When so applied, the technique consists of the removal of non-viable and infected tissue, foreign bodies or hardware, and the application of the Ilizarov external fixator (**Fig. 11-11**).

The Ilizarov fixator frame employs small wires and, with connecting bars and rings, the fixator permits gradual cor-

rection through distraction osteogenesis, de-angulation, and compression. In addition and most importantly, the system permits the active use of the limb to restore physiological function. Such reconstruction of complex non-unions may take up to 6 months. However, during that time the patient is able to ambulate moderately well.

Using this technique in human patients, a 94% union was achieved over 6 months and showed that the Ilizarov technique is superior to traditional techniques of managing non-union [55].

The Ilizarov technique has also been combined with muscle flapping in the reconstruction of bone and soft-tissue defects [56]. The combined approach provides a more reliable soft-tissue bed for the early cancellous bone grafting at the docking site and permits the accurate retention of limb strength for the very difficult problem cases.

10.4 Infected non-union with drainage present

While the basic principles outlined for infected non-union without drainage will also be used in this type of fracture, additional treatment will be necessary.
- Excise all dead bone.
- Excise the draining tract, including any adjacent fistula.
- Saucerize the surrounding bone—that is, the adjacent area is curetted, in a shallow fashion, in order to permit exposure of active healthy bone.
- The medullary cavity should be opened to permit invasion of fresh blood vessels (see **Fig. 11-9**).
- The fracture should be fixed rigidly, as previously mentioned.
- Cancellous bone should be packed liberally around the fracture site. A large number of osteoblasts will survive in an infected area.
- Control infection systemically and locally with the appropriate antibiotics, as determined by sensitivity testing.

Fig. 11-11:
Ilizarov fixation device
(Courtesy of Smith &
Nephew Richards, Inc.)
(see also **Chapter 10**)

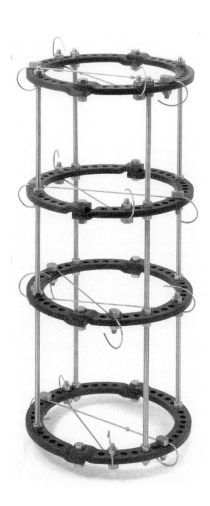
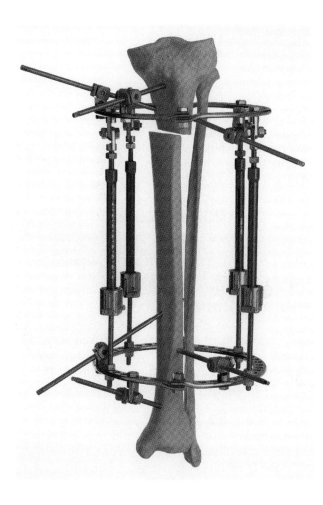

- Produce indwelling permanent irrigation drainage, as for all cases of osteomyelitis. Large volumes of fluid should be used to irrigate the site mechanically as well as to introduce chemotherapy.
- If at all feasible the operative site should be closed. Internal fixation devices should not be removed because the fracture is infected; they should be removed when the fracture is healed or if they become too loose to benefit the situation.

Healing of bone in the presence of infection has been studied and summarized by Rittmann and Perren, who demonstrated that the rigid stabilization of fracture fragments favors healing, and that the advantages of the stabilizing implant outweighs the disadvantage of its presence as a foreign body [57].

Autogenous cancellous bone grafting, using the principles of infection control, has been found to be an effective means to treat infected non-unions [58].

It has been shown by a Health Impact Analysis that infected non-union in humans represented a chronic and debilitating disorder with a lasting impact [59].

10.5 Metaphyseal fractures

- The treatment of fractures involving metaphyseal areas that fail to unite can be extremely difficult and requires particular attention to detail.
- The neighboring joint should be opened and fully examined.
- Any excessive amount of thickening of synovial membrane should be resected.
- Small loose fragments of bone or soft tissue should be removed.
- It is of paramount importance to realign the articular surface of the joint in order to bring about contiguity of the articulation.
- Internal fixation of the various segments of the fracture should be achieved by at least two-point fixation by pins and/or screws. These may well be supplemented in many cases by a buttress plate.

Early active motion of the joint and consequent ambulation of a patient is essential if "fracture disease" is to be averted. In many cases involving metaphyseal union, once the articular surfaces have been reduced it is found that the subarticular areas are deficient in cancellous bone, and consequently it becomes necessary for this area to be supported with massive cancellous bone grafts or, alternatively, by the use of "bone cement" as a supporting table. This is particularly the case in osteoporotic bone of the elderly patient.

In cases of distraction osteogenesis it has been suggested that new bone formation and mineralization are better and faster in metaphyseal than in diaphyseal sites and may sometimes lead to premature consolidation [60].

11 Electrical and electromagnetic repair of non-union

The concept that non-union might be stimulated to heal without invasive surgery has long been the desire of orthopedic surgeons and, of course, their patients. The last few decades have seen a considerable amount of research directed toward that end. There appears to be general agreement that the implantation of electrodes and the passage of current across the fracture site may well have a stimulating effect on the production of callus, although the technique is partially invasive.

The totally non-invasive technique of electromagnetic stimulation has aroused considerable interest and has resulted in two distinct schools of thought—the protagonist and the antagonist. Each technique necessitates the exact placement of electrodes or magnetic fields with particularly exact amplitudes, type, and frequency of currents. The field is complex, and the reader is referred to the bibliography of this chapter for a detailed study of the subject [61].

12 Summary of pathogenesis and treatment

Clinical experience and discussion lead one to believe that radiographed fractures are often thought not to be united when clinically the site lacks movement and the limb is sound and free of pain. The state cannot correctly be called non-union, and certainly not pseudarthrosis. The state that exists is that of a lack of mineralization of the callus. Ham et al. [23] stated that non-calcification is not non-union and bony union is judged by the organic arrangement, not by the calcification. While today the term "mineralization" is more acceptable, the concept appears to have been confirmed [42]. Ham had produced experimental fractures in animals whose diets were deranged in calcium and phosphorous [23]. The animals produced, histologically, an excellent callus at 3 weeks, but radiographically the site was not mineralized. However, the callus mineralized very rapidly in 4 days following the administration of vitamin D. It has been suggested that the organic phase is a contributor to fracture non-union, and this may well have some foundation [42, 62, 63].

The work of Cameron is pre-eminent in the field of experimental investigation into fracture non-union [15]. One of his main findings was that a fracture is able to heal in the presence of movement, provided that movement is not in the form of a torque (shear), in which case he was invariably able to produce a non-united fracture which later healed if the torque was surgically eliminated. The concept may be seen when a limb is in a cast. Disuse atrophy causes loosening of the cast and permits rotational shearing at the fracture site. Hence particular techniques are employed to combat this shear, such as including the joints above and below the site and replacement of ill-fitting casts.

This problem of torsion in fractures was recognized by Bjorck [64]. He devised a method of immobilization using pins that transfixed an external cast, passed through the limb tissue, and transfixed the bone. The pin then emerged on the opposite side to pass through the tissue and splint again.

The techniques of stabilization of fractures have been eminently described in **Chapter 10**, and many reports have been made in the last few decades concerning the stabilization of non-united fractures. All the techniques reported have as a basic principle the elimination of movement at the fracture site, particularly those creating rotational shear forces. Some fractures also require compression of bone on bone and, in long standing cases of non-union and pseudarthrosis, the "seeding" of the site with fresh osteoblastic material in the form of a bone graft and the provision of an adequate blood supply.

Section B

Robert K. Schenk, Johannes Müller, and Hans Willenegger (deceased)

13 The histology of non-union

As described earlier in this chapter, non-unions have various causes. These are exacerbated when the vascular reactive type of non-union develops after insufficient external or internal stabilization. This reactive form is characterized radiologically by a conspicuous, sometimes abundant, callus formation, and is therefore considered as being hypertrophic.

The histological study of fracture non-union in the clinical case has obvious and considerable limitations. Consequently, in order to study the phenomenon at a cellular level, an experimental model is necessary [64, 65].

14 Experiments

The experiments described in this section deal with the pathogenesis and treatment of experimentally created delayed unions and non-unions of the reactive hypertrophic form. In the first place, it was necessary to find a method of consistently reproducing non-unions in dogs which subsequently might be examined histologically to assess the process of healing after rigid internal fixation. After a number of unsuccessful attempts following recommendations made in the literature, a surprisingly simple but reliable procedure was found. The radius was osteotomized in its midshaft, a disk of 2–3 mm thickness was removed and, after

wound healing was completed, the animals were allowed full weight bearing without any external fixation of the limbs (**Fig. 11-12**).

In most animals the operation was performed simultaneously on both forelegs, resulting in almost symmetric non-unions. One hazard in this method is that of fatigue fractures of the ulna due to overload. If this occurs within the first 4–6 weeks, both foreleg bones will heal spontaneously.

The second and important condition is the age of the animals; young dogs will not develop non-unions, but simply delayed unions which finally heal spontaneously. Thus the model has good inherent healing potential and is not sensitive enough for comparing various methods of treatment, such as internal plating with and without compression, internal fixation versus plaster casts, or evaluation of electrical or electromagnetic stimulation. However, it is informative for analysis of tissue reaction following mechanical instability and the changes in the repair process that occur following stabilization [67, 68].

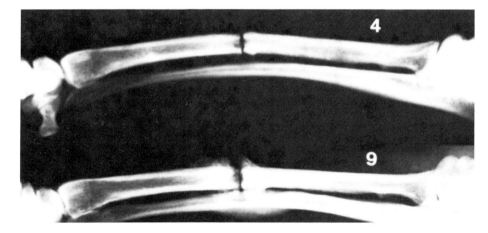

Fig. 11-12:
Radiographs of a dog's radius after transverse osteotomy and disk resection, 4–9 weeks postoperatively. Resorption of the fragment ends and abundant callus formation are seen, but no bone union.

15   Morphology of delayed union and non-union

15.1   Radiologic appearance

Radiologically, delayed unions differ from spontaneous fracture healing only in the time course of the events, which are basically identical. The dominant feature is the callus formation on the periosteal surface of the fragments. The accompanying callus formation in the medullary cavity contributes to an increase in density of the fragment ends seen in the radiographs (**Fig. 11-12** and **Fig. 11-13**). On the other hand, the interfragmentary gap remains radiolucent and even increases in width owing to osteoclastic resorption along the surfaces of the fragment ends.

15.2   Histological appearance of delayed union

Histological examination not only confirms the abundant callus formation from both the periosteum and endosteum, but also shows a tremendous stimulation of intracortical remodeling in the diaphyseal bone (**Fig. 11-14**). In addition, it provides an insight into the tissue differentiation within the fracture gap, where the original hematoma was first replaced by granulation tissue and then by fibrous tissue and fibrocartilage (**Fig. 11-15**). The collagen fibers of these intermediate connective and supporting tissues are anchored in the bony fragment ends and contribute to the increasing stiffness of the fracture area. In spontaneous and delayed union these intermediate tissues are gradually replaced by bone in an ossification process which closely resembles osteogenesis in fetal life, and during growth. In areas where fibrous tissue is present, intramembranous bone formation proceeds from osteoblasts lined up along the surface of the fragment ends (**Fig. 11-16**). They deposit osteoid, which mineralizes and thus incorporates the collagen fibrils such as Sharpey fibers into newly formed bone. The presence of blood vessels in between the collagen fiber bundles is a prerequisite for osteoblastic activity and limits this type of bone formation to areas not directly submitted to mechanical load. Actual compression sites in between the fragment ends are almost exclusively filled by fibrocartilage, an avascular tissue well suited for resistance toward compaction (**Fig. 11-17**). The presence of this tissue changes the pattern of bone formation

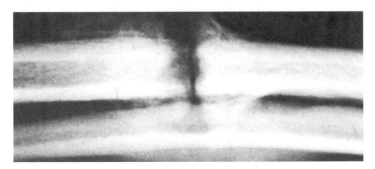

Fig. 11-13:
Radiograph of a delayed union, 14 weeks after osteotomy.

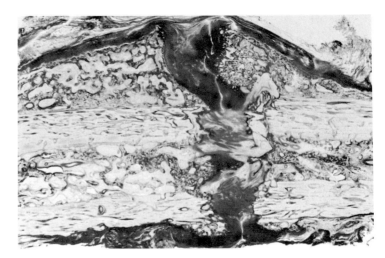

Fig. 11-14:
Corresponding undecalcified ground section. Bony callus has been formed by the periosteum and within the marrow cavity. The interfragmentary gap contains fibrous tissue and fibrocartilage. (×7)

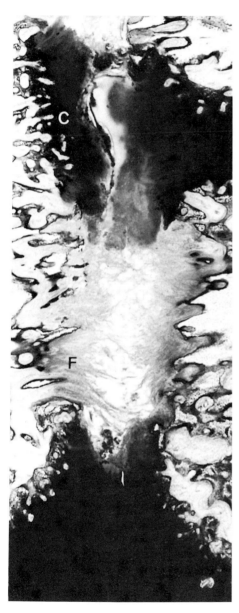

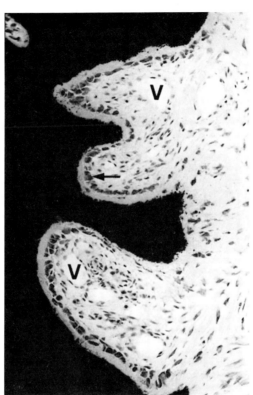

Fig. 11-16:
Intramembranous ossification in an area near F in **Fig. 11-15**. Mineralized bone (*black*) is lined by osteoid seams and osteoblasts (*arrow*). The fibrous tissue is rich in blood vessels (V). (Von Kossa reaction; ×120.)

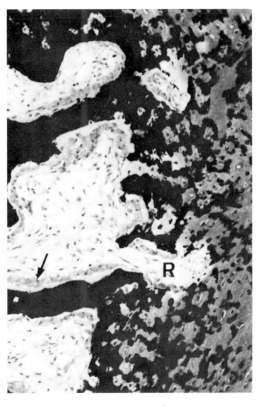

Fig. 11-17:
Chondral ossification (near C in **Fig. 11-15**) proceeding from left to right. Calcified cartilage and bone appear black after the von Kossa reaction. Resorption channels penetrate into mineralized cartilage (R), and osteoblasts (*arrow*) line the surface of newly formed trabeculae. (×120.)

Fig. 11-15:
Interfragmentary gap in a delayed union illustrating areas filled by fibrous tissue (F) and fibrocartilage (C). (Ground section; ×30.)

toward the endochondral type as it normally occurs in the growth plate. Since cartilage is avascular, bone formation is strictly dependent upon vascular ingrowth.

Capillary invasion, on the other hand, requires preliminary cartilage mineralization. The sequence of events in the bony substitution of fibrocartilage in a fracture site is therefore similar to endochondral ossification and consists of: (1) fibrocartilage mineralization, (2) the formation of resorption channels containing blood vessels, and finally (3) the deposition of new bone by osteoblasts (**Fig. 11-17**) upon the remnants of the mineralized fibrocartilage [**69–71**].

16   Non-union osteotomies

16.1   Histological appearance of non-union

As outlined before, spontaneous healing and delayed union are, as far as the histological pattern is concerned, almost identical, but differ in the time they require to establish bone union between the fragments. This again correlates with the amount of instability and the degree of motion between the

fragments which results from this instability. In the case of a non-union, the biological capacity for building up sufficient rigidity between the fragments by massive callus production and interfragmentary fibrocartilage lags behind the mechanical forces acting on the fracture site. As consequences of persisting interfragmentary instability, a further increase in mass and density of callus is observed, leading finally to a "horseshoe" or even "elephant foot-like" appearance in radiographs, with a persisting radiolucent interfragmentary gap (**Fig. 11-18**).

The fragment ends are often described as being "sclerotic", but scintigramography as well as histology reveal a tremendous turnover of bone tissue. The interfragmentary tissue consists uniformly of non-mineralized fibrocartilage and may show fissures which eventually fuse to form an equivalent of a joint space, and this classifies the late stage of non-union as a so-called pseudarthrosis. In spite of the high vitality and turnover in the fragment ends, the vascular resorptive canals are not able to penetrate into the fibrocartilage, which stays non-mineralized and impedes any further progress of the endochondral type ossification (**Fig. 11-19, Fig. 11-20**). It appears that this fibrocartilage has a barrier-like function and prevents consolidation, making attempts to remove it during surgical interventions understandable. On this background, a closer investigation of the tissue reaction in non-unions following rigid fixation is mandatory in order to establish a therapeutic concept which is biologically correct [**72**].

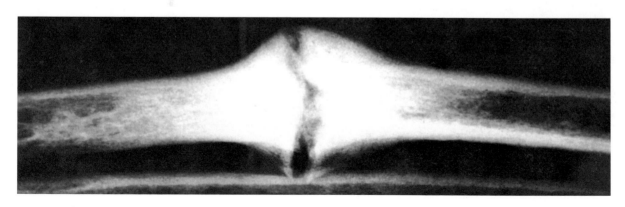

Fig. 11-18:
Hypertrophic non-union, 40 weeks after osteotomy. Radiograph shows enlarged dense fragment ends and radiolucent interfragmentary tissue.

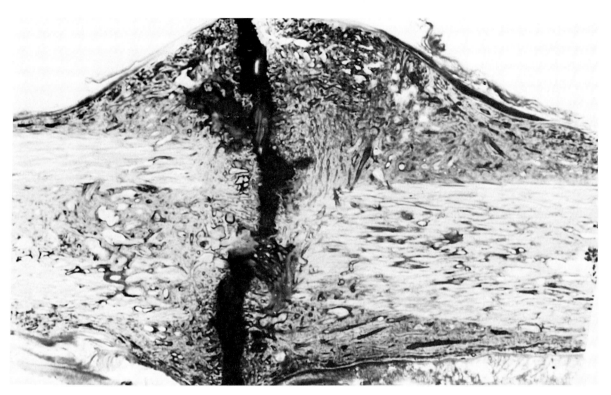

Fig. 11-19:
Ground section of the same non-union. The fibrocartilage between the fragments is intensely stained by basic fuchsin. Compact bony callus on the periosteal surface and within the marrow space. (×7.)

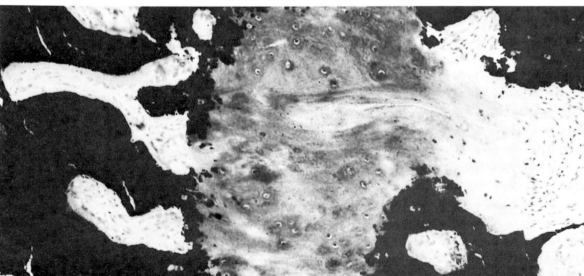

Fig. 11-20:
Unmineralized inter-fragmentary fibrocartilage, approached but not eroded by resorption channels in the fragment ends. (Von Kossa reaction; ×120.)

17   Tissue reaction in non-unions after rigid fixation

From clinical experience it is well known that reactive non-unions heal rapidly after rigid fixation. The same is true in the experimentally induced non-unions in the dog's radius when a plate is applied. In principle, the interfragmentary tissue remains untouched, except in those cases where the fitting of the plate upon the anterior convexity of the radius requires removal of some callus. In 30 dogs with symmetric non-unions, which had persisted for at least 20 weeks, plates were applied on one side without and, on the other side, with compression. There was no significant difference in the rate of healing, but there is no doubt that compression leads to a far better stability in systems more complicated than in this model [65, 73].

17.1   Radiographic appearance

In the radiographs, the radiolucent interfragmentary zone appears united by mineralized tissue after 4–6 weeks, the callus diminishes slowly and, within 5–6 months, the site of the former non-union approaches the original shape and density of compact diaphyseal bone (**Fig. 11-21**).

17.2   Histological appearance

Specimens for microscopic evaluation were collected at intervals of 2–4 weeks. The most interesting change in tissue differentiation occurs in the first 6 weeks, when the interfragmentary fibrocartilage starts to mineralize (**Fig. 11-22**, **Fig. 11-23**). This fibrocartilage mineralization can be followed in microradiographs and in thin sections stained for calcium phosphate by the von Kossa reaction. Both methods reveal that mineralization of fibrocartilage is initiated and mediated by chondrocytes (**Fig. 11-24**, **Fig. 11-25**). Thus, the first mineral deposits are always found around single chondrocytes or clusters of chondrocytes, and they appear as spherical

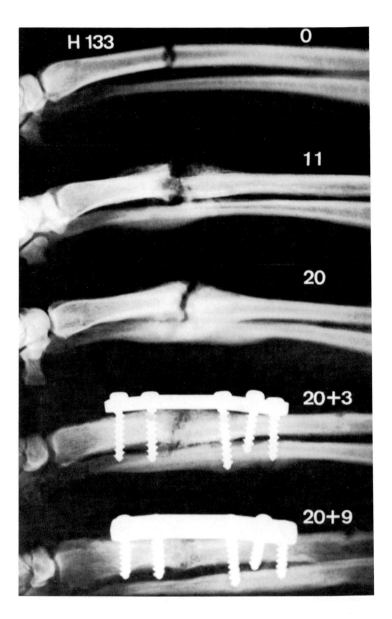

Fig. 11-21:
Radiologic changes of a non-union during development and after rigid fixation. The numbers indicate weeks after osteotomy (up to 20 weeks) and after plating (+3 and +9). Bony union is achieved within 8 to 9 weeks following rigid fixation.

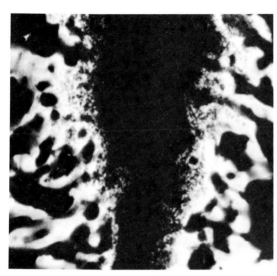

Fig. 11-22: Microradiograph of a fracture gap in a non-union. The black area consists of unmineralized fibrocartilage. (×30.)

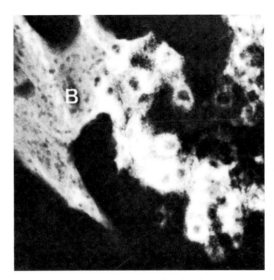

Fig. 11-24: Fibrocartilage mineralization in microradiographs is indicated by spherical calcified areas with a central black zone representing the chondrocytes. Bone (B) shows osteocyte lacunae as smaller black spots. (×150.)

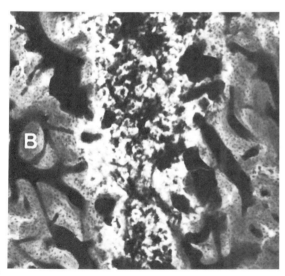

Fig. 11-23: Microradiograph of a fracture gap in a non-union 6 weeks after rigid fixation by compression plate. The heavily mineralized material represents mineralized fibrocartilage. Bone (B) appears gray. (×30.)

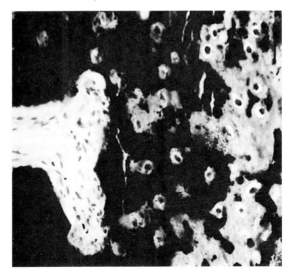

Fig. 11-25: Pericellular fibrocartilage mineralization after rigid fixation demonstrated by the von Kossa reaction. The nuclei of chondrocytes are darkly counterstained. (×150.)

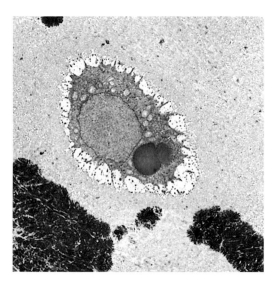

Fig. 11-26: Electron micrograph of mineralizing fibrocartilage. Coalescent clusters of apatite crystals are present in the intercellular substance close to the cells, which are surrounded by a shell of proteoglycans. Undecalcified thin section. (× 4,000.)

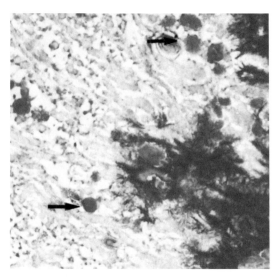

Fig. 11-27: Mineralization in fibrocartilage is mediated by cell-borne matrix vesicles *(arrow)* which seem to be involved in the initial precipitation of calcium phosphate. (× 40,000.)

hollow elements in the microradiograph. At lower magnification it also becomes obvious that mineralized fibrocartilage exhibits a high radiographic density, even surpassing the surrounding bone tissue (see **Fig. 11-23**). Disappearance of the fracture gap on the radiograph does not therefore indicate bone union but simply mineralization of fibrocartilage, which is still a rather fragile tissue. At the electron microscope level, the concept of a cell-mediated mineralization is further substantiated by the presence of matrix vesicles, which are structurally identical to those found in growth cartilage and in osteoid (**Fig. 11-26, Fig. 11-27**). It is known from numerous studies that these vesicles are of cytoplasmic origin and are always associated with the initial deposition of apatite crystals in biological calcification. It must be understood that fibrocartilage is a vital tissue and responds to changes in the mechanical condition by resuming mineralization and thus initiating its subsequent replacement by bone. It remains entirely unclear, however, why continuous motion in the gap of non-unions inhibits fibrocartilage mineralization.

Immediately after mineralization resumes, penetration of fibrocartilage by vascular channels and its replacement by bone continues and the fragments become united by bone that resembles the primary spongiosa in growing metaphyses (**Fig. 11-28**). Its trabeculae consist of remnants of mineralized fibrocartilage, entombed within layers of woven and parallel-fibered bone (**Fig. 11-29**). In the following months, this composite is remodeled and substituted by trabecular bone. Substitution occurs in discrete remodeling units (BMU's), where resorption and formation are coupled in space and time. Since the rate of osteoclastic resorption is about 50 times higher compared to lamellar bone apposition (1.5 μm/day), this results in a transient decrease in bone density, or "osteoporotic" stage (**Fig. 11-30**). Its improvement can be cotnrolled in radiographs (**Fig. 11-31**) and has to be taken into consideration in view of the decision about implant removal (**Fig. 11-32**) and full functional weight bearing [**66, 74, 75**].

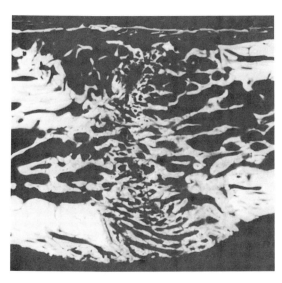

Fig. 11-28: Microradiograph of a healing non-union 12 weeks after rigid fixation. Woven bone has united the fragment ends. (×5)

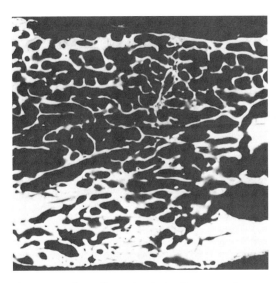

Fig. 11-30: Microradiograph of a healing non-union during the substitution of woven bone by lamellar bone about week 20 after rigid fixation. The diaphysis consists temporarily of mostly cancellous bone. (×5.)

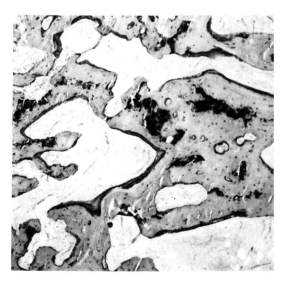

Fig. 11-29: Microtome section of the interfragmentary woven bone shown in Fig. 11-28. The stain differentiates between mineralized fibrocartilage (*dark*), mineralized bone *(light gray),* and superficial osteoid seams (*dark gray*) (×50).

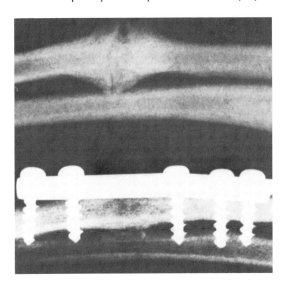

Fig. 11-31: Transitory porosis is also demonstrated in radiographs around 20 weeks after plate fixation.

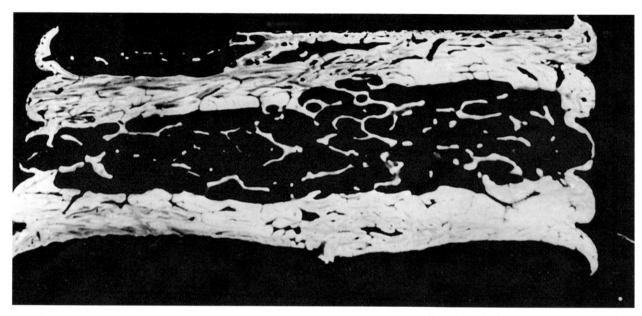

Fig. 11-32: Final reconstruction of compact diaphyseal bone 6 months after plating of a non-union shown in a microradiograph (×5). The threads of the screws and the surface facing the plate (*on top*) are both clearly visible.

18   Histological techniques employed

All the micrographs showed undecalcified sections after embedding of the bones in methylmethacrylate and block staining with basic fuchsin. From these blocks, 80–100 μm-thick ground sections were made which were used for the low-power microphotographs and for the preparation of micro-radiographs which showed the mineralized fractions in the tissue and their mineralization density exclusively. In addition, microtome sections were cut about 5 μm thick and stained by various methods, here mostly by the von Kossa reaction which revealed calcium phosphate as a black precipitate. These sections were counter-stained with pyronine and methyl green, both basic dyes that stain not only nucleic basophilic cytoplasm but also the cartilaginous matrix [76].

19 Bibliography

Blue references indicate links to abstracts of articles available online:
http://www.aopublishing.org/BONE/11.htm

1. **Moodie RL** (1923) *Paleopathology.* Urbana, IL: Univ Illinois Press.
2. **Bonnin JG** (1942) Time of union in the fractured tibia. *Lancet;* 2:439.
3. **Tippett GO** (1942) Time of union in fractured tibiae. *Lancet;* 2:439.
4. **Braschear JR** (1965) Diagnosis and prevention of nonunion. *J Bone Joint Surg [Am];* 47:174.
5. **Cave EF** (1963) Infected ununited long bone fractures with bone loss. *Am J Surg;* 113:453.
6. **Wray JB** (1965) Factors in pathogenesis of non-union. *J Bone Joint Surg [Am];* 47:168.
7. **Frost HM** (1973) Bone remodeling and its relations to metabolic bone diseases. *Orthop Frac;* 3:1.
8. **Weber H, Čech O** (1976) *Pseudarthrosis.* Bern: Hans Huber Verlag.
9. **McMurray CR** (1931) Delayed and non-union in fractures in adults. *Ann Surg;* 93:961.
10. **McMurray TD** (1942) Delay in the union of fractures. *Br Med J;* 1:8.
11. **Hobson AJ** (1942) Delayed union of fractures. *Br Med J;* 2:231.
12. **Anderson R, Burgess F** (1943) Delayed union and nonunion. *J Bone Joint Surg [Br];* 25:427.
13. **Watson-Jones R, Coltart WD** (1943) Slow union of fractures of the tibia and femur. *Br J Surg;* 30:260.
14. **Wong PC** (1965) Femoral neck fractures among the major racial groups in Singapore. Incidence patterns compared with the non-Asian communities. *Singapore Med J;* 5:150.
15. **Cameron BM** (1966) *Shaft Fractures and Pseudoarthrosis.* Springfield, IL: Charles C Thomas.
16. **Hickman J** (1966) Limb fractures in the dog and cat. VI. Complications of fractures in the dog. *J Small Anim Pract;* 7 (2):169–175.
17. **Piermattei DL** (1966) Treatment of nonunion fractures in the dog. *Anim Hosp;* 2:139.
18. **Whittick WG** (1974) *Canine Orthopedics.* Philadelphia: Lea & Febiger.
19. **Hicks JH** (1964) Rigid fixation as a treatment of nonunion. *Proc R Soc Med;* 57:358.
20. **Tisdall FF, Harris RI** (1922) Calcium and phosphorus metabolism in patients with fractures. *J Am Vet Med Assoc;* 79:884.
21. **Watt JC** (1925) The deposition of calcium phosphate and calcium carbonate in bone and in areas of calcification. *Arch Surg;* 10:983.
22. **Harris HH** (1929) The vascular supply of bone with special influence to the epiphyseal cartilage. *J Anat;* 64:3.
23. **Ham D, Tisdall FF, Drake TGH** (1938) Experimental non-calcification of callus similar to nonunion. *J Bone Joint Surg [Br];* 20:345.
24. **McKeown RM, Lindsay MK, Harvey SC, et al.** (1932) The breaking strength of healing fractured fibulas of rats, II. Observations on a standard diet. *Arch Surg;* 24:458.
25. **Said AH** (1964) Adrenal and plasma corticosteroids and ascorbic acid content during bone fracture healing. *Nature;* 204:386.
26. **Said AH** (1965) Healing of bones under oestrogens. *Nature;* 205:605.
27. **Stirling RI** (1939) Causation of delayed union and nonunion of fractures. *Br Med J;* 2:219.
28. **Bouckaert JM, Said AH** (1961) Influence of drugs on healing of fractures with reference to vitamin K, isoniazid and cortisone. *Berl Munch tierärztl Wschr;* 74:97.
29. **Kay HD** (1926) Function of phosphate in bone formation. *Br J Exp Pathol;* 7:177.
30. **Tylkowski CM, Wezeman H, Ray RD** (1976) Hormonal effects on the morphology of bone defect healing. *Clin Orthop;* (115):274–285.
31. **Laraya JSR** (1973) *Alkaline phosphatase activity in the initial stages of healing of stable and unstable canine bone fractures.* University of Guelph. Thesis. Guelph, Ontario.
32. **Pauwels F** (1935) Der Schenkelhalsbruch. Ein mechanisches Problem. *Beitr Orthop Chir;* 63:1.
33. **Pauwels F** (1940) Grundriss einer Biomechanik der Frakturheilung. *Verh Dtsch Ges Orthop;* 34th Kongress.
34. **Schenk RK, Müller J, Willenegger H** (1968) [Experimental histological contribution to the development and treatment of pseudarthrosis]. *Hefte Unfallheilkd;* 94:15–24.
35. **Sumner-Smith G, Cawley AJ** (1970) Nonunion of fractures in the dog. *J Small Anim Pract;* 11 (5):311–325.
36. **Martin B** (1920) Über experimentelle Psuedarthrosenbildung und die Bedeutung von Periost und Mark. *Arch klin Chir;* 114:664.
37. **Judet R, Judet L, Roy-Camille R** (1958) La vascularisation des pseudarthroses des os longs d'après une étude clinique et experimentale. *Rev Chir Orthop;* 55:5.
38. **Cave EF** (1963) The healing of fractures and nonunion of bone. *Surg Clin No Am;* 43:337.
39. **Blumfield I** (1947) Pseudoarthrosis of the long bones. *J Bone Joint Surg [Br];* 29:97.

40. **Henderson MS** (1938) Bone grafts in ununited fractures. *J Bone Joint Surg [Br];* 20:635.

41. **Vaughan LC** (1964) A clinical study of nonunion fractures in the dog. *J Small Anim Pract;* 5:173.

42. **Sumner-Smith G** (1969) *Study of nonunion of fractures in the dog.* University of Guelph. Thesis. Guelph, Ontario.

43. **Ebraheim NA, Skie MC, Heck BE, et al.** (1995) Metaphyseal nonunion: a diagnostic dilemma. *J Trauma;* 38 (2):261–268.

44. **Puranen J, Kaski P** (1974) The clinical significance of osteomedullography in fractures of the tibial shaft. *J Bone Joint Surg [Am];* 56 (4): 759–776.

45. **Markel MD, Bogdanske JJ, Xiang Z, et al.** (1995) Atrophic nonunion can be predicted with dual energy x-ray absorptiometry in a canine ostectomy model. *J Orthop Res;* 13 (6):869–875.

46. **Sarmiento A, Pratt GW, Berry NC, et al.** (1975) Colles' fractures. Functional bracing in supination. *J Bone Joint Surg [Am];* 57 (3):311–317.

47. **Smith JEM** (1959) Internal fixation in the treatment of fractures of the shaft of the radius and ulna in adults. The value of delayed operation in the prevention of nonunion. *J Bone Joint Surg [Br];* 41:122.

48. **Lam SJ** (1964) Amputations. *Nurs Times;* 59:1964.

49. **Smith JE** (1964) Results of early and delayed internal fixation for tibial shaft fractures. Review of 470 fractures. *J Bone Joint Surg [Br];* 56:469.

50. **Wilber MC, Evans EB** (1978) Fractures of the femoral shaft treated surgically. Comparative results of early and delayed operative stabilization. *J Bone Joint Surg [Am];* 60 (4):489–491.

51. **McKee MD** (2000) *Aseptic nonunion.* In: Rüedi TP, Murphy WM, editors. *AO Principles of Fracture Management.* Stuttgart–New York: Thieme, pp 759, 761.

52. **Rokkanen P, Slatis P** (1972) Subcortical cancellous bone grafting in the treatment of delayed union of tibial shaft fractures. *J Trauma;* 12 (12):1075–1082.

53. **Watson JT, Anders M, Moed BR** (1995) Management strategies for bone loss in tibial shaft fractures. *Clin Orthop;* (315):138–152.

54. **Ilizarov GA** (1976) *Results of Clinical Tests and Experience Obtained from the Clinical Use of the Ilizarov Compression-Distraction System.* Moscow: Med Export Moscow.

55. **DiPasquale D, Ochsner MG, Kelly AM, et al.** (1994) The Ilizarov method for complex fracture nonunions. *J Trauma;* 37 (4):629–634.

56. **Lowenberg DW, Feibel RJ, Louie KW, et al.** (1996) Combined muscle flap and Ilizarov reconstruction for bone and soft tissue defects. *Clin Orthop;* (332):37–51.

57. **Rittmann WW, Perren SM** (1974) *Cortical Bone Healing After Internal Fixation and Infection.* Berlin Heidelberg New York: Springer-Verlag.

58. **Patzakis MJ, Scilaris TA, Chon J, et al.** (1995) Results of bone grafting for infected tibial nonunion. *Clin Orthop;* (315):192–198.

59. **Toh CL, Jupiter JB** (1995) The infected nonunion of the tibia. *Clin Orthop;* (315):176–191.

60. **Aronson J, Shen X** (1994) Experimental healing of distraction osteogenesis comparing metaphyseal with diaphyseal sites. *Clin Orthop;* (301):25–30.

61. **Brighton CT, Black J, Pollock SR** (1979) *Electrical Properties of Bone and Cartilage.* New York: Grune & Stratton.

62. **Ch'ai PF, Ling LL, Kuo PF** (1965) Osteogenesis in nonunion of fractures, II. *Clin Med J;* 84:19.

63. **Frost HM** (1968) Personal communication.

64. **Bjorck G** (1952) Transfixation plaster cast in the treatment of fractures of small domestic animals. *Nord Vet Med;* 4:89.

65. **Schenk R** (1973) Fracture repair–overview. *Ninth European Symposium on Calcified Tissues.*

66. **Schenk R, Willenegger H** (1967) Morphological findings in primary fracture healing. *Symp Biol Hung;* 7:75.

67. **Johner R** (1972) [Dependence of bone healing on defect size]. *Helv Chir Acta;* 39 (1):409–411.

68. **Müller J, Schenk R, Willenegger H** (1968) [Experimental studies on the development of reactive pseudarthroses on the canine radius]. *Helv Chir Acta;* 35 (1):301–308.

69. **Schenk R, Müller J** (1972) *Histologie der Pseudoarthrose.* In: Boitzy A, editor. Osteogènese et Compression. Bern: Hans Huber Verlag, 174.

70. **Schenk RK, Perren SM** (1977) [Biology and biomechanics of fracture healing in long bones as a basis for osteosynthesis]. *Hefte Unfallheilkd;* 129:29–41.

71. **Schenk R, Willenegger H** (1964) Zur Histologie der primären Knochenheilung. *Arch Klin Chir;* 308:440.

72. **Schenk R, Willenegger H** (1963) Zum histologischen Bild der sogenannten Primärheilung der Knochenkompakta nach experimentellen Osteotomien am Hund. *Experentia;* 19:593.

73. **Rahn BA, Gallinaro P, Baltensperger A, et al.** (1971) Primary bone healing. An experimental study in the rabbit. *J Bone Joint Surg [Am];* 53 (4):783–786.

74. **Rahn BA, Perren SM** (1971) Xylenol orange, a fluorochrome useful in polychrome sequential labeling of calcifying tissues. *Stain Technol;* 46 (3):125–129.

75. **Schenk RK** (1998) Biology of fracture repair. In: Browner BD, Jupiter JB, Levine AM et al., editors. *Skeletal Trauma*. Philadelphia: WB Saunders, 33–77.

76. **Schenk RK, Olah AJ, Herrmann W** (1984) Preparation of calciefied tissues for light microscopy. In: Dickson GR, editor. *Methods for calcified tissue preparation*. Amsterdam New York Oxford: Elsevier Sciene Publishers B.V., 1–56.

12 The replacement of broken, missing, and diseased bone

Sydney Nade

1 Introduction

In the normal course of embryonic development of endo-skeletal animals, bone is laid down in those parts which form the skeletal frame of the body (see **Chapter 1**). Although there is a dynamic turnover of the constituents of bones, the shape of this framework remains relatively constant throughout life. The template for the site of bone formation is initiated in the fetus, and this template is followed until skeletal maturity. In postfetal life, apart from the growth of the predetermined skeleton, the production of bone is an unusual event. Numerous reports of bone formation in ectopic sites, some with a known stimulus and others unknown, have given some clues about bone formation and led to various ways of replacing missing and diseased bone in man.

The natural repair of a fractured bone is a unique process in which hematoma forming about the fracture site is organized, replaced by callus (often containing cartilage), and transformed to bone, which is eventually remodeled to have structure and function present before the fracture (see **Chapter 9**). In many organs, specialized cells are not replaced by similar tissues, and the return to an almost embryonic developmental state, with subsequent structural remodeling is a property only of bone. The stimulus and mechanism for fracture repair still remains an enigma.

Not all fractures, however, progress through such a pathway to union, and the orthopedic surgeon spends a considerable amount of time and expertise in trying to prevent non-union in long bones, or attempting to stimulate fracture union (see **Chapter 11**). The dental surgeon, also, has frequently wished for a means of stimulating osteogenesis in defects of the jaws, which can be so functionally and cosmetically disabling. No single form of treatment is successful, and results of treatment are so unpredictable that there is a demand for continuing investigations into the nature of osteogenesis and methods of controlling it.

Bone transplantation in man has been practiced for over 100 years [1], and in animals for even longer [2]. There are many clinical situations in which transplanted bone may be useful—correction of deformities of defective development, the treatment of non-united fractures, replacement of bone destroyed by infection or neoplasm—and many types of transplant have been used.

Replacement of broken, missing, or diseased bone when using autografts, allografts, or xenografts has been practiced and studied for a long time; modern technology has in recent years permitted such replacement to be performed using synthetic materials, such as metals, ceramics, and plastics, either alone or in combination. The greatest impetus to this type of surgery has been the development over the last 20 years of prostheses for the replacement of joints and, in a far smaller number, the trend toward limb-saving surgery for neoplasia, as chemotherapeutic drugs have become more specific and effective.

During the last 20 years there has been an enormous amount written on the subject of joint replacement surgery, particularly with regard to implant design and surgical technique. More recently, considerable effort has been turned toward means of dealing with the complications of such surgery, and particularly the augmentation of volume of bone adjacent to such failed prostheses, using previously described techniques of bone transplantation.

The author of an occasional survey published in The Lancet in 1952 wrote: "The literature on bone growth, grafting, and regeneration is now voluminous. Much of this, though forming a valuable record of advances in surgical techniques, sheds little light on the fundamental problems of bone growth and regeneration". Forty-five years on, the demand in orthopedics for replacing broken, missing, and diseased bone is greater than ever, and thereby warrants reappraisal of the subject.

The most successful results of clinical bone transplantation have occurred when the source of transplanted bone was from another site in the same patient—an autograft. Allografts (from another human) and xenografts (from an animal), both fresh and treated in some way or other, have been used with less success. The notion of having a store of easily available and useful bone has not been completely discarded; indeed there has been a great resurgence of interest since it was first introduced by Inclan [3]. He reported the successful use in 52 cases of refrigerated allografts and xenografts, and initiated a strong clinical recommendation for the concept of a "bone bank" (see **Section 3**). There are now numerous reports to suggest that the use of preserved osseous and osteochondral allografts in reconstructive surgery can be used successfully [4, 5]. A successful bone bank would have several advantages in clinical practice for both patient and surgeon.

The stimulation of bone formation is probably the most important theoretical indication for the transplantation of bone. Unfortunately, most materials that have been advocated as useful in a bone bank do not possess this property. It may, therefore, be that the premises on which the search for "bone-bank" materials are based are incorrect. Perhaps more attention needs to be concentrated on the cellular, rather than the physical configuration of the graft.

There have been numerous reports of bone transplants [6–8], and these studies have necessarily involved investigations and discussions of the source of bone cells and their fate after transplantation. Several conflicting ideas have been proposed, many at a time when the strongest tool available to the

investigator was the optical microscope. With the advent of modern technology the older theories should be re-examined, in order to attempt to confirm or refute them.

The science of molecular biology has helped the understanding of cellular differentiation. The role of the micro-environment is becoming prominent in discussions of cellular differentiation; the classical premises of development from one of the three germinal layers—endoderm, mesoderm, and ectoderm—is open to debate.

The studies of Urist [9–12] in the United States and of Burwell [8, 13, 14] in the United Kingdom, from 1960 to 1980, were a major advance. These workers looked systematically at the cellular and environmental factors involved in osteogenesis and showed how both had a part to play. The formation of bone can be induced in non-skeletal sites, in experimental animals, and in man, and some control can be had over this postfetal form of osteogenesis. In this chapter it is proposed to develop a rationale for the replacement of broken, missing, and diseased bone based on previous experience and an understanding of cellular mechanics.

2 History of autotransplants of bone

The transference of animal bone to replace defects in the human skeleton have been attempted since the earliest recorded evidence of surgical endeavor, and it is sufficient to say of these attempts that descriptions appear, no doubt vague, in Hindu, Egyptian, and Greek sources [15]. Church records, describing the excommunication from his church of Jobi Meekren, a Dutchman, are the source of the earliest report of a successful xenograft of bone. In 1682 this courageous surgeon replaced a defect in the skull of a soldier by using pieces of a dog's skull [16].

The principles of bone grafting were known to John Hunter over 200 years ago. He had studied the antlers of deer and became aware of the importance of blood supply in the formation of bone. He knew that in the healing of fractures, bone was formed by growth of a vascular, and a cellular, tissue from surrounding muscles, periosteum, and the bone ends themselves. He transplanted bone spurs of hens into the legs of young cockerels and saw them take root and grow. His transplant of a chicken's spur to its head was the first recorded autograft. Sepsis prevented Hunter from establishing bone grafting as a part of surgical technique.

At about the same time, Duhamel [17] in France was conducting similar experiments to Hunter with transplants and also looking into features involved in the growth of bones.

Studies directed at the mechanisms of bone formation, that is osteogenesis, were later carried out to a high degree of sophistication by Louis Ollier [1] in France and Sir William Macewen [18] in Glasgow. They used transplants in their experimental studies. Many others also wrote about osteogenesis in relation to transplanted bone; the historical aspects have been well covered by Orr [19] and Bick [15], and painstakingly reported by Keith [20] his book, Menders of the Maimed.

Seventy years after John Hunter's death, (Lord) Joseph Lister published his work on the control of wound infection; a few years later, in the same building in Glasgow where Lister developed his techniques, Macewen wrote a new chapter on surgical history. He was unwilling, in 1880, to amputate the arm of a boy with chronic osteomyelitis of the humerus. Bone wedges from the legs of six bow-legged rachitic boys were used as transplants to become intrinsic parts of the humerus of the seventh. The operation was successful and the patient grew to be a capable workman, with a strong, though slightly curved humerus.

Thus, in 1880 bone grafting was introduced to the wards of the Royal Infirmary, Glasgow. From the wards of Guy's Hospital in London it received a powerful impetus in 1894 when Arbuthnot Lane resolved to "treat the bones as one would the broken leg of a table or chair". He established the principles of internal fixation and set a new standard for the treatment of fractures. His methods of operative reduction were guided by rules of precision, and internal fixation was achieved by metal plates and screws.

In 1908 Axhausen [21] published his classical monograph on free bone transplants, carefully considering the morphological changes which ensued. Until 1910 the transplantation of bone, while in some instances surgically feasible, proved for the most part to be unsuccessful. The real beginning of bone graft surgery dates from 1911; Albee [22] devised the surgical armamentarium for cutting and modeling bone which at least approached that of the power-driven precision tools of the machinist or cabinet maker, and thus was able to transplant autografts of bone from a cortical diaphysis into a bed of cancellous bone prepared at the site of the lesion. Albee had noted the botanist's art of transplanting plants accurately and taken an analogy from this. He believed that accurate placement of the graft in a "physiological" site was essential and thus developed his technique of inlay grafting, for which he developed an electric motor saw [22].

The technique of closely applying and fixing the cortical graft to host bone was developed for spinal fusion and Pott disease, but later proved successful in many other parts of the skeleton for varied lesions. It used most of the carpenter's art—indeed, the art of the joiner and cabinet maker—but did not apply the sophistication of the cellular biologist.

From about 1912 the "inlay" autograft devised by Albee [22] was used almost exclusively. About 15 years later a variation called an "onlay" graft became popular: a relatively massive autograft attached to a bared bone surface and held in place by suture, wire, screws, or other fixation materials. Inlay grafts suffered some disadvantages: they could break when being "sprung" into their beds, and not infrequently the curve of bones did not allow a fit in perfect tissue apposition as Albee had advised. The onlay graft gained a period of prominent use and required less expertise than the beautifully crafted inlay grafts.

Developed from the onlay graft were: the double onlay graft, the buried graft, sliding bone grafts, split bone techniques, and the use of bone pegs, as well as intramedullary grafts. The latter quickly proved themselves to be ineffective.

All of these methods had their proponents, and, as usual, the originator of the technique could produce much better clinical results than any other surgeon. Diagrammatic representations of fine examples of the joiner's art and radiographs showing spectacularly convincing results are poor consolation to a surgeon with a practical problem to solve. The surgical development of 200 years appeared to provide some answers to the problems of slow union, delayed union, and non-union of fractures.

Since then, surgeons have acknowledged the debt to the metallurgist for stainless steel, vitallium, and other alloys, titanium, and have abandoned amateurish methods—twisted bits of wire and fragments of catgut—which any carpenter would scorn.

Since the 1930s the advances in metallurgy have ensured that a bone graft need no longer provide for internal fixation as well as osteogenesis—neither of which it achieved optimally.

However, bone graft surgery is still not fully established, even though sepsis, which was thought for 30 years to be the only problem involved, can be prevented, or treated, by careful surgical technique and antibiotics. Following the enthusiastic surge to bone grafting at the beginning of the century, interest became again centered upon the viability of the transplanted autogenous bone: Does it remain alive and become actively fused to the receptor site, or does it die and act only in the nature of a scaffold for the invasion of osseous tissue?

The question of cell viability had been considered at the end of the 19th century by Ollier [23], Axhausen [21], and Macewen [18], among others, and not resolved. Interest in cell viability had commenced a century or more before [17], and it needed further investigation. Even though the problem has not yet been entirely solved, most authorities agree that the transplanted bone dies once it has been disconnected from its blood supply.

This, then, raised the interesting question that if autografts of bone die when removed from their normal blood supply, why it is necessary to use them as a bone graft? In addition, surgeons became aware that cortical bone pieces, in the course of being incorporated, became decalcified and lost their structural rigidity in the weeks following autologous transplantation so that original strength was also lost.

The next advance came during World War II when the myriad of injured led surgeons to a greater use of autologous cancellous bone. This substance had been mentioned by Macewen [18], Gallie [24, 25], Matti [26, 27], Ghormley [28], and King [29]. Its use in maxillofacial surgery was advocated by Mowlem [30], and later in orthopedic surgery [31–33], and from that time has stemmed a greater understanding and a vast amount of investigation into the repair of bone.

Mowlem [33] made a plea for the use of cancellous bone, together with some other method for rigid fixation, in sites where bone grafts were required. He reaffirmed that cancellous grafts would survive the presence of infection. The use of cancellous bone chips had been earlier over-shadowed by the great hope that inlay and onlay grafts would supply both osteogenic capacity and mechanical structural rigidity. Over the last 50 years there has been acceptance of cancellous bone grafting, particularly the advantages of availability in fairly plentiful supply and osteogenic potential.

In 1975 Taylor, Miller, and Ham [34] heralded the introduction of a new technique of bone grafting into clinical practice; a free fibular graft, which retained its vascular pedicle, was anastomosed to a vessel in the recipient site. They took the fibula of the opposite leg and reconstructed a large tibial defect; revascularization was accomplished with microvascular anastomosis, and the medullary and periosteal circulation of the graft were preserved. During the last 20 years there has been considerable development of techniques for free vascularized bone grafts and composite grafts including bone, muscle, and skin. Free vascularized grafts with maintenance of a significant amount of original blood supply go part of the way toward solving the problem of retention of cell viability. However, such autografts are fresh and cannot be used from storage in a bone bank.

Distraction histogenesis is yet another technique of bone autograft. It was introduced in by Ilizarov [35] in Khurgan, Russia, many years ago, but has only been used in the Western world during the past decade. The term bone transport is now used for the application of the technique, described below, in which callus is stretched as it forms to fill a defect in bone. Quite large gaps can be spanned in that way (see **Chapter 10**).

The transplantation of bone—or bone grafting—has become a fundamental operative method of orthopedic surgery. This valuable addition to the armamentarium of bone surgery has been the end result of two centuries of physiological experimentation which now make it possible, in most circumstances, to replace broken, missing, and diseased bone. Fresh grafts and stored grafts still remain fundamentally different, the only common factor being their derivation from bone, and hence their architectural structure.

3 A bone bank?

The concept of creating a store of tissues for subsequent use also has a long history. Carrel [36] wrote of the storage of various tissues, including bone, and their subsequent implantation, and Gallie [24] reported the use of boiled allografts and xenografts of bone. The experiences of Lexer [37] in Germany, with the transplantation of whole joints, do not appear to have been bettered today, although he recorded very few cases. Orell [38] reported the use of an osseous substance that he called "os purum". This was bone, freed from fat, connective tissue, and proteins but not all of the collagenous matrix, by subjecting it to chemical treatment with sodium chloride, potassium hydroxide, and acetone. Inclan [3] reported 52 cases in 1942, in which refrigerated allografts or xenografts of bone had been used clinically in man. His was probably the first clinical report of the successful use of bone obtained from a bone bank.

The concept of a bone bank is considerably different from autotransplantation of bone from one part of a patient to another. It would, of course, be possible to take the bone at one time and store it until a suitable time for reimplantation to the donor; but such a graft does not have the convenience that a bone bank would allow. The bank component signifies the ability to carry out various transactions—most frequently deposits and withdrawals, but also other derivatives.

Wilson [39] suggested that the functions of bone grafts were:

- Catalytic in that their presence promoted and influenced an osteogenic reaction.
- To provide of a framework or scaffolding to guide the invading tissues of the host.
- To provide a local supply of calcium.

It is of great interest that he placed no importance on the survival of cells in the grafted material. He believed that there were definite advantages in having a bone bank when compared with the alternative clinically acceptable procedure of using fresh autologous bone.

Longmire, Cannon, and Weaver [40] stated that the difference between freeze-dried and frozen allografts of bone which had been reported, seemed to be insignificant as both seemed to serve as a scaffold, which new bone invaded and generally replaced.

If allogeneic bone is to be used widely in clinical practice, it will, of course, be helpful to have simplified methods of preparation, storage, and transportation, but the single most influential factor affecting general clinical acceptance of the tissue will always be its reliability in clinical procedures.

Although much of the very early work related to the transplantation of tissues was directed at an examination of what happens to the transplanted cells, and what effect they have on the host tissues, it is probable that bone transplantation studies began in response to a clinical need. The indications for bone transplantation have not changed since enumerated by Murphy [41]:

- To correct deformities resulting from defective development.
- To effect union in non-united fractures.
- To replace bone which has been destroyed by infection.
- To restore or supplant such parts of bone that may have been dislodged by a fracture.
- To replace bone which was removed because of its having been the seat of a neoplasm.

The advantages of having a bone bank, should the transplanted bone serve its biological purpose, include:

- Sparing the patient a second site or multiple operative sites with associated pain and risk of complications.
- Prevention of weakening of the tibia (which is often the donor site for grafted bone).
- Reduction of duration of operation.
- Reduction of blood loss.
- A constantly available source of bone.
- A greater choice of bone shapes and sizes for the surgeon.

3.1 Materials used

Mitchell and Shankwaller [42] quoted Albee and Morrison as saying, in 1900, that the following substances had been used to stimulate bone growth, without apparent success: "osmic acid, fibrin, blood, gelatin, lime salts, zinc chloride, thyroidin, glacial acetic acid, codeine tincture, adrenaline, hypophysis extract, bone marrow, copper sulfate, oil of turpentine, ammonia, lactic acid, silver nitrate solution, alcohol, carbolic acid, oak bark extract, vaccines, and sera. Many calcium salts were used with little success".

In addition to this formidable list, there are a large number of skeletally derived materials that have been, and are still being used. Included in such materials are bones which have been subjected to various processes, thus rendering it: fresh and autologous, fresh and allogeneic, refrigerated and allogeneic, plasma-stored allogeneic, merthiolate-treated and allogeneic, freeze-dried and allogeneic, deproteinized and allogeneic (using trypsin, hydrogen peroxide, ethylene diamine, or formamide), frozen xenogeneic, boiled and autoclaved and allogeneic, boiled and autologous, processed and xenogeneic, decalcified and allogeneic, "os purum", "os novum", cathode or γ-irradiated xenogeneic and allogeneic, and β-propiolactone-treated xenogeneic bone, as well as coral.

Burwell [8], in 1969, carefully reviewed the fate of such allografts. His conclusions were that there was considerable difficulty in assessing clinically the worth of any "bone-bank" material, especially when used in the spine. The effectiveness of most materials could be improved by two procedures: cleaning of soft tissues from bony spaces to facilitate revascularization, and placing the bone graft in close apposition with host tissue of high osteogenic capacity or osteogenic potential and vascularity. He separately considered xenografts and stated that fresh allografts had no place because of immunological rejection. Preserved xenografts such as ivory or cow horn were very resistant to incorporation into the host by beef bone remodeled to some extent. Frozen calf bone (at –40°C) gave unsatisfactory results. Several other chemically treated allograft bone materials were introduced and subsequently removed from the market by their manufacturers because of various problems.

3.2 Biological problems

The major biological problems of bone-bank materials are:
- Immunity: is the material foreign, or does it stimulate an immune reaction?
- Does the material permit revascularization, which is a pre-requisite for invasion, by specialized cells of the host?
- Osteogenesis: is this influenced in any way?
- Remodeling of the implant site after bone formation has occurred.
- How can the material be best sterilized?

If one were to define criteria for an ideal bone-bank material the following would be included:
- It must be accepted by the host tissue which facilitates revascularization and host new bone replacement (osteoconduction).
- It should provide a correlated function of osteogenesis (bone formation) and osteofixation (incorporation).
- Its complete remodeling should not be necessary for a successful clinical result.
- It should be catalytic in that its presence promotes and influences an osteogenic reaction (osteoinduction).
- It should provide a framework or scaffolding to guide the invading tissues of the host.
- It should be sterile, easily available, easily transported, easily handled, able to be stored long-term at room temperature, and able to be easily shaped.
- It must not be expensive to produce.

Nowadays, under circumstances of modern surgery, structural stability is not a requirement, as this can be supplied by metallic implants.

Autografts of bone, cancellous and cortical, are usually freshly implanted. Cortical grafts, whether autologous or allogeneic, at least initially, act as weight-bearing space fillers. All bone grafts are initially resorbed, but cancellous grafts may be completely replaced in time by a process described as creeping substitution, while cortical grafts remain as a mixture of necrotic and viable bone for a prolonged period of time. The 3-D framework which supports invasion of the bone graft, by capillaries and osteoblastic cells, termed osteoconduction, is another important function of bone autografts and allografts. Allografts do not provide a source of osteoprogenitor cells.

3.3 Why maintain viability in the preserved graft?

Many methods of preserving allografts are based on the necessity of preserving cell viability. These methods, as a group, have several shortcomings. They are expensive, elaborate, and are also subject to mechanical failure of equipment, power failure, contamination, and changes in temperature. The tissues so preserved have relatively short periods of storage, cannot be shipped or stockpiled, and in some cases give an unsatisfactory clinical result. Furthermore, the reliance upon humans to maintain careful records about each piece, and to follow instructions regarding storage leads to a significant number of stored pieces being discarded!

If the viability at the time of transplantation is not necessary, entirely new fields of preservation and new attacks on the problem of allografting arise. Chalmers [43] studied autografts and allografts, fresh and freeze-dried, in rats after the transplantation of bone. He concluded that bone allografts, whether living or dead, were not able to make a significant contribution of living bone tissue, and that there is no advantage of a living allograft over a preserved material, indeed, preserved bone-bank material may even be better in view of its altered antigenicity. Chalmers and Sissons [44] stated further that the choice of methods of preservation of banked bone could be governed by convenience, rather than because of any significant biological advantage of a particular method. This statement appears to be based on the assumption that some form of bone should be used as a transplant to stimulate osteogenesis.

Heiple, Kendrick, Herndon, and Chase [45], on discussing bone-bank materials, stated that: "at the present time it may well be that the best possible homograft (allograft) or heterograft (xenograft) is the one whose natural content of a hypothetical inductor substance is least reduced". A hypothetical inductor substance is, in terms of stimulation of bone formation, a substance which directs the specialization of cells toward osteogenesis. The subject of osteogenic induction will be discussed in **Section 4**.

3.4 The antigenicity of bone

Since the findings of Medawar [46] regarding the humoral and cellular responses to tissue transplants, in the form of antigen–antibody reactions, there have been numerous studies of the antigenicity of bone grafts. In the last 25 years knowledge in the field of immunology has mushroomed and techniques for studying antigenicity of transplanted tissues, and the response to such antigens, have become very sophisticated. An early worker in this field was Burwell, who concluded that the principal antigenic component of a fresh allogeneic iliac cancellous bone graft was contained within the cells of the bone marrow. He also found that treatment of marrow-free bone by boiling, freezing, and freeze-drying destroyed the capacity of the bone to elicit bone transplantation immunity. Despite this, examination of implants revealed that there was less new bone formation around allografts than autografts, even when there was no evidence of an immune response. Elves [47] continued Burwell's work, confirming how freeze-drying could almost obliterate antigenicity. Cell-mediated immunity has also been studied. Langer and Gross [48] found that articular shavings induced cellular immunity but no detectable antibody response.

Allogeneic bone excites an immune response characterized by the appearance of activated lymphocytes and cytotoxic antibodies. This is true for fresh and frozen bone, although preserved grafts require longer time periods to induce a response and the reaction is usually less intensive. The precise nature of the antigens responsible for producing this allograft reactivity is, at present, poorly characterized. Horowitz and Friedlaender [49] are of the view that allograft reactivity is at least a primary contributor to the biological fate of an allogeneic bone graft. In addition, there is reason to suspect that immunocompetent cells play a substantial role in bone resorption, and this relationship between the immune system and bone remodeling may be of considerable importance for normal bone homeostasis.

In addition to antigenicity, it is also pertinent to comment on disease transmission, particularly that which may not be easily identified. While the stocking of bone banks was originally based upon cadaveric bone, the supply of femoral heads at the time of surgery for femoral neck fracture or total hip replacement in aseptic environments has allowed for a greater quantity of bone to be stored. At present it is possible that bone removed either from cadavers or during surgery, may carry the HIV virus. Therefore, those associated with a bone bank have a great responsibility, not only to provide a supply of bone from an informed donor of appropriate blood group and free of transmissible disease, but also to follow-up the utilization of that bone and to review the experience of that bone bank in the light of relevant new developments [50].

3.5   Biomechanical considerations

The biomechanical behavior of a graft is often the most clinically important in determining success or failure, and fracture of bone allografts occurs in a significant number of cases [51]. Enneking, Eady, and Burchardt [52] found fractures in 18 out of 40 autologous cortical bone grafts used for the reconstruction of segmental skeletal defects. They concluded from their clinical experience that rigid immobilization was required to achieve union. The grafts must be protected throughout the prolonged incorporation phase until the radiographic appearance indicates that the repair process is sufficient for the extremities to resume function. At that time adequate stress must be transmitted to the grafts during this period to stimulate repair, and enough graft must be used to provide functional replacement in the major tubular bones.

In considering the physical properties of transplanted bone, it is important to include the initial properties of the grafts at the time they are removed from the donor, the effects of various preservation and sterilization procedures, and biomechanical factors influencing incorporation and remodeling of the transplant. The strength and biomechanical parameters of the new graft–host unit are dependent upon the properties of the union site between the graft and the host, as well as the properties of the graft itself, distinct from any mechanical fixation devices used. In addition, all of these characteristics are subject to change over time, as ongoing biological process has repaired and remodeled the tissues [53].

It is generally accepted that freezing bones to −20°C will result in little, if any, alteration in the physical properties. Degradation, however, is not completely arrested at this temperature. Therefore, it has become fairly routine to preserve bone grafts by freeze-drying or freezing specimens to colder temperatures (−70°C to −80°C, or in liquid nitrogen −196°C). While freezing adds little significance to the mechanical property of bone under bending loads, freeze-drying may cause a modest increase in the compression strength of rehydrated bone. The bending strength, however, is lowered to half or less of controls, and the torsion strength to one-third.

In order to ensure sterility, before implantation bone may be retrieved using aseptic technique for procurement and storage, or non-sterile grafts may be secondarily sterilized by irradiation. If more than 3 Mrad are used, there is a significant decrease in the breaking strength of irradiated bone. The strength of the graft is further compromised if the tissues are freeze-dried in addition to being irradiated.

While living vascularized bone is capable of responding, over time to changes in loading conditions by adaptive remodeling, thereby preventing fatigue or failure, the transplanted grafts do not have the potential to do so until they become revascularized. This consideration makes a vascularized bone graft superior to other forms of graft material in some circumstances, because of the abilities to prevent failure due to structural damage and to remodel, as well as providing an early opportunity of repair.

The incorporation of transplanted bone into host sites and its union at the boundary of that site, also influences its strength. The remodeling process may lead to an initial weakening of the graft if its substance is removed at a greater rate than bone is laid down.

It is concluded that the mechanical properties of the graft are affected by preservation, storage, and sterilization. Subsequent incorporation and remodeling of the graft further alters its properties. Some of these effects are predictable and others are not.

4 The concept of bone induction

The concept of induction has been an important working hypothesis in the field of experimental embryology for a century. Makin [54] defined bone induction as the mechanism by which a non-osseous tissue is induced to change its cellular structure to become osteogenic. Induction of bone takes place as a result of a close proximity or contact of the inductor substance or structure with a non-osseous connective tissue. Many experiments have been performed to test the hypothesis that osteogenic induction occurs. While the search has been continuing for specific chemical molecules as osteogenic inducers, there is much more convincing evidence for tissues behaving as such.

Just over 100 years ago, Senn [55] described his use of antiseptic decalcified bone implants in the healing of osteo-myelitis and other bone deformities. This predated any studies on the process of induction. Urist [9] discovered that implantation of freeze-dried demineralized segments of bone matrix induced new bone formation and subsequently pursued this material seeking a "bone morphogenic protein". Many studies have since been done on documenting the cellular and biochemical changes occurring during bone induction by such a matrix. The major phases are chemotaxis, mitosis, and differentiation. Chemotaxis is the direct migration of cells in response to a chemical gradient. Plasma fibronectin, a protein with a molecular mass of 450 kd, binds avidly to the implanted bone matrix and has affinity for collagen, fibrin, and heparin, the major components in the site of any skeletal trauma [56]. The major phase of bone induction is mitosis. Proliferation of newly attached mesenchymal cells indicates that the bone matrix is a local mitogen. This mitotic phase is followed by the differentiation of cartilage, vascular invasion, and bone differentiation.

In experimental studies with transplanted decalcified bone matrix it takes some 10–12 days before the first appearance of osteoblasts, bone formation, and mineralization. Multi-nucleate osteoclasts remodel the newly formed bone by days 12–18, resulting in selective dissolution of implanted matrix and the formation of an ossicle, consisting essentially of newly induced bone. Between day 16 and 21, there is further remodeling of bone, and the roughly ovoid ossicle is filled almost entirely with bone marrow elements.

While the evoked mechanisms of bone induction are not known, it would appear that the osteoinductive potential of matrix is restricted to only mineralized tissue, such as bone and teeth. Further, the mineral phase has to be removed for the organic matrix to express its biological potential. The geometry of extracellular bone matrix has a profound influence on bone induction. The process can be inhibited by chemical alteration of the matrix. Reddi [56] has the view that there is some species specificity involved in bone induction, which may be related to immunogenic or inhibitory components. It is likely that there is a family of related proteins that are involved in bone induction. Modern techniques have allowed molecular characterization of the proteins involved, called osteogenins, whose hypothetical existence was predicted by Lacroix [57] in 1945. The broad term used for such chemical messengers is cytokine.

Cytokines are soluble factors that play a critical role in mediating cell-to-cell interactions within skeletal and other tissues. They rarely exert their biological activities in isolation. The soluble factors are usually produced locally in concert with many other cytokines. The interaction of these structurally and functionally distinct factors in a highly ordered spatial and temporal sequence creates a cytokine network that ultimately determines a given tissue response. Those cytokines that appear to have the greatest effect on the stimulation of bone formation come from the transforming growth factor beta "superfamily" (TGF-β). Bone matrix acts as a storehouse for growth regulating factors, including those known as bone morphogenic proteins. Their unique property is the ability to stimulate ectopic bone in vivo. Several bone morphogenic proteins have been characterized chemically. They are now being called osteogenic proteins. Chemically they all contain a highly conserved seven cysteine transforming growth factor beta domain in their C-terminal end. There are probably more than 12 recognized, and target undifferentiated mesenchymal-type perivascular cells. Osteogenic protein 1 (BMP-7) has been described by Cook and Rueger [58], and BMP-2 by Riley et al. [59].

5   The transplantation of bone marrow

While bone marrow transplantation has taken the interest of hematologists treating for diseases in the blood, they have rarely commented on the formation of bone in transplanted marrow. The observation that extravascular allografts of bone marrow form bone was first made by Goujon [60] in 1869. For a considerable time it was thought that the bone that formed was derived from endosteal cells, or spicules of bone transplanted with the marrow. It would appear that these transplanted bone spicules die like other transplanted bone and do not contribute to osteogenesis. Therefore, it is the cells of marrow, either hematogenous or stromal, which can give rise to cells of bone. The site to which the marrow is transplanted has a considerable influence on whether bone forms or not, and perhaps the tissue with which the marrow is transported. Bone marrow autografts frequently produce bone, allografts occasionally, whereas xenografts invariably fail to make bone. Osteoblasts appear about 6 days after transplantation, and an ossicle of a bony shell with a marrow center eventually forms.

Weiss [61] believed that marrow was a vascular connective tissue, which partakes of many connective tissue functions—and not hematopoiesis alone—and this is the way in which one should consider it. Functional need and microenvironment may be the factors determining the distribution of its cellular sub-population.

It is more than just fortuitous that bone marrow and bone are found adjacent to each other; the marrow is protected by the hard bone and also has its functional blood supply controlled by surrounding muscle activity influencing blood flow.

Numerous experiments have been performed to study the response of bone marrow to injury. Repopulation of a disrupted marrow cavity is by bony trabeculae before hemopoietic elements. The removal of bone marrow, and subsequent fracture of a bone, lead to inhibition in rate and quantity of bone formation at the fracture site.

It is adduced that the bone marrow is a rich source of cells, which are closely involved in bone production. The stimulus is such that osteogenesis appears to be under the control of the microenvironment, either by direct cell contact or related to a hormonal-like substance released from nearby bone. Burwell performed an elegant series of experiments in which he separated the osseous and marrow components of bone grafts to characterize their relative contribution to osteogenesis. He attempted to produce a foreign graft capable of forming new bone as readily as a fresh autograft of iliac cancellous bone, by producing living cells of osteogenic potential and autologous type into a foreign graft. When such composite was inserted into a muscular site in rats, considerably more new bone was found than after implantation of either component alone [13]. In order to look further into the mechanisms of osteogenesis, and more particularly after implantation of a composite graft, Burwell [14] decided to treat the marrow-free allograft bone in different ways before combining it with fresh autologous bone marrow. He found a greater response in respect of bone formation, which related to the method of prior treatment of the allogeneic iliac bone. His findings constitute perhaps the best evidence for an inductive theory of osteogenesis and exclude the theory that new bone formation is from endosteal osteoblasts contained in the marrow portion of the composite. The model of an allograft and autograft composite was extended to xenografts by Salama [62] and subsequently by Nade et al. [63] who incorporated autologous marrow into a synthetic ceramic material. Both groups were able to demonstrate the osteoconductive potential of the materials they used, and the formation of bone from marrow cells, within the interstices of the non-living structural carrier for the marrow cells.

6   Biological bone replacement

Obviously, bone can be replaced by similar or different substances. I have divided these into two categories for the purpose of discussion, but often the two are combined. Bone replacement by bone, I have called biological, while **Section 8** addresses synthetic materials for bone replacement.

6.1 Autografts

The earliest clinical use of bone autografts is attributed by Lance [64] to Von Nussbaum, who in 1821 performed a sliding bone graft of the ulna in an attempt to facilitate fracture union. The surgical techniques of bone autografting are now well established. The current problems, however, relate less to technique and more to the cellular changes that occur in it after grafting. It is wise to remember that an autograft of bone contains cells of several types, and not only bone cells. The periosteum and the marrow may play an important role. Also, cancellous bone and cortical bone have different physical structures and cell populations, which may account for the dissimilarities following their use as grafts. Detailed descriptions of the fate of bone autografts can be found in Burwell [8] and Lance [64].

Once living bone is divorced from its blood supply at the time of transplantation, the cells of bone die. Vascularized autografts may be a partial solution to ensuring the viability of the bone cells. However, periosteal and bone marrow cells are also transplanted at the time of removal and insertion of autografts of bone, and these may play a role in subsequent bone formation. A third possibility is that an osteogenic inducer, perhaps in the form of a single molecule, or a family of related molecules, derived from the transplanted (and dead or dying) bone acts as a stimulus for host tissues to produce bone. The major difference between autografts and foreign grafts (allografts and xenografts) is antigenicity and stimulation of the immune responses in the recipient; therefore, the fate of autografts and foreign grafts warrant separate discussion.

The advances in metallurgy have ensured that a bone graft need no longer provide for internal fixation, as well as osteogenesis. Therefore, the most important property desired of any type of bone graft must be its ability to stimulate the formation of bone, and maintain viability of the bone that has formed.

It is cellular biology associated with techniques of bone grafting, rather than the mechanical aspects, which warrant further study and development. The cellular changes are both degenerative and proliferative and must be discussed with respect to necrosis, mitosis, revascularization, osteogenesis, remodeling, and growth.

Autografted bone is most usually freely transplanted, as a composite tissue graft, containing bone, periosteum, and marrow cells. The fate of a freely transplanted autograft to bone is followed radiologically and by clinical examination. To understand more fully the fate of a bone graft, the approach must be made at a cellular level. However, owing to the limitations of human biopsy specimens, sequential analysis is possible only in the animal, in which the variables can be reduced to a minimum. We are still largely ignorant of the mechanisms which initiate and control the changes that take place.

Cortical bone dies after transplantation. Revascularization occurs across its periosteal and endosteal surfaces into necrotic haversian canals. The first formed new bone occurs mainly on the medullary surface of the graft and is derived mainly from the graft bed. After revascularization, osteoclastic cells erode the bone and form cavities. This resorption leads to osteoporosis and adds to a weakening of the mechanical strength of the graft. Subsequently, lamellar bone is laid down in these cavities. The combined process of resorption and excretion is termed "creeping substitution" and with the reverse in remodeling leads to the full incorporation of the graft of the skeleton. The grafted area is then subjected to the mechanisms that normally control the mass of bone tissue in the body.

The fate of cancellous bone grafts is broadly similar to that of cortical bone grafts. The details differ, as surviving portions contain larger numbers of osteogenic cells, derived from the bone marrow which invade the deeper lying necrotic tissues. Revascularization is facilitated because of the texture of spongy bone, and the first formed bone is of woven type, which later matures into cortical and cancellous bone, presumably by mechanical stimuli.

It is unlikely that the amount of new bone that forms is related to the number of transplanted bone cells that survive. The survival of "cells of bone" in the graft does not appear to be an important factor, and it is likely that the newly formed bone arises from the recipient site. The stimulus to produce bone in such a site may be the result of an inductive phenomenon. The physical and chemical structure of the autograft is also of profound importance, as well as its contained population of cells.

Autografts of bone are the major osseous transplants in contemporary clinical practice. The autograft represents a comparative "gold standard" for evaluation of bone transplantation. However, the autografts are obtained at a cost to the patient, including loss of normal skeletal structure, increased morbidity, and decreased mechanical strength of the donor site. Autografts are also limited in size, shape, quality, and the type of material that can be obtained.

The word commonly used to describe repair of a bone transplant is "incorporation". This is the process of uniting the host tissue to the transplant material, as well as the envelopment and admixture of necrotic and viable new bone. The mechanisms of incorporation for cancellous and cortical bone are similar. The incidence of graft-to-host union and creeping substitution repair reflect a biological acceptance of the transplant, while later remodeling of the template ensures the subsequent functional usefulness of the transplant. The process of incorporation is primarily the function of the recipient bed and depends upon the close contact with viable donor tissues. The inherent variables for incorporation are the proliferative activities of osteoprogenitor (mesenchymal) cells, differentiation of cells, osteoinduction, osteoconduction, and biomechanical properties of the graft and site [65]. The very nature of the words used is an indication of how little is really known about the process.

The process of osteoconduction is the growth of capillaries and osteoprogenitor cells from the recipient into the transplanted material. It is the passive ingrowth of new bone by extension from the recipient bed.

Osteoinduction is the process of differentiation of fibroblast-like mesenchymal cells in contact with bone matrix. Urist [10, 11] claimed that this process is regulated by soluble polypeptides, which he has called bone morphogenic protein, and specific enzymes and enzyme inhibitors.

It is fundamental to an understanding of bone formation, and growth, that once a cell of bone has stimulated the hard tissue to form around it, and thereby changed its morphological appearance from that of an osteoblast to an osteocyte, it can no longer contribute to further growth of bone. Because bone grows by apposition, another cell must present itself to the surface of the growing bone, and contribute to the production of osseous matrix. Where do these cells come from?

The foundation of the modern approach to cell specialization involves the selective activation and repression of genes. This approach maintains that the basic mechanism of cell specialization is the same, whether it be prenatal or postnatal, temporary or permanent. A bone cell can thus specialize by turning off one set of genes and turning on another, thereby sending to its ribosomes a new set of protein templates (messenger-RNA) as the previous ones are destroyed. There must be a precisely regulated mechanism to control the selective activation and repression of integrated groups of genes. Such regulation appears to be exerted through "regulator" genes, which control the expression of "structural" genes. There must be factors which regulate the activity of the regulator genes themselves, and hence adapt the cells, by re-specialization, to the changing demands of the immediate surroundings. These factors arise in the cellular microenvironment, which comprises the sum of the chemical and physical forces impinging on the individual cells. Indeed, this is what happens in the process of induction.

In respect of formation of bone, it is likely that the crucial microenvironmental elements in a complex inductive event may well be simple metabolites or common tissue components whose role in induction is subsidiary, even unrelated to their usual role in cell metabolism.

It is further hypothesized that transplanted bone acts more in the role of a structural template, which releases chemical messages stimulating to the surrounding host tissue to become osteogenic. Perhaps one of the reasons cancellous bone is considered to be a better osteogenic stimulus than cortical bone is its retained bone marrow cells which are transplanted at the same time. In fresh autografts of bone such cells are living, while in foreign grafts they are not only antigenic but also dead. The greater surface area of cancellous bone for similar volume may also be significant.

It is also of critical importance to realize that transplantation of bone marrow cells alone, and not protected by bone, into an extra-skeletal site, also results in the formation of bone in that site.

In current orthopedic practice the most common site of procurement of autografts is the ilium. This bone lends itself to providing various shapes of graft, obtained from its anterior or posterior aspect, the outer table, the inner table, the crest, or transiliac, but preserving the crest. In this way the bone obtained can be predominantly cortical, predominantly cancellous, or a mixture of both. If necessary, bone can be harvested from both ilia. The morbidity associated with such harvest depends upon the skill of the surgeon, but pain and discomfort is not uncommon after inexpertly removed grafts that damage the crest of the ilium.

When spinal surgery is performed the spinous processes are often used as autografts. The greater trochanter is an easily accessible but not often used site for cancellous bone, while the tibia or the fibula are the most used for cortical bone. A segment of whole fibula can be removed, while a strip of cortex of the anteromedial surface of the tibia was used frequently in the past. Ribs are not uncommonly used for autografting the spine, particularly if a thoracotomy has been performed for access to the vertebral bodies.

Living cells of the bone marrow are the most important contributors to osteogenesis in bone graft surgery [66]. Nevertheless, other cells in the vicinity of the site of broken, missing, or diseased bone which has been replaced by the transplant may be induced to contribute to bone formation.

6.1.1 Vascularized autografts

Conventional techniques of bone grafting may be used successfully in a variety of situations where there are large segmental bone defects. Advances in vascular and microsurgery over several decades have made it possible to transfer bone autografts onto vascular pedicles, to reconstitute a variety of bony defects. Several potential donor sites are available.

While local transfer of the ipsilateral fibula to a tibial defect was described 80 years ago, it was not until Carrel [67] published his paper entitled "Results of the transplantation of blood vessels, organs and limbs" that the distance transfer of vascularized bone grafts became possible. The technological advances in microsurgery followed the development of the operating microscope and improvement in instruments in the 1960s. The use of free vascularized bone grafts for the treatment of long-bone defects, now frequently utilized, was first reported by Taylor, Miller, and Ham [34] in 1975. This transfer used the peroneal artery and its venae comitantes with anastomoses to leg vessels for preservation of fibular blood supply. In 1978, a one-stage osteocutaneous free flap was described by Taylor and Watson [68] using an osteocutaneous iliac-crest graft transfer, based on the superficial circumflex iliac system.

The free vascularized bone graft developed is an extension of microvascular transplantation and soft-tissue flaps to fill a need in orthopedic surgery. Blood flow through cortical bone depends on an intact medullary blood supply, which receives major contributions for nutrient arteries. Fortunately, a predominant nutrient vessel supplies most long bones. By preserving this principal vessel, a large segment of bone may be transplanted as a living graft.

In a review of vascularized bone grafts, Goldberg et al. [69] stated that vascularized bone grafts provided with both a periosteal and medullary blood study enjoy improved osteocyte survival and enhanced bony incorporation. The vascularized grafts appeared to demonstrate less bony necrosis with subsequent trabecular collapse and architectural disorganization, when compared with the non-vascularized grafts. It would appear that the usual sequel of bone graft incorporation, which includes resorption, creeping substitution, and remodeling, is not seen.

The indications for vascularized bone transfer are broad. Revascularized bone grafts offer significant advantages over conventional treatment methods in selected patients, with segmental bone defects greater than about 6–8 cm, secondary to trauma or after resection of locally aggressive or malignant bone tumors [70]. Other indications include cases of non-union with failure of conventional techniques, cases following radical resection for osteomyelitis, and congenital pseudarthrosis of the tibia or forearm. Another situation in which vascularized iliac grafts are particularly helpful is a composite defect of skin, muscle, and bone.

Free vascularized allografts will not be possible until the problems of bone antigenicity and resection are safely overcome.

In making a choice of a potential bone for vascularized transfer, the following must be taken into account. First, the donor graft must be of sufficient size to fill a recipient defect. Second, the nutrient vessels must be of adequate size for successful microvascular anastomosis. Third, the donor site morbidity must be minimized. Several bones may meet with criteria. The three that have been used most frequently in free-vascularized bone transfers are rib, iliac crest, and fibula. The application of vascularized rib graft in orthopedics is limited, because ribs are curved and malleable. Its major use, as a result, is in mandibular reconstruction. The osteocutaneous iliac flap is useful in the treatment of segmental long-bone defects with an associated soft-tissue defect. For patients with massive segmental bone loss resulting from trauma or tumor resection, a free-vascularized fibular graft is very suitable because it is a straight cortical bone that can restore continuity in long bone defects up to 25 cm. It matches the radius and ulna and fits snugly in the intramedullary canals of the humerus, femur, and tibia. Its high proportion of cortical bone and triangular cross-resection helps resist angular and rotation forces. Sowa and Weiland [70] reported that their experience with microvascular transfer of fibular grafts and composite osteocutaneous iliac flaps had shown that massive autogenous bone grafting with an intact vascular pedicle decreases the time to bony union, and the duration for immobilization required for functional reconstruction of an extremity. The technique is reliable and has also been applied for limb salvage and patients with tumors or severely traumatized extremities who were not candidates for more traditional methods of bone grafting. In many cases amputation would have been the only alternative.

6.2 Allografts

The use of cadaveric bone allografts in the reconstruction of skeletal defects has a long history in orthopedic surgery, and, due to the unpredictability of end results, it has been viewed with limited enthusiasm until relatively recently. There is little doubt that the autograft is the best graft material for management of skeletal defects. However, allografts have some advantages in that they may be used for joint reconstruction, and there is practically no limit on size, shape, or quantity. Use of allografts does not require sacrifice of normal structures, nor is there donor site morbidity.

The first large series of allograft transplantations was reported by Lexer in 1908, who performed 23 whole and 11 half-joint transplants about the knee. He subsequently evaluated the patients in 1925 and believed that 60% had successful results [37]. Subsequent case reports were sporadic until the 1960s, since which time several large series have appeared.

Several different types of allografts are possible. Fresh osteochondral allografts have been used mainly about the knee following trauma, osteoarthritis, osteochondritis dissecans, and osteonecrosis. A long-term study on the first hundred cases was reported by MacDermott et al. [71]. The allografts excised under sterile conditions were stored in Ringer lactate at 4°C and transplanted into recipients within 24 hours. One half had allografts because of traumatic injury, and the best results, 75% success, were obtained in this group of patients. The overall results were not encouraging for patients with osteoarthritis or spontaneous osteonecrosis. The authors believed that the use of corticosteroid drugs in a patient is a contraindication for allografting. In their series, union of allograft was not a problem and usually occurred in the first 6 months. There was subsequent revascularization of the allograft, which seemed to be the major factor in failure. During the first year following the allograft, most patients did well. It was not until 2 or 3 years after the allograft that they began to have problems. In all patients who had reoperations, it was possible to perform more conventional orthopedic procedure without difficulty. Because the risk-to-benefit ratio of having an allograft was found to be reasonable, the authors were of the opinion that it was an appropriate procedure to perform in selected individuals. Meyers [72] has performed fresh osteochondral allografts for femoral-head surfacing to avascular necrosis with segmental collapse of the femoral head. He also found that patients taking systemic steroids had worse outcomes. This operation must still be regarded as experimental.

In order to reduce the immunogenicity of allografts, freezing has been shown to have effect. The largest experience with this type of graft appears to be that of Mankin [51] and his staff at the Massachusetts General Hospital, who commenced allograft surgery in 1971. They took the view that fresh frozen bone could be stored for long periods, should remain strong enough in vivo to provide structural stability to the skeleton, should ultimately unite with the host bone at the anastomotic site, and should be replaced by host bone at a slow and steady rate. They also felt that allografts had a major and crucial advantage over metallic implant devices or autografts because the surrounding soft tissue could serve as anchors for reattachment of muscles and ligaments. They considered that the cartilage covering the end of the bone and serving an essential role in the joint must be seen as a different system, based on the necessity to maintain an intact surface and retain the synthetic activities of the chondrocyte, both being essential for normal joint function. Experimental studies led them to the conclusion that the bone to be used should be treated by slow freezing and rapid thawing.

They also drew attention to the fact that in order to maintain a program of allograft surgery, the procurement of tissue and maintenance of a bank of stored tissue are two major factors. This will be addressed separately. Of their first 150 patients receiving allograft bone, 130 were for tumor resection, and 17 for non-tumor conditions including trauma, Gaucher disease, pigmented villonodular synovitis, fibrous dysplasia, and osteonecrosis. 110 had an osteoarticular graft, 29 had an intercalary segmental graft, and 11 had an allograft in a combination with a prosthesis. All 150 patients were kept under review. While demonstrating that the procedure was successful as a tumor management system primarily for low-grade lesions, there were a significant number of complications including infection (13%), allograft fracture (16.5%), and non-union rate (11%). An analysis of the data suggested that the rate of complications would be reduced to an acceptable level through careful patient selection, better preoperative and post-operative attention to skin coverage, and a genuine attempt to control infection, improve internal fixation, eliminate sizing problems, and improve methods of reconstruction. They also hinted that there was a group of complications presumed to have an immunological basis. It is pertinent to note that in 1983 the authors were of the view that the procedure remains experimental, even though the results of bone allograft surgery are encouraging. In subsequent reports [5, 73], the group expanded their experience to 314 and over 870 patients respectively. These authors again drew the attention to the paradoxical situation that while bone allografting is perhaps a less than optimal solution to the patient with massive bone loss, even in its current state the system has become an important method of dealing with major skeletal defects. Despite the immune response with readily detectable cellular and humoral antibodies, allograft material is generally well tolerated and non-toxic. It has the appropriate modular structure and is relatively easily implanted. It can be infrequently incorporated by the host bone, and the supply is potentially unlimited. This controversy must be considered in view of the fact that most of the patients requiring massive replacement of bone are below the age of 30.

Mankin also drew attention to the surgical procedure for patients with tumors of the extremities. He stressed that it was important to recognize the vision of the operative procedure in two parts; firstly a marginal and wide resection of the tumor, and secondly the implantation of the graft. In planning the surgery, adequate resection should never be compromised. Overall they found that 75% had good results and 25% had not. The bad results were almost entirely accounted for by the extraordinary rate of complications, infection, fracture, and non-union. They stressed that when these grafts failed, especially by fracture, they can be treated by conventional means and rarely require a solution that seriously disables the patient.

In Russia, Volkov and Imamaliyev [74] developed a method of preserving bone in high polymer plastics. They stated that these might be stored at room temperature for several years without losing biological properties. A hammer and chisel were used to remove the allograft from the plastic. They reported 360 operations for joint and osteoarticular bone end transfers, carried out between 1957 and 1972. This technique does not seem to have been pursued elsewhere.

In France, Delepine and Delepine [75] reported their use of massive allografts, which were preserved by freezing to −30°C and sterilized by irradiation. They reported 72 cases with an average length of defect of 20.5 cm. Their patients had three deep infections, eight pseudarthroses, and eight non-unions of which four joined after a second operation, and four late fractures. They recommended that such grafts be used and put together with long-stemmed titanium prostheses, rather than massive stainless-steel prosthesis for joint replacement.

The Toronto Group [76] provided the following recommendations for fresh osteochondral grafts. The patient with the best indication is one who is under 50 years and has a posttraumatic osteoarticular defect. The unipolar graft, one condyle or plateau, yields the most predictable successful results. Graft transplantation should be performed before secondary degenerative changes occur on the opposite articular surface. Transplantation is undertaken within 24 hours of procurement, preferably within 12 hours. The osteochondral graft should have a bony component of at least 1 cm thickness. The host bed must be resected to a bed of healthy bleeding bone to accommodate the graft. The graft must be appropriately sized to fit the size and contour of the bone defect. Fixation of the graft with a host should be accomplished by interfragmentary compression screws. The graft should not be used to correct limb alignment. Limb alignment should be corrected prior to, or at the time of, transplantation by osteotomy. Damaged host menisci should be excised and replaced by intact allograft menisci. In order to decrease joint stiffness, encourage cartilage nutrition and continuous passive movement, patients are placed in an initial weight-bearing caliper for 9–12 months after the operation.

Over the past two decades the dramatic increase in implant surgery has led in turn to an increase in revision of surgery for failure of joint prostheses. Wear particles combined with loosening of the prosthesis are intimately related to progressive loss of bone. This can result in such massive bone loss that conventional methods of reconstruction are inadequate. In the hip, the alternative of revision arthroplasty is often unsatisfactory, due to instability and shortening. In other joints the salvage alternative of arthrodesis may also be very difficult to achieve due to extensive bone loss. Frozen allografts of bone are being used, in increasing numbers, to support revision prostheses. Indeed, revision total hip arthroplasty has provided

the major indication for the use of allograft bone. On the acetabular side, the medial wall may be deficient or there may be substantial loss of anterior and posterior columns. The femoral side of the joint may have lost the calcar femorale, or there may be massive osteolysis, compromising the whole proximal femur. For hip revision and reconstruction, allografts of several types are utilized: morsellized bone primarily from femoral heads, femoral-head slices, partial or whole acetabular fragment, proximal femur, distal femur, and proximal tibia. Gross et al. [76] made the following statements regarding allografts and hip reconstruction. "Fixed acetabular components should be implanted when morsellized bone or femoral head slices have been used to graft protrusion of the acetabulum. Femoral head allografts utilized for shelf reconstruction of superolateral acetabular deficiencies readily incorporated and are successful. For large pelvic defects including columns or domes, partial or whole femoral head allografts are used and provide excellent results. Femoral deficiencies can be restored using femoral tibial allografts, which are cemented to the implant but not to the host. Grafts should not be violated by drill holes. Any host allograft interface should be augmented with autograft cancellous bone to enhance union. Cement should be avoided where possible in host bone and care should be taken to clear cement from the allograft host interface. Rotational stability is provided by a step osteotomy of healthy diaphyseal recipient bone".

While allografts of bone offer a means of bone replacement, only a few groups have published substantial experiences. Their advice should be followed until the real place for such material and the methods of using it are widely experienced.

6.3   Xenografts

There are a number of bone products available commercially, made from animal bones; they are treated in various ways to remove cellular material and soft tissue, cut to a range of sizes, sterilized, and packed for storage at room temperature.

As animal tissue is readily available, its role in surgery, in the preserved state, has been extensively studied. Such tissues include ivory, deer antler, and bovine bone and horn. Ivory and bovine horn are very resistant to incorporation into the host and are currently not used, but bovine bone does remodel more rapidly. Nevertheless, ivory has been used for femoral-head replacement, and after resection of giant cell tumors, in those countries where it is readily available, such as Myanmar (Burma). Fresh bone xenografts, of course, have no place in orthopedic surgery. Among the materials that have been used and subsequently discarded are: frozen calf bone; freeze-dried calf bone (Boplant); decalcified ox bone; various types of deproteinized bone; os purum—which is bone that is mechanically freed from soft tissue and soaked in warm potassium hydroxide, acetone, and salt solutions; an organic bone from which the organic material is extracted by ethylene diamine; and Oswestry bone, which is fully deproteinized bovine cancellous bone prepared by double extraction, using both hydrogen peroxide and ethylene diamine.

Probably the only xenograft of bone available commercially at present is Kiel bone, which consists of partly deproteinized bone prepared from freshly killed calves. The bone is washed in water, extracted with hydrogen peroxide, treated with fat solvents and dried with acetone. It is then sterilized by ethylene dioxide. It appears to be weakly antigenic and does not possess active bone inducing properties. Kiel bone has been used clinically in Europe for several years with varying success rates. Salama [62] reported his experience in humans in 110 operations on 98 patients.

Using Burwell's method of combining autologous bone marrow with a treated foreign bone, Salama [62] believed that xenograft bone might be good bone-bank material provided it was deproteinized and either impregnated with living autologous marrow as a composite graft or placed in a bed of bleeding cancellous bone. Although his experimental work suggested that Oswestry bone gave the best results, he used partially deproteinized Kiel bone in the human clinical situation because:

- It was more easily available.
- It had better mechanical properties than Oswestry bone, which was very brittle and when mixed with marrow became paste-like.
- There was some evidence to suggest it enhanced osteogenesis over a longer period.
- It appeared less antigenic.

The appropriate size of Kiel bone was chosen for the clinical situation. Autologous bone marrow was aspirated from the iliac crest using a wide bore sternal puncture needle and an ordinary syringe. 6–8 mm were aspirated at a time, and the aspirate rapidly mixed with Kiel bone in order to prevent premature clotting and to ensure the greatest possible proportion of marrow to blood in the aspirate. Multiple punctures 2 cm apart in the iliac crest were used to obtain as much marrow as was necessary to ensure thorough impregnation of all bone grafts. In 25 operations the xenografts were placed in a bed of bleeding cancellous bone. In 85 operations, xenografts were impregnated with fresh marrow. The clinical indications were fracture of the tibial plateau (18), excision of benign bone lesions (25), arthrodeses (three), spinal fusion (four), pseudarthroses (52), traumatic bone defects (two), and following leg-lengthening procedures (two). He described his results as very satisfactory, except in those of femoral and tibial pseudarthroses. Sepsis was responsible for failure in three patients. Salama [62] stated "The advantage of the method is obvious. It is almost atraumatic. It also saves time: it obviates the need for additional operation to procure autografts and the laborious procurement at operation of suitable allografts. It is easier, practical, and safe, avoiding the numerous complications at the donor site. It is economical because it obviates the need for a sophisticated bone bank. Unlimited supplies of xenograft are available, and it would seem rendered osteogenic by a simple procedure. This is particularly important in children and the elderly osteoporotic patients, especially when large amounts of bone graft are needed but are not easily available". Despite his advocacy of the technique it seems that current endeavor, especially in North America, is directed toward allografts rather than xenografts.

7   Bone-banking procedures

Bone banks should provide safe tissues, with predictable biological and biomechanical properties, compatible with their intended clinical applications. They must be free of potentially harmful transmissible diseases. Depending on the specific application, loads on bone grafts may be substantial or insignificant, and such load is a major determinant of surgical technique and the selection of bone replacement material.

In the establishment of a bone bank the pertinent issues are donor selection, tissue recovery, preservation techniques, long-term storage, and record keeping. The American Association of Tissue Banks has produced guidelines and standards, and specific application to bone banking has been reviewed by Friedlaender [4]. Those guidelines are now used regularly, at a national level in the United States, and are readily available. The current situation of the guidelines is to protect the recipient. They also serve to protect the tissue banks, and provide a reasonable and commonly accepted basis on which grafts may be shared among institutions.

Selection of donors aims to exclude the potentially harmful transmissible diseases, or those systemic or localized disorders of the skeleton that might influce the properties of the graft when transplanted. Donors are eliminated if medical history includes a generalized infection or infection of the tissues to be collected at transplantation. Bacterial and fungal pathogens are all of concern, with specific attention placed on the possibility of transmitting hepatitis, venereal disease, or acquired immune deficiency syndrome. Patients with malignant disease are usually excluded as donors as are those with metabolic bone diseases, those on corticosteroid treatment, and those who might have toxic substances accumulated in bone. Cadaveric donors offer the opportunity to remove large segments of bone, including the femur. The screening of live and cadaveric donors is similar. Bacteriological cultures are used liberally during the procurement of bone.

Consent or authorization must be obtained prior to tissue donation. This can be accomplished for cadaveric donors where antemortem agreement consisting of the donor's signature on a uniform donor card, or obtaining authorization from the appropriate relative. Recovery and banking of femoral heads, during reconstruction surgery, can be authorized by pre-operative informed consent obtained from the patient and noted by the surgeon on the operative consent form.

Recovery of tissue can be accomplished under sterile and non-sterile conditions, both of which have their advantages and problems. Removal of tissues under sterile conditions is clearly demanding. However, osteochondral allografts can be excised only under sterile conditions, because all sterilizing procedures will severely damage cartilage. Non-sterile recovery requires that effective sterilization be accomplished without jeopardizing the graft's biological potential. In general, preservation and storage methods which safely and reliably retain biological and biomechanical properties are required [77].

Supplying patients with allografts excised from cadaveric donors constitutes professional activity, and surgeons who excise and prepare such allografts assume the joint responsibility for the care of the patients with the surgeons who operate on the recipient.

In the case of cadaveric donors, tissue may be recovered in a clean, but non-sterile environment, or in a customary sterile fashion. Non-sterile tissue recovry requires a method of secondary sterilization, usually high-dose radiation or chemical sterilization using agents such as ethylene oxide. It is important to know that whatever method is chosen is effective and does not substantially interfere with biological potential. It is also important that toxic by-products of the sterilization procedure be eliminated from the graft before transplantation. Recovery of tissues in a sterile fashion uses the same techniques that apply in a conventional operating suite. Although more time consuming while the bone is being procured, it avoids the need for secondary sterilization.

There are numerous approaches used for long-term preservation of bone. Those methods most commonly used are deep freezing, freeze-drying, demineralization with hydrochloric acid, or combinations of those. This variety of techniques reflects the fact that bone does not have to retain its cellular viability in order to be biologically useful.

It is not known how long bone may be stored at various temperatures, but it appears that temperatures in the $-20°C$

range are compatible with storage for several months, and that temperatures of −70°C to −80°C are consistent with long-term preservation for years. Deep freezing is relatively easy and convenient, and is also compatible with cryopreservation of cartilage. Freeze-drying is compatible with long-term preservation of bone. This method permits indefinite storage in evacuated containers at room temperature. The process is initially more costly than deep freezing, but prolonged storage without the need to maintain low temperatures is an advantage. Cartilage cannot be preserved in this way. Freeze-drying also causes structural change in the form of cracks and makes bone less useful for segmental replacement, unless the bone graft is adequately protected by internal fixation. Demineralized bone has high osteogenic potential with reduced structural resistance. Grafts, stored deep frozen, can be wrapped in sterile plastic and then either an additional layer of sealed plastic or a double layer of cloth may be added. Femoral heads can be similarly stored or placed in two glass containers, one inside the other. Freeze-dried grafts remain in vacuum-sealed containers of glass or plastic.

Regardless of the method of long-term storage, the packaging material must be a barrier to contamination, and the integrity of the container must not be compromised by storage conditions.

It is also important to keep accurate records of the medical history of the donor and the results of all tests to confirm sterility and the absence of transmissible disease. Random cultures should be obtained periodically to ensure maintenance of sterility.

Detailed reports of experience with bone banking of massive articular allografts used as intercalary bone allografts over a 12-year period have been provided by Mallinin, Martinez, and Brown [78] and the Boston workers [79]. They concluded that bone banks large enough to support an allograft program required dedicated medical personnel to manage them. A large potential donor population, extensive financial resources, and modern storage facilities are also necessary. Infected donors and contamination of procured bones during storage and revival must be avoided at all costs. Detailed record keeping is of major importance to clinical investigations especially for evaluating complications. These considerations must be taken into account before embarking on an institutional bone-banking program, to provide satisfactory allogeneic bone for clinical use.

Several different types of bone banks have evolved. Friedlaender [4] described these as casual, institutional, and large regional banks. Casual bone banks are those small individual hospital projects based on the needs of a limited number of surgeons within the institution. In general, the methods rely on freezing in household refrigerators or freezers. There are probably 300 or 400 hundred such banks in the USA. Figures for other countries are not available. Not all bone banks will survive because of the difficulties of adherence to rigid methods of bone procurement and storage. Institutional bone banks are usually found in large medical centers and are viable as the result of academic programs. These banks occasionally send tissues to other hospitals but generally exist for support of those surgeons within a single medical center. They follow vigorous methodology and usually depend on deep freezing for long-term preservation. There are probably 30 or 40 of this type of bank in the USA, and other countries are following this idea.

Large regional banks are often available for different tissues to be stored and provide a number of users with those tissues. They provide grafts to large geraphic segments of the country and often serve as a national resource. They are meticulous about the bone-banking methodology and respond to the needs of their clientèle. There are probably 12 to 18 such banks in the USA which are evolving toward cooperative and integrated networking programs. These banks tend to be loosely affiliated with large medical centers and academic institutions. They often use several different methodologies for preservation. The growth of institutional banks and particularly the establishment of expanded network and cooperation at regional level would appear to be a reasonable approach to provide safe and efficacious bone grafts in an increasing and sufficient supply.

It must always be remembered that even if allogeneic bone is available in optimal form from a bone bank, there must be an appropriate and satisfactory recipient site with healthy bone and soft tissue free from infection if success is to be achieved.

8   Synthetic materials for bone replacement

The internal fixation of fractures has been practiced for about 100 years. Unfortunately the steels that were initially used were subjected to corrosion and rusting, and could not be retained in the body for long periods. Although Lane was one of the earliest users of mild steel for internal fixation and responsible for design of a plate and screws used for many years [80], Northfield [81] was reluctant to publish the results of his operations because of such corrosion. The developments in metallurgical sciences has now given orthopedic surgeons a range of materials which can be used for the rigid immobilization of fractures and are highly resistant to the effects of the moist, salty, and warm environment which surrounds them when implanted in the body. It is only natural that the development of the polymer and plastics industry in the last 50 years would have its energies directed toward the replacement of human parts. In the last 30 years technical developments have given opportunities for close association among materials scientists, orthopedic surgeons, dentists, and veterinarians, and have led to more rapid progress in the use of synthetic materials for bone and joint replacement. The problems of procurement of biological products and their preservation, storage, immunogenicity, and potential for infection can already be overcome by materials scientists. The materials used for the replacement of broken, missing, and diseased bone fit into the categories of metals, ceramics, and plastics.

8.1   Metals

The most common use of metals in orthopedic surgery is for the apposition of fragments and temporary replacement of bone strength following fracture of the bone. Most fractures heal without any form of treatment due to normal physiological reparative processes. Surgical interference, using various techniques of internal fixation, is a means of providing mechanical stability of bone during the fracture healing process, and maintaining the pieces of bone in anatomical alignment.

Under most circumstances, once the fracture has healed, the reinforcing and re-aligning metals can be removed.

The purpose of this section is to address the use of metals in those conditions in which the natural replacement of bone is not envisaged, either by virtue of the disease process preventing such healing involving the bone or the eradication of neoplasia by the resection of bone and surrounding tissues.

In this respect, the replacement of large segments of bone harboring neoplasms is being performed more commonly. Such surgery usually requires a prosthesis, usually incorporating at least one joint, to be manufactured individually for the patient, so that the correct size of prosthesis can be available at the time of bone resection. Modular systems are also available now. The use of computed tomography in building up a model of the bone shape, and utilization of this model for design and fabrication of the prosthesis, is a sequel of modern technology [82].

Probably the largest series of massive metallic implants of this nature was reported by Bradish et al. in 1987 [83]. Among their patients, a number have lived for many years with the prostheses, which have provided good function. Indeed, whole bones can be replaced in this way. The principal problems of metallic implants are at the point of attachment to normal bone. Usually some sort of intramedullary stem, with or without transverse fixation through the stem and encircling diaphyseal bone, is used.

Any metal retained within the body for a long time is subject to corrosion; therefore, the choice of metals is limited. Those that are acceptable are surgical grade stainless steel (316L), chrome cobalt and molybdenum alloys, pure titanium, and titanium alloys.

Many years of experience have shown that metals placed in the body for skeletal support can often fatigue and break. The continuous remodeling of natural bone, as a consequence of stresses placed on it, give it resilience and resistance to fatigue which is unobtainable in artificial implants.

Furthermore, the effects of metals on surrounding tissues cannot be ignored, as none of the metals used is inert. In order to achieve biological acceptability metals must fulfill the criteria of:

- Negligible toxicity and destructiveness to surrounding tissues.
- Resistance to corrosion.
- Maintenance of tensile strength.
- Acceptable electrochemical characteristics.
- The desired combination of mechanical strength, ductility, and hardness.

Implants must be properly designed and placed to most effectively carry a load and perform functionally. Because of weight and size limitations of the human musculoskeletal system, many implants cannot be designed for high load-carrying capacity.

Stainless steel (316L) is fabricated by annealing or cold reduction to be strong and corrosion resistant. It is widely used and has stood the test of time. Pure titanium is not as strong as 316L but has excellent corrosion resistance. It is weldable, machinable, and can be cold-worked. Chrome-cobalt-molybdenum alloy has good corrosion resistance and adequate strength but it is difficult to machine, and it is fabricated by casting. When metals are used as implants, it is important to ensure that retaining screws or bolts are made of the same material as the implant to avoid electrolytic reactions. Care must be taken to avoid implanting two dissimilar metals in the same surgical site, for example, when treating a fracture close to a prosthetic joint.

8.2 Ceramics

The emergence of technical ceramics has been linked to the evolution of materials from the stone age, through the bronze and iron ages, and more recently in the plastics age. Although "old ceramics" of much earlier times, such as bricks and tiles, were clay-based, the "new ceramics" are essentially non-clay ceramics. The new technical ceramics are materials that deliver superior mechanical, electrical, magnetic, and optical properties in performance. Many are based on readily available materials such as the oxides, nitrides, or carbides of silicon, aluminum, zirconium, or iron. The technical ceramics industry can be classified as one of high technology. The exciting properties of

ceramics include wear resistance, hardness, stiffness, corrosion resistance, and relatively low density. One of their main attractions is their high melting point for mechanical strength at high temperature. A consequence of the high melting point of technical ceramics is that they must generally be fabricated from powders. The growing use of ceramics as biocompatible materials for dental implants and orthopedic surgical prostheses is now leading to their emergence as a significant replacement for traditional devices. Ceramics offer a number of advantages. The ceramics may be made porous to permit bone ingrowth and bonding. Such a bond is strong, permanent, and natural. Ceramics chosen for biological use can be highly resistant to corrosion.

Initially the ceramic material most used for biological application was alumina (aluminum oxide, Al_2O_3), but a number of ceramics based on minerals naturally occurring in bone have also been used: calcium and phosphorus in the form of synthetic hydroxyapatite and tricalcium phosphate. Currently under trial are partially stabilized zirconium and silicon nitride. Silicon nitride has excellent engineering properties, such as machinability, tensile and compressive strength, and electrical insulation. Such engineering ceramics are approximately half the density of steel. Silicon nitride has outstanding resistance to thermal shock, fatigue and creep, hardness, wear resistance, and deformation.

A combination of ceramics with metals can also be used. A number of prosthetic hip joints use an articulation of a ceramic femoral head in a plastic acetabulum, or a metal head in a ceramic acetabulum, or a ceramic coating on a metallic femoral stem. Furthermore, metals can be surface coated with ceramics, such as hydroxyapatite, allowing for fixation of an implant far superior to cemented or cementless current techniques [84].

While considerable effort has gone into the development of ceramic articulations in artificial joints, there seems to have been less interest shown in their use for bone replacement. Hanley [85] used porous tricalcium phosphate in experimental animals to determine suitability of synthetic bone graft for reconstruction of anterior spinal column defects. Gudeshauri et al. [86] reported their experience in 38 patients, in whom they had replaced segments of bone resected for tumors of the limbs with corundum (alumina) ceramic. In 23 patients the joint portions of long bones were replaced, in four patients, diaphyseal defects, and in 11 patients various bones of the hand and foot were replaced. The latter were mainly for enchondromas, and most of the others had either osteoclastoma or chondrosarcoma. Contact surfaces were polished to a high degree of purity. Most of their ceramic prostheses had protruding metallic stems sprayed with ceramic dust in order to obtain stable fixation and to isolate the metal from the surrounding tissues. Apart from their own cases, they cited only six other contributions to the literature in which there was the same application of ceramic endoprostheses in bone tumors.

There are numerous reports of experimental use of tricalcium phosphate for diaphyseal replacement in animals, with a cylinder of ceramic usually supported by an intramedullary nail.

Howlett, McCartney, and Ching [87] examined the replacement of a segment of a femoral diaphysis in rabbits with silicon nitride. Each implant was enclosed within a stable cuff of bone within 4 months of implantation and remained unchanged throughout the rest of the animal's life. Tissue apposition to each prosthesis was morphologically normal, making it clear that silicon nitride has the potential of an important ceramic for use in bone reconstruction.

Another way in which ceramic materials have been used has been in the form of large or small granules to fill a cavity in bone. Because of their shape such granules, usually of tricalcium phosphate or hydroxyapatite, form a porous filling for the cavity and allow ingrowth of vessels and fibrous connective tissue. Uchida and colleagues [88] reported clinical experience with about 60 patients in whom bone grew in to the pores surrounding the ceramic granules, thereby reconstituting the defect with an integrated mixture of calcium and phosphate and normal bone.

It is possible to make porous ceramics of solid form, which also allow for ingrowth of vascular fibrous tissue. Bone-marrow cells with osteogenic potential can be introduced in to such pores, between 100 μm and 300 μm in diameter, and eventually the pores become filled with bone. If a biode-gradable ceramic could be developed, then it might be replaced over time by further growth of bone, a process not dissimilar to creeping substitution about autografts and allografts of cancellous bone.

One problem with porous ceramic materials is their mechanical strength if the pore sizes are to be of the optimum diameter for bone ingrowth. An alternative to porous ceramics are solid ceramics, which act to permanently replace bone. Using a variable number of alumina rings threaded over an intramedullary nail, Huckstep [89] has replaced large segments of long bones and also incorporated such a design into joint prostheses.

It would seem that ceramic materials offer a great potential for bone replacement in the future, because of their versatility in terms of size, shape, chemical structure, resistance to corrosion, and mechanical properties. Furthermore, they overcome the current problems of storage and sterilization.

As with all other implants it is essential to consider: (1) the effect of the biological environment on the implant, and (2) the effect of the material on its surrounding environment. There may be debris around a ceramic implant, either inorganic or small particles broken off from the implant, or cellular debris from surrounding tissue affected by the ceramic implant, usually because of chemical toxicity. Such debris must be removed or engulfed by a phagocytic mechanism, thereby altering the cellular population about an implant. The release of ions or radicals into the tissues may react with them and denature proteins—hence rendering them antigenic, which the ceramic material, itself, is not. An implant may be "rejected", however, if an abscess forms around it subsequent to the inflammatory process of normal healing following the surgery for its insertion. Obviously, neoplasia stimulated by implants is a cause for serious concern, and would prevent approval of the particular ceramic that was associated with it. Neoplasia about implants often takes many years to appear, and to date our experience is insufficient.

For a review of the use of ceramics as surgical implants the reader is referred to Hulbert and Young [90].

8.3 Plastics

Prostheses in the form of acrylic plastics have been used in medicine and dentistry for a number of years. False teeth in the form of dentures are made from acrylic plastics. Progress in the replacement of joints was hastened by Charnley's use of acrylic cement to seat a prosthetic acetabulum and femoral stem in his development of an artificial hip.

So called "bone cement", an acrylic plastic made up from a mixture of monomer and polymer together with appropriate catalysts, provides the surgeon with a malleable and ductile plastic material which can be implanted into the body. It then hardens quickly, retaining shape at the site where it was placed. Following the introduction of this material to orthopedic surgery, it was then used for bone replacement, because of its availability. There are numerous reports of the use of poly-methylmethacrylate (cement) for replacement of vertebrae, particularly those removed for primary or secondary neoplasm, either alone or as augmentation to autologous bone graft. There are also numerous reports of filling of cavities with methacrylate cement, particularly in association with metallic stabilization of bone harboring metastatic neoplasms. Acrylic bone cements have also been used to augment osteopenic bone requiring internal fixation, and following curettage of neoplasms such as giant cell tumors. Acrylic plastics are also used for replacement of skull bone following craniectomy.

Another group of polymers that have been used are short chain compounds of lactic acid, glycolic acid, or a combination. Polylactates and polyglycolates were introduced as resorbable suture materials, to replace catgut, and have subsequently been fabricated in larger sizes as pegs, or screws for fixation of fractures. The rationale behind their use is that they secure the bone during the fracture healing process, and as the bone regains its intrinsic strength the polymer is resorbed. They are very slowly gaining popularity. One reason for that slowness may be their radiolucency, so that their site can not always be detected by radiological examination. An alternative use has been in the fabrication of complex shapes, such as an arrow shape, for the arthroscopic fixation of meniscal splits or as suture anchors for inaccessible sites with a conventional needle on a holder.

Although plastics have long been considered as materials for bone replacement, they have not yet proved to be a panacea, and medical polymers, including plastics, are more often used in soft-tissue implantation than in bone (or were until successful litigation was widespread about breast prostheses). Pure plastic materials generally cause little local tissue reaction. Monomers and low molecular weight polymers do cause tissue sensitivity. Compound plastics, and those with added stabilizers, antioxidants, curing agents, and residual catalysts are capable of exerting toxic effects on the host. Non-conductive materials, notably Teflon, Dacron, some silicones, polyethylene, polypropylene, and certain polyurethanes, are sufficiently inert and non-toxic to be used in prostheses. They are encapsulated by a fibrous scar and do not often excite unfavorable responses.

Nevertheless, chemical degradation can occur leading to a loss of strength and fragmentation of structure, allowing a polymer plastic to become more brittle, subject to fatigue, and liable to crack under stress. The loss of mechanical characteristics, subsequent to such chemical change, leads to malfunction of prostheses. Polysiloxane silicon materials have been used for replacement of small bones and joints, particularly in the hands and feet. In recent times there has been some concern about their safety and longevity for the above reasons, and because of the formation of phagocytic granulation and inflammatory tissue surrounding them. The manufacturers have voluntarily withdrawn their supply for this reason and replaced them with titanium implants of the same shapes!

9   Stimulating osteogenesis without transplantation

9.1   Chemical methods

Mention has been made of Urist's concept of a bone morphogenic protein (BMP) as a diffusible substance, which stimulates the formation of osteoprogenitor cells. He maintained that the protein could be isolated from cortical bone, dentine, and various bone tumors, being one or more acidic proteins with a relative migration rate of 17.5–19 kd, a pI of 4.9–5.1, and a blocked N terminal amino acid. Its purification has proved difficult. Analysis of Urist's BMP showed the presence of several distinct proteins that either alone, or in combination with other regulatory molecules, induce bone formation. Partial purification of these proteins has permitted an osteogenic protein gene to be recovered from host-conditioned media. To date seven potentially osteogenic recombinant proteins have been produced, and three have been proven to have osteogenic activity in animals. Cook et al. [91] recently evaluated the effectiveness of recombinant human Bone Morphogenic Protein-7 (rhOP-1) as a composite with bovine bone collagen carrier for the restoration of an osteoperiosteal diaphyseal defect in a canine segmental model. They found that more bone was found to fill the defect than in control animals and claimed to have done the first tests of human BMP in dogs. It is postulated that BMP release recruits cells for an osteoprogenitor pathway of development and therefore adds new cells to the pool of predifferentiated cells in bone marrow stroma, endosteum, and periosteum. Perivascular cells with inherited osteogenic competence (a not-yet-activated state of readiness to differentiate into osteoprogenitor cells) are the target for BMP [12]. BMP by itself, in more or less purified forms, does not stimulate the formation of bone and requires either the simultaneous implantation of bone marrow cells or an environment adjacent to those cells. Bone regeneration may be augmented but not caused directly by BMP. It has not found use clinically, although demineralized bone matrix was used by Senn [55] a century ago and has had sporadic use since then. Cook et al. [91] also stated that for effective osteoinduction, osteogenic proteins must be implanted with an appropriate carrier since the proteins are water soluble and readily diffusible. The differentiation of cells may be controlled in part by "morphogenic fields" (analogous to electrical fields) but the nature of such fields has not been explored or identified. Hulth [92] postulated, from observations of clinical fracture healing, that damaged tissues could stimulate the formation of bone. It appears unlikely that a single molecule will control bone formation, which is a very complex mechanism. It is also clear that many of the steps along the way to bone formation can be inhibited by chemical compounds, and in order to stimulate osteogenesis just as much effort will have to be invested into recognition of inhibitors and controlling them. Preliminary studies, using partially purified human BMP in the management of non-unions, have been reported by Johnson et al. [93, 94]. Refractory femoral, tibial, and humeral non-unions were treated with human BMP on a carrier of gelatin or polylactic or polyglycolic acid with various internal fixations and autografts or allografts of bone. Union was achieved but there were no controls for comparison, so the value of the study is only that it points the way to the future. An animal study in sheep with appropriate controls [95] also supported the use of recombinant human BMP (rhBMP-2) when inserted on a carrier of inactive bone matrix.

9.2   Physical methods

As bone is a tissue that adjusts its architecture to its functional environment (a modern paraphrase of Wolff's Law), the strains encountered during functional activity reflect the response of bone and surrounding tissues to loading. It is well known that bone mass is lost if the bone is inactive for even a short period, and increased activity may stimulate an osteogenic response. There probably exists a population of cells sensitive to "strain" which can initiate an adaptive response if required [96].

9.2.1 Mechanical methods

It is clear that the interaction between physical loads and fracture healing mechanisms is of great importance in the treatment of fractures. McKibbin [97] elegantly described a hypothesis which links cellular behavior to movement at a fracture site at different times after the injury. We also know from experience that immobilization of fractures is required at a specific time in their management, while movement of the limb may be beneficial at a later time in the healing process. Kenwright et al. [98] showed that cyclic compression of a fracture can significantly accelerate fracture stiffness, presumably by stimulating osteogenesis or a component of it (e.g., mineralization). To date this concept, using a mechanically driven "shaker" as part of an external fixation frame, has not gained clinical acceptance as the precise loading parameters have not been established. It is of interest to note that animals in the wild rarely have non-union of fractures and self regulate their levels of activity in a limb after fracture. It may be that some of our treatment methods for humans inhibit the fracture-healing process rather than stimulate osteogenesis!

(While the comment is true for an animal in the wild, it is not true for domesticated animals which have been treated, incorrectly, by the veterinary orthopedist. Also, it should be appreciated that even though fractures of long bones of feral animals usually heal, they do so as a malunion. Editor)

One method of stimulating osteogenesis in non-union after fracture is to subject the fracture to rigid immobilization with a plate and screws inserted under compression at the non-union site, or to insert an intramedullary nail. The first procedure is effective in securing union where there is a hypertrophic non-union and does not require an additional bone graft. The latter probably provides its own bone-marrow graft in the process of intramedullary reaming. However, both show the application of a change in mechanical state of the bone to convert a non-union to union of a fracture by promoting bone formation.

The technique of distraction histogenesis of bone was evolved in Siberia by Ilizarov [35] in the post-World-War-II era and has been under animal and clinical investigation in the western hemisphere since 1984. Distraction histogenesis means that limbs can be regenerated by gradual tension force. This revolutionary technique has directly influenced clinical methods of limb lengthening, while introducing new solutions for the treatment of chronic osteomyelitis, non-unions, malunions, and soft-tissue contractures. With these phenomenal innovations came intense curiosity mitigated by appropriate skepticism. In some centers there was an enthusiastic surge to apply the complicated biological and mechanical methods, and much had to be learned about technique [35]. The ways of exploiting distraction histogenesis to stimulate osteogenesis are time consuming, often frustrating, and frequently associated with complications, and some have become disenchanted with their use.

Green [99] compared open bone-graft technique (Papineau) with Ilizarov's intercalary bone transport to manage segmental skeletal defects and came to the conclusion that a combination of the two helped reduce the number of problems associated with the bone transport method alone, although bone was stimulated to form within the deficient segment. Chronic infected tibial non-unions were treated by Marsh et al. [100], who found that conventional treatment and distraction osteogenesis gave similar rates of union, but leg-length discrepancy could be minimized by the bone transport mechanism. Much is yet to be learned about the control of osteogenesis by this potentially exciting method, such as the rate of distraction, the forces that need to be applied, and the prevention of complications. Overall, it is not really stimulating osteogenesis, but exploiting the normal response of injured bone and periosteum to form bone and incrementally increasing the bony gap that needs to be bridged.

9.2.2 Electrical and magnetic fields

The effects of the mechanical environment on healing have been accepted for many years. Mechanisms were not really postulated until piezoelectricity in bone, the electrical potentials generated by mechanically stressing crystalline substances of which bone mineral is an example, was detected by Yasuda [101]. This provided an explanation of the mechanism by which physical stress or strain could alter the cellular environment and thus affect cell proliferation and function. Friedenberg and Brighton [102] measured electrical potentials in different parts of growing bones and around fractures and suggested that biopotentials are a stimulus for bone formation. Electrical stimulation of delayed or non-union has raised much interest, although enthusiasm for its use seems to be on the decrease despite encouraging reports of clinical success.

There are three general methods used:

• Direct current through implanted electrodes.
• Alternating currents induced by time-varying electromagnetic fields.
• Constant or pulsed capacitatively coupled fields [103].

The results in fresh fractures are mixed. Large, well-designed randomized and blinded studies need to be performed. Constant direct current can be supplied by electrodes (cathodes) in the form of needles passed percutaneously into the non-union site, and a skin surface cathode, with power pack interposed between and carried on the patient's belt [104, 105], or with a fully implanted system. The advocates of such systems assert that the results are equal to, or better than, those obtained with autologous bone grafting. Pulsing electromagnetic fields can be made to traverse a site of non-union by the application of specially designed coils incorporated in rigid splints surrounding the limb. The aim is to produce similar electrical fields in the non-union site to that provided by implanted, or percutaneous, electrodes. The manufacturers of the equipment can produce coils and electromagnetic characteristics suitable to achieve bone stimulation after a study of the patient's radiographs. Bassett, Mitchell, and Gaston [106] reported in 1981 that they had used this method in 127 non-united fractures, achieving union in 87%. The results from another center [107] were not as encouraging.

9.3   Ectopic ossification

The formation of bone in non-skeletal sites is not an infrequent radiological observation. Ectopic ossification is different from ectopic calcification. It may occur in abdominal scars (particularly after bladder surgery), or follow trauma within hematomas. It is also frequently seen after hip replacement surgery, or after pelvic fracture surgery, and may reflect migration of large quantities of bone marrow into the surrounding muscle. The final cellular pathway is no doubt the same as in normal bone formation. If the stimulus to ectopic osteogenesis could be recognized, it might be exploited. Marrow cells lodging at those sites might be the osteoprogenitors.

9.4   Accelerating fracture union

While delay in fracture union is common, accelerated union is not often identified. There is physiological acceleration of union in children when compared to adults. The acceleration may be apparent rather than real, as in the child a smaller volume of repair bone is needed to restore mechanical strength required for normal activity. It is well known that refracture in children, particularly of the forearm bones, is common and usually occurs due to another fall. The definition of fracture healing is unclear, but the logical end point is to achieve the same strength that the bone had before fracture. As the strength before fracture is not known in precise terms, and non-destructive strength tests are not performed in clinical practice, it is experience more than anything else, which determines fracture healing to such a state as to allow unprotected activity.

Attempts made to accelerate fracture healing include venous tourniquets, drugs, sympathectomy, hormones, exercise, and electrical stimulation. Most of these attempts have not produced consistent enough results to be clinically useful.

Clinicians have long recognized that patients who have multiple injuries, including brain injury or spinal cord injury, frequently and quickly produce abundant amounts of new bone about fractures. The reasons for this are not known, nor does it occur in all cases. The apparent abundance of bone has been shown to be real [108, 109]. There is no doubt that osteogenesis is stimulated under those circumstances, but little has been gleaned as to how it happens. Perhaps that is an enterprise for the near future.

10 The future

Much of our knowledge about bone formation, either physiological or pathological, has been based on morphological examination by optical microscopy or clinical radiology. There exists a voluminous amount of such observations. Yet we understand the subject poorly at a molecular level. We have accumulated much knowledge by trial and error from treating patients who have need for bone repair or replacement, and we perform our clinical duties with skill. The reward for the enormous cost and effort of research to date has been minuscule. The few major advances have been made by a few courageous and thoughtful surgeons empirically pursuing an idea, probably stimulated by clinical observation! The future advances lie in exploitation of the techniques of molecular biology and biochemistry to uncover the factors which program the DNA in the nucleus of every cell surrounding the site of deficient bone and direct those cells to make bone in preference to any other tissue. Nature has evolved mechanisms for the ordered growth and repair of bones, and we should be able to discover the key to those mechanisms and exploit them. For the present we can do little better than to teach ourselves not to interfere too much with the natural process of repair of bone unless we are confident that we are not inhibiting that natural process. Medical practitioners, whether physicians or surgeons, tend to intervene in most circumstances on the basis that "something should be done". We must realize that surgical intervention most certainly affects the repair process in bone by altering blood supply and electrical environment, interfering with appropriate differentiation of pluripotent cells, and producing motion at fracture sites that may inhibit the bone-forming process. It is my guess that the transfer of autologous bone marrow, obtained by aspiration and injected into a site where osteogenic stimulation is required, will be a commonly used technique before long as the trend to minimally invasive surgery increases.

In this chapter, I have attempted to draw the attention of the reader to the ways in which courageous and ingenious surgeons have undertaken the task of replacement of broken, missing, and diseased bones.

While broken bones normally replace themselves by an orderly sequence of cellular behavior, the stimuli which recruit cells to produce bone at a fracture site are not clearly defined.

Where bone is missing, diseased, or both, and the normal healing process fails, in most cases, and sites, bone must be replaced. The ways of doing so are either to try and mimic or stimulate the physiological mechanisms of bone growth and repair after injury, or to replace the bone with a synthetic substitute.

The synthesis of experiences gained by courageous surgeons pioneering new methods of treatment on an empirical basis, and the painstaking and tedious collection of data by experimental and inquisitive surgeons and biologists are slowly but surely leading to the selection of techniques most likely to be successful for bone replacement. From current clinical experience there seems little doubt that the former method is preferable if it can be achieved, while modern technological development and the close cooperation of surgeons, biologists, engineers, and materials scientists hold great hope for the latter. If the future could be predicted, the likely solution is a combination of both.

What we have at present is a collection of different methods, of varying levels of predictability of success, which provide the surgeon, dentist, and veterinary surgeon with an armamentarium from which an appropriate technique may be chosen to suit the particular clinical problem which he or she faces.

This chapter will have achieved its aim if the reader is now more familiar with the historical evolution of currently used techniques of bone replacement, aware of those which have been discarded, cognizant of the problems which must be addressed if a higher level of successful surgery is to be gained, and stimulated to think logically about better methods for the replacement of broken, missing, and diseased bone. There will always be a need for bone replacement.

It is the hope of the author of this chapter that the reader has been stimulated to think about bone formation in a different way from that which presents itself in the clinic each day. The combination of clinical need and an inquiring mind will be the best stimulus to exploit nature to the fullest in skeletal biology.

11 Bibliography

Blue references indicate links to abstracts of articles available online:
http://www.aopublishing.org/BONE/12.htm

1. **Ollier L** (1858) De la production artificielle des os an moyen de la transplantation de periose et des greffes osseuse. *Comptes rendues des seances de la Societe de Biologie et des ses filiales;* 5:145.
2. **de Boer HH** (1988) The history of bone grafts. *Clin Orthop;* (226): 292–298.
3. **Inclan A** (1942) The use of pre-served bone graft in orthopaedic surgery. *J Bone Joint Surg [Am];* 24:81.
4. **Friedlaender GE** (1987) Bone banking. In support of reconstructive surgery of the hip. *Clin Orthop;* (225):17–21.
5. **Mankin HJ, Gebhardt MC, Jennings LC, et al.** (1996) Long-term results of allograft replacement in the management of bone tumors. *Clin Orthop;* (324):86–97.
6. **Chase SW, Herndon CH** (1955) The fate of autogenous and homogenous bone grafts. *J Bone Joint Surg [Am];* 37:809.
7. **Bassett CAL** (1954) Bibliography of bone transplantation. *Transplantation Bulletin;* 1:167.
8. **Burwell RG** (1969) The fate of bone grafts. In: Apley AG, editor. *Recent Advances in Orthopaedics.* London: Churchill Livingstone, 115.
9. **Urist MR** (1965) Bone: formation by autoinduction. *Science;* 150 (698): 893–899.
10. **Urist MR, Dowell TA, Hay PH, et al.** (1968) Inductive substrates for bone formation. *Clin Orthop;* 59: 59–96.
11. **Urist MR, Mikulski A, Boyd SD** (1975) A chemosterilized antigen-extracted autodigested alloimplant for bone banks. *Arch Surg;* 110 (4): 416–428.

12. **Urist MR** (1989) Bone morpho-genetic protein, bone regeneration, heterotopic ossification and the bone-bone marrow consortium. In: Peck WA, editor. *Bone and Mineral Research.* Amsterdam: Elsevier Science Publishers Biomedical Division, 57.
13. **Burwell RG** (1964) Studies in the transplantation of bone: VII. The fresh composite-homograft-autograft of cancellous bone. *J Bone Joint Surg [Br];* 46:110.
14. **Burwell RG** (1966) Studies in the transplantation of bone. 8. Treated composite homograft- autografts of cancellous bone: an analysis of inductive mechanisms in bone transplantation. *J Bone Joint Surg [Br];* 48 (3):532–566.
15. **Bick EM** (1948) *Source Book of Orthopaedics. 2nd ed.* Baltimore: Williams & Wilkins.
16. **Janeway HH** (1910) Autoplastic transplantation of bone. *Ann Surg;* 52:217.
17. **Duhamel HL** (1842) Sur le development et la crue des os des animaux. *Hist Acad Inscr Paris;* 2:481.
18. **Macewan W** (1912) *The Growth of Bone.* Glasgow: J. Maclehose.
19. **Orr CW** (1939) The history of bone transplantation in general and ortho-pedic surgery. *Am J Surg;* 43:547.
20. **Keith A** (1919) *Menders of the Maimed.* London: Henry Frowde & Hodder & Stoughton.
21. **Axhausen G** (1908) Histologische Untersuchungen über Knochen-transplantation am Menschen. *Dtsche Zschr Chir;* 91:388.
22. **Albee FH** (1915) *Bone Graft Surgery.* Philadelphia: WB Saunders.
23. **Ollier L** (1867) *Traite experimental et clinique de la regeneration des os et de la production artificielle du tissu osseus.* Paris: Masson et fils.
24. **Gallie WE** (1918) The use of boiled bone in operative surgery. *Am J Orthop Surg;* 16:373.

25. **Gallie WE** (1931) The transplan-tation of bone. *Brit Med J;* 2:840.
26. **Matti H** (1932) Über freie Trans-plantation von Knochenspongiosa. *Langenbeck's Arch Chirurg;* 168:236.
27. **Matti H** (1936) Technik und Resultate meiner Pseudarthrosen Operation. *Zntrlbl Chirurg;* 25:142.
28. **Ghormley RK** (1933) Back pain with special reference to the articular facets with presentation of an opera-tive procedure. *JAMA;* 101:1773.
29. **King T** (1938) Matti's spongiosa bone transplantation for ununited fractures. *Med J Aust;* 1:526.
30. **Mowlem AR** (1941) Bone and cartilage transplants. *Brit J Surg;* 29:182.
31. **Abbott LC, Saunders JB, Bost FC** (1942) Arthrodesis of the wrist with the use of grafts of cancellous bone. *J Bone Joint Surg [Br];* 24:883.
32. **Abbott LC** (1944) Lectures on reconstruction surgery. *Instructional Course Amer Acad Orthop Surg;* 2.
33. **Mowlem AR** (1944) Cancellous chip grafts for the restoration of bone defects. *Proc Royal Soc Med;* 38:171.
34. **Taylor GI, Miller GD, Ham FJ** (1975) The free vascularized bone graft. A clinical extension of micro-vascular techniques. *Plast Reconstr Surg;* 55 (5):533–544.
35. **Ilizarov GA, Lediaev VI** (1969) [Replacement of defects of long tubular bones by means of one of their fragments]. *Vestn Khir Im I I Grek;* 102 (6):77–84.
36. **Carrel A** (1912) The preservation of tissues and its application to surgery. *JAMA;* 59:523.
37. **Lexer E** (1925) Joint transplantation and arthroplasty. *Surg Gyn Obstet;* 40:782.
38. **Orell S** (1938) The use of os purum in bone implantation. *Surg Gyn Obstet;* 66:23.

39. **Wilson PD** (1951) Follow-up study of the use of refrigerated homogenous transplants in orthpaedic operations. *J Bone Joint Surg [Am]*; 33:307.

40. **Longmire WP, Cannon JA, Weaver RA** (1954) General surgical problems with tissue transplantation. In: Wolstenholme GW, O'Connor M, editors. *Preservation and Transplantation of Normal Tissues*. London: Churchill Livingstone.

41. **Murphy JB** (1913) Osteoplasty. *Surg Gyn Obstet*; 16:492.

42. **Mitchell DF, Shankwaller GE** (1958) Osteogenic potential of calcium hydroxide and other materials in soft tissues and bone wounds. *J Dent Res*; 37:1157.

43. **Chalmers J** (1959) Transplantation immunity in bone homografting. *J Bone Joint Surg*; 41:160.

44. **Chalmers J, Sissons HA** (1959) An experimental comparison of bone grafting materials in the dog. *J Bone Joint Surg*; 41:209.

45. **Heiple KG, Kendrick RE, Herndon CH, et al.** (1967) A critical evaluation of processed calf bone. *J Bone Joint Surg [Am]*; 49 (6):1119–1127.

46. **Medawar PB** (1944) The behavioural fate of skin allografts and skin homografts in rabbits. *J Anat*; 78:176.

47. **Elves MW** (1976) Newer knowledge of the immunology of bone and cartilage. *Clin Orthop*; (120):232–259.

48. **Langer F, Gross AE** (1974) Immunogenicity of allograft articular cartilage. *J Bone Joint Surg [Am]*; 56 (2):297–304.

49. **Horowitz MC, Friedlaender GE** (1987) Immunologic aspects of bone transplantation. A rationale for future studies. *Orthop Clin North Am*; 18 (2):227–233.

50. **Johnson EE, Urist MR, Finerman GA** (1988) Bone morphogenetic protein augmentation grafting of resistant femoral nonunions. A preliminary report. *Clin Orthop*; (230):257–265.

51. **Mankin HJ, Doppelt S, Tomford W** (1983) Clinical experience with allograft implantation. The first ten years. *Clin Orthop*; (174):69–86.

52. **Enneking WF, Eady JL, Burchardt H** (1980) Autogenous cortical bone grafts in the reconstruction of segmental skeletal defects. *J Bone Joint Surg [Am]*; 62 (7):1039–1058.

53. **Pelker RR, Friedlaender GE** (1987) Biomechanical aspects of bone autografts and allografts. *Orthop Clin North Am*; 18 (2):235–239.

54. **Makin M** (1962) Osteogenesis induced by vesical mucosal transplant in the guinea pig. *J Bone Joint Surg [Br]*; 44:165.

55. **Senn N** (1889) On the healing of aseptic bone cavities by implantation of antiseptic decalcified bone. *Amer J Med Sci*; 98:219.

56. **Reddi AH, Wientroub S, Muthukumaran N** (1987) Biologic principles of bone induction. *Orthop Clin North Am*; 18 (2):207–212.

57. **Lacroix P** (1945) Recent investigations of the growth of bone. *Nature*; 156:176.

58. **Cook SD, Rueger DC** (1996) Osteogenic protein-1: biology and applications. *Clin Orthop*; (324):29–38.

59. **Riley EH, Lane JM, Urist MR, et al.** (1996) Bone morphogenetic protein-2: biology and applications. *Clin Orthop*; (324):39–46.

60. **Goujon E** (1869) Recherches experimentales sur les proprietes physiologique de la moelle des os. *Journal Anat Physiol*; 6:399.

61. **Weiss L** (1967) The histophysiology of bone marrow. *Clin Orthop*; 52:13–23.

62. **Salama R** (1983) Xenogeneic bone grafting in humans. *Clin Orthop*; (174):113–121.

63. **Nade S, Armstrong L, McCartney E, et al.** (1983) Osteogenesis after bone and bone marrow transplantation. The ability of ceramic materials to sustain osteogenesis from transplanted bone marrow cells: preliminary studies. *Clin Orthop*; (181):255–263.

64. **Lance EM** (1972) Bone and cartilage. In: Najarian JS, Simmons RL, editors. *Transplantation*. Philadelphia: Lea and Febiger.

65. **Burchardt H** (1987) Biology of bone transplantation. *Orthop Clin North Am*; 18 (2):187–196.

66. **Nade S** (1979) Clinical implications of cell function in osteogenesis. A reappraisal of bone-graft surgery. *Ann R Coll Surg Engl*; 61 (3):189–194.

67. **Carrel A** (1908) Results of the transplantation of blood vessels, organs and limbs. *JAMA*; 51:1662.

68. **Taylor GI, Watson N** (1978) One-stage repair of compound leg defects with free, revascularized flaps of groin skin and iliac bone. *Plast Reconstr Surg*; 61 (4):494–506.

69. **Goldberg VM, Shaffer JW, Field G, et al.** (1987) Biology of vascularized bone grafts. *Orthop Clin North Am*; 18 (2):197-205.

70. **Sowa DT, Weiland AJ** (1987) Clinical applications of vascularized bone autografts. *Orthop Clin North Am*; 18 (2):257–273.

71. **McDermott AG, Langer F, Pritzker KP, et al.** (1985) Fresh small-fragment osteochondral allografts. Long-term follow-up study on first 100 cases. *Clin Orthop*; (197): 96–102.

72. **Meyers MH** (1985) Resurfacing of the femoral head with fresh osteochondral allografts. Long-term results. *Clin Orthop*; (197):111–114.

73. **Mankin HJ, Gebhardt MC, Tomford WW** (1987) The use of frozen cadaveric allografts in the management of patients with bone tumors of the extremities. *Orthop Clin North Am;* 18 (2):275–289.

74. **Volkov MV, Imamaliyev AS** (1976) Use of allogenous articular bone implants as substitutes for autotransplants in adult patients. *Clin Orthop;* (114):192–202.

75. **Delepine G, Delepine N** (1988) [Preliminary results of 79 massive bone allografts in the conservative treatment of malignant tumors in adults and children]. *Int Orthop;* 12 (1):21–29.

76. **Gross AE, Rudan JF, McAulty JP, et al.** (1988) The use of allografts in orthopaedic surgery. *Current Orthop;* 236:22.

77. **Doppelt SH, Tomford WW, Lucas AD, et al.** (1981) Operational and financial aspects of a hospital bone bank. *J Bone Joint Surg [Am];* 63 (9): 1472–1481.

78. **Malinin TI, Martinez OV, Brown MD** (1985) Banking of massive osteoarticular and intercalary bone allografts—12 years' experience. *Clin Orthop;* (197):44–57.

79. **Tomford WW, Doppelt SH, Mankin HJ, et al.** (1983) 1983 bone bank procedures. *Clin Orthop;* (174): 15–21.

80. **Hicks J** (1970) The influence of Arbuthnot Lane on fracture treatment. *Injury;* 1:314.

81. **Northfield DWC** (1936) On the fate of metallic foreign bodies introduced into the tissues in treatment of fractures. *Guys Hosp Repts;* 86:159.

82. **Macdonald W, Thrum CB, Hamilton SG** (1986) Designing an implant by CT scanning and solid modelling. Arthrodesis of the shoulder after excision of the upper humerus. *J Bone Joint Surg [Br];* 68 (2):208–212.

83. **Bradish CF, Kemp HB, Scales JT, et al.** (1987) Distal femoral replacement by custom-made prostheses. Clinical follow- up and survivorship analysis. *J Bone Joint Surg [Br];* 69 (2):276–284.

84. **Geesink RG, de Groot K, Klein CP** (1987) Chemical implant fixation using hydroxyl-apatite coatings. The development of a human total hip prosthesis for chemical fixation to bone using hydroxyl-apatite coatings on titanium substrates. *Clin Orthop;* (225):147–170.

85. **Hanley EN** (1985) The suitability of porous tricalcium phosphate as a synthetic bone graft for reconstruction of segmental column defects. *Pro Int Soc Lumbar Spine;*111.

86. **Gudushauri ON, Gagulashvili AD, Chkhatarashvili ML, et al.** (1987) The use of corundum ceramic implants after excision of tumours of the extremities. *Int Orthop;* 11 (2): 125–128.

87. **Howlett CR, McCartney E, Ching W** (1989) The effect of silicon nitride ceramic on rabbit skeletal cells and tissue. An in vitro and in vivo investigation. *Clin Orthop;* (244):293–304.

88. **Uchida A, Araki N, Shinto Y, et al.** (1990) The use of calcium hydroxyapatite ceramic in bone tumour surgery. *J Bone Joint Surg [Br];* 72 (2):298–302.

89. **Huckstep RL** (1987) Stabilization and prosthetic replacement in difficult fractures and bone tumors. *Clin Orthop;* (224):12–25.

90. **Hulbert SF, Young FA** (1978) *Use of Ceramics in Surgical Implants.* New York: Gordon and Breach Scientific Publishers.

91. **Cook SD, Baffes GC, Wolfe MW, et al.** (1994) Recombinant human bone morphogenetic protein-7 induces healing in a canine long-bone segmental defect model. *Clin Orthop;* (301):302–312.

92. **Hulth A** (1980) Fracture healing. A concept of competing healing factors. *Acta Orthop Scand;* 51 (1):5–8.

93. **Johnson EE, Urist MR, Finerman GA** (1988) Repair of segmental defects of the tibia with cancellous bone grafts augmented with human bone morphogenetic protein. A preliminary report. *Clin Orthop;* (236):249–257.

94. **Johnson EE, Urist MR, Finerman GA** (1992) Resistant nonunions and partial or complete segmental defects of long bones. Treatment with implants of a composite of human bone morphogenetic protein (BMP) and autolyzed, antigen-extracted, allogeneic (AAA) bone. *Clin Orthop;* (277):229–237.

95. **Gerhart TN, Kirker-Head CA, Kriz MJ, et al.** (1993) Healing segmental femoral defects in sheep using recombinant human bone morphogenetic protein. *Clin Orthop;* (293):317–326.

96. **Rubin CT** (1984) Skeletal strain and the functional significance of bone architecture. *Calcif Tissue Int;* 36 (Suppl 1):S11–18.

97. **McKibbin B** (1978) The biology of fracture healing in long bones. *J Bone Joint Surg [Br];* 60 (2):150–162.

98. **Kenwright J, Goodship AE, Evans M** (1984) The influence of intermittent micromovement upon the healing of experimental fractures. *Orthopaedics;* 7:481.

99. **Green SA** (1994) Skeletal defects. A comparison of bone grafting and bone transport for segmental skeletal defects. *Clin Orthop;* (301):111–117.

100. **Marsh JL, Prokuski L, Biermann JS** (1994) Chronic infected tibial nonunions with bone loss. Conventional techniques versus bone transport. *Clin Orthop;* (301):139–146.

101. **Yasuda L** (1954) On the piezo-electric activity of bone. *J Jap Orthop Surg Comm;* 28:267.

102. **Friedenberg ZB, Brighton CT** (1966) Bioelectric potentials in bone. *J Bone Joint Surg [Am];* 48 (5):915–923.

103. **Brighton CT** (1981) The treatment of non-unions with electricity. *J Bone Joint Surg [Am];* 63 (5):847–851.

104. **Brighton CT, Black J, Friedenberg ZB, et al.** (1981) A multicenter study of the treatment of non-union with constant direct current. *J Bone Joint Surg [Am];* 63 (1):2–13.

105. **Heppenstall RB** (1983) Constant direct-current treatment for established nonunion of the tibia. *Clin Orthop;* (178):179–184.

106. **Bassett CA, Mitchell SN, Gaston SR** (1981) Treatment of ununited tibial diaphyseal fractures with pulsing electromagnetic fields. *J Bone Joint Surg [Am];* 63 (4):511–523.

107. **Sedel L, Christel P, Duriez J, et al.** (1982) Results of non unions treatment by pulsed electromagnetic field stimulation. *Acta Orthop Scand Suppl;* 196:81–91.

108. **Perkins R, Skirving AP** (1987) Callus formation and the rate of healing of femoral fractures in patients with head injuries. *J Bone Joint Surg [Br];* 69 (4):521–524.

109. **Spencer RF** (1987) The effect of head injury on fracture healing. A quantitative assessment. *J Bone Joint Surg [Br];* 69 (4):525–528.

13 Determinants of bone strength and mass: A summary and clinical implications

Harold M. Frost

1 Abstract

A common mechanism that controls bone strength and bone "mass" is involved in osteoporosis, traumatic and spontaneous fractures, the healing of fractures and bone grafts, the service lives of load-bearing bone implants, and some aspects of homeostasis. Some of the mechanism's features are:

- Modeling by drifts can increase bone strength and "mass" where mechanical strains exceed a modeling threshold; it turns OFF where strains stay below that threshold. BMU-based (basic multicellular unit) remodeling can remove bone where strains stay below its smaller threshold; it begins to retain bone where strains exceed its threshold.
- Loads on a bone cause those strains. When they continually increase (as during growth), or decrease, the adaptations in bone strength would usually lag behind the need.
- Muscles place the largest loads on bones; muscle strength increases during growth, plateaus in young adults, and declines slowly after 30–40 years of age.

That means:
- During growth, increasing body weight and muscle strength would make modeling increase bone strength and "mass" and make remodeling retain the added bone.
- In young adults the bone loads and strains would plateau, so adaptations of bone strength could "catch up" and turn modeling OFF. Remodeling would still conserve bone, so bone strength and "mass" would plateau too.
- In aging adults, decreasing muscle forces on bones adapted to stronger young-adult muscles would put the bones in mild disuse, to turn modeling OFF and make remodeling slowly reduce bone strength and "mass".

Therefore:
- More arduous exercise could readily increase the already active modeling in children, to further increase bone strength and "mass", aided by growth hormone and related factors. In young adults modeling would turn OFF, but increased muscle strength from weight-lifting-type activities could turn it back ON.
- To turn it ON in older adults would require more increase in muscle strength than they can achieve.
- Physical exercise helps to retain bone at all ages, but it can increase bone strength and "mass" better in children than in young adults, and seldom in older adults.
- Failures of those adaptations could lead to too little bone for ordinary mechanical usage and cause bone pain and/or spontaneous fractures, usually of the spine.

2 Introduction

The physiology that determines bone strength and "mass" provides a common mechanism that many bone features and problems depend upon. The problems include osteopenia, osteoporosis, and the service lives of load-bearing implants such as artificial joints, bones, and teeth. They include the healing of fractures, bone grafts and arthrodeses, the susceptibility of bone to traumatic and fatigue fractures, and homeostasis. Our understanding of that physiology changed dramatically after 1960 and led to a new paradigm of skeletal physiology based on multidisciplinary evidence. It concerns joints and collagenous tissues as well as bone [1–6]. In part, it proposes that mechanical-usage effects on bone strength and "mass" would dominate most non-mechanical ones. The latter could help or hinder the former effects but could not replace them, a view that now has strong support. This summary of that physiology in humans and animals depends upon some vocabulary and ideas taught in few schools, so the text appends explanatory notes (**Section 8**) and a glossary.

3 Physical determinants of bone strength

Bone strength depends upon four things: its materials properties, the amount of bone tissue (bone "mass"), its architecture, and the amount of fatigue damage in it.

3.1 Material properties, "mass", and architecture

- Bone's materials properties include stiffness, specific gravity, and ultimate strength. Those properties differ relatively little with age, sex, species, and most diseases (osteomalacia excepted) when compared to the "mass", architectural, and microdamage determinants [7].

- The amount of bone in a cross-section (the "mass" determinant) affects the strength of a whole bone. Usually, the more bone, the greater the strength.
- The size and shape of a bone and the distribution in its cross-section of its spongiosa and compacta (the architectural determinant) also affect a bone's strength. As an example, doubling the diameter of a hollow bone while retaining the same amount of bone in its cross-section increases its bending strength eight times [7–9].

With the exception of osteomalacia, genetic instructions mainly determine the materials properties, while bone modeling and remodeling (see below) mainly determine the "mass" and architectural features.

3.2 Microdamage

Microscopic fatigue damage in bone is caused by repeated load–unload cycles. It can reduce bone strength to below 20% of normal, without affecting bone architecture or "mass" [1, 10–12]. It can cause stress and spontaneous fractures of whole bones and trabeculae, and pseudofractures in osteomalacia. It can loosen load-bearing bone implants, including artificial joints and teeth, and spine instrumentation and other internal fixation devices [13]. Excessive microdamage can increase bone fragility in true osteoporosis, an old idea [14] that caused diminishing controversy [15].

Bone has an operational microdamage threshold range of strain. Under loads that originally cause 2,000 microstrain, bone endures about 10 million loading cycles before it breaks, but under loads that cause 4,000 microstrain, it can break in less than 20,000 cycles. As loads and strains only double in that range, microdamage increases phenomenally, well over 400 times [16]. Its repair by BMUs can normally keep up with any microdamage caused by strains below 2,000 microstrain. Larger strains can cause too much to permit repair, so it can accumulate to cause fatigue fractures of trabeculae or whole bones. The 2,000–4,000 microstrain region can define an operational microdamage threshold range or MESp [17]. Its center should lie near 3,000 microstrain.

3.3 Age-related effects

The strength and "mass" of whole bones usually increase during growth and plateau in young adults. In humans around 35 years of age they begin slow decreases that go on for the rest of life. By 80 years of age, only 60–70% of the young-adult bone "mass" can remain [18].

4 Vital biomechanical determinants of bone strength and "mass"

Longitudinal bone growth excepted, a bone's architecture, "mass", and its microdamage burden depend mainly on two biological mechanisms: remodeling by BMUs and modeling by

drifts [6, 19]. Bone exists mainly to serve mechanical needs without breaking or hurting, and for life. Since it cannot predict its mechanical usage, remodeling and modeling adapt it to its past and ongoing mechanical usage and loads in ways summarized next.

4.1 Basic multicellular units (BMUs) and bone remodeling

Global BMU-based remodeling (not osteoclasts alone) can conserve or reduce bone strength and "mass" but seldom, if ever, increases them [1, 19] (Fig. 13-1). In an activation "resorption" formation sequence that takes 3 or more months, BMUs turn bone over in small "packets" on most bone surfaces for life. Next to marrow, completed BMUs usually remove

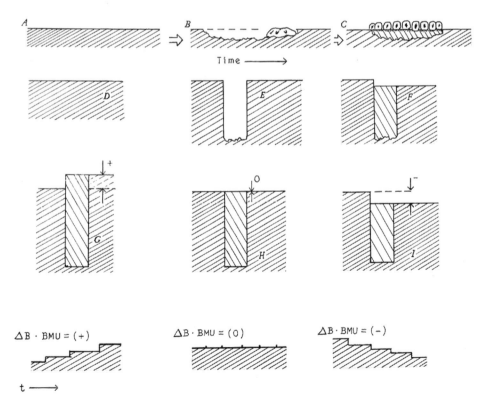

Fig. 13-1: Bone remodeling BMUs.
Top row: An activation event on a bone surface at (A) causes a packet of bone resorption at (B), then replacement of the resorbed bone by osteoblasts at (C) on the right. The BMU makes and controls the new osteoclasts and osteoblasts that do this.
Second row: Idealize those events to emphasize the amounts of bone resorbed (E) and formed (F) by completed BMUs.
Third row: In these "BMU graphs" (after Frost), (G) on the left shows a small excess of formation over resorption as, perhaps, on periosteal surfaces. (H) shows equalized resorption and formation as on haversian surfaces, and as in "conservation-mode" remodeling. (I) on the right shows a net deficit of formation, as on cortical-endosteal and trabecular surfaces, and as in "disuse-mode" remodeling.
Bottom row: These "stair graphs" (after PJ Meunier) show the effects on the local bone balance and "mass" of a series of BMUs of the kind immediately above. Healthy adult human skeletons probably create and complete around 3 million BMUs annually, along with corresponding numbers of new but short-lived osteoclasts and osteoblasts. BMUs are created when and where they are needed, and include a capillary, precursor and "supporting" cells, and some wandering cells. They are multicellular entities in the same sense as renal nephrons and hepatic lobules. (Reproduced by permission from Frost, 1987, [123].)

more bone than they form, to cause life-long trabecular and cortical-endosteal bone losses. In cortical bone, BMUs resorb and form nearly equal amounts while they make new haversian systems or osteons. "Global" means averaged over a whole bone or skeleton. This remodeling is slow.

Where bone strains stay below a remodeling threshold range, the MESr centered near 50–100 microstrain, "disuse-mode" remodeling increases permanent bone loss, usually next to marrow [2, 20]. This reduces bone strength and "mass" and can cause an osteopenia. Where strains exceed that threshold, "conservation-mode" remodeling reduces bone turnover and begins to preserve existing bone strength. This tends to prevent an osteopenia.

Microdamage repair: Remodeling BMUs also repair bone microdamage by removing the damaged bone and replacing it with new bone [14, 17, 21–23]. When detection and/or repair of microdamage is impaired, it can accumulate and eventually cause spontaneous fractures, or loosen a load-bearing implant.

Remodeling's two-stage disuse pattern in adults [20, 24–30]— the initial tissue dynamics: Acute disuse-mode remodeling has two variants, one for acute partial disuse, the other for acute total disuse (**Fig. 13-2**). But both increase bone loss where bone touches marrow, and both cause an osteopenia characterized by losses of spongiosa, increased marrow-cavity diameter, thinned cortex, normal outside bone diameter, and reduced bone strength and "mass".

The final (chronic) tissue dynamics: Several years of those activities would cause an osteopenia. Its severity would correspond to the severity of the disuse. Then conservation-mode remodeling begins to minimize further losses of bone strength and "mass". Gradual-onset disuse causes partial disuse effects so slowly, that it can take years to clearly see the bone effects. This should happen in most aging human adults and other aging mammals due, at least, partly to their declining muscle strength. It should also occur in people developing chronic debilitating problems like those in **Table 13-1**.

Nota bene: As and after they develop, the pattern of bone loss and the tissue dynamics in the medically important osteopenias and osteoporoses strongly resemble the acute and chronic disuse patterns [1]. This suggests that the medical causes of those affections act on the same mechanisms that control mechanical usage effects.

Tab. 13-1: Some conditions that cause acute and chronic partial disuse in humans (and related osteopenia).*

Asthma	Emphysema	Pulmonary fibrosis
Renal failure	Hepatic failure	Cardiac failure
Malnutrition	Anemia	Polyarthritis
Metastatic cancer	Depression	Stroke
Muscular dystrophy	Multiple sclerosis	Alzheimer's disease
Organic brain syndrome	Huntington's chorea	Myelomeningocele
Lou Gehrig disease	Paralyses	Leukemia
Cystic fibrosis	Still's disease	Alcoholism
Drug addiction	Nursing home residence	Myasthenia gravis

*   In causing bone loss and an osteopenia, the relative importance of the mechanical disuse and the biochemical-endocrine abnormalities accompanying some of these entries is uncertain at present. Past studies of the matter did not really evaluate the mechanical usage effects. In view of the paradigm, the mechanical effects probably dominate most biochemical-endocrine ones, which of course opens the matter for discussion (modified from Frost) [1].

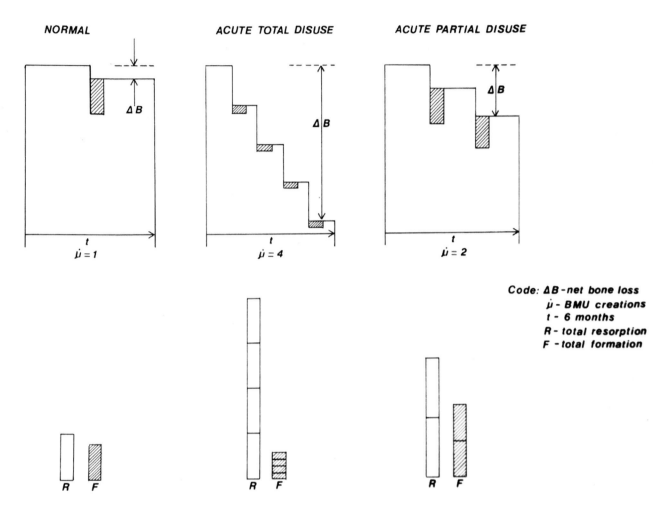

Code: ΔB - net bone loss
μ̇ - BMU creations
t - 6 months
R - total resorption
F - total formation

Fig. 13-2: On complete and partial disuse.
Top row: These "stair-BMU graphs" look at part of a trabecular surface from the side. In idealized form they show how much bone a typical completed trabecular BMU resorbed (R) and formed (F). Since each BMU resorbed more than it made here, each permanently removed a small amount of bone. *Left column:* The adapted state during normal mechanical usage. Since this is a trabecular surface next to marrow, the BMU resorbs a bit more bone than it makes. *Middle column:* In acute total disuse, increased BMU creations combine with a marked decrease in total formation by each completed BMU. *Right column:* In acute partial disuse, and compared to total disuse, a smaller increase in BMU creations accompanies an even smaller decrease in formation. The horizontal arrows (*t*) mean each column

models the same time period, say 6 months. A dot above μ means the number of new BMUs created in the above time period (μ̇ = dμ/dt). Bar graphs below: These show the total resorption (R) and formation (F), and net bone losses as the difference between (R) and (F), in the "*t*" time period for each mechanical usage situation above. In acute partial disuse and compared to normal, net bone loss and total resorption and formation can each increase. In acute total disuse, total resorption and net bone loss increase further, but now total formation falls below normal. As a result, global bone formation could increase in acute partial disuse but decrease markedly in acute total disuse. This occurs in life and has confused interpretation of some clinical and experimental data. (Reproduced by permission from Frost, 1994, [124].)

4.2   Bone modeling by drifts

Global modeling (not osteoblasts alone) can increase bone strength and "mass" but rarely, if ever, reduces them [1, 6, 7, 19] (**Fig. 13-3**). Formation and resorption drifts use osteoblasts and osteoclasts respectively to determine the cross-sectional shape and size of bones and trabeculae and their longitudinal shape, and to increase bone strength and "mass". This modeling works best during growth. It can affect trabeculae for life but it becomes inefficient on adult cortical bone. It is another slow process. Formation drifts initially create all cortical bone, and secondary osteons can then slowly replace it [19].

Where bone strains enter or exceed a modeling threshold range, the MESm centered near 1,000 microstrain, modeling begins to strengthen the bone and reduce later strains toward the bottom of that range (see **Note 1**, i.e., **Section 8.1**) [2]. In juveniles, this increases bone strength and the cross-sectional

bone "mass". In older adults it has minimal effects on cortical modeling, but it can strengthen trabeculae throughout life (as in the medial-compartment subchondral spongiosa of a varus knee). Where strains stay below the modeling threshold, mechanically con-trolled modeling turns OFF. Bone fractures at 25,000 microstrain [7], while modeling tries to make bones strong enough to keep their strains from exceeding 1,000 microstrain (the MESm threshold). That relationship would make bones stronger than needed for their usual mechanical usage. Their strength would have a safety factor [31].

Overly vigorous mechanical usage (as in weight lifting, USA-style football, hard physical labor, but not marathon running) [1, 32, 33]: Sudden such usage increases bone loads and strains. In juveniles this can increase bone modeling, additions of spongiosa and compacta, bone strength and "mass". Meanwhile conservation-mode remodeling keeps the added bone. In adults this acute usage has little effect on

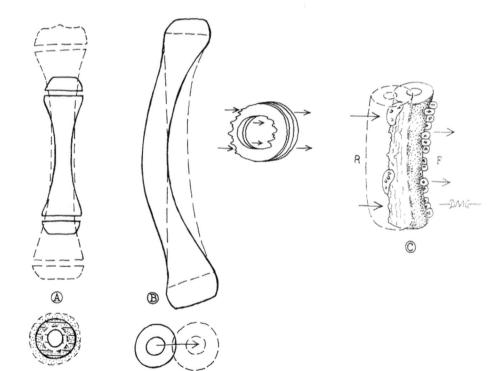

Fig. 13-3: Bone modeling drifts.
A: Diagram of an infant's long bone with its original size and shape in solid line. To keep this shape as it grows in length and diameter, its surfaces must move in tissue space as the dashed lines suggest. Formation drifts make, and control, new osteoblasts to build some surfaces up. Resorption drifts make, and control, new osteoclasts to remove bone from other surfaces.
B: A different drift pattern can correct the fracture malunion in a child, shown in solid line. The cross-sectional view to the right shows the cortical-endosteal as well as the periosteal drifts.
C shows how the drifts in B would move the whole segment to the right. Large forces from voluntary activities as in weight lifting make modeling strengthen bone far better than smaller voluntary forces, no matter how frequent, as in marathon running. Drifts are created anew when and where they are needed, and also include capillaries, precursor and "supporting" cells and some wandering cells. They are multicellular entities in the same sense as renal nephrons and hepatic lobules. (Reproduced by permission from Frost, 1987, [123].)

cortical bone modeling, but conservation-mode remodeling still retains existing bone [32]. After some years such adults can have more bone than others because it was better retained [34]. In chronic hypervigorous mechanical usage in adults, bone strength would usually have increased enough to reduce bone strains to the bottom of the modeling threshold range and turn modeling OFF, while conservation-mode remodeling would keep the bone added previously. "Chronic" would mean adapted well enough (strong enough) to keep bone strains from exceeding the modeling threshold, which would also keep them well below the microdamage threshold [1, 17].

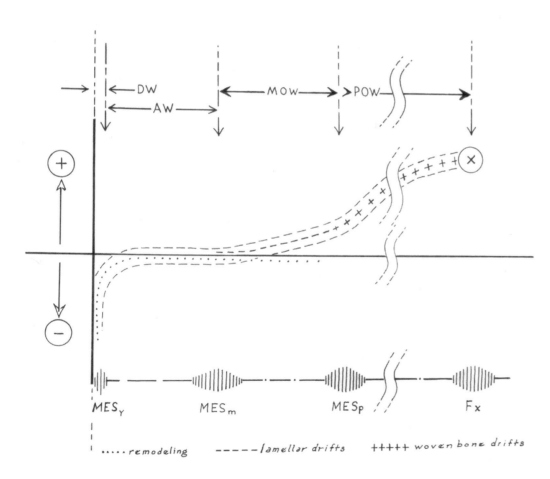

Fig. 13-4: Modeling and remodeling effects on bone strength and "mass". The horizontal line at the bottom of this graph suggests typical peak bone strains from zero on the left, to the fracture strain on the right (Fx), plus the location of the remodeling, modeling, and microdamage thresholds (MESr, MESm, MESp). The horizontal axis represents no net gains or losses of bone strength or "mass". The lower dotted-line curve suggests how remodeling would remove and weaken bone where strains fall to, or below, the MESr range and stay there, but otherwise would tend to keep existing bone and its strength. The upper dashed-line curve suggests how modeling drifts would begin to increase bone strength and "mass" where strains enter or exceed the MESm range. The dashed outlines suggest the combined modeling and remodeling effects on bone strength and "mass". DH Carter originally suggested such a curve. At and beyond the MESp range, woven bone formation drifts usually replace lamellar bone formation drifts.

Fx = fracture strain near 25,000 microstrain; DW = disuse window; AW = adapted window or "comfort zone" as in normally adapted adults; MOW = mild overload window as in healthy growing mammals; POW = pathological overload window [20].

In the nearly flat region between the MESr and MESm, bone strength and "mass" change little as typical strains change. In juveniles, increasing body weight and muscle loads on bone cause bone strains in or above the MESm range. In most aging adults the strains would tend to downshift toward the MESr region, due to decreasing muscle strength. For such reasons, more vigorous mechanical usage should make modeling increase bone strength and "mass" more in children than in aging adults. In the latter, raising bone strains to the MESm range would require more increase in muscle strength than most aging adults can achieve; bicycling and running, for example, would not achieve this. Many studies reviewed by Forwood and Burr [32] and Smith and Gilligan [51] support this explanation. (Adapted from Frost, 1994, [56].)

4.3 Combined modeling–remodeling effects

Fig. 13-4 and **Note 2** (i.e., **Section 8.2**) explain the combined effects on bone strength and "mass" of modeling and remodeling, and their thresholds. In general, when strength and "mass" increase, modeling drifts are responsible (not osteoblasts alone). When strength and "mass" decrease, remodeling BMUs are responsible (not osteoclasts alone).

4.4 The mechanostat

Skeletal tissues and organs normally endure their voluntary mechanical usage without breaking or hurting, and for life. This occurs in all large and small amphibians, birds, mammals, and reptiles of either sex and all ages. Some mechanisms must orchestrate the adaptations of skeletons to their voluntary mechanical loads in ways that achieve that situation, so it was named the mechanostat [1, 7, 35, 36]. Its disorders can cause disease. Illustrative examples include: true osteoporoses, arthroses, spontaneous bone and tendon ruptures, scoliosis, congenital hip dislocation, joint contractures, genu valgum, dwarfism, and many healing problems in hard and soft tissues [1].

4.5 A "vital" biomechanical equation

Bone's remodeling threshold (MESr) lies below the modeling threshold (MESm), which lies below the microdamage threshold (MESp), which lies far below its ultimate strength (Fx). If "E" signifies the usual strains of any properly adapted bone, they tend to stay within the range bounded by the MESr and the MESm, which has been called the "adapted window" [17, 20].

Thus: $MESr < "E" < MESm \ll MESp \ll Fx$

That relationship seems to exist in all small and large bones of all healthy small and large amphibians, birds, mammals, and reptiles. If so, it would define a fundamental property of living lamellar bone. The mechanostat should orchestrate the modeling and remodeling activities that make it happen. Satisfying it would tend to minimize microdamage and spontaneous fractures. With different strain values, the relationship may also apply to cartilage, joints, tendons, ligaments, and fascia [1].

5 Muscle strength as a determinant of bone strength and "mass"

Mechanical loads cause the bone strains that strongly influence bone strength and "mass". A summary of the source(s) of those loads and some relevant physiology follows.

5.1 The largest loads on bones

With the exception of trauma, the largest loads on bones come from muscles. For example, when walking, running, and jumping, muscles must fight the resistance of the body's weight multiplied by the bad lever arms against which most muscles work [7, 37]. Therefore, it takes more than 2 kp of muscle force on bones to move each kilogram of body weight around during work and play. For that reason, the voluntary total load on a player's femur during a football or soccer game can briefly exceed five times body weight [7, 38].

5.2 Muscle strength

In view of the paradigm, muscle forces dominate most (not all) non-mechanical influences on postnatal bone strength and "mass". This old idea [39] still troubles some, but nevertheless it has very strong support. Genetic effects aside, postnatal muscle strength depends on two general factors.

- The growth-dependent factor:
  Endocrine and related elements control muscle growth before maturity [40. 41]. In children, they can increase muscle strength without requiring weight-lifting-type exercises. Muscle strength depends partly upon growth

hormone and somatomedins [42–45], and upon androgens after puberty in males [46]. Increased muscle strength from this factor correspondingly increases bone loads, strains, modeling, and bone strength and "mass" (see **Note 3**, i.e., **Section 8.3**). This factor would plateau in young adults and would decline in aging adults [47].

- The mechanical usage factor:
  Increasing the resistance against which muscles work (as in weight lifting) can increase muscle strength at any age [48–50], but more so in children than in adults, probably due to help from the above mentioned growth-dependent factor. As the resistance that muscles work against increases during growth, their strength and the loads they put on bones increase correspondingly. In young adults, weight-lifting-type exercises or activities can further increase muscle strength, but less markedly than in children and adolescents [32, 51, 52].

- On muscle strength and endurance:
  Weight lifting can increase muscle strength, while marathon running can increase muscle endurance; but excelling at one seems to prevent excelling at the other. Good weight lifters make poor marathon runners, and vice versa. Marathon running puts far more numerous but smaller loads on bones than weight lifting [33].

- Muscle strength and aging:
  Usually muscle strength increases during general growth. It plateaus in most young human adults, and after 30 years of age slowly declines [47, 53–55]. This steadily decreases muscle forces on aging bones that had adapted to stronger young-adult muscles, so such bones would begin a gradual-onset partial disuse [18, 34]. At 80 years of age, less than half the young-adult muscle strength can remain [53]; 60–70% of their young-adult bone strength and "mass" usually remains at that age. Aging adults who retain most of their young-adult muscle strength usually retain most of their young-adult bone strength and "mass", too. Such adults usually do arduous physical work, and include lumberjacks, farmers, steelworkers, and weight lifters [18, 51].

5.3 The adaptational "lag and catch up" [4, 56, 57]

During growth, body weight and muscle strength keep increasing. Modeling tries to increase bone strength and "mass" to satisfy those increasing loads, but it is sluggish so it lags behind. This lets bone strains exceed the modeling threshold and turn modeling ON (see **Notes 2** and **4**, i.e., **Sections 8.2** and **8.4**). In young adults, body weight and muscle strength usually plateau, so the adaptations can "catch up" to the need, down-shift bone strains below the modeling threshold range, and turn modeling OFF. Then bone strength and "mass" should plateau too [32]. As a result, bone strains from voluntary activities during growth should exceed those in adults (see **Note 1**, i.e., **Section 8.1**).

During growth this adaptational lag should cause a modest bone-strength deficit relative to the needs of muscle strength, body weight, and physical activities. If growth increases for a while, this strength deficit should increase, leading to a higher likelihood of fractures. Indeed, fractures do increase during our adolescent growth spurt [58–60]. They decrease in young adults as the "catch up" occurs.

5.4 Two meanings of "vigorous" mechanical usage

Exercise to exhaustion by adults, as in marathon running, jogging, aerobics, or swimming, is one meaning of "vigorous". It does not increase adult bone strength and "mass" [32, 61]. Such exercises cause relatively small loads on bones, creating enough strain to turn conservation-mode remodeling ON, but not enough to turn modeling ON [33] (**Fig. 13-4**). Since the largest voluntary bone loads and strains control bone modeling, and since weight lifters have stronger muscles than marathon runners, weight lifters should have the greater bone strength and "mass" [33, 62–64]. Activities such as weight lifting provide another meaning of "vigorous" (see **Note 1**, i.e., **Section 8.1**).

6　A synthesis
(of the normal determinants of bone strength and "mass")

6.1　In juveniles

In juveniles, steadily increasing body weight and muscle loads on bones, plus the adaptational lag, would let strains exceed the modeling threshold and turn modeling ON to increase bone strength and "mass", while conservation-mode remodeling would retain the added bone. Aided by the growth-dependent factor(s), more strenuous activities could further up-shift bone strains to increase bone strength and "mass" faster than before (see **Note 5**, i.e., **Section 8.5**).

6.2　In young adults

In young adults, bone loads and the growth-dependent factor usually plateau to allow modeling to "catch up" and make bones strong enough to down-shift strains below the modeling threshold. This would turn modeling OFF but leave conservation-mode remodeling ON; so bone strength and "mass" also plateau. For physical exercise to increase bone strength and "mass", muscle strength should increase enough to up-shift strains into the modeling threshold. Weight lifting could do this, but not activities that cause smaller loads and strains, no matter how exhausting. Lacking the juvenile's growth-dependent factor, young adults should find it harder than juveniles to increase their bone strength and "mass" through physical exercise [32, 51, 52].

6.3　In aging adults

In aging adults, decreasing muscle strength, plus bones adapted to young-adult muscle strength, should put their bones into gradual-onset disuse. Strains would down-shift into the re-modeling threshold to turn modeling OFF and disuse-mode remodeling ON; thus bone strength and "mass" should decrease.

Up-shifting their bone strains into the modeling threshold could require doubling or tripling their muscle strength, which few aging adults can achieve. In humans, walking, running, cycling, swimming, and aerobics do not suffice, but they can cause large enough strains to make conservation-mode remodeling minimize further bone losses.

6.4　Aging and remodeling

An age-related inability to create formation drifts cannot explain the inability of physical exercise to turn modeling ON in older adults, because cortical modeling drifts can appear in adult acromegaly, lues, Paget disease of bone, some infections, osteoid osteomas, and fracture malunions [65–68]. Here, any separate aging effect should mainly affect the rate of such drifts, and perhaps their starting and end points, instead of preventing them completely [69].

7　Comments

Mentioned here are a few things of clinical interest that the "common mechanism" (mentioned in the Introduction and described above) participates in. Cited references contain more information.

7.1　Remodeling functions [1, 10, 19, 20]

The known functions of BMU-based remodeling include removing mechanically bone that is not required (usually that next to marrow) and repairing microdamage, as described above. They include replacing fracture callus with lamellar bone and replacing the primary spongiosa beneath growth plates with the permanent secondary spongiosa made of lamellar bone [19]. Failure of these functions can contribute to osteopetrosis [70], spontaneous fractures [10, 17], failures of bone healing [25, 71], and failures of bone allografts [72] (see **Section 7.7**). Remodeling can also help in calcium homeostasis.

7.2 Homeostasis

BMU-based remodeling and osteoclasts were long viewed as essential in controlling calcium homeostasis. That was also often assumed to be their main function [73–75]. But, both ideas seem to be untrue.

- Remodeling and BMUs are essential for the functions mentioned in **Section 7.1** as well as in **Sections 7.5** and **7.7**, but,
- Bone's role in homeostasis can usually work quite well in their absence; at least in the short term. While this is not yet generally known in the skeletal basic science community, **Note 8**, i.e., **Section 8.8**, mentions some proof of this. Still, remodeling (not osteoclasts alone) does help to maintain homeostasis during prolonged periods of severe calcium deprivation or malabsorption.

7.3 Modeling functions [1, 7, 19]

The known functions of bone modeling by drifts include adjusting bone architecture and "mass" in order to make bones strong enough to prevent normal mechanical usage and physical activities from breaking them or making them hurt. Failure to do this causes some osteoporoses and contributes to osteogenesis imperfecta [1]. Its functions also include reshaping healing fractures and bone grafts so they provide enough strength to meet the mechanical demands put on them by an individual's usual physical activities. Failure to do this leads to some late failures of bone grafts, spinal fusions and other arthrodeses, and of fracture healing [71] (see **Section 7.7**).

7.4 Roles of non-mechanical agents and factors

With the exception of longitudinal bone growth and bone's signaling mechanisms, knowledge of the cell-biological and molecular-biological factors in bone increased rapidly after 1960, but it mainly concerned osteoblasts, osteoclasts, and their immediate precursor cells [73, 74]. It emphasized biochemistry, endocrinology, cytokines, and other cell-level factors (**Tab. 13-2**). It did not study how non-mechanical agents affect the tissue-level responses of modeling and remodeling to mechanical challenges, or their effects on bone strength and "mass". Consequently we do not yet know how such agents affect those responses, nor do we know the cell and molecular biology on which those responses depend. Further research must determine this [76] (see **Note 6**, i.e., **Section 8.6**). Important mechanical challenges include microdamage, acute and chronic disuse, and acute and chronic hypervigorous mechanical usage. The few such studies done so far were unusually informative [77–88]. At present, poor interdisciplinary communication in skeletal science causes some controversy in these matters (see **Note 7**, i.e., **Section 8.7**).

7.5 Some implications for osteoporosis

- Lowering the modeling and remodeling thresholds should increase bone strength and "mass", while raising the thresholds would reduce them [35, 89]. Modeling's responses to overly vigorous mechanical usage could cure osteopenia, remodeling's responses could prevent it, and disuse-mode remodeling can cause it. To cure osteopenia, research should seek things that turn modeling ON, as some prostaglandins and intermittent parathyroid hormone treatment can do [82, 86, 90–93]. To prevent osteopenia in adults, research should seek things that turn conservation-mode remodeling ON, which estrogen and some bisphosphonates can do [30, 94–96]. To prevent osteopenia in children, research should seek things that turn both modeling and conservation-mode remodeling ON.
- A normal mechanostat would lead to physical inactivity and decreased muscle strength causing corresponding osteopenia, in which the individual's usual activities would not cause spontaneous fractures or bone pain. Of course, the osteopenia would increase the likelihood of falls and other injuries causing fractures, mainly of

Tab. 13-2: Some non-mechanical agents that can influence skeletal physiology (modified from Frost [1]).

Natural agents		
Estrogen	Androgens	Growth hormone
Calcitonin	Somatomedins	Insulin
Parathormone	Thyroxine	Vitamin D
D metabolites	Vitamin A	Other vitamins
Dietary calcium	Magnesium	Iron, copper
Growth factors	Morphogens	Mitogens
Membrane pumps	Ligands	Membrane receptors
Apoptosis	Other cytokines	Paracrine effects
Autocrine effects	Cell–cell interactions	ACTH, FSH, TSH
Amino acids	Lipids	Prolactin
SER, RER	DNA, RNA	Genes
Cell–intercellular matrix interactions	others	

Drugs and other artificial agents		
Hormone analogs	Vitamin analogues	Bisphosphonates
Electric fields	Magnetic fields	Fluoride
All other synthetic or chemically modified natural agents	Non-steroidal anti-inflammatory agents	others

extremity bones (wrist, hip) [1, 34]. This should explain most of the bone loss in most aging humans, even if other age-related factors also contribute. This condition occurs often. It was recently called a "physiologic osteopenia" [97].

- A mechanostat disorder could reduce bone strength and "mass" so that a patient's usual physical activities and muscle strength cause spontaneous fractures and/or bone pain. However, the fractures and pain affect the spine more than extremity bones [97]. Here too, injuries such as falls could fracture extremity bones. This condition was recently called a "true osteoporosis".

- Such observations suggested that comparing muscle strength to absorptiometric estimates of bone strength might help to classify, evaluate, and manage osteopenia and osteoporoses better than absorptiometric measurements of bone mineral "density" and content alone [3, 5, 8, 9, 25, 98].

7.6   Implications for implant design

Clearly, the design of load-bearing implants should try to satisfy the above "vital biomechanical equation", firstly to prevent strains in the bone supporting the implants from exceeding the modeling threshold, and thus to keep them well below the microdamage threshold [13]. Equally clearly, the design should keep strains in the supporting bone from approaching or falling below the remodeling threshold, since this would cause local bone loss. Burr et al. [99] suggested a microdamage threshold in 1983 and Carter demonstrated one in 1984 [100]. Yet no such implant marketed in 1997 was specifically designed to keep bone strains below that threshold. However, the dental implant system designed by Branemark appears to have done so incidentally [101].

7.7 Implications for fracture and bone-graft healing

Implications for fracture and bone-graft healing are that healing occurs in broad and partly overlapping callus, remodeling and modeling phases, aided by a regional acceleratory phenomenon [1, 66, 71, 102].

- First, a fracture callus forms. It contains newly created vessels, supporting and precursor cells, osteoblasts that make woven bone, and often chondroblasts that make hyaline cartilage. In a fracture the callus fills the gap(s) and surrounds the fragments. In a bone graft the callus embeds and surrounds the graft material. The callus is chiefly isotropic (it lacks long-range order) with respect to any loads on it.
- Then BMU-based remodeling begins to replace the callus (and any graft material) with packets of new lamellar bone, the grain of which is parallel to the largest strains of the callus.
- In response to, and guided by, strains of the callus, modeling drifts begin to modify its shape and size to make it strong enough for the loads on it. Completion of these phases in humans can take 1 year in a child and over 5 years in adults, and longer in large than in small bones.

It has become clear that small strains help to guide the remodeling and modeling phases of bone healing [1, 103, 104]. Lacking any strains, disuse-mode remodeling tends to remove the callus, while modeling remains OFF. This can cause failed or inadequate healing. Excessive strains (i.e., gross motion) can also impair or prevent healing. The permissible strains may lie in the adapted and mild overload "windows" shown in **Fig. 13-4**; between 50–100 and 3,000 microstrain, they are small. Note that it takes very small loads to cause such small strains in compliant, still healing fractures or bone grafts.

The regional acceleratory phenomenon begins at the time of the fracture or bone-grafting operation. It is normal, and it speeds up the above healing processes. When it fails to develop, a delayed union or a "biological failure" of bone healing can occur.

8 Notes

8.1 On bone strains in vivo

Before in vivo strain studies were available, clinical-pathological evidence suggested that

- Modeling drifts provide additions of bone strength and "mass".
- Bone strains from voluntary activities control the drifts.
- The drifts respond to the average of those strains instead of responding to rare or single ones.
- A few large strains have a far greater effect than small ones, no matter how numerous.
- Changing, as opposed to constant, strains control the drifts.
- Some minimum effective strain (MES) switches these drifts ON, otherwise they stay OFF.
- Modeling drifts are rate-limited; they cannot exceed a certain maximum speed. While controversial at the time [105], subsequent studies in many animal species and humans verified all those ideas, and current work concerns their values and how to express them [10, 22, 32, 36, 50, 89, 106–112].
- Those studies show that peak bone strains from voluntary effort can rise to around 2,000–4,000 microstrain in most rapidly growing subjects, but peak around 800–1,300 microstrain in most adults. Strains above 3,000 microstrain tend to cause woven bone formation instead of lamellar bone [107, 113].

Nota bene: The strain values quoted in this text apply to longitudinal tension and compression. They need more study; shear, strain gradients, their rates and frequencies, strain energy density, etc. may also help to control a bone's architectural adaptations [7, 114, 115]. Until these matters are resolved, the longitudinal strains can provide useful indices, and reliable evidence of the loads on a bone. For such reasons, wherever this article mentions strain as an influence on a biological activity, the qualifier, "or equivalent stimulus", always applies.

8.2 On the combined modeling and remodeling effects on bone strength and "mass"

It may help to look at the "comfort zone" or adapted window in **Fig. 13-4** in the following way:

*   Where bone strains from voluntary activities stay in the middle of that zone, conservation-mode remodeling retains bone strength and "mass" but modeling is OFF, so bone strength and "mass" would plateau. This "adapted window" would apply to most healthy young adults.
*   Where strains down-shift into the remodeling threshold range, disuse-mode remodeling begins reducing bone strength and "mass", while modeling remains OFF. This would apply to most aging older adults and would cause an osteopenia relative to the bone strength and "mass" in young adult life.
*   Where strains up-shift to, or above, the modeling threshold, modeling turns ON to increase bone strength and "mass", while conservation-mode remodeling retains existing bone. This "mild overload window" would apply to healthy children and other growing mammals. To repeat, mainly the size of the strains matters here. The size of the loads on a bone combined with the bone's strength (not its bone "mass" alone) would mainly determine the size of the strains.
*   The true aim of modeling would lie in adjusting bone stiffness to keep strains from exceeding the modeling threshold. But, given nearly constant materials properties, increasing a bone's stiffness usually also requires increasing its strength, so strength can provide a surrogate for stiffness that non-engineers can understand more easily. Accordingly, this text refers to bone strength instead of stiffness.

8.3 On the role of growth hormone in bone's vital biomechanics

According to current general belief, growth hormone (and/or related somatomedins) enables and stimulates osteoblastic activity to cause the increased bone strength and "mass" in gigantism and acromegaly [42–44, 116, 117]. For this reason, some readers might wonder why this text places more emphasis on vital biomechanics than endocrinology. Several factors are involved:

*   Growth hormone increases muscle strength [41, 118], which increases the bone strains that can turn modeling-associated osteoblastic activity ON.
*   The hormone stimulates longitudinal bone growth in children [19, 118]. Increased bone length increases the bending strains of bones that can turn cortical bone modeling ON, so it tends to potentiate muscle-force effects on a child's bone strains and modeling. Growth plates close at skeletal maturity, so adults lack this strain-increasing effect.
*   In hypophysectomized young rats, the osteoblastic activity, associated with modeling, stopped, while that associated with remodeling continued in the same bone [77, 88]. This is part of the acute partial disuse pattern described in **Section 3.1**. Longitudinal bone growth, muscle weight, and body weight stopped increasing too, and the hypophysectomized animals became inactive in their cages so that their bones entered partial disuse. This could explain the varied osteoblastic activity while hormonal control at the cellular level could not.
*   In another experiment, adult rats suspended by the tail, to prevent weight bearing on the hind limbs, received added growth hormone. Their hind-limb muscles could still contract freely, but without the resistance of body weight multiplied by bad lever arms. Muscle weight increased in the hind limbs, but modeling-associated osteoblastic activity in hind-limb bones did not increase [78]. Direct stimulation of osteoblasts by the hormone cannot easily explain

these facts, as opposed to the hormone's effects on muscle strength and bone loads.

- Previous analyses of this matter did not account for the effects of muscle strength, longitudinal bone growth, and physical activities on bone strains, or for how these strains can affect both modeling and remodeling.
- It is still possible that this hormone increases the responsiveness of modeling and remodeling to mechanical influences.

8.4   The role of large bone strains

Body weight, muscle strength, and bone length steadily increase during growth [40], which increases bone loads and strains. The magnitude of a bone's strain depends upon the relationship between a its strength and the loads imposed upon it [1, 7]. Strains above the modeling threshold would determine the location, type, and degree of any strength deficit.

8.5   On the locations of small and large bone strains

- While bone strains from voluntary activities can exceed the modeling threshold in children and other rapidly growing mammals, this does not happen in all parts of a given bone at any one time. In some parts (e.g., most metaphyseal secondary spongiosa) the strains could stay below that threshold [1, 57]. Where they exceed the threshold (e.g., most diaphyseal compacta), modeling would switch ON to increase the local bone strength and "mass". The excess of such increases over the losses provides the global increases in bone strength and "mass" that normally occur during growth [56, 57]. Compact bone comprises about 80% of the total bone "mass" [119].
- As evidence that the above-described mechanical usage "story" is still incomplete (should anyone want such evidence), our cranial vault and turbinates do not carry large enough loads to explain their strength,

architecture, and bone "mass" in the same terms that seem to apply to femurs, radii, and vertebral bodies. This article summarizes more about such matters than we understood even 10 years ago, but still not all. Nevertheless, a better understanding of the roles of non-mechanical and mechanical influences on the skeleton did crystallize after 1990, based on evidence and ideas from many fields of skeletal science.

8.6   On roles of non-mechanical agents

Tab. 13-2 lists a few non-mechanical agents. Many of them can help, or hinder, the effects of mechanical usage and muscle strength on bone strength and "mass", but none can replace those effects in paralyzed or otherwise amyotonic limbs. To explain:

- At birth the initial conditions (baseline conditions) of bone architecture already exist, as do the biological mechanisms that can adapt bones to their postnatal mechanical usage and loads. In addition, the "game-rules" that govern the responses of those mechanisms to mechanical and non-mechanical influences also exist.
- After birth, bone architecture and strength differ predictably in congenitally or neonatally paralyzed, or otherwise amyotonic, limbs and in the contralateral limbs with normal muscles and neuromuscular function.
- The features of the neonatally paralyzed limb show the baseline conditions, unaffected by normal post-natal mechanical usage.
- The differences between the paralyzed and normal limbs show the mechanical usage and loading effects added to the baseline conditions in the normal limb. This article concerns those differences [1].
- During growth, heavier loads on bones make bones bigger; this also applies to joints, tendons, ligaments, and fascia.

These differences need systematic study. Clinical and pathological observations, from times when polio residuals were common, suggest that postnatal mechanical usage in normal limbs could account for 80% of their bone strength and "mass".

8.7 On perspective and controversy

Applications of the new paradigm are currently in flux in the skeletal science, medical, and surgical communities, and some readers might like to know more.

Up to 1990, vital biomechanics had few clear applications in the management of clinical problems. Many applications became apparent after 1990, but poor interdisciplinary communication left many in skeletal science and medicine unaware of, or perhaps unsure about them. Thus, most reviews explained bone physiology mainly on non-mechanical, cell and molecular biological grounds (biochemistry, genetics, diet, endocrinology, cell and molecular biology, etc.) and ignored, or paid lip service to, the tissue and organ-level vital biomechanics. The uniquely seminal Hard Tissue Workshops, sponsored annually by the University of Utah since 1965, provide an outstanding exception.

While the non-mechanical factors are clearly essential, they are not sufficient, and the equally essential but belatedly perceived vital biomechanics supplements them. The non-mechanical and vital-biomechanical "faces" of skeletal physiology are as essential to health and as dependent upon each other as lungs and hearts in all air-breathing vertebrates. Conflict arises when people, used to thinking the non-mechanical face was "the whole thing", confront the idea that it is not and the need to learn the vital-biomechanical face to understand how both faces collaborate in life. Also, this conflict stems far less from the vital-biomechanical evidence than from its meanings or implications, which can modify some former ideas about the pathogenesis, nature, and management of disease. The meanings reveal the indissoluble dependence of cell and molecular biology on tissue and organ-level physiology and vital biomechanics. Like other scientific controversies, this one will resolve and skeletal science, surgery, and medicine will be all the better for it.

8.8 Remodeling and homeostasis

The statements in **Section 7.2** may disturb some skeletal scientists, since after Fuller Albright's pioneering ideas [120] the idea that remodeling and osteoclasts are essential for homeostasis became a bone-physiological dogma [73–75]. However, experiments with adult dogs in the 1970s with the bisphosphonate known as Didronel showed that large enough doses of the agent eliminated detectable functioning osteoclasts (and osteoblasts) for the duration of the treatment (9 months). Yet none of the 20 animals developed hypercalcemia or hypocalcemia, tetany, acidosis, or alkalosis [121]. Parenthetically, the dose also caused spontaneous fractures that did not heal until treatment with the agent stopped [94]. For these reasons, research must show that bisphosphonates, intended for human use, do not cause spontaneous fractures or impair bone healing.

Bone has at least three other cell-driven mechanisms that contribute to homeostasis, but so far have received little attention from interested physiologists. They seem to provide bone's main defense against short-term challenges to that homeostasis [1].

A natural experiment supports the above statements and initially led the author to consider them in the 1960s. While osteoclasts are absent or profoundly reduced in number and function in osteopetrosis, problems with calcium homeostasis, tetany, and acid-base physiology are not common in this disease [122]. Yet if those cells were essential for homeostasis, such problems would be common.

9 Bibliography

Blue references indicate links to abstracts of articles available online:
http://www.aopublishing.org/BONE/13.htm

1. **Frost HM** (1995) *Introduction to a New Skeletal Physiology.* Pueblo, CO: The Pajaro Group.
2. **Frost HM** (1996) Bone development during childhood: Insights from a new paradigm. In: Schönau E, editor. *Paediatric Osteology. New Trends and Developments in Diagnostics and Therapy.* Amsterdam: Elsevier Science Publishers.
3. **Frost HM, Ferretti JL, Jee WS** (1998) Perspectives: some roles of mechanical usage, muscle strength, and the mechanostat in skeletal physiology, disease, and research. *Calcif Tissue Int;* 62 (1):1–7.
4. **Jee WSS, Frost HM** (1992) Skeletal adaptations during growth. *Triangle* (Ciba Geigy); 31:77.
5. **Schönau E, Werhahn E, Schiedermaier U, et al.** (1996) Bone and muscle development during childhood in health and disease. In: Schönau E, editor. *Paediatric Osteology. New Developments in Diagnostics and Therapy.* Amsterdam: Elsevier, 147.
6. **Takahashi HE** (1995) *Spinal Disorders and Growth and Aging.* Berlin Heidelberg New York: Springer-Verlag.
7. **Martin RB, Burr DB** (1989) *Structure, Function and Adaptation of Compact Bone.* New York: Raven Press.
8. **Ferretti JL** (1995) Perspectives of pQCT technology associated to biomechanical studies in skeletal research employing rat models. *Bone;* 17 (4 Suppl):353S–364S.
9. **Gasser JA** (1995) Assessing bone quantity by pQCT. *Bone;* 17 (4 Suppl): 145S–154S.
10. **Burr DB, Forwood MR, Fyhrie DP, et al.** (1997) Bone microdamage and skeletal fragility in osteoporotic and stress fractures. *J Bone Miner Res;* 12 (1):6–15.
11. **Carter DR, Caler WE, Spengler DM, et al.** (1981) Fatigue behavior of adult cortical bone: the influence of mean strain and strain range. *Acta Orthop Scand;* 52 (5):481–490.
12. **Schaffler MB, Choi K, Milgrom C** (1995) Aging and matrix microdamage accumulation in human compact bone. *Bone;* 17 (6):521–525.
13. **Frost HM** (1992) Perspectives on artificial joint design. *J Long Term Eff Med Implants;* 2 (1):9–35.
14. **Frost HM** (1966) *Bone Dynamics in Osteoporosis and Osteomalacia.* Springfield, MA: Charles C Thomas.
15. **Heaney RP** (1993) Is there a role for bone quality in fragility fractures? *Calcif Tissue Int;* 53 (Suppl 1):S3–5; discussion S5–6.
16. **Pattin CA, Caler WE, Carter DR** (1996) Cyclic mechanical property degradation during fatigue loading of cortical bone. *J Biomech;* 29 (1):69–79.
17. **Kimmel DB** (1993) A paradigm for skeletal strength homeostasis. *J Bone Miner Res;* 8 Suppl 2:S515–522.
18. **Riggs BL, Melton LF, III,** (1995) *Osteoporosis. Etiology, Diagnosis and Treatment.* 2nd ed. Philadelphia: Lippincott-Raven Publishers.
19. **Jee WSS** (1989) The skeletal tissues. In: Weiss L, editor. *Cell and Tissue Biology. A Textbook of Histology.* Baltimore: Urban and Schwartzenberg, 211.
20. **Frost HM** (1992) Perspectives: bone's mechanical usage windows. *Bone Miner;* 19 (3):257–271.
21. **Burr DB, Martin RB, Schaffler MB, et al.** (1985) Bone remodeling in response to in vivo fatigue microdamage. *J Biomech;* 18 (3):189–200.
22. **Burr DB** (1993) Remodeling and the repair of fatigue damage. *Calcif Tissue Int;* 53 (Suppl 1):75–80; discussion 80–71.
23. **Mori S, Burr DB** (1993) Increased intracortical remodeling following fatigue damage. *Bone;* 14 (2):103–109.
24. **Jee WSS** (1995) Proceedings of the International Conference on Animal Models in the Prevention and Treatment of Osteopenia. Cairns, Australia, February 11–13, 1995. *Bone;* 17 (4 Suppl):113S–469S.
25. **Schönau E** (1996) New developments in diagnostics and therapy.
26. **Wronski TJ, Morey ER** (1983) Effect of spaceflight on periosteal bone formation in rats. *Am J Physiol;* 244 (3):R305–309.
27. **Wronski TJ, Morey ER** (1983) Inhibition of cortical and trabecular bone formation in the long bones of immobilized monkeys. *Clin Orthop;* (181):269–276.
28. **Wronski TJ, Walsh CC, Ignaszewski LA** (1986) Histologic evidence for osteopenia and increased bone turnover in ovariectomized rats. *Bone;* 7 (2):119–123.
29. **Wronski TJ, Schenck PA, Cintron M, et al.** (1987) Effect of body weight on osteopenia in ovariecto-mized rats. *Calcif Tissue Int;* 40 (3): 155–159.
30. **Wronski TJ, Dann LM, Qi H, et al.** (1993) Skeletal effects of withdrawal of estrogen and diphosphonate treatment in ovariectomized rats. *Calcif Tissue Int;* 53 (3):210–216.
31. **Currey JD** (1984) *The Mechanical Adaptations of Bones.* Princeton: Princeton University Press.
32. **Forwood MR, Burr DB** (1993) Physical activity and bone mass: exercises in futility? *Bone Miner;* 21 (2):89–112.
33. **Frost HM** (1997) Perspectives: Why do long distance runners not have more bone? A vital biomechanical explanation and an estrogen effect. *J Bone Min Res;* 15:9.
34. **Avioli LV** (1993) *The Osteoporotic Syndrome.* 3rd ed. New York: Wiley-Liss.

35. **Frost HM** (1987) Bone "mass" and the "mechanostat": a proposal. *Anat Rec;* 219 (1):1–9.

36. **Turner CH, Forwood MR** (1995) Bone adaptation to mechanical forces in the rat tibia. In: Odgaard A, Weinans H, editors. *Bone Structure and Remodelling.* London: World Scientific, 65.

37. **Nordin M, Frankel VH** (1989) *Basic Biomechanics of the Musculo-skeletal System. 2nd ed.* Philadelphia: Lea and Febiger.

38. **Crowninshield RD, Johnston RC, Andrews JG, et al.** (1978) A bio-mechanical investigation of the human hip. *J Biomech;* 11 (1–2): 75–85.

39. **Thompson DW** (1917) *On Growth and Form.* Cambridge: University of Cambridge Press.

40. **Vaughn VC, McKay RJ, Nelson WE** (1975). *Nelson Textbook of Pediatrics. 10th ed.* Philadelphia: WB Saunders Co.

41. **Wilson JD, Foster DW** (1992) *William's Textbook of Endocrinology. 8th ed.* Philadelphia: W. B. Saunders Co.

42. **Inzucchi SE, Robbins RJ** (1994) Clinical review 61: Effects of growth hormone on human bone biology. *J Clin Endocrinol Metab;* 79 (3):691–694.

43. **Ohlsson C, Isgaard J, Tornell J, et al.** (1993) Endocrine regulation of longitudinal bone growth. *Acta Paediatr Suppl;* 82 Suppl 391:33–40; discussion 41.

44. **Raisz LG** (1988) Hormonal regula-tion of bone growth and remodelling. *Ciba Found Symp;* 136:226–238.

45. **Venable JH** (1966) Morphology of the cells of normal, testosterone-deprived and testosterone-stimulated levator ani muscles. *Am J Anat;* 119 (2):271–301.

46. **Bhasin S, Storer TW, Berman N, et al.** (1996) The effects of supra-physiologic doses of testosterone on muscle size and strength in normal men. *N Engl J Med;* 335 (1):1–7.

47. **Buckwalter JA, Woo SL, Goldberg VM, et al.** (1993) Soft-tissue aging and musculoskeletal function. *J Bone Joint Surg [Am];* 75 (10):1533–1548.

48. **Colletti LA, Edwards J, Gordon L, et al.** (1989) The effects of muscle-building exercise on bone mineral density of the radius, spine, and hip in young men. *Calcif Tissue Int;* 45 (1): 12–14.

49. **Heinonen A, Sievanen H, Kannus P, et al.** (1996) Effects of unilateral strength training and detraining on bone mineral mass and estimated mechanical characteristics of the upper limb bones in young women. *J Bone Miner Res;* 11 (4):490–501.

50. **Sievanen H, Heinonen A, Kannus P** (1996) Adaptation of bone to altered loading environment: a biomechanical approach using x-ray absorptiometric data from the patella of a young woman. *Bone;* 19 (1):55–59.

51. **Smith EL, Gilligan C** (1989) Mechanical forces and bone. *J Bone Min Res;* 6:139.

52. **Tsuji S, Katsukawa F, Onishi S, et al.** (1996) Period of adolescence during which exercise maximizes bone mass in young women. *J Bone Min Res;* 14:89.

53. **Faulkner JA, Brooks SV, Zerva E** (1990) Skeletal muscle weakness and fatigue in old age: Underlying mechanisms. In: Cristofalo VJ, Lawton MP, editors. *Annual Review of Gerontology and Geriatrics.* Berlin Heidelberg New York: Springer-Verlag, 147.

54. **McCarter RJ** (1990) Age-related changes in skeletal muscle function. *Aging (Milano);* 2 (1):27–38.

55. **Young A, Stokes M, Crowe M** (1984) Size and strength of the quadriceps muscles of old and young women. *Eur J Clin Invest;* 14 (4): 282–287.

56. **Frost HM, Jee WS** (1994) Perspectives: a vital biomechanical model of the endochondral ossification mechanism. *Anat Rec;* 240 (4): 435–446.

57. **Frost HM, Jee WS** (1994) Perspectives: applications of a biomechanical model of the endochondral ossification mechanism. *Anat Rec;* 240 (4): 447–455.

58. **Frost HM** (1997) Perspectives: On increased fractures during the human adolescent growth spurt. Summary of a new vital-biomechanical explanation. *J Bone Min Res;* 15:115.

59. **Parfitt AM** (1986) Cortical porosity in postmenopausal and adolescent wrist fractures. In: Uhthoff H, editor. *Current Concepts of Bone Fragility.* Berlin Heidelberg New York: Springer-Verlag, 167.

60. **Rockwood CA, Jr., Green DP** (1991) *Fractures in Children. 3rd ed.* Philadelphia, PA: J.B. Lippincott.

61. **Murray MP, Gardner GM, Mollinger LA, et al.** (1980) Strength of isometric and isokinetic contractions: knee muscles of men aged 20 to 86. *Phys Ther;* 60 (4):412–419.

62. **Karlsson MK, Johnell O, Obrant KJ** (1993) Bone mineral density in weight lifters. *Calcif Tissue Int;* 52 (3): 212–215.

63. **Micklesfield LK, Lambert EV, Fataar AB, et al.** (1995) Bone mineral density in mature, premeno-pausal ultramarathon runners. *Med Sci Sports Exerc;* 27 (5):688–696.

64. **Robinson TL, Snow-Harter C, Taaffe DR, et al.** (1995) Gymnasts exhibit higher bone mass than runners despite similar prevalence of amenorrhea and oligomenorrhea. *J Bone Miner Res;* 10 (1):26–35.

65. **Bogomil GP, Schwamm HA** (1984) *Orthopaedic Pathology: A synopsis with clinical and radiographic correlation.* Philadelphia: WB Saunders Co.

66. **Damjanov I, Linder J** (1996) *Anderson's Pathology.* St. Louis: C. V. Moseby Co.

67. **Jaffe H** (1972) *Metabolic, Degenerative and Inflammatory Diseases of Bones and Joints.* Philadelphia: Lea and Febiger.

68. **Jubb KVF, Kennedy PC, Palmer N** (1985) *Pathology of Domestic Animals.* New York: Academic Press:135–145.

69. **Turner CH, Forwood MR, Rho JY, et al.** (1994) Mechanical loading thresholds for lamellar and woven bone formation. *J Bone Miner Res;* 9 (1):87–97.

70. **Milgram JW, Jasty M** (1982) Osteopetrosis. A morphological study of twenty-one cases. *J Bone Joint Surg [Am];* 64 (6):912–929.

71. **Frost HM** (1989) The biology of fracture healing. An overview for clinicians. Part I. *Clin Orthop;* (248): 283–293.

72. **Aho AJ, Ekfors T, Dean PB, et al.** (1994) Incorporation and clinical results of large allografts of the extremities and pelvis. *Clin Orthop;* (307):200–213.

73. **Bilezikian JP, Raisz LG, Rodan GA** (1996) *Principles of Bone Biology.* San Diego: Academic Press.

74. **Favus MJ** (1996) *Primer on the Metabolic Bone Diseases and Disorders of Mineral Metabolism. 3rd ed.* New York: Lippincott-Raven Press.

75. **McLean FC, Urist MR** (1961) *Bone. 2nd ed.* Chicago: University of Chicago Press.

76. **Kalu DN** (1995) Evolution of the pathogenesis of postmenopausal bone loss. *Bone;* 17 (4 Suppl):135S–144S.

77. **Chen MM, Yeh JK, Aloia JF** (1995) Skeletal alterations in hypophysectomized rats: II. A histomorphometric study on tibial cortical bone. *Anat Rec;* 241 (4):513–518.

78. **Halloran BP, Bikle DD, Harris J, et al.** (1995) Skeletal unloading induces selective resistance to the anabolic actions of growth hormone on bone. *J Bone Miner Res;* 10 (8): 1168–1176.

79. **Jee WS, Li XJ** (1990) Adaptation of cancellous bone to overloading in the adult rat: a single photon absorptiometry and histomorphometry study. *Anat Rec;* 227 (4):418–426.

80. **Jee WS, Li XJ, Schaffler MB** (1991) Adaptation of diaphyseal structure with aging and increased mechanical usage in the adult rat: a histomorphometrical and biomechanical study. *Anat Rec;* 230 (3):332–338.

81. **Jee WSS, Li XJ, Ke HZ** (1991) The skeletal adaptation to mechanical usage in the rat. *Cells Mater;* S1:131.

82. **Jee WS, Ke HZ, Li XJ** (1991) Long-term anabolic effects of prostaglandin-E2 on tibial diaphyseal bone in male rats. *Bone Miner;* 15 (1):33–55.

83. **Li XJ, Jee WS** (1991) Adaptation of diaphyseal structure to aging and decreased mechanical loading in the adult rat: a densitometric and histomorphometric study. *Anat Rec;* 229 (3):291–297.

84. **Li XJ, Jee WS, Chow SY, et al.** (1990) Adaptation of cancellous bone to aging and immobilization in the rat: a single photon absorptiometry and histomorphometry study. *Anat Rec;* 227 (1):12–24.

85. **Li XJ, Jee WS, Li YL, et al.** (1990) Transient effects of subcutaneously administered prostaglandin E2 on cancellous and cortical bone in young adult dogs. *Bone;* 11 (5):353–364.

86. **Ma YF, Ferretti JL, Capozza RF, et al.** (1995) Effects of on/off anabolic hPTH and remodeling inhibitors on metaphyseal bone of immobilized rat femurs. Tomographical (pQCT) description and correlation with histomorphometric changes in tibial cancellous bone. *Bone;* 17 (4 Suppl): 321S–327S.

87. **Tang LY, Cullen DM, Yee JA, et al.** (1997) Prostaglandin E2 increases the skeletal response to mechanical loading. *J Bone Miner Res;* 12 (2):276–282.

88. **Yeh JK, Chen MM, Aloia JF** (1995) Skeletal alterations in hypophysectomized rats: I. A histomorphometric study on tibial cancellous bone. *Anat Rec;* 241 (4): 505–512.

89. **Burr DB, Martin RB** (1989) Errors in bone remodeling: toward a unified theory of metabolic bone disease. *Am J Anat;* 186 (2):186–216.

90. **High WB** (1987) Effects of orally administered prostaglandin E-2 on cortical bone turnover in adult dogs: a histomorphometric study. *Bone;* 8 (6):363–373.

91. **Jerome CP** (1994) Anabolic effect of high doses of human parathyroid hormone (1-38) in mature intact female rats. *J Bone Miner Res;* 9 (6): 933–942.

92. **Tada K, Yamamuro H, Kasai R, et al.** (1990) Therapeutic effects of h-PTH (1-34) on skeletons of osteoporotic rats with parathyroidectomy. In: Takahashi H, editor. *Bone Morphometry.* Tokyo: Springer Verlag, 448.

93. **Takahashi HE, Tanizawa T, Hori M, et al.** (1991) Effect of inter-mittent administration of human parathyroid hormone (1-34) on experimental osteopenia of rats induced by ovariectomy. *Cells Mater;* S1:113.

94. **Fleisch H** (1995) *Bisphosponates in Bone Disease. From the laboratory to the patient.* London: The Parthenon Publishing Group.

95. **Jee WS, Ma YF, Chow SY** (1995) Maintenance therapy for added bone mass or how to keep the profit after withdrawal of therapy of osteopenia. *Bone;* 17 (4 Suppl):309S–319S.

96. **Lindsay R, Tohme JF** (1990) Estrogen treatment of patients with established postmenopausal osteoporosis. *Obstet Gynecol;* 76 (2):290–295.

97. **Frost HM** (1997) On defining osteopenias and osteoporoses: Problems! Another view (with insights from a new paradigm). *Bone;* 20:385.

98. **Schiessl H, Ferretti JL, Tysarczk-Niemeyer G, et al.** (1996) Noninvasive bone strength index as analyzed by peripheral quantitative computed tomography (pQCT). In: Schönau E, editor. *Paediatric Osteology. New Developments in Diagnostics and Therapy.* Amsterdam: Elsevier, 141.

99. **Burr DB, Martin RB, Radin EL** (1983) Threshold values for the production of fatigue microdamage in bone in vivo. *Orthop Res Soc Abstr;* 69.

100. **Carter DR** (1984) Mechanical loading histories and cortical bone remodeling. *Calcif Tissue Int;* 36 (Suppl 1):S19–24.

101. **Branemark PI** (1988) Tooth replacement by oral endoprostheses: clinical aspects. *J Dent Educ;* 52 (12): 821–823.

102. **Woodard JC, Riser WH** (1991) Morphology of fracture nonunion and osteomyelitis. *Vet Clin North Am Small Anim Pract;* 21 (4):813–844.

103. **Aspenberg P, Goodman SB, Wang JS** (1996) Influence of callus deformation time. Bone chamber study in rabbits. *Clin Orthop;* (322):253–261.

104. **Blenman PR, Carter DR, Beaupre GS** (1989) Role of mechanical loading in the progressive ossification of a fracture callus. *J Orthop Res;* 7 (3):398–407.

105. **Frost HM** (1973) *Bone Modelling and Skeletal Modelling Errors.* Springfield: Charles C Thomas.

106. **Burr DB, Schaffler MB, Yang KH, et al.** (1989) The effects of altered strain environments on bone tissue kinetics. *Bone;* 10 (3):215–221.

107. **Burr DB, Schaffler MB, Yang KH, et al.** (1989) Skeletal change in response to altered strain environments: is woven bone a response to elevated strain? *Bone;* 10 (3):223–233.

108. **Burr DB, Milgrom C, Fyhrie D, et al.** (1996) In vivo measurement of human tibial strains during vigorous activity. *Bone;* 18 (5):405–410.

109. **Kannus P, Sievanen H, Vuori I** (1996) Physical loading, exercise, and bone. *Bone;* 18 (1 Suppl):1S–3S.

110. **Lanyon LE** (1996) Using functional loading to influence bone mass and architecture: objectives, mechanisms, and relationship with estrogen of the mechanically adaptive process in bone. *Bone;* 18 (1 Suppl):37S–43S.

111. **Nunamaker DM, Butterweck DM, Provost MT** (1990) Fatigue fractures in thoroughbred racehorses: relationships with age, peak bone strain, and training. *J Orthop Res;* 8 (4):604–611.

112. **Torrance AG, Mosley JR, Suswillo RF, et al.** (1994) Noninvasive loading of the rat ulna in vivo induces a strain-related modeling response uncomplicated by trauma or periostal pressure. *Calcif Tissue Int;* 54 (3):241–247.

113. **Raab-Cullen DM, Akhter MP, Kimmel DB, et al.** (1994) Periosteal bone formation stimulated by externally induced bending strains. *J Bone Miner Res;* 9 (8):1143–1152.

114. **Rubin C, McLeod K** (1995) Endogenous control of bone morpho-logy via frequency specific low magnitude functional strain. In: Odgaard A, Weinans H, editors. *Bone Structure and Remodeling.* London: World Scientific, 79.

115. **Skerry TM** (1997) Mechanical loading and bone: what sort of exercise is beneficial to the skeleton? *Bone;* 20 (3):179–181.

116. **Andreassen TT, Jorgensen PH, Flyvbjerg A, et al.** (1995) Growth hormone stimulates bone formation and strength of cortical bone in aged rats. *J Bone Miner Res;* 10 (7):1057–1067.

117. **Bouillon R** (1991) Growth hormone and bone. *Horm Res;* 36 (Suppl 1):49–55.

118. **Ullman M, Oldfors A** (1989) Effects of growth hormone on skeletal muscle. I. Studies on normal adult rats. *Acta Physiol Scand;* 135 (4):531–536.

119. **Parks NJ, Jee WS, Dell RB, et al.** (1986) Assessment of cortical and trabecular bone distribution in the beagle skeleton by neutron activation analysis. *Anat Rec;* 215 (3):230–250.

120. **Albright F, Reifenstein EC, Jr.** (1948) *The parathyroid glands and metabolic bone disease. Selected Studies.* Baltimore: Williams and Wilkins Co.

121. **Florta L, Hassing GSD, Parfitt AM, et al.** (1980) Comparative skeletal effects of two diphosphonates in dogs. *Metab Bone Dis Rel Res;* 2:389.

122. **Key LL, Ries W** (1996) Osteopetrosis. In: Bilezikian JP, Raisz LG, Rodan GA, editors. *Principles of Bone Biology.* New York: Academic Press, 941.

123. **Frost HM** (1987) Osteogenesis imperfecta. The set point proposal (a possible causative mechanism). *Clin Orthop;* (216):280–297.

124. **Frost HM** (1994) Wolff's Law and bone's structural adaptations to mechanical usage: an overview for clinicians. *Angle Orthod;* 64 (3):175–188.

14 Cytokines, inflammatory mediators, and matrix-degrading enzymes in normal and diseased articular cartilage and bone

Brigitte von Rechenberg

1 Introduction

With the development and advances of molecular biology during the last two decades, knowledge regarding the role of local factors in extracellular matrix (ECM) has been exploding. Complicated mechanisms of ECM formation, homeostasis and degradation, as well as interactions between cells localized within the ECM have been partially elucidated.

1.1 Importance of local factors

In bone, as well as cartilage, local factors such as cytokines, inflammatory mediators, and matrix-degrading enzymes are produced by the resident cells of the ECM. Others may be transported to the site by vascular mechanisms or migration of inflammatory cells. The resident cells usually play "in concert" to maintain homeostasis of ECM. These local factors stimulate, or inhibit, matrix breakdown or formation by transmitting signals between cells. Their effect may be exhibited through specific surface receptors of cells, or through activating cell metabolism, such as the formation of cAMP (cyclic adenosine monophosphate). These mechanisms trigger the recipient cells to express or deregulate gene expression, synthesize proteins, or secrete enzymes into the ECM. In physiological conditions, the cascade of "the concert" is finely tuned. However, if disturbances occur through local trauma, mechanical overload,

or incongruency between joint surfaces, the "local orchestra" may fail with one of the factors becoming too prominent resulting in excessive ECM breakdown. In fortunate cases, repair can be achieved if all factors play well together, such as in bone fractures; in unfortunate cases, such as osteoarthrosis, the matrix breakdown is beyond repair. Overall, besides systemic hormones, local factors play a major role not only in normal but also in diseased articular cartilage and bone.

2 Cytokines

Cytokines comprise a group of molecules that are capable of intracellular signal transduction. The term "cytokines" was used for substances responsible for cell–cell interactions, while the term "growth factors" was applied for substances eliciting mitogenic activity in other cells. Since the effects of these substances can be either one, the term "cytokines" is now used for both groups [1, 2]. The interleukins are probably the most important cytokines involved in ECM breakdown of cartilage [3] and bone [4, 5], whereas growth factors stimulate cell replication, differentiation, and activation to form new cartilage [6] or bone [7].

2.1   Interleukins

These molecules are peptides, also called monokines or lymphokines, that are produced by many cell types after stimulation [2]. IL-1 and IL-6 were found to be the most important representatives of this group for ECM of articular cartilage and bone; therefore the description of interleukins in this text will be limited to those two molecules. Both IL-1 and IL-6 were found to be associated with pathological cartilage degradation [8] and bone resorption due to malignancies, Paget disease, and postmenopausal osteoporosis [1, 5, 9].

Initially called "catabolin", interleukin-1 (IL-1) was shown to be one of the most potent molecules initiating ECM breakdown, and to be produced by almost all cell types, except erythrocytes and T-lymphocytes [10]. This peptide has two related isoforms, IL-1α and IL-β, which show 30% homology in their amino-acid sequence. They are located on two non-allelic genes [11]; however, their biological function is very similar and equally potent on the resident cells of ECM [4]. Specific receptors for IL-1 are located on cell surfaces, where the interleukins bind and exhibit their action directly. A second messenger is not required [12].

IL-1 is not constitutively produced by cells, but rather stimulated by various triggers, such as trauma, ECM components, other cytokines, or bacterial products [13].

Specific IL-1-receptor antagonists (IL-1ra) that are synthesized parallel and located on the same gene as IL-1, naturally inhibit the effect of IL-1 by blocking the receptor sites. Although, IL-1ra is a specific inhibitor of IL-1, it is relatively weak, and if local IL-1 production exceeds production of IL-1ra, pathological ECM breakdown will occur. Besides IL-1ra, IL-4 seems to be a true antagonist of IL-1 in vivo [10, 14].

One of the major effects of IL-1 was shown to be stimulating synthesis of nitric oxide (NO) [12], prostaglandin E2 (PGE2), matrix metalloproteases (MMPs) [3, 15], IL-6 [16, 17], and, although indirectly, IL-11 [18] by ECM resident cells. All of these substances play a major role in ECM remodeling and pathological breakdown of cells [3, 12].

Furthermore, IL-1 was proven to affect proteoglycan, collagen, DNA and alkaline phosphatase synthesis, dose-dependently, in chondrocytes and osteoblasts [1, 10, 11, 19, 20].

Through a combination of these effects on cell metabolism, IL-1 was shown to increase bone resorption as well as inhibit bone formation [13, 21], and to initiate articular cartilage breakdown [3, 12].

As IL-1, IL-6 is produced by many cell types. Its role in the physiology of articular cartilage is less clear than it is in bone. In contrast to other cytokines, IL-6 is not only regulated by local effects, such as stimulation by IL-1, but also systemically by parathyroid hormone (PTH), PTH–related protein, and vitamin D3 [1].

IL-6 has similar effects on bone as IL-1, supporting bone resorption by suppressing osteoblast differentiation, recruiting osteoclasts and stimulating their differentiation from precursor cells [1]. In cartilage, IL-6 stimulated the production of tissue inhibitor of metalloproteinases (TIMP) without affecting collagenase activity or PGE2 production, hence suggesting a more protective role for cartilage. Since IL-6 is required for T-cell activation and antibody production (including RhF), it may play a role in immune-mediated joint diseases (rheumatoid arthritis) [8].

2.2   Tumor necrosis factor (TNF) and interferon (IFN)

TNF-α and β (also called lymphotoxin or cachectin) are polypeptides (17 kd) exhibiting effects not only on tumors but also on non-neoplastic tissue [2, 10]. Predominantly, macrophages and PMN-leukocytes produce TNF, but also other cells, such as synoviocytes, chondrocytes [19], and osteoblasts [1, 22]. In cartilage, TNF-α is not as potent as IL-1 inducing ECM breakdown by stimulating MMP synthesis. However, it acts synergistically with IL-1 [23], and its effects on articular cartilage are almost identical [17]. TNF-α may partly exhibit its effects through stimulation of PGE2 [2].

Although both isoforms of TNF were shown to inhibit replication of tumor cells, while stimulating it in normal cells, it seems that overall at least TNF-α has a more catabolic effect on ECM of cartilage and bone. Besides other stimuli, TNF production in synoviocytes could be triggered with the inflammatory mediator, nitric oxide. The effects of TNF can be inhibited by calcitonin and γ-interferon (γ-IFN) [1, 2].

Bone resorption is increased after stimulation with TNF-α by inducing proliferation and differentiation of osteoclast-like precursor cells, while bone formation by osteoblasts is inhibited. Furthermore, the synthesis of collagen, alkaline phosphatase, and osteocalcin is inhibited, as well as ectopic bone formation in vivo [1, 2, 10].

γ-Interferons (γ-IFN) are glycosylated peptides (26 kd) [10] produced by activated lymphocytes, monocytes, fibroblasts, synoviocytes, and chondrocytes. The metabolic effects of IFN are complex and somewhat controversial in ECM homeostasis, but overall it was proven that it is an important inhibitor of catabolic activities induced by other cytokines in cartilage and bone [2, 10, 19]. Although its synthesis by osteoblasts could not be demonstrated, it inhibits differentiation of osteoclast precursors and increases alkaline phosphate activity, thus inhibiting bone resorption and promoting bone formation [2]. In articular cartilage, γ-IFN was found to "down-regulate" the synthesis of matrix degrading metalloproteinases, as well as "up-regulate" the synthesis of their naturally occurring inhibitor (TIMP) [19].

2.3 Growth factors

Growth factors counterbalance the catabolic effect of cytokines in many instances by increasing synthesis of matrix macromolecules. There are many members to this family (**Tab. 14-1**), of which some are produced systemically and/or locally by the resident cells of the ECM. The systemic growth factors (GF), such as platelet derived GF (PDGF), endothelial GF (EGF), transforming GF (TGF-α and β), fibroblast GF (FGF), and insulin GF (IGF-1 and IGF-2), mainly encourage DNA synthesis and proliferation of resident cells. However, this effect may be cell-type dependent. Although in individual cases they may enhance ECM resorption synergistically with other catabolic enzymes (e.g., TNF-α on bone), they support local repair mechanisms by aiding in revascularization through their angiogenic activity [4, 10]. In this text, only the locally produced GF of ECM will be outlined in more detail.

Skeletal GF (SGF), bone-derived GF (BDGF), and cartilage-derived GF (CDGF) may stimulate cell replication and matrix synthesis by ECM resident cells, at least in bone. They do not have any effect on inducing mesenchymal cells to differentiate into mature bone or cartilage cells [10]. In contrast, the bone

Tab. 14-1: Cytokines and their effect on ECM [2, 10].

Cytokine group	Cytokine name	Abbreviation	Molecular weight in kd	ECM degradation	Matrix synthesis	Cell replication
Systemic GF	Endothelial GF	EGF	6	–	–	+
	Fibroblast GF	FGF	13	–	–	+
	Platelet derived GF	PDGF	30	–	+	+
	Transforming GF-α and β	TGF-α and β	7–10	–	+	+
	Bone morphogenetic protein	BMP	various	–	–	–(+)
	Insulin GF	IGF	7.5–7.7	–	+	+
Monokines	Tumor necrosis factor-α	TNF-α	17–19	+	–	?
	Interleukin-1	IL-1	17–19	+	+(low)/–(high)	+
Lymphokines	Interferon-γ	IFN-γ	26	–	+	?
	Tumor necrosis factor-β	TNF-β	17–19	+	–	?
	Interleukin-6	IL-6	26	+	–	(+)

morphogenetic proteins (BMP) are capable of inducing bone or cartilage formation in vitro and also at ectopic sites in vivo [7, 10]. Most of the BMPs now belong to the TGF-β supergene family, revealing predominant sequence homology [4, 10]. BMPs are thought to contribute to fracture healing, as well as to the enhancing effect of various autogeneic, allogeneic, and heterogeneic bone grafts in orthopedic surgery [7]. BMPs can be extracted from mineralized matrix, where they were found to be localized along collagen fibers of normal bone and in periosteal cells. Several isoforms of BMP were identified, of which BMP-2 and BMP-7 are the most important for bone and cartilage induction [7, 10].

Various growth factors have been demonstrated to contribute to fracture healing, with sequential appearance during the different stages of callus formation. In the early stages, while hematoma formation is still prominent, PDGF has been shown to be abundant within the fracture area, shortly thereafter followed by FGF. When mesenchymal cells move into the area of the hematoma and start to remodel the callus with organized fibrous tissue, IGF becomes more important in stimulating proliferation and differentiation of chondrocytes. Later, when the cells are differentiating into cells of the osteoblastic lineage, TGF could be demonstrated to be mostly within the callus area [24].

3 Inflammatory mediators

Inflammatory mediators, such as free radicals and the eicosanoids, play an important role in ECM formation, homeostasis, and degradation. Nitric oxide (NO) and PGE2 are prominent members of these groups. Their effects may be dose dependent, either protecting or damaging ECM homeostasis. Free radicals were shown to damage endothelium, cell membranes, DNA strands, or other matrix macromolecules [12], while PGE2 has long been acknowledged as a mediator in local inflammation, generating local pain and increasing vascular permeability [15]. Concentrations of both mediators are increased not only in inflammatory arthritis and osteoarthritis in humans and animals [15, 25], but also in diseases involving pathological bone resorption [5, 26, 27].

3.1 Nitric oxide

NO is identical with the endothelial-derived relaxing factor (EDRF) that has been found to be produced by endothelial cells of vessels causing dilatation of the adjacent smooth muscle cells. NO in vivo is a dissolved non-electrolyte with the capability of diffusing through tissue without any need for specific cell receptors to be effective [12]. NO is an intermediate in the oxidation process of L-arginine to citrulline catalyzed by the enzyme NO synthase (NOS), and has a high affinity to hemoglobin and other Fe^{2+}-containing enzymes [28]. It oxidizes readily into the stable end-product nitrite (NO_2^-) and nitrate (NO_3) [23]. NO activates guanylate cyclase, leading to increased concentrations of intracellular cGMP levels [28].

NO synthesis was demonstrated in macrophages, hepatocytes and synoviocytes, chondrocytes, osteoblasts, and osteoclasts [12, 23, 29]. Specific inhibitors are not available in the body system. Since the substrate, L-arginine, is easily available in cells and is not the limiting factor, it seems that NO is regulated on the one hand by the quantity of enzyme present, and on the other hand by stimulation of the trigger cytokines. However, structural analogues of L-arginine can inhibit production of NO, such as N^G-monomethyl-L-arginine (L-NMA) or N^G-dimethylarginine [28].

Stimulation with cytokines, mainly IL-1, leads to synthesis of NO in synoviocytes, chondrocytes, osteoblasts, and osteoclasts [12, 30]. Human [28] and equine [31] chondrocytes produced more NO compared to synoviocytes. There is evidence that NO activity is related to the synthesis of PGE2. Its effects seem to be dose dependent and its role has a twofold character in the ECM metabolism. On the one hand NO is protective in ECM homeostasis by inhibiting in high dosages PGE2 synthesis, osteoclastic function, and, it seems, also in MMP synthesis [12, 23, 32, 33]. On the other hand, its function may be damaging, while at the same time inhibiting synthesis of important macromolecules or cell replication, such as proteoglycan, collagen, DNA synthesis, or IL-1ra on cell surfaces [12].

3.2 Prostaglandins

Of all prostaglandins, the E-series were found to be the most important members of this group in relation to ECM metabolism of articular cartilage and bone. The basic structure of prostaglandins consists of a cyclopentane ring, with the ß-hydroxy-ketone ring of the E-series being the most effective [34]. Two enzymes are involved in the synthesis of PGE2. Phospholipase-A2 (PLA$_2$) releases arachadonic acid from phospholipids of cell membranes. Prostaglandin G/H synthase (PGHS-2), also called cyclo-oxygenase, converts arachadonic acid to prostaglandin peroxides [17, 35, 36]. PLA$_2$ alone seems to be involved in mineralization of bone [36]. Indomethacin and other non-steroid anti-inflammatory drugs, as well as corticosteroids, are very potent inhibitors of PGE2 by blocking PGHS-2 or PAL$_2$ [17, 26, 35].

PGE2 induces intracellular cAMP, thus increasing synthetic activity in many cell types, probably by activating protein kinase [26, 37]. Furthermore Ca^{2+} shifts, increases of calcitonin receptors on osteoclasts, release of IL-11 by osteoblasts stimulating osteoclast activity, and inhibition of collagen and proteoglycan synthesis were noted dose dependently parallel to increased PGE2 concentrations [15, 23, 26]. In low doses, PGE2 stimulated collagen synthesis as well as bone formation [26].

IL-1, TNF-β, and LPS were demonstrated to be very potent triggers of PGE2 synthesis in synoviocytes, chondrocytes, and osteoblasts [15, 23, 26].

PGE2 concentrations were elevated in inflammatory joint disease, synovial fluid of joints affected with osteoarthrosis, pathological bone resorption due to malignancy, rheumatoid arthritis, periodontal disease, and unicameral bone cysts in humans [15, 17, 26].

4 Matrix-degrading enzymes and their inhibitors

Proteinases are enzymes that are classified in four groups, according to their active catalytic sites: the aspartic, cysteine, serine, and matrix metalloproteinases (MMPs). They are produced in cells and either stored in lysosomes or secreted into the ECM [3, 38]. Those enzymes stored in lysosomes can be released immediately upon demand, whereas synthesis of the others has to be induced on demand. This mechanism explains the lag phase of several hours until these enzymes can be detected after stimulation with triggers [3, 38, 39]. The aspartic and cysteine proteinases are usually lysosomal and function optimally at acidic pH conditions; whereas the serine and metalloproteinases are not stored in lysosomes and prefer neutral pH conditions [3, 35]. Proteinases have to be converted from the latent to the active form by proteolytic cleavage [39]. All proteinases play a role in bone resorption mediated by osteoclasts, whereas the MMPs are the most important enzymes in ECM degradation of articular cartilage [3].

Proteinase activities in ECM are regulated either by their secretion upon stimulation through triggers, and/or activation by converting latent enzymes into their active form, and/or by naturally occurring inhibitors of endogenous proteinases. The ubiquitous plasma globulin, α-macroglobulin (α$_2$M), is the only inhibitor capable of stochiometrically interacting with the enzymes of all four groups. They can irreversibly bind the active forms of the proteinases building complexes that are then removed from body fluids by macrophages or endocytosis [39]. The limiting factor of α$_2$M activity is its size that only allows to act on surfaces of ECM, but not penetrate into deeper layers of the matrix [3]. Besides α$_2$M, there are specific α-cysteine inhibitor and cystatins as inhibitors for cysteine proteinases, serpins for serine proteinases and tissue inhibitor of metalloproteinases (TIMP) for MMPs. These inhibitors are either provided by plasma, as α$_2$M, or simultaneously synthesized by the same resident cells producing the enzymes within the ECM [3, 38–40].

4.1 Aspartic proteinases

Cathepsin D is probably the most important representative of the aspartic proteinases, belonging to the same group as pepsin and renin. It is found in lysosomes of phagocytic cells, and can cleave proteoglycans and native collagen at acid pH conditions (pH 4) [3, 38, 39].

4.2 Cysteine proteinases

The best known enzymes of this group are cathepsin B and L, which are both demonstrated to be excreted by lysosomes and, once activated, can cleave the N-terminal of collagen fibrils and the site of the link protein of cartilaginous proteoglycan [39, 41]. Even though they function best at an acidic pH, cathepsin B and L have been found to be elevated in human articular cartilage of patients suffering from arthritic joints [3].

4.3 Serine proteinases

In contrast to the aspartic and cysteine proteinases, the serine proteinases unfold their activity extracellularly, at about a neutral pH, and belong to the most important proteinases in the body system. Members of this family are plasminogen activator, bradykinin, plasmin, plasma kallikrein, PMN-elastase, cathepsin G, mast cell proteinases (trypsin, chymotrypsin), and serine esterases of lymphocytes; all of which play a role either directly by cleaving matrix molecules or, very importantly, by activating latent proteinases by proteolytic cleavage [3, 38, 39].

4.4 Matrix metalloproteinases

The family of matrix metalloproteinases (MMPs) consists of nine recognized members, that belong to the endopeptidases-degrading macromolecules of the ECM (**Tab. 14-2**)[4, 40]. MMPs differ in their substrate specificity, although some of their activities overlap [39, 40]. They all have a role to play in ECM degradation in articular cartilage and bone, although in bone their activity is restricted to unmineralized matrix, like in the embryonic development of skeletal tissue, unmineralized osteoid, or growth plates.

Their most important representatives are the collagenases, gelatinases, and stromelysins [40, 42]. A newer member, the putative metalloproteinase (PUMP-1), has been detected and is involved in ECM breakdown, although its role is still unclear [3, 40]. MMPs are secreted into the ECM as latent enzymes and need activation. This is usually achieved by proteolytic cleavage through other proteinases, such as: trypsin, chymotrypsin, plasmin, kallikrein, cathepsin B, and neutrophil elastase.

The collagenases consist of fibroblast-type (MMP-1) and PMN-type collagenases (PMN-CL) [40]. Their main difference is that PMN-CL is only present in polymorphonuclear leukocytes and can be released immediately. In addition, it cannot cleave gelatin as a substrate [39]. MMP-1 is produced by many cells, such as synoviocytes, fibroblasts, macrophages, chondrocytes, osteoblasts, and endothelial cells [40]. For both collagenases, the main substrate is collagen, of which they have been shown to cleave collagen type I, II, III, VII, VIII, and X at a specific site of the a-chain of the triple helix [38, 39].

The gelatinases also have two representatives, the 72 kd (MMP-2) and the 92 kd (MMP-9) molecule. MMP-2 has been also referred to as type IV collagenase or matrilysin, the MMP-9 as type V collagenase or invasin [3, 17]. As with PMN-CL, MMP-9 is mainly produced by leukocytes or monocytes and can be released immediately. Whereas MMP-2 is produced by many cell types on demand, such as: fibroblasts, synoviocytes, keratinocytes, endothelial cells, macrophages, osteoblasts, and chondrocytes [40]. Their substrates are gelatin (identical to denatured collagen) [43], collagen type IV, V, VIII, X, elastin, and fibronectin for MMP-2, and gelatin, collagen type IV, V, and elastin for MMP-9 [17]. Thus, the most important activity of gelatinases in ECM degradation is post-collagenase breakdown of collagen [43].

The stromelysins (earlier called proteoglycanase) are very important members of the MMP family, since their main substrate is cleavage of proteoglycans (mainly aggrecanes) at the level of the link protein [17] in articular cartilage and bone (especially growth plate) [3, 38–40]. In addition, they have been shown to contribute to the degradation of fibronectin, laminin, elastin, and collagen type IV, V, IX, X, and XI and are very important in activating procollagenase [3]. Three mem-

Tab. 14-2: Overview of matrix metalloproteinases [3, 17, 40].

Enzyme	Abbreviation	MMP No.	Molecular weight in kDa	Source	Substrate	Inhibitor
Fibroblast-type CL	FIB-CL	MMP-1	57/52	synoviocytes fibroblasts macrophages chondrocytes osteoblasts endothelial cells	collagen types I, II, III, VII, VIII, X gelatin (proteoglycan)	TIMP TIMP-2 α-macroglobulins
PMN-type CL	PMN-CL	MMP-8	75	PMN-leukocytes	types I, II, III, VII, VIII X collagens (gelatin)	TIMP α-macroglobulins
72kDa gelatinase	Mr 72K GL	MMP-2	72	fibroblasts keratinocytes endothelial cells macrophages osteoblasts synoviocytes chondrocytes	gelatin collagen types IV, V, VII, X elastin fibronectin	TIMP TIMP-2 α-macroglobulins
92kDa gelatinase	Mr 92K GL	MMP-9	92	PMN-leukocytes macrophages keratinocytes (fibroblasts)	gelatin collagen type VI, V elastin	TIMP α-macroglobulins
Stromelysin-1	SL-1	MMP-3	60/55	stromal cells include chondrocytes synoviocytes osteoblasts	proteoglycans (aggrecan, decorin, fibromodulin) fibronectin laminin, elastin collagen type IV, V, IX, X, XI procollagenase	TIMP α-macroglobulins
Stromelysin-2	SL-2	MMP-10	60/55	unknown fibroblasts	fibronectin I, II, III, VII, VIII, X	TIMP α-macroglobulins
Stromelysin-3	SL-3	MMP-11	unknown	mammary carcinoma embryonic fibroblasts	unknown	unknown
Putative metalloproteinase-1	PUMP-1	MMP-7	28		fibronectin, laminin collagen type IV procollagenase gelatin, protein proteoglycan core	TIMP

bers of this group have been detected, namely stromelysin-1 (MMP-3), stromelysin-2 (MMP-10 or transin), and stromelysin-3 (MMP-11). Although it seems that MMP-3 is the most important in ECM degradation. Stromal cells have been shown to produce stromelysins constitutively or after induction by cytokines [3, 15, 38, 40], but expression could not be demonstrated in keratinocytes or PMN-leukocytes [39, 40].

5   Regulation of extracellular matrix by local factors

Homeostasis of articular cartilage and bone is maintained by complex mechanisms involving turnover and remodeling of ECM resident cells and macromolecules. As discussed in **Chapters 1**, **3**, **4**, and **7**, important systemic factors, such as mechanical load and endocrine influences, regulate this mechanism on a general basis. However, as became evident with the description of the various cytokines and matrix-degrading enzymes, the local factors play an equally important part in that regulation by fine tuning this "orchestra", sometimes by additionally modulating the effect of the systemic factors on a local basis.

5.1   Physiological remodeling in articular cartilage and bone

Bone and cartilage are structures well suited to adapt compressive, shearing, and torsional forces, mainly through the structure of the macromolecules of their ECM, including the collagens, proteoglycans, and hyaluronan [35]. Their rate of turnover is relatively slow and has to be coordinated between function, growth, degradation, and renewal by the resident cells. Physiological stimuli, such as movement at various speeds and gaits, will either stimulate or inhibit resident cells to increase or deregulate gene expression, increase or decrease the synthesis of the various macromolecules or the secretion of the matrix-degrading enzymes through the release of cytokines and/or inflammatory mediators. These may be brought to the local sites by vascular transport, by migration of cells, as in a joint; but also by production of local resident cells. Mechanical factors were shown to influence the synthesis and production of IL-1, IL-6, NO, and PGE2 and "up or down-regulate" their expression [3, 36, 44]. Elevated concentrations of these cytokines and inflammatory mediators exhibit their effects on the secretion and activity of matrix-degrading enzymes, which then start to degrade the matrix macromolecules. Fragments of those, such as collagen or fibronectin fragments, may elicit cell responses by stimulating cells to secrete even more cytokines. The degradation of ECM molecules also liberates growth factors, such as BMP in bone, that have been secreted by the resident cells and embedded in the ECM. As growth factors and inhibitors counterbalance these effects, and stimuli under normal conditions subside before causing damage, physiological homeostasis under normal conditions can be maintained (**Fig. 14-1**).

5.2   Extracellular matrix degradation in disease

Correlation between the activities of cytokines, growth factors, and matrix-degrading enzymes have been demonstrated in many in vitro and in vivo studies, permitting visualization of a cascade of how ECM degradation in disease of articular cartilage and bone may occur. Different tissues and cells were stimulated with cytokines and growth factors elucidating the effects on synthesis or degradation of ECM macromolecules. However, not all of the studies undertaken produced identical results and, what is even more intriguing, in many instances the opposite effects were seen. Accepting that these differences may be due to study design, species differences, and techniques applied, also proves the complexity of these mechanisms. It must be taken into account that these local factors act in concert, meaning that their effect can be to counteract each other, or to be synergistic in their anabolic or catabolic effects. Furthermore, the same cytokines, or inflammatory mediators,

Fig. 14-1: Diagram of the cascade of cytokines, inflammatory mediators, and MMPs on extracellular matrix.

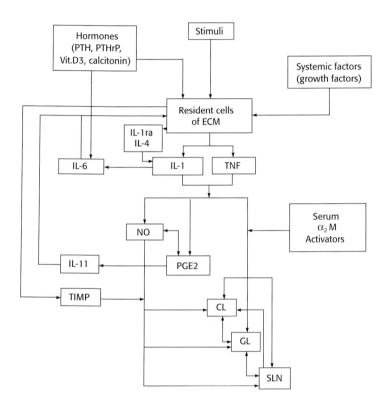

Abbreviations:

PTH	=	Parathyroid hormone
PTHrP	=	Parathyroid-hormone–related protein
ECM	=	Extracellular matrix
IL	=	Interleukin
TNF	=	Tumor necrosis factor
NO	=	Nitric oxide
PGE2	=	Prostaglandin
CL	=	Collagenase
GL	=	Gelatinase
SLN	=	Stromelysin
TIMP	=	Tissue inhibitor of metalloproteinases
α_2M	=	α - Macroglobulin

can elicit different reactions depending upon the cell type and/or doses applied. As bone is composed of different cells, such as the osteoblastic or osteoclastic cell lineage, including undifferentiated bone mesenchymal cells and the vascular system within the bone marrow, the local effect of these factors may be very different in the various compartments. Although articular cartilage seems to be more homogenous with regards to the cell population, the chondrocytes vary in their responses to stimulation according to their localization in either the superficial, middle, or deep zone [45]. Furthermore, articular cartilage, especially in the superficial zone, is also exposed to the activity of these local factors in the synovial membrane and synovial fluid and thus indirectly to plasma content in cases of inflammation, when vascular permeability is increased and macromolecules of the blood get released into the joint space [3]. In the area of subchondral bone, or at the zone of calcification of cartilage to bone, cell populations of articular cartilage and bone, including vessels, are the target of local cytokines, inflammatory mediators, and matrix-degrading enzymes .This complexity has to be kept in mind when attempting to outline schematic diagrams of ECM formation and degradation.

6 Methods to study the effects of local mediators in bone and cartilage

The complexity of the interactions of local factors in ECM homeostasis, formation, and pathological breakdown makes it very difficult to study these effects in experimental in vivo conditions, since it is almost impossible to look at isolated effects of each individual factor at any one time. Although modern molecular biology permits manipulation of genetic material and breeding animals that lack certain genetic information, such as the so-called "knock-out mice", it still is very difficult to study the exact mechanisms in these systems [46]. Fortunately, to the benefit of the study design and the reduction of the use of experimental animals, in vitro experiments can mostly overcome these shortcomings in that they facilitate focusing on the effect of one individual factor, with or without stimulation with various triggers, under standardized conditions. In vitro experiments can be performed with tissue stemming from normal or diseased animals. Only the most important techniques will be mentioned in this text.

6.1 Cell cultures

Cell cultures of synovial membrane, articular cartilage, and bone can be performed either as explant cultures, or isolated as pure cell populations that have been received by enzymatic digestion (trypsin, hyaluronidase, or collagenase) of tissue [45]. These cell cultures can be maintained for long periods of time under specific, sterile conditions using special culture media, additional substances such as serum, antibiotics and fungicidal medication, and incubation facilities. The cell cultures are normally kept at a constant temperature (37°C), with humidification in a special atmosphere with oxygen and 5% CO_2. The definite advantage of explanted cultures is that cells can be studied in their natural environment. Whereas isolated cell cultures allow one to investigate the effects of local factors on an isolated cell population. Both systems have their justification, although isolated cell populations may change their phenotype and cell metabolism in this new artificial environment, especially in chondrocytes [35, 45].

6.2 Biochemistry and molecular biology

Another method for the study of the effects of local factors is to measure the content of the various macromolecules of ECM. This can be done either with tissue stemming from clinical cases, cell cultures, or with media of cell cultures. Macromolecules, such as proteoglycans, are released into culture media after the cells are stimulated with various triggers, and they can be measured. Release or up-take studies, with labeled radioisotopes added to cell cultures exposed to local factors, facilitate the study of increased or decreased synthesis of ECM

macromolecules. The methods of molecular biology permit semi-quantitative studies with several hybridization methods, such as Northern for mRNA, Southern for DNA, or Western blots for protein determinations.

6.3 Histology techniques

Special histological methods, such as histochemistry, immunohistochemistry, or in-situ hybridization have the advantage of being able to demonstrate the presence or absence of macromolecules, cytokines, or proteins within histological sections of tissue. Special staining techniques indicate the presence of proteoglycans, and antibody preparations can demonstrate the localization and distribution of proteins. Last but not least, molecular probes can prove the up or down-regulation of mRNA of certain substances (enzymes, macromolecules).

7 Bibliography

Blue references indicate links to abstracts of articles available online:
http://www.aopublishing.org/BONE/14.htm

1. Lorenzo JA (1991) The role of cytokines in the regulation of local bone resorption. *Crit Rev Immunol;* 11 (3–4):195–213.

2. **Zengh MH, Wood DJ, Papadimitriou JM** (1992) What's new in the role of cytokines on osteoblast proliferation and differentiation? *Path Res Pract;* 188:1104.

3. **Evans CH** (1991) The role of proteinases in cartilage destruction. In: Parnham MJ, Bray MA, van den Berg WB, editors. *Drugs in Inflammation.* Basel Boston Berlin: Birkhauser Verlag, 135.

4. **Goldring MB, Goldring SR** (1990) Skeletal tissue response to cytokines. *Clin Orthop;* (258):245–278.

5. **Mundy GR** (1991) Inflammatory mediators and the destruction of bone. *J Periodontal Res;* 26 (3 Pt 2): 213–217.

6. **Guerne PA, Sublet A, Lotz M** (1994) Growth factor responsiveness of human articular chondrocytes: distinct profiles in primary chondrocytes, subcultured chondrocytes, and fibroblasts. *J Cell Physiol;* 158 (3):476–484.

7. **Kirker-Head CA** (1995) Recombinant bone morphogenetic proteins: novel substances for enhancing bone healing. *Vet Surg;* 24 (5):408–419.

8. **Tatakis DN** (1993) Interleukin-1 and bone metabolism: a review. *J Periodontol;* 64 (5 Suppl):416–431.

9. **May SA, Hooke RE, Lees P** (1991) Late-stage mediators of the inflammatory response: identification of interleukin-1 and a casein-degrading enzyme in equine acute inflammatory exudates. *Res Vet Sci;* 50 (1):14–17.

10. **Girasole G, Passeri G, Jilka RL, et al.** (1994) Interleukin-11: a new cytokine critical for osteoclast development. *J Clin Invest;* 93 (4): 1516–1524.

11. **Stashenko P, Dewhirst FE, Rooney ML, et al.** (1987) Interleukin-1 beta is a potent inhibitor of bone formation in vitro. *J Bone Miner Res;* 2 (6):559–565.

12. **Palmer JL, Bertone AL** (1994) Joint structure, biochemistry and biochemical disequilibrium in synovitis and equine joint disease. *Equine Vet J;* 26 (4):263–277.

13. **Mundy GR** (1992) Cytokines and local factors which affect osteoclast function. *Int J Cell Cloning;* 10 (4): 215–222.

14. **Stadler J, Stefanovic-Racic M, Billiar TR, et al.** (1991) Articular chondrocytes synthesize nitric oxide in response to cytokines and lipo-polysaccharide. *J Immunol;* 147 (11): 3915–3920.

15. **McIlwraith CW** (1996) General pathobiology of the joint and response to injury. In: McIlwraith CW, Trotter G, editors. *Joint Disease in the Horse.* Philadelphia: WB Saunders Co, 40.

16. **Bourque WT, Gross M, Hall BK** (1993) Expression of four growth factors during fracture repair. *Int J Dev Biol;* 37 (4):573–579.

17. **Yasui T, Akatsuka M, Tobetto K, et al.** (1992) The effect of hyaluronan on interleukin-1 alpha-induced prostaglandin E2 production in human osteoarthritic synovial cells. *Agents Actions;* 37 (1-2):155–156.

18. **Raisz LG, Dietrich JW, Simmons HA, et al.** (1977) Effect of prostaglaidin endoperoxides and metabolites on bone resorption in vitro. *Nature;* 267 (5611):532–534.

19. **Dickson IR** (1992) Bone. In: Royce PM, editor. *Connective Tissue and its Heritable Disorders: Molecular, Genetic, and Medical Aspects.* New York: Wiley-Liss, 286.

20. **Evans CH, Stefanovic-Racic M, Lancaster J** (1995) Nitric oxide and its role in orthopaedic disease. *Clin Orthop;* (312):275–294.

21. **von Rechenberg B, McIlwraith CW, Akens M, et al.** (1997) Spontaneous production of nitric oxide and protaglandin E2 in media of explant cultures of equine synovial membranes and articular cartilage. *Vet Surg;* 26:258.

22. **Dietrich JW, Goodson JM, Raisz LG** (1975) Stimulation of bone resorption by various prostaglandins in organ culture. *Prostaglandins;* 10 (2):231–240.

23. **Todhunter RJ** (1992) Synovial joint anatomy, biology, and pathobiology. In: Auer JA, editor. *Equine Surgery.* Philadelphia: WB Saunders Co, 844.

24. **Kumei Y, Shimokawa H, Katano H, et al.** (1996) Microgravity induces prostaglandin E2 and interleukin-6 production in normal rat osteoblasts: role in bone demineralization. *J Biotechnol;* 47 (2–3):313–324.

25. **Norrdin RW, Jee WS, High WB** (1990) The role of prostaglandins in bone in vivo. *Prostaglandins Leukot Essent Fatty Acids;* 41 (3):139–149.

26. **Sellers A, Murphy G** (1981) Collagenolytic enzymes and their naturally occurring inhibitors. *Int Rev Connect Tissue Res;* 9:151–190.

27. **Werb Z** (1989) Proteinases and matrix degradation. In: Kelley WN, Harris ED, Ruddy S, editors. *Textbook of Rheumatology.* Philadelphia: WB Saunders Co, 300.

28. **Seltzer JL, Adams SA, Grant GA, et al.** (1981) Purification and properties of a gelatin-specific neutral protease from human skin. *J Biol Chem;* 256 (9):4662–4668.

29. **Zaman G, Rawlinson SCF, Pitsillides AA, et al.** (1996) Mechanical strain enhances NO production and upregulates nNOSmRNA levels. In: Society I, editor. *Sixth Workshop on Cells and Cytokines in Bone and Cartilage.* Davos: Elsevier Science Inc., 576.

30. **Platt D** (1996) Isolated chondrocytes and cartilage explant culture systems as techniques to investigate the pathogenesis of equine joint disease. In: McIlwraith CW, Trotter G, editors. *Joint Disease in the Horse.* Philadelphia: WB Saunders Co, 441.

31. **May SA** (1996) Animal models and other experimental systems in the investigation of equine arthritis. In: McIlwraith CW, Trotter G, editors. *Joint Disease in the Horse.* Philadelphia: WB Saunders Co, 421.

32. **Henrotin YE, De Groote DD, Labasse AH, et al.** (1996) Effects of exogenous IL-1 beta, TNF alpha, IL-6, IL-8 and LIF on cytokine production by human articular chondrocytes. *Osteoarthritis Cartilage;* 4 (3):163–173.

33. **Manolagas SC, Jilka RL, Girasole G, et al.** (1993) Estrogen, cytokines, and the control of osteoclast formation and bone resorption in vitro and in vivo. *Osteoporos Int;* 3 (Suppl 1):114–116.

34. **Watrous DA, Andrews BS** (1989) The metabolism and immunology of bone. *Semin Arthritis Rheum;* 19 (1): 45–65.

35. **Tyler JA, Benton HP** (1988) Synthesis of type II collagen is decreased in cartilage cultured with interleukin 1 while the rate of intra-cellular degradation remains unchanged. *Coll Relat Res;* 8 (5):393–405.

36. **Evans CH, Watkins SC, Stefanovic-Racic M** (1996) Nitric oxide and cartilage metabolism. *Methods Enzymol;* 269:75–88.

37. **Evans CH, Robbins PD** (1994) The interleukin-1 receptor antagonist and its delivery by gene transfer. *Receptor;* 4 (1):9–15.

38. **Nietfeld JJ, Wilbrink B, Helle M, et al.** (1990) Interleukin-1-induced interleukin-6 is required for the inhibition of proteoglycan synthesis by interleukin-1 in human articular cartilage. *Arthritis Rheum;* 33 (11): 1695–1701.

39. **Platt D, Bayliss MT** (1994) An investigation of the proteoglycan metabolism of mature equine articular cartilage and its regulation by interleukin-1. *Equine Vet J;* 26 (4):297–303.

40. **Hukkanen M, Hughes FJ, Umeda T, et al.** (1992) Murine, rat, and human osteoblasts express inducible nitric oxide synthase which in turn mediates the cell function. In: Moncada S, Feelisch M, Bussse R, editors. *Proc 2nd Mtg Biol Nitric Oxide.* London: Portland Press, 328.

41. **Umeda T, Gross SS, Cudd A, et al.** (1992) Osteoclasts contain both inducible and constitutive nitric oxide synthase isoforms: A key role in bone resorption? In: Moncada S, Feelisch M, Busse R, editors. *Proc 2nd Mtg Biol Nitric Oxide.* London: Portland Press, 328.

42. **Ralston SH, Grabowski PS** (1996) Mechanisms of cytokine induced bone resorption: role of nitric oxide, cyclic guanosine monophosphate, and prostaglandins. *Bone;* 19 (1):29–33.

43. **von Rechenberg B, McIlwraith CW, Akens M, et al.** (1999) Spontaneous production of nitric oxide (NO), prostaglandin E2 (PGE2) and matrix metalloproteinases (MMPs) in media of explant cultures of equine synovial membrane and articular cartilage. *Equine Vet J.*

44. **Birkedal-Hansen H** (1993) Role of matrix metalloproteinases in human periodontal diseases. *J Periodontol;* 64 (5 Suppl):474–484.

45. **Nguyen Q, Mort JS, Roughley PJ** (1990) Cartilage proteoglycan aggregate is degraded more extensively by cathepsin L than by cathepsin B. *Biochem J;* 266 (2):569–573.

46. **Birkedal-Hansen H** (1993) Role of cytokines and inflammatory mediators in tissue destruction. *J Periodontal Res;* 28 (6 Pt 2):500–510.

15 The evolving concept of indirect fracture fixation

John R. Field

1 Introduction

The use of internal fixation devices for fracture repair induces profound changes in the bone to which they are applied. Both vascular and structural changes have been observed in bone, following the application of bone plates with the subsequent development of cortical osteopenia (**Fig. 15-1**). The phenomenon appears to be biphasic with an initial osteonecrosis (8–12 weeks), proposed to be the result of cortical vascular insufficiency followed by osteopenia (24–36 weeks), induced by changes to the mechanical environment within the bone [1].

Surgical trauma, screw placement, and the rigidity of the fixation device, act singly or in conjunction with vascular insufficiencies, related to the bone–plate interface contact area and pressure distribution, to bring about pathogenic changes. The end result is a thinning of the diaphyseal cortices. Should bone plate removal be deemed necessary, such osteopenia is a cause for concern in view of the bone's predisposition to refracture following plate removal.

Indirect fracture fixation aims to redress these problems; the use of new concepts in bone plate design, the implantation of reduced amounts of hardware, the utilization of the mechanical environment of the plate–bone construction to stimulate indirect fracture repair through callus formation, and the limitation of surgical exposure and soft-tissue trauma through prudent surgical technique.

2 Ischemic osteonecrosis

Much effort has gone into defining the vascular response to the application of various implants using microangiography [2, 3], radiolabeled microspheres [4, 5], laser Doppler flowmetry (LDF) [6], strontium uptake and clearance [7, 8], intravascular vital dyes [9–11], and radionuclide angiography [12, 13].

Rhinelander [2] first described the blockade of the centrifugal movement of blood, as a direct response to the application of a bone plate. It was further proposed that the screws traversing the medullary cavity did not significantly disturb the circulation.

Other studies support the development of an alternate route for venous outflow, observed following the placement of cerclage bands, in intact canine femora [14, 15]. The numerous anastomoses between the centrifugal afferent arterial and centripetal efferent venous vessels appear capable of permitting flow in either direction depending on the physiological or pathological status of the bone [3, 15].

2.1 Plate–bone interface and vascularity

Using disulfine blue vital stain in intact sheep tibiae, the vascular effects of the application of a semi-tubular plate and a dynamic compression plate (DCP) were investigated [16]. The

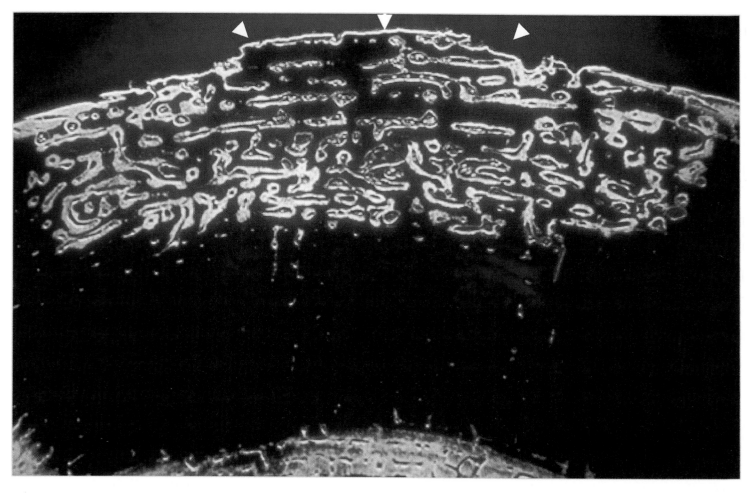

Fig. 15-1: Cortical osteopenia subsequent to the application of a bone plate. Note the dramatic bone remodeling in the vicinity of bone–plate contact and regions remote from contact (provided by courtesy of the AO Research Institute, Davos, Switzerland).

semi-tubular plate, having a greater interface contact with the bone, induced significant ischemia at both low and high level application forces. The DCP produced significant ischemia only at high application forces. The conclusion drawn was that plate rigidity and interface contact area were significant factors in the increased avascularity apparent, particularly when the semi-tubular plate was applied.

Several other studies employing disulfine blue [9–11, 17] have concluded that the overall contact area and extent of vascular disturbance corresponds well with the zone of remodeling and porosis observed. The vascular impairment is believed to be short lived with revascularization following plate application observed at 4 weeks and markedly increased by 8 weeks.

The effect of applying plates with variable surface contour has been examined using intact sheep tibiae for periods up to 20 weeks following plate application [9, 18]. A significant correlation was found between the width of the plate–bone contact and the area of intracortical perfusion deficiency. Fluorochrome bone labeling did not reveal any differences in the distribution or amount of bone remodeling. The conclusion drawn was that the area of remodeling depends on the width of plate interface contact and not on implant rigidity.

Radiologic, histological, and histomorphometric techniques have been utilized in attempts to correlate bone necrosis of vascular origin with cortical porosis attributed to the application of bone plates [19, 20]. Two plates having different interface contact areas were applied to intact canine femora with measurements recorded between 8 and 24 weeks post-implantation. A correlation between necrosis of vascular origin and porosis could not be shown. In fact, it was the inner endosteal envelope, far removed from the plate–bone interface, where porosis appeared most prominent in the absence of necrosis.

2.2 Surgical trauma

Strontium-labeled microspheres have been used to measure blood flow in both intact and osteotomized canine tibiae, in which various fixation devices had been implanted [21]. Blood flow was analyzed at 4 and 48 hours, and 14 and 90 days postapplication. Common levels of structural changes were observed with all forms of fixation methods (plating, external fixation, and intramedullary nails) in the face of differing levels of blood flow. Blood flow to the cortex appeared related not to biomechanical factors but rather to the physiologic factors existing at the time of fracturing and fixation. It was commented upon that disulfine blue, as a marker for vascular supply, appeared more representative of interstitial fluid flow driven by hydrostatic pressure and not by blood flow.

A later study [7] reported that the increased blood flow observed in the early postoperative period was due to the trauma of drilling screw holes. At 1 and 2 months a continued elevation in blood flow appeared related to the continued

presence of the screws. Histologically, cortical thinning and porosity were observed although the histological changes were not correlated with the increased strontium clearance [22]. The development of implant-induced osteopenia, it was concluded, showed a regional orientation as evidenced by the different histomorphometric appearance of bone following implant fixation. The histomorphometric appearance was also observed to change over time and may be indicative of a link with Frost's Regional Acceleratory Phenomenon (RAP) [23].

3 Adaptational osteopenia

Stress protection or stress redistribution occurs if two or more components having different elastic moduli form one mechanical system. An apparent association between cortical osteopenia and rigid internal fixation has been demonstrated using clinical and mathematical models.

3.1 Clinical models

Research in dogs has provided qualitative information about structural changes in bone following the application of rigid internal fixation. This was based principally on the radiographic, gross, and histological appearances [24]. A decrease in cortical porosity was observed when a graphite-fiber-reinforced methyl methacrylate resin composite plate was used in a comparison with a stainless-steel plate. The resin plate had a modulus of elasticity approximately ten times lower than that of the stainless steel. In skeletally mature dogs a plate of each type was applied to intact femora for periods of 9 and 12 months. It appeared that the cortical bone remodeled according to the functional stress demands placed on it and that the osteopenia observed beneath rigid stainless-steel plates was at least partially avoidable when less rigid plates were used. By collating the results of radiology, histology, histomorphometry, and fluorescence bone labeling, the following conclusions were drawn:

- The continued presence of plates (60 weeks), regardless of plate composition, delayed remodeling with a concurrent reduction in bone mass.
- The loss in bone mass is significantly greater in stainless-steel plated bones.
- The removal of plates at 8 weeks led to a widespread structural remodeling and return to normal bone mass, regardless of the plate composition.
- Remodeling was more active with titanium-plated bones.
- Later removal of plates (60 weeks) produced a less active and more limited remodeling response [25].

3.2 Mathematical models

Mathematical modeling has also been utilized to assess the influence of bone–plate fixation on the resultant stress fields in bone. By applying bone plates to plexiglass, a three-dimensional finite element model of compression plate fixation (composite beam theory) was formulated [26, 27]. This study concluded that osteopenia should, in theory, be limited to the region between the central screws. This mathematical model assumed that strain continuity was present across the bone plate interface and at the screw thread–bone interface.

Other studies [28] suggest that the assumptions of this particular mathematical model are incorrect and that modeling with plexiglass, utilizing an ideal geometric form, is not analogous to bone. The composite rigidity of plated bone was shown to differ significantly from the finite element model originally described. Discontinuity was observed between the screw, the bone, and the plate while the plexiglass assumptions were only able to show discontinuity between plate and bone.

Screw torque has also been shown to be a major contributor in establishing the rigidity of the final construction [28]. Minor screw torque changes in plate placement have been shown to cause significant differences in bone strain distribution. Minimal loosening of screws causes metal plates to become ineffective in the stress shielding of bone [29]. Mathematical modeling has determined that plate fixation to bone does not achieve ideal interface conditions and that the amount of redistribution of stress that actually occurs may be significantly less than previously thought [28].

The inability to apply metal plates in a consistent manner only adds to the variability of the bone-plate construction rigidity and therefore the ability to shield stress. The effect of applying plates designed to cause less shielding of strain on intact canine femora has been examined [29]. Observations were made at 8 weeks after implantation, and it was concluded that the plates induced increased bone flexural rigidity. With plating that significantly shielded strain, a decrease in bone midplate rigidity was observed along with an increase in bone deposition around the outer screws. This suggested that the surgical implantation of any plate (polymer or metal) provided a net stimulus for bone formation, with increasing structural rigidity observed at 8 weeks in the face of increased cortical porosity.

If a plate were to significantly reduce normal stress distribution, then a net stimulus for bone resorption would occur, resulting in a loss of midplate structural rigidity as early as 8 weeks after implantation.

4 Indirect fracture fixation

Historically, orthopedic surgeons have relied upon rigid internal fixation and, where possible, absolute anatomical reduction for the repair of diaphyseal fractures. In this manner fragments were brought into close (< 0.5 mm) and stable apposition. As a consequence, direct osteonal or haversian remodeling of the bone occurs across the fracture gap with minimal callus formation [30].

In order to achieve these goals, considerable soft-tissue dissection and surgical trauma was often inflicted, resulting in even greater disruption to the blood supply and of the fracture hematoma. As a consequence, impairment of the bone's ability to repair and remodel occurs.

In recent years, the technique of "indirect fracture fixation" or "biological fracture repair" has gained acceptance. This technique centers on the maintenance of the soft-tissue attachments and the blood supply to the fractured bone [31, 32]. Absolute anatomical reduction is not critical, with the fragments brought into approximate reduction providing a scaffold for indirect osteonal bone formation. The judicious use of fragment distractors and/or the implantation of less hardware lead to a decrease in the amount of vascular disruption, while at the same time maintaining fracture reduction and stability.

4.1 Concepts of fracture fixation

4.1.1 Bone plate design

The utilization of fixation devices which minimize the amount of vascular impairment may be achieved through new concepts in bone plate design or changes to the structural rigidity of currently used designs.

The notion that interface contact area between a plate and the underlying bone might precipitate vascular disruption in bone has led to the development of the limited contact dynamic compression plate (LC-DCP) and the point contact Fixator (PC-Fix). These plates combine the benefits of a reduction in potential plate contact area and minimal vascular impairment with ease of handling, improved healing in the zone of contact, and diminished tissue responsiveness [31, 33, 34].

Using LDF in intact sheep tibiae, the benefits of the LC-DCP appear to have been supported [6]. In a comparison between the DCP and LC-DCP it was concluded that contact pressure from bone plates elicited the ischemia observed in cortical bone. It appears that the limited-contact plate reduces this effect through diminished vascular impairment. Correlation was made between flowmetry values and contact-pressure film with areas lacking contact having flowmetry values within the normal range. Another study [35], looking at the effect of the limited contact design, saw a small but significant increase in perfusion beneath the LC-DCP, although it did not result in a difference in strength at 12 weeks after implantation.

As a means of better defining the mechanical characteristics of the interface between plate and bone, a number of elements involved in bone plate application have been quantified [36–38].

This included screw torque, object radius of curvature, mode of loading, location within the bone and bone plate design, and the effect of each on the interface contact area and force between plate and bone.

To accomplish this, Fuji prescale pressure-sensitive film was used. The film was interposed between the bone plate and object prior to screw insertion and bone plate fixation and enabled the generation of an image that reflected the mechanical features of the interface.

The film chosen allowed quantitation of pressure in the range 100–500 kg force per cm^2. The stains produced were then digitized, resulting in a tabulation of mean gray levels versus applied pressure. A polynomial equation was used to fit a calibration curve to the data allowing conversion of gray level in the digitized patterns to units of pressure.

Each interface image was scanned into a digital format with parameters of interest extracted using computerized image analysis.

Cadaveric studies

Human femora and humeri, and equine third metacarpi were used to evaluate the effect of bone plate design, bone surface topography, and implant location within a given bone on the interface features.

The LC-DCP was designed to provide a reduction in interface contact area [9, 10, 33]. This claim was evaluated in a comparison with the DCP. At two locations within either the femora or metacarpi there was no advantage, in terms of a reduction of the interface contact area, using the LC-DCP. When applied to the posterior humeral diaphysis, a comparatively flat surface, the LC-DCP showed a reduced interface contact when compared to the DCP. However, when applied to the medial humeral diaphysis there were no significant differences between plate types.

This suggested that plate–bone interface contact is as much determined by surface topography and location, within a given bone, as by bone plate design. In assessing the digitized interface patterns, it was readily apparent that contact between a plate and the underlying bone varied dramatically along the length of the interface (**Fig. 15-2**). This fact, in conjunction with relatively low values for interface contact area, casts some doubt on the previously described effect of plate–bone interface contact and the development of ischemic osteonecrosis as a direct consequence.

Surprisingly high values of interface force were recorded in all plate sizes and bone specimens. For example, the average force at the interface in femora ranged from 850–1,200 kg of force. Considerably higher values were recorded in equine metacarpi (2,000 kg). Static forces of this magnitude, it was proposed, must have some effect in the distribution of both interstitial and vascular space fluid and, by implication, the development of osteopenia.

Plexiglass studies

Subsequent studies using plexiglass models evaluated the influence of applied screw torque, object radius of curvature, plate dynamization (compression or neutral loading), and bone plate design on plate–bone interface mechanical features.

A significant relationship, between the level of applied screw torque and the average force at the interface, was defined. It was proposed that this feature, and not interface contact area, may be the predominant factor in the development of the observed vascular insufficiency following bone plate application. The clinical implications of screw torque, and average force, are yet to be defined. However, these studies have highlighted the need for more accurate control of the applied screw torque, at the least in experimental studies.

The DCP and LC-DCP responded differently to dynamization. The DCP, when applied in compression loading mode, was lifted off the object between the two compressing central screws when compared to the same plate in neutral loading mode. Conversely, in the LC-DCP, an increase in the overall contact area was observed when applied in compression loading mode. This, and the reverse effect in the LC-DCP, may relate to the differing screw-plate mechanics or different material characteristics. Increasing the object radius of curvature to which the plates were applied saw an increase in

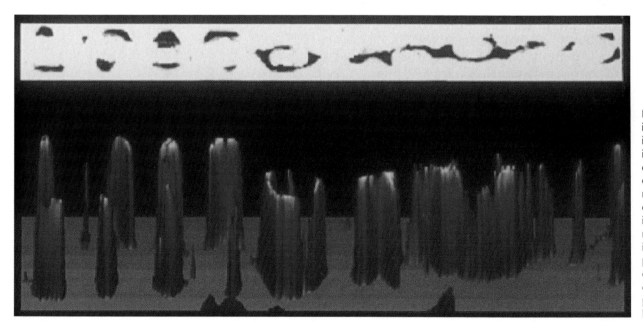

Fig. 15-2: Bone–plate interface contact image. The upper image represents the digital form of an edited Fuji film stain representing points of contact. The lower image is a 3-D representation of image intensity at each point. Note the discontinuity of contact between the plate and underlying bone.

contact area and average force become apparent, compounding the belief that surface topography is also a major factor in determining interface characteristics.

For the LC-DCP, at the larger object radius of curvature (20 mm), a significant advantage in terms of decreased contact area was apparent for both neutral or compression loading. This fact correlates with the findings in bone that the LC-DCP adopts a more point-contact configuration when applied to the flatter posterior surface of the humerus. The point-contact pattern at the plate–bone interface is, it is believed, what the designers of the LC-DCP were attempting to achieve.

At 13-mm object radius of curvature, the advantage of the LC-DCP was diminished. Following dynamization of the DCP (compression loading) in which the DCP was lifted off the object, the resultant decrease in contact area aligns it very closely with the increased interface contact of the LC-DCP following dynamization. It was concluded that other variables, as well as bone plate design, significantly influence the interfacial mechanical characteristics of bone plate fixation. The benefit of interface contact area reduction in bone plate design may not be as clear as previously thought.

Applied screw torque

Using the description "fracture stability" synonymously with rigidity and stiffness, it has been shown that stability can be enhanced by maximizing the amount of friction at the plate–bone interface. Several factors are key to this: the holding power of the screws, the applied screw torque, the relative strength of the bone, and the extent of the plate–bone interface [28, 39]. It is the axial force generated within the screw that dictates the efficiency of the screw in compressing the fragments together or compressing the plate to the bone surface [40, 41]. The axial force generated (F_z) is directly proportional to the amount of torque applied to the screw (M_z). As a consequence, the amount of slippage that occurs between a plate and the bone, is dependant upon the friction arising at the plate–bone and the screw–plate interfaces, which are dictated by the level of screw torque.

In immature or osteoporotic human bone, even at low screw torque (M_{max}), unexpected stripping of the thread within the bone can occur. This can vary from hole to hole and bone to bone and precludes the use of torque-limiting devices in fracture repair. Surgeons adapt to what they perceive as the optimal torque (M_{opt}) depending on the bone quality [42, 43].

The forces acting at the interface between a plate and the underlying bone are influenced by the interaction between the screw head and the plate [28, 29, 44]. It has been inferred that a reduction in the force present at the screw head-plate interface will bring about a decrease in the plate–bone interface force over time [29].

There are a number of pathological consequences apparent in exceeding the "optimal" screw torque applied. These included an increase in plate–bone contact [16] implicated in osteopenia and the destruction of the screw thread with subsequent implant failure [42, 44–46].

As the applied level of screw torque can induce significant effects on both vascular and mechanical attributes of the plated bone, the perceived level of optimal applied screw torque was quantitated using cadaveric bone. Furthermore, the composite rigidity and distribution of strain were evaluated at different levels of screw torque and were also quantified using cadaveric bone specimens.

Perceived optimal applied screw torque

Orthopedic surgeons were surveyed to establish what was perceived as the optimal level of applied screw torque for bone plate fixation using cadaveric bones. The torque applied to screws (perceived optimal applied screw torque—M_{opt}) was measured using a torque-limiting device as was the torque at point-of-failure (M_{max}).

Significant variations in the level of applied screw torque were found between and within individual surgeons. A gender–related variation was also apparent with women applying lower levels of screw torque. In diaphyseal bone there were no effects of cortical thickness or location on the level of applied screw torque. However, the application of screws in distal diaphyseal, epiphyseal, and metaphyseal regions did highlight significant differences in the level of applied torque, which were obviously related to the quality of the bone.

The reports indicated that torque control is an important factor in determining plate–bone interface mechanical features, construction rigidity, and bone strain distribution [17].

Construction rigidity and strain distribution

The impact of the level of applied screw torque on composite stiffness and bone strain were evaluated using cadaveric bones.

Plate-bone composite specimens were subjected to either four-point bending (gap closed) or torsional loading, following the application of a 10-hole DCP, using a Materials Testing System. Following the placement of screw holes, strain-gauge sites were prepared at five locations, encompassing the length of the plate.

Force displacement histories were recorded at a sampling rate of 100 Hertz (Hz) with strain outputs simultaneously measured at all five locations.

The findings indicated that adverse effects (repair failure) did not occur following screw application at lower levels of applied torque. In both four-point bending and torsional loading the rigidity of the final plate-bone constructions were not significantly diminished, whilst the inherent bone strain was augmented throughout, particularly in regions removed from the fracture gap.

These reports have implications in amelioration of osteopenia following bone plate fixation. At lower levels of screw torque, the plate interface mechanics are changed; lower contact area and average force at the plate–bone interface were observed, which may decrease the pathological side effects of higher interface contact. It has been suggested that the use of torque-limiting devices [42, 45] has severe limitations, particularly in immature or osteoporotic bone. The use of lower levels of applied screw torque appears advantageous in order to avoid stripping of the thread and implant failure. At lower torque levels the differential between M_{opt} and M_{max} is also increased, avoiding the osseous disintegration that occurs at currently used levels of applied screw torque.

Selective omission of screws

Using an idealized plated bone model [47], the issue of structural adaptation to changes in bone strain following the selective removal of screws was reported as a means of counteracting osteopenia following internal fixation. Removal of 25–50% of the total number of screws was shown to appreciably increase strain per load in the bone model. As a result, it was recommended that selective screw removal be considered as a means of limiting bone mass reduction by staging of screw removal (selective screw removal at various periods) following internal fixation.

Subjecting a laboratory model of a plated fracture to either cantilever or four-point bending revealed that fewer, more widely spaced screws resulted in an increase in yield strength of a given plate fixation when compared to the same plate with all the screws applied [48]. This complemented a similar study in which osteotomized cadaver ulnae were repaired using a longer plate with fewer screws. The end result was an increase in the amount of elastic deformation of the plate–bone composite [49].

In light of the desire to implant less hardware, the effect of the selective omission of screws on bone–plate interface mechanical features (contact area and average force), and the inherent bone characteristics of rigidity and strain distribution have been evaluated.

Interface mechanics

In a report, employing pressure-sensitive film was used to quantify the effect of selective omission of screws on the resultant plate–bone interface mechanics. Testing was performed using 10-hole DCP 4.5 applied to equine cadaveric third metacarpal bones. The resultant digitized bone plate patterns enabled computation of the interface contact area (%) and the average force (Newtons—N) at the interface [15]. This work showed that it was possible to dramatically reduce the number of screws applied to a given plate and not unduly effect the interfacial features. This was dependent upon the patterns of screw omission which produced significant differences in the interface mechanics in some combinations, while in others the effects of screw omission were much less than was expected.

A number of implications have been postulated from these findings; Interface contact area was observed to decrease with the selective omission of screws, presumably resulting in a reduction of the impairment of vascular outflow observed following bone plate fixation. The use of fewer screws in bone plate fixation may serve to augment the inherent bone strain and thereby stimulate callus formation and remodeling.

Construction rigidity and strain distribution with screw omission

The impact of selective omission of screws on plate bone construction stiffness and bone strain have also been reported [38]. Cadaveric long bones were used in a manner similar to that previously described. For each load regime (four-point bending and torsion) bone surface strain and the construction stiffness were quantitated. Using the terms "stiffness" and "rigidity" synonymously, it was reported that the omission of screws, in certain treatment patterns, did not bring about a significant decrease in the rigidity of the final construction. Through the application of strain gauges along the plate–bone interface, the pattern of bone surface strain was also quantitated. The results concurred with those of others [25, 28, 50], in that bone strain was redistributed following the application of bone plates.

The report [38] concludes that the omission of screws in certain defined locations appeared to meet the criteria for indirect or biological fracture repair without deleterious effects on composite structural rigidity. In diaphyseal fracture repair, without the need for absolute anatomical reduction, it was suggested that selective omission of screws may provide major advantages by the following means:

- A reduction in the amount of hardware implanted, thereby limiting the surgical exposure and trauma. In so doing, the vascular integrity of the fracture hematoma and surrounding soft tissues would be preserved.

- The augmentation of bone strain away from the fracture may result in the earlier stimulation of callus formation and bone remodeling.

4.2 Surgical trauma

A significant amount of evidence supports the theory that ischemic osteonecrosis is a consequence of the application of bone plates, and that it is primarily a response to the impairment of vascular outflow, precipitated by the interface contact area between the plate and the underlying bone.

A reduction in the amount of soft-tissue trauma through prudent surgical technique assures the maintenance of a vascular supply to the bone and reduces the amount of disruption to the fracture hematoma. In conjunction with reduced soft-tissue trauma, "bridge plating" of diaphyseal fractures is becoming popular. Plates are applied in a subfascial manner employing fluoroscopy with minimal, or without any, contouring; hence limiting the surgical exposure and disruption to the fracture hematoma. They are held in position with a significantly reduced number of screws [51]. The desired end point is a comparatively well-vascularized fracture site which enters the remodeling phase earlier because of an augmented remodeling environment.

The use of "first pass" radionuclide angiography and intravascular vital dye disulfine blue have been reported to provide dynamic and static appraisals of the effect of surgical trauma (drilling and tapping screw holes) on bone vascularity (blood flow and distribution) [38].

4.2.1 Surgical protocol

Using a sheep model, the anteromedial aspect of the tibia was surgically approached. The cranial tibialis muscle was transected distally, and reflected proximally, to reduce any artifacts from the angiographic images. Strict hemostasis was maintained to reduce contamination of the field with extraneous radionuclide.

4.2.2 Radionuclide angiography

The effects of surgical intervention were reported in the immediate postapplication time period (30 minutes) [29]. Technetium 99m diethylenetriamine pentaacetic acid (^{99m}Tc-DTPA) was injected into the descending aorta. Flow activity was recorded as a dynamic acquisition by gamma camera at three frames per second for one minute. Background radioactivity was accounted for and subtracted from each activity curve.

By integrating the time activity curves (TAC), derived from regions of interest (ROI), the ratio of the slopes of the smoothed and integrated femoral and smoothed tibial curves were measured. The relative maximum of the two curves is the relative blood flow. A static image of disulfine blue distribution was then compared to the dynamic images acquired with radionuclide angiography.

Blood flow in bone has been shown to vary according to region [52, 53], while changes in blood flow produced by physical events appears irregular throughout the bone; regional changes are manifest and most apparent in areas immediately adjacent to traumatized bone. This was the appearance observed in tibiae perfused with disulfine blue following the surgical trauma of drilling and tapping screw holes (**Fig. 15-3**). A "segmental ischemia" was apparent, particularly in the region immediately adjacent to the drilled screw hole.

This response seems to fit the criteria for what Frost [22] termed the "Regional Acceleratory Phenomenon" (RAP) which centers on a localization or regionalization of occurrences in bone. The results were for the acute posttrauma period (30 minutes) and do not correspond with the findings of others [8, 10] which suggest a localized increase in blood flow at 4 and 48 hours posttrauma. Differences in the timing of analyses may account for the apparent dissimilarity of results.

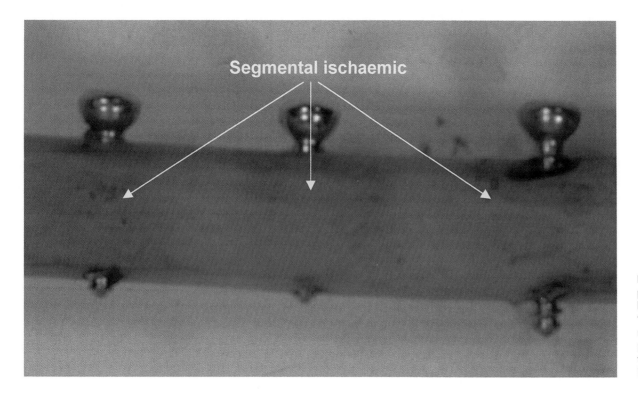

Fig. 15-3: Disulfine blue perfusion of traumatized bone, highlighting the "segmental ischemic response". Screws are placed merely to indicate the location of screw holes.

Fig. 15-4: An angiographic image depicting the pattern of vascular perfusion in response to surgical trauma. "Gaps", representing the location of drill holes, are indicated and reflect the "segmental ischemic response".

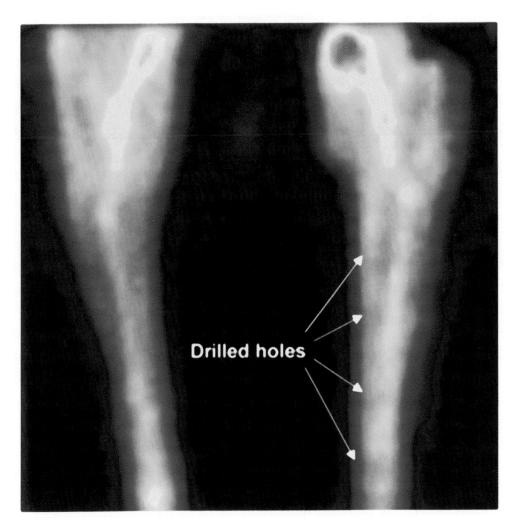

Drilled holes

The findings with disulfine blue perfusion were supported qualitatively and quantitatively by the radionuclide angiographic images obtained. Qualitatively, a similar pattern of segmental ischemia was observed in the images obtained for all operative tibiae. "Gaps" appeared in the angiographic images, which were directly related to the location of drilled and tapped screw holes (**Fig. 15-4**). When these regions were quantitatively assessed, in a comparison with the contralateral leg, it was confirmed ($P < .0050$) that the region of each screw hole had a lower relative rate of blood flow. Interestingly, quantitative assessment of the relative rate of blood flow through the distal femoral/proximal tibial region reference organ ($P < .0306$) and the entire operated tibiae ($P < .0099$) showed significantly higher rates of blood flow than the non-operated contralateral control. This apparent overall increase in the rate of blood flow in the operative tibiae complements the findings of others [8].

5 Summary

The occurrence of osteopenia following internal fixation appears to have a multifactorial pathogenesis. Implant rigidity and shape dramatically effect the construction stiffness and distribution of strain within the bone. Technical inconsistency in the application of plates, both individual and among surgeons, and the variable nature of the level of applied screw torque are also implicated in alterations to construction stiffness, strain distribution, and the interface features of contact area and average force.

Using conventional plates (DCP, LC-DCP) with bicortical screw fixation, in which plate contouring and contact are current practice, there is mounting evidence to refute previous claims that interface contact between plate and bone are the cause of the ischemia and osteonecrosis observed. It now appears that interface contact is as much dependent upon bone surface topography and plate positioning as it is on implant design [36, 37].

With radionuclide angiography and intravascular vital dye it has been shown that a substantial ischemic event occurs in the acute period (30 minutes) after the drilling of screw holes. Moreover, the inconsistencies cited earlier which have confused the development of a clear picture of the pathogenesis of implant-induced osteopenia may have some relationship with the reported findings and the "Regional Acceleratory Phenomenon" of Frost [22].

One is left to reflect as to the role which drilling and tapping of screw holes has in the pathogenesis of osteopenia, previously determined to be the sole response to bone-plate contact vascular interference.

All of the factors cited, bone plate design, applied level of screw torque, number of screws, and degree of surgical trauma appear capable of being modified in order to provide a more biological environment in which fracture healing can occur.

6 Bibliography

Blue references indicate links to abstracts of articles available online:
http://www.aopublishing.org/BONE/15.htm

1. **Field JR** (1997) Bone plate fixation: Its relationship with implant induced osteoporosis.
    Vet Comp Orthop Traum; 10:88–94.

2. **Rhinelander FW** (1968) The normal microcirculation of diaphyseal cortex and its response to fracture.
    J Bone Joint Surg [Am]; 50 (4):784–800.

3. **Rhinelander FW, Wilson JW** (1982) Blood supply to developing, mature, and healing bone. In: Sumner-Smith G, editor. *Bone in Clinical Orthopaedics.* Philadelphia: WB Saunders Co, 81–158.

4. **Reichert IL, McCarthy ID, Hughes SP** (1995) The acute vascular response to intramedullary reaming. Microsphere estimation of blood flow in the intact ovine tibia.
    J Bone Joint Surg [Br]; 77 (3):490–493.

5. **Tothill P** (1984) Bone blood flow measurement.
    J Biomed Eng; 6 (4): 251–256.

6. **Swiontkowski MF, Senft D, Taylor S, et al.** (1991) Plate design has an effect on cortical bone perfusion. *Trans 37th Orthop Res Soc;* 387.

7. **Daum WJ, Simmons DJ, Chang SL, et al.** (1985) Effect of fixation devices on radiostrontium clearance in the intact canine femur.
    Clin Orthop; (194):306–312.

8. **Gautier E, Cordey J, Mathys R, et al.** (1983) Porosity and remodelling of plated bone after internal fixation: Result of stress shielding or vascular damage?
    Proc 4th European Conf Biomat Biomech; 195–200.

9. **Gautier E, Rahn BA, Perren SM** (1986) Effects of different plates on internal and external remodelling of intact bones.
    Trans 32nd Orthop Res Soc; 322.

10. **Dueland R, Rahn BA, Perren SM, et al.** (1986) Morphological effect on bone with standard and experimental plate conformations.
    Trans 32nd Orthop Res Soc; 323.

11. **Nutton RW, Fitzgerald RH, Jr., Kelly PJ** (1985) Early dynamic bone-imaging as an indicator of osseous blood flow and factors affecting the uptake of ^{99m}Tc hydroxymethylene diphosphonate in healing bone.
    J Bone Joint Surg [Am]; 67 (5):763–770.

12. **Early PJ, Sodee DB** (1995) *Principles and Practice of Nuclear Medicine.* New York: Moseby: 339–350.

13. **Kirby BM, Wilson JW** (1991) Effect of circumferential bands on cortical vascularity and viability.
    J Orthop Res; 9 (2):174–179.

14. **Trias A, Fery A** (1979) Cortical circulation of long bones.
    J Bone Joint Surg [Am]; 61 (7):1052–1059.

15. **Jacobs RR, Rahn BA, Perren SM** (1981) Effects of plates on cortical bone perfusion.
    J Trauma; 21 (2):91–95.

16. **Perren SM, Cordey J, Rahn BA, et al.** (1988) Early temporary porosis of bone induced by internal fixation implants. A reaction to necrosis, not to stress protection?
    Clin Orthop; (232):139–151.

17. **Dueland R, Varga JS, Rahn BA, et al.** (1986) Early morphological effect on bone with standard and experimental plates.
    Trans 32nd Orthop Res Soc; 391–392.

18. **Uhthoff HK, Foux A, Yeadon A, et al.** (1993) Two processes of bone remodeling in plated intact femora: an experimental study in dogs.
    J Orthop Res; 11 (1):78–91.

19. **Uhthoff HK, Boisvert D, Finnegan M** (1994) Cortical porosis under plates. Reaction to unloading or to necrosis?
    J Bone Joint Surg [Am]; 76 (10):1507–1512.

20. **Smith SR, Bronk JT, Kelly PJ** (1990) Effect of fracture fixation on cortical bone blood flow.
    J Orthop Res; 8 (4):471–478.

21. **Simmons DJ, Daum WJ, Calhoun JH** (1988) Regional alterations in long bone 85Sr clearance produced by internal fixation devices. Part II. Histomorphometry.
    J Orthop Trauma; 2 (3):245–249.

22. **Frost HM** (1983) The regional acceleratory phenomenon: a review.
    Henry Ford Hosp Med J; 31 (1):3–9.

23. **Uhthoff HK, Dubuc FL** (1971) Bone structure changes in the dog under rigid internal fixation.
    Clin Orthop; 81:165–170.

24. **Uhthoff HK, Finnegan M** (1983) The effects of metal plates on posttraumatic remodelling and bone mass.
    J Bone Joint Surg [Br]; 65 (1):66–71.

25. **Cheal EJ, Hayes WC, White AA, et al.** (1983) Stress analysis of a simplified compression plate system for fractured bones.
    Comput Struct; 17:845–855.

26. **Cheal EJ, Hayes WC, White AA, 3rd, et al.** (1985) Stress analysis of compression plate fixation and its effects on long bone remodeling.
    J Biomech; 18 (2):141–150.

27. **Beaupre GS, Carter DR, Orr TE, et al.** (1988) Stresses in plated long-bones: the role of screw tightness and interface slipping.
    J Orthop Res; 6 (1): 39–50.

28. **Carter DR, Shimaoka EE, Harris WH, et al.** (1984) Changes in long-bone structural properties during the first 8 weeks of plate implantation.
    J Orthop Res; 2 (1):80–89.

29. **Rahn BA, Gallinaro P, Baltensperger A, et al.** (1971) Primary bone healing. An experimental study in the rabbit. *J Bone Joint Surg [Am]*; 53 (4):783–786.
30. **Ganz R, Mast J, Weber BG, et al.** (1991) Clinical aspects of "biological" plating. *Injury*; 22:4–8.
31. **Gerber C, Mast JW, Ganz R** (1990) Biological internal fixation of fractures. *Arch Orthop Trauma Surg*; 109 (6):295–303.
32. **Perren SM, Klaue K, Pohler O, et al.** (1990) The limited contact dynamic compression plate (LC-DCP). *Arch Orthop Trauma Surg*; 109(6): 304–310.
33. **Miclau T, Remiger A, Tepic S, et al.** (1995) A mechanical comparison of the dynamic compression plate, limited contact-dynamic compression plate, and point contact fixator. *J Orthop Trauma*; 9 (1):17–22.
34. **Kowalski M, Schemitsch EH, Senft D** (1993) Comparative evaluation of the effect of plate design on fracture healing with special reference to cortical bone blood flow and biomechanical properties. *Trans 39th Orthop Res Soc*; 569.
35. **Korvick DL, Monville JD, Pijanowski GJ, et al.** (1988) The effects of screw removal on bone strain in an idealized plated bone model. *Vet Surg*; 17 (3):111–116.
36. **Field JR** (1998) *Elements of bone plate fixation* [Diss/Uppsala]. Swedish University of Agricultural Sciences. Veterinary. Uppsala.
37. **Field JR, Hearn TC, Caldwell CB** (1997) Bone plate fixation: an evaluation of interface contact area and force of the dynamic compression plate (DCP) and the limited contact-dynamic compression plate (LC-DCP) applied to cadaveric bone. *J Orthop Trauma*; 11 (5):368–373.

38. **Cordey J, Martin D, Schlaepfer F, et al.** (1980) Interaction between screw and plate in internal fixation: Torque components in cortical bone screws. In: Uthhoff HK, editor. *Current Concepts of Internal Fixation of Fractures*. Berlin Heidelberg New York: Springer-Verlag, 235–243.
39. **von Arx C** (1975) Force transmission through friction in plate osteosynthesis. *AO Bulletin*.
40. **Frandsen PA, Christoffersen H, Madsen T** (1984) Holding power of different screws in the femoral head. A study in human cadaver hips. *Acta Orthop Scand*; 55 (3):349–351.
41. **Cordey J, Rahn BA, Perren SM** (1980) Human torque control in the use of bone screws. In: Uhthoff HK, editor. *Current Concepts of Internal Fixation of Fractures*. Berlin Heidelberg New York: Springer-Verlag, 235–243.
42. **Cordey J, Florin P, Veihelmann D, et al.** (1978) The control of torque applied to screws and the compression achieved in self-compression plates. In: Asmussen P, Joregensen L, editors. *Biomechanics V*. Baltimore: University Park Press, 281–293.
43. **Matter P, Brennwald J, Perren SM** (1975) The effect of static compression and tension on internal remodelling of cortical bone. *Helv Chirurg Acta*; S12.
44. **Cordey J, Martin D, Schlaepfer F, et al.** (1980) Torque components in cortical bone screws. In: Uhthoff HK, editor. *Current Concepts of Internal Fixation of Fractures*. Berlin Heidelberg New York: Springer-Verlag, 235–243.
45. **Gotzen L, Haas N, Hutter J** (1980) Biomechanical studies of torque and force of the 4.5 mm AO cortex screw as a lag screw. In: Uhthoff HK, editor. *Current Concepts of Internal Fixation of Fractures*. Berlin Heidelberg New York: Springer-Verlag, 259–267.

46. **van Riet YE, van der Werken C, Marti RK** (1997) Subfascial plate fixation of comminuted diaphyseal femoral fractures: a report of three cases utilizing biological osteosynthesis. *J Orthop Trauma*; 11 (1):57–60.
47. **Tornkvist H, Hearn TC, Schatzker J** (1996) The strength of plate fixation in relation to the number and spacing of bone screws. *J Orthop Trauma*; 10 (3):204–208.
48. **Dennis J, Sanders R, Milne T** (1993) Minimal vs. maximal compression plating of the ulna: A biomechanical study of indirect reduction technique. *J Orthop Traum*; 7:152–153.
49. **Cheal EJ, Mansmann KA, DiGioia AM, 3rd, et al.** (1991) Role of interfragmentary strain in fracture healing: ovine model of a healing osteotomy. *J Orthop Res*; 9 (1):131–142.
50. **Jones LC, Niv AI, Davis RF, et al.** (1982) Bone blood flow in the femora of anesthetized and conscious dogs in a chronic preparation, using the radioactive tracer microsphere method. *Clin Orthop*; (170):286–295.
51. **Woo SL, Lothringer KS, Akeson WH, et al.** (1984) Less rigid internal fixation plates: historical perspectives and new concepts. *J Orthop Res*; 1 (4): 431–449.
52. **Okubo M, Kinoshita T, Yukimura T, et al.** (1979) Experimental study of measurement of regional bone blood flow in the adult mongrel dog using radioactive microspheres. *Clin Orthop*; (138):263–270.
53. **Field JR, Hearn TC, Caldwell CB** (1998) The influence of screw torque, object radius of curvature, mode of bone plate application and bone plate design on bone-plate interface mechanics. *Injury*; 29 (3):233–241.

G Glossary

absorpiometry: Measurements of how much of one or more x-ray beams absorbed by bone mineral can provide an index of its amount, often expressed as bone mineral content and "density". While this estimates the "mass" contribution to bone strength, it does not account for the architectural contribution. With suitable software, peripheral quantitative computed tomography can account for both.

acceleration: The rate of increase of an object's velocity (meters or feet/second^2).

anisotropic: The directionality of mechanical properties (i.e., the material does not behave the same in all directions).

anode: In a battery or corrosion situation, the more-reactive metal that dissolves (ionizes) and gives up electrons.

architecture: The size, shape, and orientation of a bone, the amount of bone tissue in it, and the arrangement of the tissue in longitudinal and cross-sectional anatomical space. In this context, the cross-sectional size and shape of a bone, its length, and longitudinal shape, and the amounts and spatial distribution of its cortical and trabecular bone. As an example of its effect on bone strength, doubling the diameter of a hollow bone, while keeping the same amount of bone in its cross-section, increases its bending strength eight-fold. Given a constant bone "mass", changing a bone's architecture can make it stronger or weaker.

area moment of inertia: The relative resistance to bending of a given cross-section. The stress due to bending at any point is proportional to the bending moment and inversely proportional to the area moment of inertia.

arthrosis: A joint in which articular cartilage, and particularly its Type II collagen, has broken down physically. This final cause of an arthrosis could have many first causes. Other definitions exist for this still debated matter. (Osteoarthritis, degenerative arthritis.)

bending: Induction of curvature in the long axis of an object by the application of an eccentric force or bending moment.

bending moment: Measure of the bending intensity created by a force; (moment of force) obtained by multiplying a force by its lever arm.

BMU: basic multicellular unit of bone remodeling. In 4 months, and in a biologically coupled activation/resorption/formation or ARF sequence, it turns over 0.05 mm^3 of bone. When it makes less bone than it resorbs, this tends to remove bone permanently. Adult humans may create about three million new BMUs annually, and about a million may function at any moment in the whole skeleton.

bone "density": The true physical density of bone as a material varies little with age, sex, bone, and species. "Density", as absorptiometrists use the term, only provides an estimate of the total amount of bone tissue (as bone mineral) in the path of one or more x-ray beams. Here, one can assume gamma rays and x-rays are the same. While many still believe otherwise, true bone density is normal in most

osteoporoses and osteopenias. When in quotes, "density" is as defined in absorptiometry.

bone "mass": The amount of bone tissue in a bone or skeleton, preferably viewed as a volume, minus the marrow cavity. It does not mean mass as used in physics. Absorptio-metric estimates of bone mineral content and "density" do not always provide reliable indices of bone strength, particularly under the bending and torsional loads that help to cause hip and wrist fractures due to falls.

boundary lubrication: The separation of bearing surfaces by a film of lubricant that adheres to the surfaces themselves. Also "dry friction", where asperities or high points of the two bearing surfaces touch when rubbed. The latter definition is in a strict engineering sense and does not apply to a joint that always contains a film of fluid lubricant.

brittle: Sustains little or no permanent deformation prior to fracture.

buckling: Bending produced by vertical forces along the long axis of an object.

casting: Fabrication of parts by melting and pouring into molds.

cathode: In a battery or corrosion situation, the lesser reactive metal. It does not corrode.

center of gravity: For analytical purposes, the point at which the mass of an object is thought to be concentrated. The point at which any object is exactly balanced.

coefficient of friction: A parameter used to relate frictional resistance of two objects rubbing on each other as determined by dividing the frictional force by the compressive load across the bearing.

components of force: The portion of a force acting in a particular direction or directions. The vector sum of all force components is just equal to the original force. Thus deformation and reaction to force components are the same as to the original force.

compression: Application of force tending to squeeze or crush an object.

CGFRC: The chondral growth–force response curve, a hypothesis that can explain many known responses of growing joints to mechanical loading.

corrosion: Destruction of metal by electrochemical action.

critical load: A vertical force that begins to produce buckling.

deceleration: The rate at which a moving object is slowed (same units as acceleration).

disuse: For a bone, "disuse" would be the relationship between the bone's strength and its usual loads. The resulting strains and the remodeling threshold would provide criteria that recognize disuse.

drift: see modeling.

ductile: May be deformed permanently without fracture (i.e., can be drawn into a wire or rolled into a sheet).

elastic: Deformation that disappears when the stress is removed.

elastic (Young's) modulus: The ability to return ("destrain") to the exact shape and size after a load strains or deforms

the tissue, regardless of how quickly or slowly that happens. An elastic material that destrains promptly with little loss of mechanical energy (like rubber) is resilient. A material that destrains slowly with considerable loss of mechanical energy (like wet articular cartilage, or an orange) is usually viscoelastic instead of resilient. But, both are elastic. Elasticity differs from stiffness.

elasticity: Deformation of an object when the stress depends only on the magnitude of the strain, independent of the rate at which the object is being strained or deformed. When the stress is removed, the strain disappears.

elastohydrodynamic: The friction-lowering advantage obtained when the bearing surfaces are elastic in nature.

elongation at fracture: Permanent (percentage) deformation remaining at fracture; ductile material has a larger elongation at fracture than does brittle material.

extreme fibers: Outermost fibers on the convex and concave sides of bent object.

fatigue: Progressive weakening of a structure by accumulating microscopic physical damage.

fatigue fracture (failure): Structural failure caused by repetitive tensile stresses that, although below the ultimate strength, cause a slowly propagating crack to cross the material. Microscopic damage in a structure caused by one or more load applications, each of which stays below the structure's ultimate strength: the damage reduces the strength and stiffness of the affected structure.

fatigue failure: A structural failure caused by two or more loading episodes when all loads lie below the structure's ultimate strength: Typically such failures occur after thousands or millions of loading episodes.

fatigue life: A measure of strength in fatigue. Usually expressed as the number of loading cycles at a given load, strain, or stress that cause a complete fatigue failure of a material or structure. It can vary from two to many millions of loading cycles.

forging: Fabrication by mechanical deformation.

fracture: Failure caused by growth of a crack.

fragility-increased: More easily fractured by normal activities or an injury: weaker, less strong.

free body analysis: The method of determining forces acting on a body by isolating that body and ensuring that it is in static equilibrium.

gradient: When the unit load is the same on two adjacent square millimeters of an articular cartilage, no loading gradient would exist. But, if the unit loads differ, a spatial gradient would exist from one area to the adjacent one. Temporal gradients occur as well.

growth: General body and longitudinal bone growth excepted, here "pure" growth increases the number of cells and the amounts of intercellular materials. When modified by various influences to produce functionally and biomechanically purposeful architecture and organization, it is called modeling.

hydrodynamic lubrication: A situation in which the two bearing surfaces are separated by a fluid film held in place by the relative motion of the two bearing surfaces.

hydrostatic lubrication: The creation of a fluid film by pressurizing the fluid.

hydrostatic pressure: A stress produced by forces acting equally in all directions.

inertia: The tendency of a mass to resist changing velocity.

kinetic energy: Energy achieved by the motion of an object, determined by multiplying one-half of the mass by the square of the velocity.

load: Any external mechanical force applied to a skeletal organ or tissue. Loads come in at least two categories: The total load on a whole bone or joint, and the unit load (see **unit load**).

maintenance: Activities that help to keep existing tissues mechanically competent during their voluntary mechanical usage. It must affect at least the tissue's cells, composition, and materials properties, and involve detecting and repairing some microdamage.

mechanical competence: The ability to endure voluntary physical activities for life without developing spontaneous fractures or bone pain. Sometimes called "biomechanical competence". The antonym: mechanical incompetence.

mechanical energy: Energy stored in the form of elastic stresses and strains; originally, this energy was work done by applied forces.

mechanical usage: All of the loads applied to bones by usual physical activities of the body. The largest voluntary loads come from muscles.

MESm: minimum effective strain threshold (or equivalent stimulus) for switching mechanically controlled bone modeling "ON". This genetically determined "modeling threshold" range seems to lie in a region centered near 1,000–2,000 microstrain in most young human adults, which one could view as its "set point". Non-mechanical agents, drugs, age, and disease might modify it.

cMESm: The modeling threshold for articular cartilage (cMESm = minimum effective stimulus for cartilage modeling). Its value is unknown at present.

MESp: The operational microdamage threshold range for bone (MESp = minimum effective stimulus or strain for pathological-mode behavior). It seems to center near 3,000 microstrain, which would correspond to a stress of approx. 60 mPa. Investigators in biomechanics now study it and how to express it mathematically.

MESr: The minimum effective strain threshold (or equivalent stimulus) for mechanically controlled BMU-based remodeling. Above it, BMU creations begin to decrease, and resorption and formation incompleted BMUs tend to equalize. This genetically determined "remodeling threshold" may center near 50–100 microstrain in most human adults, which one could view as its set point. Non-mechanical agents, drugs, age, and disease might modify it.

metabolic energy: The processes by which a living organism creates energy from its food.

microdamage (MDx): Microscopic fatigue damage in a structural tissue. It weakens the affected tissue or structure without changing its size, shape, density, or appearance. It usually begins at the ultrastructual level, progresses to visibility in the light microscope, and then to naked-eye visibility.

microstrain: see **strain**.

modeling: The biological activities that shape and size skeletal organs, and help to organize their components usually to promote mechanical competence. Modeling drifts usually do so in bone, and chondral modeling does so for structures made of cartilage. This can involve holding growth back in some places and increasing it in others. If bone's modeling threshold range centers near 1,000 microstrain, that would correspond to a "typical peak unit load" (or stress) of about 20 MPa or 20 N/mm^2 ($\approx$ 2 kp/mm^2).

moment arm: Shortest distance between the line of application of a force and the point of interest around which the moment of the force is being taken.

momentum: Mass of the object multiplied by its velocity.

muscle strength: The maximum momentary contractile force exerted by a muscle. It can be expressed in Newtons, kiloponds (the attraction of earth's gravity for a mass of one kilogram), or pounds-force (the attraction of earth's gravity for a mass of one pound avoirdupois). Or, it can be measured as the peak torque in Newton-meters produced by muscles

across joints like the hip, elbow, knee, and fingers. It differs from endurance, which concerns how long and often submaximal muscle forces can be exerted, as in marathon running. It differs from mechanical work or energy, which can be expressed in accumulated foot-pounds, Newton-meters, Joules, or kilowatt-hours. It differs from power, which concerns how rapidly muscles perform mechanical work and is usually expressed in foot-pounds/sec, Newton-meters/sec, or Joules/sec. Since bones seem to adapt their strength and stiffness to the typical peak momentary loads they carry, accounting for these distinctions can minimize errors in interpreting mechanical usage effects on bone strength and "mass".
Nota bene: Increasing momentary muscle strength usually increases muscle mass and maximum cross-sectional area, but increasing muscle endurance need not do either. Increasing muscle power can also modestly increase muscle mass and momentary strength, but often not enough to make bone strains reach the modeling threshold in aged adults.

neutral axis: The plane in a bent object at which zero stresses and strains occur.

Newton's First Law: Every body continues in its state of rest or of uniform motion in a straight line, except as it is compelled by force to change that state.

Newton's Third Law: Every action has an equal and contrary reaction; i.e., the mutual actions of two bodies on each other are always forces equal in amount and opposite in direction.

osteopenia: The presence of less bone than usual for most healthy people of the same age, height, weight, sex,

and race. It can also be relative, as when older adults are compared to their young-adult status. It need not represent a disease.

osteoporosis: An osteopenia in which an individual's usual physical activities cause spontaneous fractures (usually in the spine) and/or bone pain. The condition usually stems from a mechanostat disorder.

partial body mass: The mass of part of the body. For example, the mass acting on the hip joint on the "swing" side in gait is a partial body mass, as the weight of the "swing" leg distal to that hip is not being supported by that hip.

piezoelectric: A solid that responds to applied stresses by becoming electrically polarized. A voltage is produced when forces are applied.

plastic flow: The deformation caused by shear stress, resulting in permanent changes in the shape of any solid.

Poisson's ratio: A ratio of the strain perpendicular to the line of force application divided by the strain parallel to the line of force application.

polar moment of inertia: The resistance of a given cross-section to twisting; the stress caused by twisting (torsion) is proportional to the torque and inversely proportional to the polar moment of inertia.

potential energy: The energy created by work done against the force of gravity (e.g., an increase in the height of the center of mass).

power: The work or energy per unit of time.

principal strains or stresses: These are compression, tension, and shear.

remodeling: The turnover of bone in small packets by BMUs. Pre-1964 literature lumped modeling and remodeling together as remodeling. While drifts and BMUs create and use what seem to be the same kinds of osteoblasts and osteoclasts to do their work in different parts of the same bone at the same time, the osteoblasts and osteoclasts in drifts and BMUs can even respond oppositely to the same mechanical or non-mechanical factor. In disuse-mode remodeling, BMU creations increase and completed BMUs next to the marrow make less bone than normal. This accelerates the loss of bone next to the marrow. In conservation-mode remodeling, completed BMUs tend to equalize their bone resorption and formation, and BMU creations usually decrease, unless increased microdamage increases them. This reduces, or stops, bone losses.

resorption: The removal of bone by osteoclasts. Few true anti-resorption agents exist and they do not include estrogen, or presently known and studied bisphosphonates, which are anti-remodeling agents that chiefly decrease BMU creations. Due to the ARF (see BMU) sequence, this reduces global resorption first, and then formation, both about equally. A true anti-resorption agent would produce the equivalent of osteopetrosis.

resultant force: The sum of force components.

safety factor for bone strength: The amount by which bone is stronger than needed to carry the typical largest voluntary loads placed upon it. One can define it as the ultimate strength divided by the modeling threshold when each is expressed as a stress.

self-tapping screw: A screw that cuts its own threads as it turns.

shear and shear stress: The force applied parallel to an object's surface (e.g., rubbing force). Shearing forces can also exist deep within the material itself.

static equilibrium: The state at which the sum of the forces acting on a body is zero (Newton's first law is satisfied).

stiffness: The resistance of a material or structure to being deformed by a load. Often expressed as the stress divided by the strain that caused it, so that larger values of "Young's modulus of elasticity" would mean stiffer. Within the loading ranges and rates found in life for healthy bones and joints, their stiffness and strength are reasonably proportional to each other, so stronger by a certain per-centage would usually mean stiffer by the same percentage. Accordingly, strength can often substitute for stiffness in ordinary discourse.

strain: The deformation, or change, in dimensions and/or shape caused by a load on any structure or structural material. Loads always cause strains, even if very small ones (see ultimate strength).

strength: The maximum resistance to stress before failure. The lowest load or strain that, when applied once, usually fractures a bone or an articular cartilage, or ruptures a tendon or ligament. This is also called the "ultimate strength". Normal lamellar bone's fracture strength, expressed as a strain, is a range centered near 25,000 microstrain. In ordinary conversation, strength can provide a useful surrogate for an organ's stiffness.

stress: The elastic resistance of the intermolecular bonds in a material to being stretched by strains. Loads cause strains, which then cause stresses. Three "principal" stresses (and strains) include tension, compression, and shear. We cannot measure stress directly but must calculate it from other information that can, but need not include strain. The stress–strain curves of bone and cartilage are non-linear.

stress concentration: The point at which the stress is appreciably higher than elsewhere due to the geometry of the stressed object or the point of application of the force.

surface energy: The energy required to create new surfaces; essentially the energy of broken chemical bonds.

tensile stress: The tensile (stretching) force divided by the cross-sectional area.

tension: The application of force tending to elongate an object (a pull).

tension band: A member that is put in tension in order to compress other portions of the structure (e.g., a guy wire).

thixotropy: Viscosity that is shear rate-dependent.

torque: A twisting moment (force × lever arm).

torsion: An applied force that tends to rotate an object about its long axis (a twist).

toughness: Energy necessary for fracture. A soft, ductile material may be relatively tough.

turnover: The amount of older bone replaced by new bone; often expressed as percent per year. Other definitions were suggested in the past.

typical peak loads: Visualize a histogram that plots the sizes of a bone's strains (or loads) on one axis, and on the other axis the number of times strains of a given size occur during a week. The strains large enough to turn bone modeling on would comprise less than 0.01% of all strains in that week. For example, counting each systolic pulse pressure in the marrow cavity as a loading event on a hollow bone like the femur, in a week it would strain over 725,000 times from each event. Only about 50 caused by peak muscle forces could be large enough to reach or exceed bone's modeling threshold. The bone would adapt its strength and "mass" to those 50 strains and chiefly ignore the others. This model might also apply to the modeling of growing cartilage.

ultimate strength: Load or strain that, when applied once, causes failure.

ultimate tensile stress: The maximum tensile stress sustainable by a given material.

unit load: The part of the total load on a bone carried by, say, one mm^2, one cm^2, or one $inch^2$, of its cross-section area. It would cause corresponding principal strains and stresses. One could state it as kp/mm^2 or $kp/inch^2$, N/m^2 (= 1 Pa, 1 Pascal) or megapascals (millions of Newtons per $meter^2$). The unit compression (or tension) load usually equals the unit compression (or tension) stress it causes.

vector: The graphic representation of a force as an arrow. The direction of the arrow is the line of action of the force; the length of the arrow is proportional to the magnitude of the force.

vigorous exercise: The literature reveals some confusion about the meaning of this term. The biomechanically important distinctions between low-force exercise, power, and high-force exercise are often not acknowledged or made, although their different effects on bone strength and "mass" reveal the need to make that distinction. That difference explains why weight lifters have more bone strength and "mass" than marathon runners, even though the muscles of the latter may exert far more mechanical energy, joules, or "horsepower hours" per month than the former.

viscoelasticity: When stress depends on the rate of strain as well as on the magnitude of the strain. A perfect spring would strain instantly under a load and destrain instantly upon removing the load, and its strain would be the same no matter how briefly the load was applied or how long it was maintained. Viscoelastic materials strain slowly under a load, and the longer the load is applied the more they strain, although more slowly with increasing time. Upon deloading they destrain slowly too. Bone and articular cartilage are viscoelastic. Rubber and oranges are both elastic (see **elasticity**), but the former is resilient, the latter is viscoelastic.

vital biomechanics: A biomechanics subfield that is concerned with how the skeleton's biologic mechanisms respond to mechanical and non-mechanical influences, in order to fit skeletal tissues to their mechanical usage.

weeping lubrication: A special form of hydrostatic lubrication in which the interstitial fluid of cartilage is extruded into the joint space by the deformation of cartilage under load.

work: Force multiplied by the distance over which it acts.

yield strength: The stress necessary to cause plastic flow, also known as yield stress.

Index

Page numbers in *italics* refer to figure captions/illustrations.

H

O